Practical Handbook
of
Advanced Interventional Cardiology

Second edition

edited by

Thach N. Nguyen, MD, FACC, FACP, FSCAI
Editorial Consultant, *Journal of Interventional Cardiology*;
Co-editor, *Journal of the Institute of Geriatric Cardiology*;
Professor of Medicine (Hon.)
Capital University of Medical Sciences
Beijing, China;
Director of Cardiology, Community Health Care System
St Mary Medical Center, Hobart, IN

Dayi Hu, MD
Professor of Medicine
Peking University and Capital University of Medical Sciences;
President, The Institute of Cardiovascular Diseases;
Chief of Cardiology, People and Beijing Tong Ren Hospital
Beijing, China

Shigeru Saito, MD, FACC, FSCAI, FJCC
Chief of Division of Cardiology and Catheterization Laboratories
Heart Center of Shonan Kamakura General Hospital
Heart and Great Vessel Center of Beijing You-Yi Friendship Hospital
Beijing, China

Cindy L. Grines, MD
Director, Cardiac Catheterization Laboratories
William Beaumont Hospital
Royal Oak, MI

Igor Palacios, MD
Director of Cardiac Catheterization Laboratories
and Interventional Cardiology
Massachusetts General Hospital
Boston, MA

Blackwell
Publishing

Futura, an imprint of Blackwell Publishing

© 2001, 2003 by Futura, an imprint of Blackwell Publishing

Blackwell Publishing, Inc./Futura Division, 3 West Main Street, Elmsford,
    New York 10523, USA
Blackwell Publishing, Inc., 350 Main Street, Malden, Massachusetts 02148-
    5018, USA
Blackwell Publishing Ltd, 9600 Garsington Road, Oxford OX4 2DQ, UK
Blackwell Publishing Asia Pty Ltd, 550 Swanston Street, Carlton, Victoria
    3053, Australia

03 04 05 06 5 4 3 2 1

First published 2001
Second edition 2003

ISBN: 1-4051-1731-1

Library of Congress Cataloging-in-Publication data

Practical handbook of advanced interventional cardiology /
        [edited by] Thach Nguyen ... [*et al.*]. – 2nd ed.
        p. ; cm.
    Includes bibliographical references and index.
    ISBN 1-4051-1731-1
        1. Heart – Surgery. 2. Heart – Endoscopic surgery. 3. Heart
    – Diseases – Treatment. I. Nguyen, Thach.
        [DNLM: 1. Cardiac Surgical Procedures – methods – Hand-
    books. 2. Cardiovascular Diseases – surgery – Handbooks.
    WG 39 P895 2003]
    RD598.P65 2003
    617.4'12–dc21

                                                    2003013912

A catalogue record for this title is available from the British Library

Acquisitions: Jacques Strauss
Production: Charlie Hamlyn
Typesetter: Sparks Computer Solutions Ltd
Printed and bound by MPG Books Ltd, Bodmin, Cornwall, UK

For further information on Blackwell Publishing, visit our websites:
www.futuraco.com
www.blackwellpublishing.com

CONTRIBUTORS

Gérald Barbeau, MD
Laval Hospital, Institute de Cardiologie de Quebec, St Foy, Quebec, Canada

Sarana Boonbaichaiyapruck, MD, FACC, FSCAI
Associate Professor of Medicine, Director, Cardiac Catheterization & Intervention Service, Ramathibodi Hospital, Mahidol University, Bangkok, Thailand

Tan Huay Cheem, MD
Director, Coronary Intervention, The Heart Institute, Singapore

Buxin Chen, MD
Vice-President, Chief, Cardiology Department, Beijing Diali Hospital, Beijing, China

Zhang Shuang Chuan, MD
Director of Pediatric Department of Peking University Shenzhen Hospital, Professor of Pediatric Cardiology of Peking University Hospital, Guest Professor of Shenzhen Children's Hospital, Shenzhen, China

Herbert Cordero, MD
Phoenix Heart Center at St Joseph Hospital and Medical Center, Phoenix, AZ

Alain Cribier, MD
Department of Cardiology, Charles Nicolle Hospital, University of Rouen, France

Vijay Dave, MD
Chairman, Department of Medicine, Director of Medical Education, Community Health Care System, St Mary Medical Center, Hobart, IN

Edward Diethrich, MD
Medical Director, Arizona Heart Institute and Arizona Heart Hospital, Phoenix, AZ

John S. Douglas, MD
Director of the Cardiac Catheterization Laboratories, Emory University Hospital, Atlanta, GA

Ho Thuong Dzung, MD, PhD
Cardiology Department, Thong Nhat Hospital, Ho Chi Minh City, Vietnam

Helene Eltchaninoff, MD
Department of Cardiology, Charles Nicolle Hospital, University of Rouen, France

Quan Fang, MD
Chief, Cardiology Department, Peking Union Hospital, Beijing, China

Ted Feldman, MD, FACC, FSCAI
Professor of Medicine, Evanston-Northwestern Hospital, Evanston IL

Kirk Garratt, MD
Interventional Cardiology, Mayo Clinics, Rochester, MN

C. Michael Gibson, MS, MD
Director TIMI Data Coordinating Center and Angiographic Core Laboratory, Brigham and Women's Hospital; Associate Chief of Cardiology for Academic Affairs, Beth Israel Deaconess Medical Center, Harvard Medical School, Boston, MA

Cindy Grines, MD
Director, Cardiac Catheterization Laboratories, William Beaumont Hospital, Royal Oak, MI

Lee Guterman, PhD, MD
Assistant Professor, Department of Neurosurgery, and Co-Director, Toshiba Stroke Research Center, School of Medicine and Biomedical Sciences, University at Buffalo, State University of New York, Buffalo, NY

Richard Heuser, MD
Phoenix Heart Center at St Joseph Hospital and Medical Center, Phoenix, AZ

Nguyen Lan Hieu, MD
Interventional Cardiologist, Vietnam Heart Institute, Hanoi, Vietnam

L. Nelson Hopkins, MD
Professor and Chairman, Department of Neurosurgery; Professor, Department of Radiology; and Director, Toshiba Stroke Research Center; School of Medicine and Biomedical Sciences, University at Buffalo, State University of New York, Buffalo, NY

Jay Howington, MD
Assistant Clinical Instructor of Neurosurgery and Neuroendovascular Fellow, Department of Neurosurgery and Toshiba Stroke Research Center, School of Medicine and Biomedical Sciences, University at Buffalo, State University of New York, Buffalo, NY

Dayi Hu, MD
Professor of Medicine, Peking University and Capital University of Medical Sciences; President, The Institute of Cardiovascular Diseases; Chief of Cardiology, People and Beijing Tong Ren Hospital, Beijing, China

Do Quang Huan, MD
Director, Cardiac Catheterization Laboratories, The Heart Institute, Ho Chi Minh City, Vietnam

Jui Sung Hung, MD
Professor of Medicine, China Medical College, Taichung, Taiwan

Pham Manh Hung, MD
Associate Director, Cardiac Catheterization Laboratories, Vietnam Heart Institute, Bach Mai Hospital, Hanoi Medical University, Hanoi, Vietnam

Greg L. Kaluza, MD, PhD
Scientific Director, Institute for Research in Cardiovascular Interventions, The Methodist DeBakey Heart Center and Baylor College of Medicine, Houston, TX

Huynh Tuan Khanh, MD
Pediatric Cardiologist, Pediatric Hospital #2, Ho Chi Minh City, Vietnam

Moo-Huyn Kim, MD
Director, Cardiac Catheterization Laboratory, Dong-A University Hospital, Busan, Korea

Rajiv Kumar
Illinois Institute of Technology, Chicago IL

Kean Wah Lau, MB, FACC
Singapore Heart Institute, Singapore

Wang Lei, MD
Director, Catheterization Laboratories of the Heart & Blood Vessel Center, Beijing Friendship Hospital, Beijing, China

Elad Levy, MD
Assistant Clinical Instructor of Neurosurgery and Neuroendovascular Fellow, Department of Neurosurgery and Toshiba Stroke Research Center, School of Medicine and Biomedical Sciences, University at Buffalo, State University of New York, Buffalo, NY

Rijie Li, MD
Vice-President, Chief, Cardiology Department, Chui Yang Liu Hospital, Beijing, China

Meilin Liu, MD
Chief, Cardiology Department, Beijing Tongren Hospital, Capital University of Medical Sciences, Beijing, China

Do Doan Loi, MD, PhD
Director of the Echocardiography Laboratories, Vietnam Heart Institute, Hanoi, Vietnam

Caiyi Lu, MD
Professor and Vice-Director of Institute of Geriatric Cardiology, Chinese PLA General Hospital, Beijing, China

Nithi Mahanonda, MD, FRACP, FACC, FSCAI, FACA
Associate Director, Bangkok Heart Institute, Bangkok General Hospital, Bangkok, Thailand

Kazuaki Mitsudo, MD
Chief of Cardiology, Department of Cardiology, Kurashiki Central Hospital, Japan

Phillip Moore, MD
Associate Professor of Pediatrics, Director of Pediatric Congenital Heart Disease Program, UCSF, San Francisco, CA

Nguyen Thuong Nghia, MD
Interventional Cardiology Unit, Cho Ray Hospital, Ho Chi Minh City, Vietnam

Thach Nguyen, MD, FACC, FACP, FSCAI
Editorial Consultant, *Journal of Interventional Cardiology*; Co-editor, *Journal of the Institute of Geriatric Cardiology*; Professor of Medicine (Hon.), Capital University of Medical Sciences, Chao Yang and Friendship Hospital, Beijing, China; Director of Cardiology, Community Health Care System, St Mary Medical Center, Hobart, IN

Phong Nguyen-Ho, MD
Interventional Cardiology Fellow, University of Toronto, University Health Network – Toronto General Hospital Campus, Toronto, Canada

Vo Thanh Nhan, MD, PhD
Deputy Head of the Department of Cardiology, Head of the Interventional Cardiology Unit, Cho Ray Hospital, Ho Chi Minh City, Vietnam; Senior Lecturer, Faculty of Medicine, University of Medical Sciences, Ho Chi Minh City, Vietnam

Igor Palacios, MD
Director of Cardiac Catheterization Laboratories and Interventional Cardiology, Massachusetts General Hospital, Boston, MA

Seung Jung Park, MD
Chief, Division of Cardiology, Asan Medical Center, University of Ulsan, Seoul, Korea

Ta Tien Phuoc, MD
Cardiology Consultant, Vietnam Heart Institute, Hanoi, Vietnam

Devan Pillay, MD
Consultant Interventional Cardiologist, Gleneagles Medical Centre, Kuala Lumpur, Malaysia

Nguyen Ngoc Quang, MD
Interventional Cardiologist, Vietnam Heart Institute, Hanoi, Vietnam

Kasja Rabe, MD
Med. Cand., Cardiovascular Center, Frankfurt, Germany

Mark Reisman, MD
Director of Cardiovascular Research, Swedish Medical Center, Seattle, WA

Gianluca Rigatelli, MD, FSCAI, FCCP, FESC
Interventional Cardiologist, Endovascular Therapy Research, Legnago, Verona, Italy

Shigeru Saito, MD, FACC, FSCAI, FJCC
Chief of Division of Cardiology and Catheterization Laboratories, Heart Center of Shonan Kamakura General Hospital, Heart and Great Vessel Center of Beijing You-Yi Friendship Hospital, Beijing, China

Jia Sanqing, MD, PhD
Director, Heart & Blood Vessel Center, Beijing Friendship Hospital, affiliated to Capital University of Medical Sciences, Beijing, China

Lihua Shang, MD
Director, Cardiac Catheterization Laboratories, The People's Hospital, Beijing, China

Samuel J. Shubrooks, Jr, MD
Associate Professor of Medicine, Harvard Medical School, Co-Director of the Cardiac Catheterization Laboratories, Beth Israel Deaconess Medical Center, Boston, MA

Horst Sievert, MD
Professor of Medicine, Cardiovascular Center, Frankfurt, Germany

Krishna Rocha Singh, MD
Director Vascular Medicine Program, Clinical Assistant Professor of Medicine, Southern Illinois University, School of Medicine, Springfield, IL

Yan Songbiao, MD
Vice Director, Heart & Blood Vessel Center, Beijing Friendship Hospital, affiliated to Capital University of Medical Sciences, Beijing, China

Pham Hoan Tien, MD
Cardiology Consultant, Vietnam Heart Insitute, Hanoi, Vietnam

David Teitel, MD
Professor of Pediatric, Chief of Pediatric Cardiology, UCSF, San Francisco, CA

Damras Tresukosol, MD
Associate Professor of Medicine, Director of Cardiac Catheterization Laboratories, Faculty of Medicine, Siriraj Hospital, Bangkok, Thailand

Christophe Tron
Department of Cardiology, Charles Nicolle Hospital, University of Rouen, France

Nguyen Quang Tuan, MD
Interventional Cardiologist, Vietnam Heart Institute, Hanoi, Vietnam

Mintu Turakhia, MD
Internal Medicine Resident, Brigham and Women's Hospital, Harvard Medical School, Boston, MA

Lefeng Wang, MD
Deputy Director of the Cardiology Center, Director of the Catheterization Laboratories and Associate Professor, Chaoyang Red Cross Hospital, Beijing, China

Shiwen Wang, MD, MCAE
Member of Chinese Academy of Engineering, Professor and
Director of the Institute of Geriatric Cardiology, Chinese PLA
General Hospital, Beijing, China

Guy Weigold, MD
Fellow, Division of Cardiology, Washington Hospital Center,
Washington, DC

Neil J Weissman, MD
Director, Cardiac Ultrasound, Cardiovascular Research Institute, Washington Hospital Center, Washington, DC

Hong Zhao, MD
Cardiology Department, The People's Hospital, Peking University, Beijing, China

Mingzhong Zhao, MD
Cardiology Department, The People's Hospital, Peking University, Beijing, China

FOREWORD

Interventional cardiovascular medicine has evolved from an extremely crude method of opening femoral arteries initiated by Dotter, to a field that has now been recognized as having a sufficient fund of knowledge to require boards sanctioned by the American Board of Internal Medicine. From Andreas Gruentzig's development of the noncompliant balloon method, we have seen an explosion of bioengineering technology. The discipline of interventional cardiovascular medicine has perhaps initiated more registries and clinical trials than any other discipline in medicine. Indeed, the whole emphasis on evidence-based medicine has evolved during the era of interventional cardiology. Many basic science breakthroughs have been stimulated by the advances produced in interventional cardiology, as well as the problems and complications created by the new technologies.

However, no matter how advanced the science becomes, the success of solving a patient's problem with interventional techniques usually depends on the operator's technical ability. This ability springs from the wealth of experience the operator has acquired to deal with routine situations as well as complex and almost unique problems that may present themselves. Because of the large number of interventional cardiologists and the rapidly expanding number of procedures that can be performed, it is difficult for many cardiologists to experience all of the situations that can be helpful in building this database.

Dr Thach Nguyen has prepared a remarkable book, rich with tips and tricks for performing interventional cardiovascular medicine procedures. He has enlisted numerous experts on various aspects of interventional cardiovascular medicine to describe their areas of expertise. Rather than let them recite the evidence from registries and trials that are available elsewhere, he forces the contributors to provide the practical tips that they have learned. It is almost as though Dr Nguyen is trying to simulate the type of scenarios that exist in the catheterization laboratories with new cardiology fellows or less experienced operators. It is the type of advice that he has often given to cardiologists in developing countries who are bringing interventional techniques to help cope with the rapidly expanding new threat in these countries, vascular disease. Since new techniques are constantly appearing, all operators, experienced or not, can benefit from these tips. Whereas every operator will not agree with every approach to a problem or a complication, it is always instructive to understand many potential approaches. In this regard, the book does a masterful job of collecting not only the authors' experiences, but those of many others collected from the published literature, from numerous postgraduate courses, and from one-on-one demonstrations throughout the world.

This book should be a valuable resource to trainees in formal programs that have now evolved in the United States and other countries, as well as the many preceptorships that are the major means of training in other countries. In addition, operators of all levels of experience will find many useful pearls of wisdom. Dr Nguyen and his colleagues are to be congratulated for compiling this most practical guide.

Spencer B. King III, MD
Atlanta, Georgia

PREFACE

ADVANCED INTERVENTIONAL CARDIOLOGY: ART OR SCIENCE?

In 2003, more than 20 years after its humble beginning, interventional cardiology is a mature and major player in the management of complex cardiovascular problems. Its goals are to improve the symptoms, sustain the positive acute gains, and prolong life. The politically correct challenge is how to apply it at a universally affordable price to the American elderly patient population living on retirement benefits (without bankrupting Medicare) or to the financially struggling patients in developed or developing countries.

The technique of any procedure is formulated as a sequence of rigorously controlled maneuvers. They can be taught to fellows or staff, or programmed into robots. To understand and explain the physical, chemical, or biologic mechanism of any of these techniques or maneuvers is a science. To perform a procedure cost- and time-effectively in a humane manner is an art. In any interventional laboratory, a lesion could be dilated with one guide, one wire, one balloon, and/or one stent (if no predilation). A similar lesion can finally be dilated by a beginner after using any number of guides, wires, balloons, or stents. This is what experience is for. The bottom line is how to perform the procedure without wasting equipment, the patient's, the physician's, and staff's time, and causing no further harm (e.g. radiation). The goals of any procedure are highlighted in Table 0-1.

Which is the best option applying to this real-life situation?

While performing a procedure, every operator has the luxury to select, to change, or to delete a strategy, a device, or a drug (or be forced to use ones because the others are not available) from many options in order to achieve a procedural or clinical success. These options are listed plentifully and available anywhere in the printed or electronic media. However, the main question is always: which one is the best option applying to this real-life situation, with the equipment available here? In the second edition of this handbook, the authors try to answer that question and give practical suggestions derived from their own daily labor in the cardiac catheterization laboratories (or, as we call it intellectually, "experience"). So we highlight these practical heart-to-heart suggestions as Best Method, along with First Maneuver, Second Maneuver, or Caveat or Take-Home Message with all of the dramatic colorings or ups and downs – reminiscent of an Italian opera – which

---

Table 0-1 Strategic goals during interventions

---

1. **Effectiveness:** Problems controlled and results sustained
2. **User-friendly performance:** Simple manipulations, single operator, low-profile device, and no complex and costly set-up
3. **Cost- and time-effective selection of device:** A device should be selected appropriately to achieve its goal at the first try
4. **Cost- and time-effective approach:** In an attempt to fix or reverse a problem, it is more cost- and time-effective to manipulate devices currently in place rather than exchange them for new equipment
5. **Low complication rate:** Anticipation of complications, rigorous prevention, early detection, and prompt damage control.

---

happen many times in every cardiac catheterization laboratory. However, we hope the outcome is always as beautiful as any Chinese kung-fu movie.

In this way, the authors try to show how to select an appropriate device (best choice among many) so it can achieve its goal on the first attempt. Once a device does not function as it ideally should, there are many simple maneuvers (best methods among many) whereby the operators try to exhaust the full potential of a device before throwing it away or replacing it. In the end, the success rate is high due to improvements of technology, drugs, operator experience, and effort, and so are the expectations of the patient and family. The complication rate may be lower due to prevention and vigilant attention of the operators, or higher due to case selection (more high-risk patients and complex lesions). In any situation, once complications occur, they should be recognized early and damage control protocol should be promptly applied. This is why, in this second edition, we have the Caveats or Take-Home Messages to remind the young and old, beginner or experienced operators, of what to do in stressful situations or how to prevent them arising.

To the readers, who are all friends and colleagues

The authors and editors, who are all your friends and colleagues, labor every day in the cardiac laboratories like you. We write from our limited experience and our heart, during many sleepless nights. This handbook contains practical heart-to-heart advice aimed at you, the readers, and at us, the authors ourselves: we practice what we preach. These pieces of advice are applied daily in our laboratories or from those of authors we quote, and hopefully in your laboratories. They are not from an ivory tower. They are practiced by the experienced and the beginners, by the young and old, by men and women, so there is no question of class, age or sex or race division here, all of us are equal in striving to achieve procedural or clinical success.

Acknowledgements

As editors and authors, we hope we achieve our role as effective communicators to our readers who are all friends and colleagues. For the completion of this handbook, we owe much to our families, friends and colleagues. From the rural cornfields of northwest Indiana, I (TNN) am indebted for the invaluable encouragement of SJ Morales (Chicago), my parents, Mr Nguyen Ngoc Sau and Mrs Tran Thi Hong Hanh (Laporte IN); and Mr Milt Triana, Administrator of Health Community System, St Mary Medical Center, Hobart IN. It has been a privilege having the special support of Mr Jacques Strauss, Vice-President of Blackwell.

We really appreciate the help and efforts of the staffs at St Mary Medical Center (Hobart IN), Cheryl Anderson RT, Manager, Suzi Emig RN, Jennifer Fraley RT, Jennifer Gould RT, Karen Filko RT, Char King RN, Pat Robinson RN, Kris Shocaroff RN, and Debbie Smith RN; at Methodist Hospital, Southlake and Northlake campuses (Merrillville and Gary IN) Susan Slivka RT, Thomas Thegze RT, Lynetter Taylor RT, Patt Patzke RN, Judy Rataczak RN, Kim Grantsaris RT, Brad Johnson RT, and Erica Myller RT; and at St Anthony Hospital and Medical Center, Linda Rempala RN, BSN, BC, Tom Swendenberg RN, BSN, Suzan Taylor RN, Jim Campagna RT, Penny Ballestero RT, and Darlene Cusick RN. Many angiographic figures and technical tips are taken from cases in the cardiac catheterization laboratories of: Beijing Tong Ren Hospital; Beijing Friendship Hospital; Shonan Kamakura Hospital in Kamakura, Japan; China Medical College Hospital in Tai Chung, Taiwan; Vietnam Heart Institute, Hanoi, Vietnam; The Heart Institute, Ho Chi Minh City, Vietnam; The National University Hospital, Singapore; and Dong A Medical Center, Busan, Korea.

Above all, we are indebted to our patients, the purpose of our care, the source of our quests, and the inspiration of our daily works. To them, we give our heartfelt thanks.

CONTENTS

Abbreviations Used in This Book

ACS = acute coronary syndrome
ACT = activated clotting time
AP = anteroposterior
ASD = atrial septal defect
ATM = atmosphere(s)
AVF = arteriovenous fistula
BP = blood pressure
CABG = coronary artery bypass graft
CAD = coronary artery disease
CBF = coronary blood flow
CCA = common carotid artery
CEA = carotid endarterectomy
CFA = common femoral artery
CHD = congenital heart disease
CTO = chronic total occlusion
DCA = directional coronary atherectomy
DES = drug-eluting stent
ECA = external carotid artery
ECG = electrocardiogram
Gy = gray
IABP = intra-arterial balloon pump
ICH = intracranial hemorrhage
IMA = internal mammary artery
IRA = infarct-related arteries
ISMN = isosorbide mononitrate
ISR = in-stent restenosis
IVUS = intravascular ultrasound
LA = left atrium; left atrial
LAD = left anterior descending artery
LAO = left anterior oblique
LCX = left circumflex coronary artery
LIMA = left internal mammary artery
LM = left main
LMWH = low molecular weight heparin
LUPV = left upper pulmonary vein
LV = left ventricle
MACE = major acute cardiovascular event
MCA = middle cerebral artery
MI = myocardial infarction
MLD = minimal lumen diameter
OM = obtuse marginal
PA = pseudoaneurysm
PCI = percutaneous coronary intervention
PCWP = pulmonary capillary wedge pressure
PDA = posterior descending artery
PET = positron-emission tomography
PFA = profunda femoral artery
PICA = posterior inferior cerebellar artery

PMMC = percutaneous mechanical mitral commissurotomy
POBA = plain balloon angioplasty
psi = pounds per square inch
PT = prothrombin time
PTA = peripheral transluminal angioplasty
PTCA = percutaneous transluminal coronary angioplasty
PTRA = percutaneous transluminal rotational atherectomy
PTT = partial thromboplastin time
PWI = perfusion weighted imaging
RAO = right anterior oblique
RCA = right coronary artery; radial artery compression
ROTA = rotational atherectomy
RUPV = right upper pulmonary vein
RV = right ventricle; right ventricular
SCA = single coronary artery
SFA = superficial femoral artery
SVG = saphenous vein graft
TEE = transesophageal echocardiography
TLA = translumbar access needle
TLR = target lesion revascularization
TMR = transmyocardial revascularization
TRA = transradial approach
TVR = target vessel revascularization
VBT = vascular brachytherapy
VT = ventricular tachycardia

Chapter 1
Vascular Access

Thach Nguyen, Rajiv Kumar

Femoral access: Standard technique
 *Preparations in obese patients
 *Directing the needle
 *If the wire cannot be inserted
 *Sequential order for arterial and venous puncture
 **Puncture of pulseless femoral artery
 ***Puncture in cyanotic patients
 **Insertion and removal of IABP through diseased iliac artery
Puncture of femoral bypass graft
 **Puncture location
 **Angle of introduction
 **Sequential dilation
 **Kinked wire
Closure devices
 ***Pre-closure of large arterial access
 ***Non-surgical removal of the AngioSeal device
 TAKE-HOME MESSAGE: What to do if collagen is inserted intra-arterially
 ***When to suspect intra-arterial deployment of collagen plug
Antegrade puncture
 **Antegrade puncture
 **Manipulation of wire
 **Puncture of CFA with high bifurcation
 **Puncture with abduction and external rotation of the thigh
Brachial approach
Translumbar approach
 ***Reverse image
Transseptal approach
 ***Manipulation of catheter

---

*Basic; **Advanced; ***Rare, exotic, or investigational.

From: Nguyen T, Hu D, Saito S, Grines C, Palacios I (eds), *Practical Handbook of Advanced Interventional Cardiology*, 2nd edn. © 2003 Futura, an imprint of Blackwell Publishing.

Complications
>> **Mechanical thrombectomy for acute thrombosis
>> **Thrombolytic therapy for acute thrombosis
>> **Different patterns of ultrasound in the differential diagnoses of access site swelling
>> BEST METHOD: Best choice for management of pseudoaneursym

FEMORAL ACCESS: STANDARD TECHNIQUE

Locate the femoral artery and inguinal ligament that runs from the anterior superior iliac spine to the pubic tubercle. The true position of the inguinal ligament is 1–2 cm below that line.[1] The femoral pulse at the inguinal crease is not a reliable landmark for the common femoral artery (CFA), particularly in obese patients.[2] Ninety-seven percent of patients have the femoral artery lying on the medial third of the femoral head. Only 3% have the artery totally medial to the femoral head.[3]

TECHNICAL TIPS

*Preparations in obese patients: The femoral pulse at the inguinal crease is not a reliable landmark for the common femoral artery (CFA), particularly in obese or elderly patients, whose crease tends to be much lower than the inguinal ligament.[2] The protruding abdomen and panniculus should be retracted, and taped to the chest with 3- to 4-inch tapes that are in turn secured to the sides of the catheterization table. Keep the tissue layer above the artery as thin and as taut as possible, so the needle will not be deflected outside the projected angle and selected pathway.

*Directing the needle: Once the needle tip is near the artery, it tends to pulsate except in patients with severe local scarring (after many prior remote femoral artery cannulations, ilio-femoral bypass, after total hip replacement, etc.). If the hub inclines to the right, the needle should be withdrawn by 1 or 2 cm and the tip redirected to the left before advancing forward. If the hub inclines to the left side, the reverse maneuver is used to change the course. If the needle pulsates on the vertical axis, it just needs to be inserted more deeply.[3]

*If the wire cannot be inserted: Most often, this is because the needle hit the contralateral wall. Just move the needle by a slight pull or rotate it a little, and the wire may be able to be inserted. If there is difficulty, it is better to withdraw the needle and re-puncture the artery rather than dissect the artery.[4] After the sheath is inserted and the wire is not able to negotiate the tortuous iliac artery then a diagnostic Judkins right catheter can be advanced to the tip of the wire in order to help steer the wire tip. A gentle injection of contrast may help to delineate the anatomy and determine the reason why the wire could not be advanced. The use of hydrophilic wires for the initial introduction through the needle should be avoided because they can easily travel subintimally and cause later dissection. Also, they can be easily cut by the sharp needle tip.

*Sequential order for arterial and venous puncture: The order of arterial and venous access is often a matter of personal preference. We prefer to puncture the vein first and insert a wire inside the vein to secure the access. Then, less than 1 minute later, after puncturing the artery, we would insert the sheath into the artery and the vein. Because there is only a wire in the vein, we do not disturb the anatomic landmark of the common femoral artery, which we try to locate and puncture. Less than 1 minute without a sheath will not produce a hematoma at the venous site. If the artery is inadvertently punctured first, we would cannulate the artery, then puncture the vein under fluoroscopy, with the needle medial and parallel to the arterial sheath.

**Puncture of pulseless femoral artery: As usual, the artery should be punctured over the middle of the medial third of the femoral head. Localize the skin puncture site by fluoroscopy just below the inferior border of the femoral head in order to prevent high punctures that may lead to uncontrollable bleeding. However, these proportions are valid only in the AP, neutral position (Figure 1-1). Internal or external rotation of the femur can considerably change the relationship of the femoral artery to the femoral head.[5] Doppler guidance is very helpful in puncturing an artery with very weak pulse or a pulseless artery, especially when the standard anatomy is deranged by a large hematoma, or thick scar after surgery. The most common cause of weak pulse is hypovolemic hypotension, heavy calcification, and is only rarely due to narrow pulse pressure such as in constrictive pericarditis (in contrast to aortic regurgitation).

***Puncture in cyanotic patients: In children with cyanotic heart disease, especially those weighing less than 15 kg and with severe polycythemia, the blood flow from a femoral puncture can resemble a venous sample: a gentle flow of dark blood. This color is due to arterial desaturation and hyperviscosity secondary to polycythemia. If there is doubt, confirm the arterial puncture by attaching the needle to a pressure transducer or by making a small contrast injection into the arterial lumen.[6]

***Insertion and removal of IABP through diseased iliac artery: When an IABP needs to be inserted and an

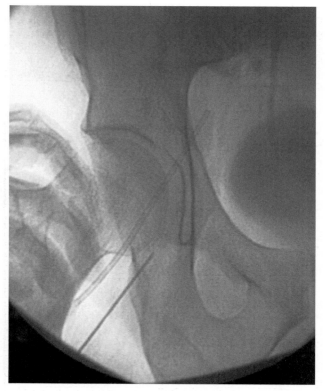

Figure 1-1: Needle position on the femoral head for arterial and venous puncture and cannulation.

iliac lesion is found, the lesion should be dilated first. Insert the balloon pump, then perform stenting of the lesion later after the IABP is removed. When a balloon pump is to be inserted through a previously stented iliac artery, do it under fluoroscopy to be sure the balloon does not get stuck on the stent struts. To remove the IABP deflated balloon, insert a large femoral sheath and withdraw the winged balloon into the sheath so the folds of the winged balloon are not caught by struts at the stent edges. Chronic endothelialization of the stent struts should diminish this problem.

PUNCTURE OF FEMORAL BYPASS GRAFT

The problems involving puncture of an old vascular graft in the femoral area include: uncontrollable bleeding and hematoma formation because of the non-vascular nature of the punctured graft; disruption of the anastomotic suture line with subsequent false aneurysm formation; infection of the graft site; and catheter damage, kinking, and separation due to scar tissue in the inguinal area and firmness of the healed graft material.[7] Inadvertent entry to the native arterial system may lead to the dead-end stump in the common femoral or iliac artery.

TECHNICAL TIPS

**Puncture location: Because the exact location of the suture line is not known, to avoid puncture of the anastomotic site, it is best to puncture the proximal end of the inguinal incision site or as close to the inguinal ligament as possible.

**Angle of introduction: To avoid kinking of the catheter at the puncture site, it is better to introduce the needle at an angle of approximately 30° to 45° to the estimated long axis of the graft.[7]

**Sequential dilation: Sometimes, because of severe scarring, the entry site has to be prepared by sequential dilation with progressively larger dilators up to 1F size larger than the sheath selected for the procedure.

**Kinked wire: It is not unusual that the wire will pass into the lumen easily but attempts to advance any dilator over the wire will result in kinking of the wire at the point of entry. Instead of exchanging the wire, if the wire is not too crooked we would advance the wire farther, so we use the dilator to dilate the entry site on a straight and stiff segment of the wire. If the wire is too soft, then it should be exchanged for a stiffer wire over a smallest size 4F dilator.[7]

CLOSURE DEVICES

The choice between collagen plugs and suture closure is largely a matter of personal preference and experience. The time needed to deploy the various devices is unique to each system. When physicians' time to utilize the device and staff time for adjunctive compression or puncture site management are considered together, sealing devices do not provide an advantage over manual pressure in decreasing complications.[8] Current arteriotomy closure devices were found to be independent predictors of major hematoma as body surface area (BSA). Infection has been reported with all of these devices.[8] Thorough training of operators in how to use any device is warranted to reduce vascular access complications. When deploying an AngioSeal device (St Jude Medical Devices, Minneapolis, MN), an iliac angiogram needs to show the artery diameter is at least 4 mm and there is no bifurcation within 2 cm of the arterial entry site.

TECHNICAL TIPS

***Pre-closure of large arterial access:** In cases of need of large size sheath (e.g. for valvuloplasty), preplacement of untied sutures using the Closer percutaneous suture delivery system (Abbotts Vascular, Redwood City, CA) prior to placement of a large intended sheath can be done. A 5F to 6F sheath may be used for arterial angiography to identify appropriate anatomy, and then a suture delivery system is used to place untied sutures. At the end of the procedure, the existing "purse string" is then closed around the arteriotomy.[9]

***Non-surgical removal of the AngioSeal device:** After PCI, many closure devices can be used to close the puncture site. In a case reported by Stein et al., a possible intra-arterial deployment of the collagen plug was suspected during an AngioSeal deployment. At that time, while inserting the tamper tube more deeply, it was observed that it could be inserted much deeper than is usually found during routine AngioSeal deployment. The patient continued to bleed. A tension spring was placed as usual. At that time, the author used a hemostat to secure the end of the suture, and a FemoStop compression device (Femostop, Radi Medical Systems AB, Sweden) was applied above the AngioSeal to stop bleeding. Then the author waited for 4 hours, so that the anchor, composed of an absorbable polymer material, would become softened and thus pliable. A hemostat was placed on the suture at the level of skin. If the suture were to break during traction, the hemostat would prevent the anchor and the collagen plug from embolizing. Then steady traction was applied to the suture, perpendicular to the femoral artery. The pressure should not be excessive. After 20 minutes, the plug was removed. The FemoStop was reapplied and hemostasis was achieved. The Take-Home Message is summarized below. [10]

TAKE-HOME MESSAGE

What to do if collagen is inserted intra-arterially:
1. Prevent the problem: always maintain tension on the suture and avoid tamping with excessive force.
2. Recognize the problem: absence of resistance during tamping and inadequate hemostasis are clues.

3. Duplex ultrasound can document intra-arterial collagen.
4. Apply tension string in the usual fashion; secure suture with hemostat at skin level to add security.
5. **Do not cut suture:** embolization of the anchor and plug may occur.
6. If there are signs of embolism and thrombosis, obtain vascular surgery consultation.
7. Wait at least 4 hours to allow softening of the anchor.
8. Steady vertical traction on suture with approximately 10 lbs of force.
9. If removal of the device is achieved, maintain manual compression to achieve hemostasis.
10. Femo-Stop device should be ready for rapid deployment after device is removed.

***When to suspect intra-arterial deployment of collagen plug:** During deployment of an AngioSeal device, intra-arterial deployment of the collagen plug can be due to inadequate tension on the suture, vigorous tamping, too deep insertion of the device into the artery, so that the anchor is caught in the posterior wall, etc. Suspicion of the problem is aroused when there is a long travel distance of the tamper tube or continued bleeding.[10] Precaution tips during deployment of the AngioSeal device are summarized in Table 1-1.

ANTEGRADE PUNCTURE

A contralateral femoral artery puncture is used to reach lesions in the profunda femoral (PFA) and proximal SFAs. An antegrade puncture is used to reach more distal lesions for interventions in the superficial femoral, popliteal, tibial, and peroneal arteries.

Optimal preparation: The antegrade femoral puncture can be greatly simplified and more successful if the tissue thickness between the skin surface and the artery is as thin as possible. This may be achieved by placing a pillow under

Table 1-1
Tips during deployment of AngioSeal device

1. Insert the insertion sheath exactly 1.5 cm after seeing squirt of blood.
2. After that, pull back the whole device, feel that the anchor is tightly apposed to the arterial wall.
3. Advance the tamper tube while keeping steady traction on the suture.
4. Be sure there is no severe blood oozing.

the buttocks. The hyperextension of the hip joint caused by this maneuver stretches the skin taut over the puncture site and tremendously decreases the tissue thickness. In obese patients, fatty panniculus may have to be retracted away from the puncture site manually and taped in position before the puncture is attempted.[5]

Standard puncture: The next step is to localize the CFA and its bifurcation under fluoroscopy. The CFA usually over-lies the medial third of the femoral head and the bifurcation occurs below the lower border of the femoral head.[4] Once the landmark is located, to make the puncture, the needle may be directed toward the superior aspect of the femoral head, under fluoroscopy. The purpose of this maneuver is to prevent the inadvertent puncture of either or both the superficial femo-ral or the profunda femoral arteries. It is important to puncture the femoral artery as high above the bifurcation as possible so that there will be enough space between the puncture site and the bifurcation for catheter exchanges and manipulation of catheters into the SFA.

TECHNICAL TIPS

**Antegrade puncture: Using fluoroscopy, the site of the intended arterial puncture is identified (upper or middle third of the femoral head). The femoral pulse is palpated against the femoral head. Local anesthetic is infiltrated 2–3 cm cranial to the intended site of puncture. An 18 gauge needle is advanced at 45–60° directed caudally, aiming at the intended site of arterial puncture. Once pulsatile flow is obtained, a soft tip wire is inserted toward the SFA. The wire should follow a straight caudal course into the SFA. Lateral deviation indicates entry into the profunda femoral artery. The wire can be withdrawn and the needle tip deflected me-dially to redirect the wire into the SFA.

**Manipulation of wire: If the wire was inserted into the PFA, it can be withdrawn and redirected by angling the tip of the needle medially toward the SFA. The other option is to have a wire with a curved tip and manipulate it so the tip points toward the SFA. The needle may be exchanged for a short dilator with a gently curved tip, which can be directed toward the SFA. This dilator can be withdrawn slowly from the PFA while injecting the contrast agent. Once the orifice of the SFA is seen under fluoroscopy, it can be selectively catheterized or it can be used to direct a wire into the SFA.[5]

**Puncture of CFA with high bifurcation: In patients with high bifurcation, one single puncture can result in entries of both the SFA and PFA. When this occurs, the first spurt of blood may indicate that the PFA is punctured. Do not re-move the needle completely. Instead, withdraw it slowly and watch for a second spurt of blood. At this point, the contrast injection may show that the needle is in the SFA. In the rare cases of high bifurcation, it may not be possible to puncture the CFA that is excessively high in the pelvic area.[5]

**Puncture with abduction and external rotation of the thigh: Another option to cannulate the SFA is with the thigh in abduction and external rotation. The goal of this maneuver is to facilitate a more mediolateral puncture site in the CFA. In the usual AP puncture, the needle is seen to point more toward the PFA that is lateral to the SFA. In the abduction and external rotation position, the needle points more toward the SFA, and the PFA is seen medial to the SFA. This relationship is important when observing the course of the wire during its intended selective entry into the SFA. If the patient is punctured in this position, after the procedure, the local compression of the artery should be in the abduction and external rotation of the thigh because the puncture site is more mediolateral than usual.[5]

BRACHIAL APPROACH

Even though the radial artery is the most common location used in the upper extremity, the brachial artery is still the access site of choice for procedures requiring a large sheath: subclavian artery stenting, renal stenting, or aortic aneurysm exclusion. The radial access is discussed in Chapter 2.

TRANSLUMBAR APPROACH

In patients with total occlusion of arteries to lower and upper extremities, PCI can still be performed through the translumbar approach.[11] This problem occurs rarely, only once in 6000 to 9000 cases. However, if the lumbar approach is the only access available in those rare circumstances in which conventional sites are not available, then it is worth offering the option to the patient.[12]

Technique
The patient is placed in the prone position. Utilizing the left flank approach, an appropriate puncture site is selected, which is approximately 4 finger breadths lateral to the midline and 2 finger breadths below the left 12th rib margin. Verification that this position is below the posterior sulcus of the lung is made by fluoroscopy. After local anesthesia, a small skin incision is made with a blade and enlarged by the hemostat. The tip of the translumbar access needle (TLA) and the outer Teflon sheath (Cook, Bloomington, IN) are placed in the skin incision and directed toward the T12 vertebral body. Three

successive attempts are made, with each increasing the vertical degree of the pass in order to "step off" of the vertebral body. When the needle tip abuts the aorta, pulsation can be felt against the fingertip. The TLA needle is then given a short thrust until the initial resistance is not felt. The tip of needle is watched closely and should never cross the midline of the body. The inner stylet of the TLA needle is removed, and blood is seen at the hub. A floppy J wire is inserted and an introducer sheath is inserted in the usual fashion. Coronary angiogram and angioplasty are performed by the standard technique. After documentation of ACT less than 150 sec, the sheath is removed without complication while the patient is in the prone position.[11]

TECHNICAL TIP

***Reverse image:** Given the prone position of the patient, the fluoroscopic images appear in reverse, compared to standard images. This problem can be corrected by using the sweep reversal mode on the video monitor.[11]

TRANSSEPTAL APPROACH

Femoral and radial access is universally used for interventional procedures. However, in some patients with pulseless disease (Takayasu's arteritis), there are no arterial pulses in four extremities, then the PCI has to be done through the femoral vein approach. Tips and tricks for puncturing the septum are discussed and illustrated extensively in Chapters 24 and 25.

Technique

A transseptal puncture was performed through the femoral vein with a modified Brockenbrough technique. A 7F pulmonary artery balloon-tipped catheter was advanced through the mitral valve, looped around the LV apex, and passed out of the aortic valve successfully to the ascending aorta. An 8F Mullins transseptal sheath (USCI, C.R. Bard, Galway, Ireland) was advanced into the LA. Heparin was given. The pulmonary artery catheter was exchanged for a 6F AL-1 (Cordis Europa, Roden, The Netherlands), then to a 6F Multipurpose catheter (Cordis) over a 0.038" exchange wire. The LM was engaged easily and selective coronary was performed. Selective right coronary selection was unsuccessful with the AL, JR, or Multipurpose catheters. At the end, selective opacification of the right coronary artery (RCA) was achieved with the JL4. There were no complications, except for asymptomatic intermittent nonsustained VT due to the wire.[13]

TECHNICAL TIP

*****Manipulation of catheter:** At all times, care was taken to maintain a loop of catheter or wire in the left ventricular apex. Shortening of this loop to the straight path between the mitral and aortic valves could result in trauma to the anterior mitral leaflet.[14] There were few problems cannulating the LM; however, it was difficult to cannulate the RCA because the catheters kept dropping into the ventricle when manipulated.[13] The total procedure time was 120 minutes with 42 minutes for the RCA engagement, compared with 12 minutes for a complete coronary angiography through the femoral approach.

COMPLICATIONS

Hematoma: Frequency is 1–3% and increases with the increasing size of the sheath, the higher level of anticoagulation, and the obesity of the patient.[8] Surgical evacuation is not required even for large hematomas, unless there is undue tension on adjacent structure or in the case of a truly huge hematoma. Surgical evacuation and arterial repair are required when the hematoma is pulsatile and expanding, an indication of communication between the hematoma and the femoral artery and the presence of a false aneurysm.[15]

Arteriovenous fistula (AVF): This happens rarely (<0.4%) when the puncture is made where the artery overlies the vein.[16] Most small AVFs are asymptomatic and usually close spontaneously. A large AVF with symptoms of high output failure needs to be corrected surgically.

Acute arterial thrombosis: Occlusion of the femoral artery may occur due to thrombosis or local arterial injury. It happens rarely, mostly in women with small femoral arteries that are completely blocked by the catheter during the procedure and in patients whose SFA is catheterized rather than the CFA. The management includes rapid clinical assessment, prompt initiation of anticoagulant to reduce or prevent thrombus propagation and protection against further embolization, pain control and rapid initiation of therapy to re-establish perfusion of the affected limb. Unlike in acute myocardial infarction, where intravenous bolus of fibrin-specific plasminogen activators (PA) dosing is necessary to rapidly achieve high concentration of plasmin activity at the site of thrombosis and facilitate rapid lysis of a relatively small thrombus, lysis of larger diameter and longer peripheral thromboses is best achieved with catheter-directed infusion of specific PAs over several hours to days.[16] Compared with urokinase, which was recently re-introduced in the US market, bolus doses of the PAs may be associated with excessive risk of bleeding or cardiopulmonary complications, necessitating transfer to intensive care units when followed by long continuous infusion. [17]

TECHNICAL TIPS

**Mechanical thrombectomy for acute thrombosis: If thrombosis of the femoral artery is suspected, access is obtained from the contralateral side and 5000 units of heparin are given. A 6F crossover sheath is placed in the external iliac artery over a 0.035" stiff Amplatz guidewire. The occluded/thrombosed/embolized segment of the artery is crossed with a 0.014" or 0.018" wire. An AngioJet catheter (Possis Medical, Minneapolis, MN) is then introduced over the wire for thrombectomy. If normal distal flow is established without any residual stenosis, the procedure is terminated. If there is still residual thrombus, then the segment is dilated with a peripheral balloon, and if the post-PTA result is not optimal, a self-expanding stent may be deployed.[18]

**Thrombolytic therapy for acute thrombosis: If heavy thrombotic burden still persists after mechanical thrombectomy, then tPA 0.05 mg/kg can be given along with heparin through a multi-hole delivery catheter (e.g. 5Fr Mewissen of Boston Scientific, Quincy, MA). Four hours later, an angiogram can be done to check the progress and if there is thrombus, the patient can undergo longer infusion (12–18 hours).[18]

Infection: The incidence is 0.2%. The risk factors include puncture of the groin area after a very recent procedure at the same site and with a fresh hematoma present and prolonged (>24 hours) sheath placement. Localized infection at a vertebral artery in the lumbar region proved to be due to injection of infectious material from the long-indwelling femoral sheath.[19]

Neuropathy: When there is a large inguinal hematoma compressing the femoral nerve, the patient feels numb at the anterior medial aspect of the thigh. Sometimes the patient has difficulty walking due to weakness of the quadriceps, the extensors of the knees. These problems should be resolved within 24 hours.

Retroperitoneal hematoma: The incidence was high at 3%[20] and is much lower now. Clinical clues include hypotension without apparent reason, blood loss without possible source, supra-inguinal tenderness and fullness, and ipsilateral (or rarely contralateral) flank discomfort. A small hematoma is not able to cause any hemodynamic disturbances or any increase of the retroperitoneal cavity pressure to cause neurologic symptoms. Only a huge hematoma compressing the lumbar plexus can really produce numbness and weakness of the muscles below the knee. Usually, bleeding into the retroperitoneal site is self-limiting unless the patient is

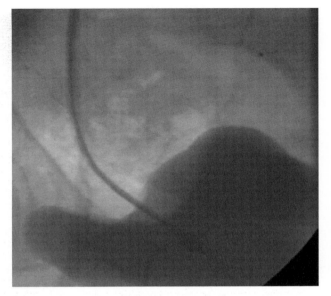

Figure 1-2: A dented bladder due to retroperitoneal hematoma. It looks different from the round shape of the bladder in Figure 1-1.

anticoagulated.[21] Just an AP view of the pelvic area under fluoroscopy may give a clue to the problem. Usually, during an interventional procedure, the bladder is seen filled with dye. In contrast, if the opacified bladder is seen displaced and its round shape is dented, retroperitoneal hematoma is strongly suspected (Figure 1-2).[21] However, significant blood needs to be sequestered before unilateral external compression occurs. The management includes stopping heparin and reversing anticoagulation with protamine, then rapid fluid resuscitation to reverse hypovolemia. Transfusion may be needed. If the above treatment fails, surgical exploration is required.

Perforation: If a balloon bursts and perforates a peripheral artery below the inguinal ligament, the local bleeding can be controlled by direct pressure. In the case of higher perforation, a large peripheral balloon should be inflated above or at the rupture site to stop the bleeding and to seal the puncture site.[21]

TECHNICAL TIP

**Different patterns of ultrasound in the differential diagnoses of access site swelling: Pseudoaneurysms are characterized by the presence of a to-and-fro blood flow across the PA neck during systole and diastole.

Hematomas are seen as hypoechoic collections without any Doppler flow movement. Deep vein thrombosis (DVT) is characterized by a lack of venous compressibility, obstruction of venous return, and a hypoechoic or isoechoic signal.[22]

Pseudoaneurysm (PA): The incidence of PA is 1–3% by clinical examination or 6% by ultrasound.[23] The main cause is inadvertent puncture of the SFA. Femoral PA forms when the puncture site does not close and there is continuous flow into a small perivascular space contained by the surrounding fibrous tissue and hematomas. It is suspected by the presence of a laterally pulsatile mass, an arterial bruit, and tenderness at the vascular access site. Confirmation is made by ultrasound, which shows a hypoechogenic cavity with flow through a neck directly visible by color Doppler, and pulsed Doppler evidence of to-and-fro flow between the cavity and the arterial lumen during systole and diastole.[23] Indications for aggressive management include: large size of the PA, whether it has increased in size, and the need for continued anticoagulation. Usually the small PAs (<3 cm in diameter) will close spontaneously, presumably due to thrombosis. A follow-up ultrasound 1–2 weeks later often demonstrates spontaneous thrombosis and obviates need of surgical repair. The >3 cm diameter PAs are less likely to close spontaneously. When PAs persist beyond 2 weeks or expand, the risk of femoral artery rupture necessitates correction. In the past, the simplest method of treatment was to use a mechanical compression device (Femostop, Radi Medical Systems AB, Sweden). The success rate is 74% with a mean compression of 33 minutes.[23] The failed patients underwent successful compression guided by ultrasound. Contraindications to mechanical compression are listed in Table 1-2. Ultrasound-guided compression is commonly used with success related to the anticoagulation status and a PA that can be readily visualized and compressed.[23]

BEST METHOD

Best choice for the management of pseudoaneurysm: The newest mode of treatment is to inject thrombin into the PA under the guidance of ultrasound.[24] With more experience in the past few years, it has become the treatment of choice.

Table 1-2
Contraindications to mechanical compression for PA

1. Sign of local infection
2. Critical limb ischemia
3. Large hematoma with overlying skin necrosis
4. Injuries above the inguinal ligament

1. Best method: injection of thrombin under guidance of ultrasound, because it is simple, quick, and painless.
2. If there is no experience with injection of thrombin, then mechanical compression device is the next step.
3. If empiric compression fails to close the PA, then mechanical compression under ultrasound guidance.
4. Surgery is rarely necessary.
5. Other investigational techniques become obsolete: coil embolization (disadvantage: coils may fall through the skin or irritate when moving the leg) and covered stent (disadvantage: 12% risk of stent occlusion and more costly).

REFERENCES

1. Kandarpa K, Gardiner GA. Angiography: general principles. In: Kandarpa K, Aruny JE. *Handbook of Interventional Radiologic Procedures*, 2nd edn. Little, Brown and Company, 1996: 8–9.
2. Grier D, Hatnell G. Percutaneous femoral artery puncture: Practice and anatomy. *Br J Radiol* 1990; **83**: 602–4.
3. Abhyankar AD. "Dancing needle sign" for obtaining access to the femoral artery. Letter to the editor. *Cathet Cardiovasc Diagn* 1995; **35**: 378.
4. Fajadet J, Hayerizadeh B, Ali H *et al*. Transradial approach for interventional procedures. In: Fajadet J, ed. *Syllabus for EuroPCR*, 2001: 11–28.
5. Gerlock AJ, Mirfakhraee M. *Essentials of Diagnostic and Interventional Angiographic Techniques*. W.B. Saunders, 1985.
6. Mehan VK. Doubtful arterial puncture during cardiac catheterization in cyanotics. *Cathet Cardiovasc Diagn* 1990; **19**: 148–9.
7. Chisholm RJ. Femoral artery catheterization in patients with previous bifemoral grafting. *Cathet Cardiovasc Diagn* 1993; **30**: 313.
8. Feldman T. Percutaneous vascular closure: Plugs, stitches, and glue. *Cathet Cardiovasc Diagn* 1998; **45**: 89.
9. Feldman T. Femoral arterial preclosure: Finishing a procedure before it begins. *Cathet Cardiovasc Interv* 2001; **53**: 448.
10. Stein B, Terstein P. Non-surgical removal of Angio-Seal Device after intra-arterial deposition of collagen plug. *Cathet Cardiovasc Interv* 2000; **50**: 340–2.
11. Chandler AH, Johnson M, Routh WD *et al*. Angioplasty of a coronary artery via the translumbar approach in a patient with severe peripheral vascular disease. *Cathet Cardiovasc Diagn* 1996; **38**: 202–4.
12. Grollman J. Back to our roots. *Cathet Cardiovasc Diagn* 1996; **38**: 205.

13. Farah B, Prendergast B, Garbarz E *et al*. Antegrade transseptal coronary angiography: An alternative technique in severe vascular disease. *Cathet Cardiovasc Diagn* 1998; **43**: 444–6.

14. Mullins CE. Transseptal left heart catheterization: Experience with a new technique in 520 pediatric and adult patients. *Pediatr Cardiol* 1983; **4**: 239–246.

15. King III SB, Douglas JS. *Management of Complications in Coronary Arteriography and Angioplasty*. McGraw-Hill, 1985: 311.

16. Dietcher S, Jaff M. Pharmacologic and clinical characteristics of thrombolytic agent. *Rev Cardiovasc Med* 2002; **3** (suppl 2): S25–33.

17. Ouriel K, Gray B, Clair DG *et al*. Complications associated with the use of urokinase and recombinant tissue plasminogen activator for catheter-directed peripheral arterial and venous thrombosis. *J Vasc Interv Radiol* 2000; **11**: 295–8.

18. Samal A, White C. Percutaneous management of access site complications. *Cathet Cardiovasc Interv* 2002; **57**: 12–23.

19. Oriscello RG, Fineman S, Vigario JC *et al*. Epidural abscess as a complication of coronary angioplasty: A rare but dangerous complication. *Cathet Cardiovasc Diagn* 1994; **33**: 36–8.

20. Muller DW, Shamir KJ, Ellis SG *et al*. Peripheral vascular complications after conventional and complex percutaneous coronary interventional procedures. *Am J Cardiol* 1992; **69**: 63–68.

21. Chambers CE, Griffin DC, Omarzai RK. The "dented bladder": Diagnosis of a retroperitoneal hematoma. *Cathet Cardiovasc Diagn* 1993; **34**: 224–226.

22. Polak JF. Peripheral vascular system. In: McGahan JP, Goldberg BB, eds. *Diagnostic Ultrasound*. Philadephia: Lippincott-Raven, 2000: 1004–5.

23. Zahn R *et al*. Pseudoaneurysm after cardiac catheterization: Therapeutic interventions and the sequelae: Experience in 86 patients. *Cathet Cardiovasc Diagn* 1997; **40**: 9–15.

24. Chatterjee T, Meier B. You broke it, you fix it: More cards up the sleeve of the catheter man. *Cathet Cardiovasc Interv* 1999; **47**: 165–6.

Chapter 2
Transradial Approach

Gérald R. Barbeau

General overview
The radial artery access
    **Right or left TRA?
    **Difficulty in accessing the ascending aorta
    **Spasm
    **Avoiding bleeding complications
Selection of guides
    **LAO angulation
    **Deep seating of guide
    **Use of Amplatz left
    **Stent loss or dislodgement

GENERAL OVERVIEW

Screening for transradial approach

To avoid ischemic complications of the hand, the percutaneous transradial approach (TRA) can be performed only in patients with patent palmar arterial arch, usually evaluated with the modified Allen's test. This test measures the amount of time to achieve maximal palmar blush after compression release of the ulnar artery with continuing occlusive pressure of the radial artery. Patients with hand blushing in 9 seconds or less are candidates for TRA. To maximize blushing, the hand is forcefully closed in a fist before arterial compression and opened before release of the ulnar artery compression. This modified Allen's test is subjective at best and should be performed by a physician.

Another method is to evaluate the palmar arch patency with plethysmography and oxymetry tests. Plethysmography readings during radial artery compression (RAC) are divided in four types and are listed in Table 2-1.

*Basic; **Advanced; ***Rare, exotic, or investigational.

From: Nguyen T, Hu D, Saito S, Grines C, Palacios I (eds), *Practical Handbook of Advanced Interventional Cardiology*, 2nd edn. © 2003 Futura, an imprint of Blackwell Publishing.

Table 2-1
Classification of pulse tracing

A. no dampening of pulse tracing
B. dampening of pulse tracing
C. loss followed by recovery of pulse tracing within 2 min
D. loss of pulse tracing without recovery

Oxymetry was either positive or negative during RAC. Patients were considered suitable for TRA with modified Allen's test 9 seconds or less or plethysmography type A,B,C and positive oxymetry readings (Figure 2-1). Using this technique, in a series of 1010 consecutive patients, only 1.5% of patients were excluded for either right or left PTRA. The clear advantage of this *objective* test is that it can be performed by personnel from the cardiac interventional laboratory after a very short period of training.[1]

THE RADIAL ARTERY ACCESS[2]

Right TRA: The right arm is placed in an abducted position with slight wrist overextension, without constraint. Right radial and bilateral femoral entry sites are disinfected with povidone-iodine and prepared for possible access. Local skin anesthesia is obtained by 2% lidocaine injected subcutaneously with a 25-gauge needle, and a small (1 mm) incision is made with #11 surgical blade. The radial artery is punctured with a 19–21-gauge open needle to obtain a pulsatile blood flow. The artery is cannulated with a 45-cm 0.019–25" straight non-Teflonized wire, which advances without resistance. A short (15 cm) or long (23 cm) 4–5F sheath is then inserted. The arm is then positioned alongside the patient. Verapamil (2.5 mg) is injected through the side arm of the sheath. Heparin sulfate (50–100 units/kg) is mandatorily given, usually IV to avoid pain. A diagnostic (4–5F) catheter is inserted with a 0.035" Teflonized J wire. In case of difficult wire progression, a Terumo™ hydrophilic wire or a coronary wire is used. After the diagnostic angiography, if the anatomy is suitable for intervention, the diagnostic catheter is exchanged over the wire for the appropriate 5–8F sheath and guide so the intervention can be performed immediately.

Left TRA: The procedure is the same as for the right TRA procedure except that the left arm is flexed over the abdomen *after* sheath and wire insertion (a small cushion is placed under the arm and elbow). The operator is positioned on the right side of the patient as usual.

Post-procedure care: Once the procedure is completed, the arterial sheath is immediately removed and a pressure dressing is applied over the puncture site with a compression

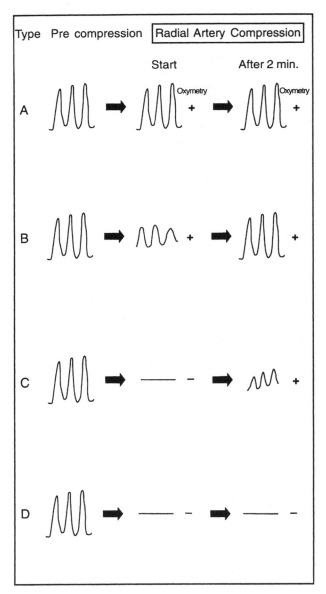

Figure 2-1: Drawing representing the four types of palmar arch patency findings with plethysmography and oxymetry as recorded with the finger clamp applied on the thumb.

band (Hemoband™). The pressure dressing is checked every 30 minutes until hemostasis. Following hemostasis, a non-compressive dressing is applied over the puncture site. A slightly elastic dressing bandage (ACE) can be applied for prevention of bleeding or in case of discrete hematoma and for patient comfort. To encourage ambulation immediately after the procedure, we remove all the intravenous lines in the catheterization laboratory and encourage liberal fluid intake.

Results of previous studies: The transradial approach is successful in approximately 93–99%. Predictors of failure are female gender, higher age, low BMI, and lack of experience in performing TRA.[3] Causes of failure include inability to puncture, anatomic variation, and vascular tortuosity, spasm, and pain. Radial artery thrombosis is seen in 3–6% of procedures. Predictors of radial thrombosis are larger sheath size and lower dose of heparin.[4] Omission of heparin results in a very high rate of thrombosis (70%).[5] Radial artery thrombosis is asymptomatic in patients with patent arterial arch.[6,7] In a large series of 7049 procedures, vascular complications, such as hematoma under tension and compartment syndrome, were extremely rare (<1/3000) despite immediate sheath withdrawal under full heparinization, thrombolytics, and platelet inhibitors.[5]

The transradial approach was not associated with increased radiation when compared with transfemoral and transbrachial approaches.[8,9] Success rate was also similar with the above two approaches.[9] The radial approach was also perceived as ideal for outpatient PTCA and stenting.[10] In a randomized study of transradial and femoral approaches, Cooper *et al.* have demonstrated a strong patient preference for the transradial approach associated with a significant reduction in total hospital cost.[11]

Advantages and limitations of transradial approach: The extremely low complication rate remains the most obvious advantage of the transradial approach. The possibility of immediate sheath withdrawal and ambulation after coronary procedures is appealing for both the physician and the patient and is ideal for outpatient procedures. Some disadvantages include necessity for a patent palmar arterial arch, a mandatory learning curve, spasms, and occasional, although asymptomatic, radial artery thrombosis. Pain on sheath pullback was seen in a significant number of patients, especially female patients with smaller body size; however, the availability of hydrophilic-coated sheaths have considerably reduced the discomfort associated with sheath withdrawal. Finally, the possibility of radial artery atherosclerotic progression after transradial cannulation remains an unresolved question, especially in diabetics in whom coronary bypass with a radial artery is considered.

TECHNICAL TIPS

**Right or left TRA? Right TRA is usually more convenient to the physician, especially if the physician is right-handed or if the patient is very obese. Most radial guides are designed for right TRA (Barbeau curve, Fajadet curve, Ochiai curve, etc.). Also, it leaves the left radial artery intact to serve as a conduit in case of coronary artery bypass graft surgery (CABG). Left TRA is preferred for left internal mammary artery (LIMA) angiography, in case of highly positioned left coronary venous or radial bypass, in patients with right pneumonectomy, in very old or hypertensive patients with extreme aortic tortuosity, and is sometimes the patient's preference.

**Difficulty in accessing the ascending aorta: Ask the patient to take a deep breath; it will ease the access to the ascending aorta and coronary cannulation. Working in a 45° LAO view helps the physician direct the wire toward the ascending aorta and also for selective left or right coronary cannulation.

**Spasm: The radial artery is prone to spasm triggered by fear, anxiety, failed puncture, pain, or rough manipulation of the wire or introducer sheath. In case of spasm encountered while manipulating the guide, remove the guide while leaving a wire in place, then inject verapamil 2–7.5 mg intra-arterially, nitrates, or intravenously fentanyl, midazolam HCl, or morphine. Sometimes, using a smaller guide (4F) for diagnostic purposes or a hydrophilic-coated wire would help the guide manipulation. Spasm can also be severe during sheath removal; analgesia combined with slow but steady pullback usually works. If the spasm is too extreme, general or regional anesthesia may be needed to resolve the problem. Spasm is never a problem when using a hydrophilic-coated introducer sheath.

**Avoiding bleeding complications: It is of utmost importance to have well-trained personnel who are familiar with the transradial approach and able to recognize early potential complications of this approach. If severe forearm bleeding should occur, especially if distant from the puncture site, apply pressure at suspected bleeding sites, lower blood pressure, reverse heparin with protamine, monitor finger oxymetry, and massage the site to diffuse the hematoma under tension. If a compartment syndrome develops associated with hand ischemia, a fasciotomy for pressure release may become necessary.

SELECTION OF GUIDES

Right TRA: Almost all specially designed guides are for right transradial approach. Because TRA implies working with smaller guides, i.e. 5F and 6F, the backup is a composite of passive and active support. The passive support comes from the curve used, usually taking advantage of the contralateral side of the aorta. Active support is facilitated by the smooth transition of angles allowing almost coaxial advancement of the guiding catheter within the coronary. For left coronary angioplasty, especially LAD, we prefer the extra-backup curves (or XB, Voda, GL, Kimny, Fajadet, ML, or Q curves). In case of circumflex angioplasty, the extra-backup curves or Amplatz left 2 or 3 are preferred in acute or wide takeoff, respectively. For the right coronary artery, regardless of upper, mid-, or downsloping orientation, the Barbeau, Multipurpose, MR, and Fajadet curves are favored.

Left TRA: Judkins curved guides are better used from the left approach, although not ideal. For left coronary angioplasty, especially LAD, we prefer extra-backup curves (or XB, Voda, GL, or Q curves). In case of circumflex angioplasty, extra-backup curves, or Amplatz left 2 or 3 are preferred. For the right coronary artery, JR4 or Barbeau curves are favored.

Angiography: For 4F angiography, guides taking advantage of support from the contralateral side of the aorta such as AL1 and AL2 are preferred; these guides have less tendency towards backing off with forceful injection obtained with a small (5 cc) syringe. These guides can even be used without an introducer sheath but at the expense of incurring somewhat more spasm. In 5F, Multipurpose or Barbeau curves have the advantage of using only one guide for both right and left coronary angiography as well as left ventriculography. The Judkins guides can also be used, usually in smaller size when using the right TRA (JL3.5 instead of JL4).

Guide size: Our approach is to use the smallest size necessary to avoid possible trauma. Angiography is usually performed with 4F–5F diagnostic catheters. Angioplasty can be performed with some wide-lumen 5F guides. Bifurcation angioplasty necessitating kissing balloon technique can be done with a 6F guide. Wide-lumen 7F allows up to 2.0-mm Rotablator burrs, and 2.25-mm burrs can be used in 8F guides. Some intravascular ultrasound (IVUS) catheters are now compatible with 6F guides. An interesting study of Japanese patients showed radial artery sizes accepting 6F, 7F, and 8F, respectively, in 81%, 73%, and 42% of male and 60%, 40%, and 21% of female patients.[12]

TECHNICAL TIPS

**LAO angulation: In our experience, the LAO view with deep inspiration is the most useful view for proper guide positioning for either left or right coronary angioplasty. This is especially true when inserting an EB type curve (XB, EBU, Voda, Fajadet, Kimny) for left coronary angioplasty: the guide's tip is directed toward the left cusp, the wire is pulled back slowly into the guide, and a small counterclockwise rotation is performed while advancing the guide until ostial engagement. At the release of the inspiration, the guide is slightly pulled back to avoid collapse of the tip.

**Deep seating of guide: Deep seating of a guide within the coronary artery is best performed in deep inspiration with the wire and the balloon already advanced and sometimes inflated inside the coronary artery. This technique is usually atraumatic, especially if the guide's tip is soft. The balloon catheter is then removed and the stent is advanced at or beyond the lesion without repositioning the guide. With the stent in place, the guide is slowly pulled back before injecting contrast media to avoid trauma with a wedged guide.

**Use of the Amplatz left: This curve provides a strong passive support, taking advantage of the contralateral side of the aorta. However, this advantage may become dangerous while cannulating right or left coronary arteries because of abrupt and deep engagement into the ostia. Active support is possible only with deep inspiration and is usually not controlled, resulting too often in collapse of the primary curve and fall into the LV. This catheter is unfortunately often responsible for proximal dissection and associated with stent dislodgement, when the stent is pulled back into the guide. This curve is usually a second or third choice except for the circumflex angioplasty; in fact, deep inspiration may bring the tip of the guide directly into the circumflex, allowing stent advancement bypassing the left main/left circumflex angle.

**Stent loss or dislodgement: This problem occurs considerably less with the new generation of premounted stents but may be seen more often with the growing popularity of direct stenting and smaller guides. In our experience, it usually occurs after failed attempts at advancing a stent across a tight lesion or in tortuous anatomy, and trying to retrieve the stent into the guide. Although many good retrieval techniques have been described, it remains a time-consuming complication. We usually leave the wire in place across the lesion and withdraw the stent and balloon as well as the guide up to the radial sheath. There, a snare, a smaller balloon, or a biotome can be used to retrieve the stent into the sheath. Sometimes, a bigger sheath is exchanged to facilitate the retrieval. Occasionally, the stent is deployed in the radial artery, as proximal as possible, avoiding late asymptomatic radial artery occlusion.

REFERENCES

1. Barbeau GR, Arsenault F, Larivière MM, Dugas L. *A new and objective method for transradial approach screening: comparison with the Allen's test in 1010 patients.* Data on file.

2. Barbeau GR, Letourneau L, Carrier G, Ferland S, Gleeton O, Larivière MM. Right transradial approach for coronary procedures. *J Invasive Cardiol* 1996; **8** (Suppl D): 19D–21D.

3. Barbeau GR, Gleeton O, Roy L *et al*. Predictors of failure of transradial approach: a multivariate analysis of a large series. *Circulation* 1999; **100**: I-306.

4. Barbeau GR, Bilodeau S, Carrier G *et al*. Predictors of radial artery thrombosis after transradial approach: a multivariate analysis of a large series. *J Am Coll Cardiol* 2000; **35**: A-32.

5. Spaulding C, Lefevre T, Funck F *et al*. Left radial approach for coronary angiography: results of a prospective study. *Cathet Cardiovasc Diagn* 1996; **39**: 365–70.

6. Barbeau GR, Gleeton O, Roy L *et al*. Transradial approach for coronary interventions: procedural results and vascular complications of a series of 7049 procedures. *Circulation* 1999; **100**: I-306.

7. Stella PR, Kiemeneij F, Laarmann GJ, Odekerken D, Slagboom T, van der Rieken R. Incidence and outcome of radial artery occlusion following transradial artery coronary angioplasty. *Cathet Cardiovasc Diagn* 1997; **40**: 156–8.

8. Tift Mann III J, Cubeddu G, Arrowood M. Operator radiation exposure in PTCA: Comparison of radial and femoral approaches. *J Invasive Cardiol* 1996; **8** (Suppl D): 22D–25D.

9. Kiemeneij F, Laarmann GJ, Odekerken D, Slagboom T, van der Rieken R. A randomized comparison of percutaneous transluminal coronary angioplasty by the radial, brachial and femoral approaches: the access study. *J Am Coll Cardiol* 1997; **29**: 1269–75.

10. Kiemeneij F, Laarmann GJ, Slagboom T, van der Rieken R. Outpatient coronary stent implantation. *J Am Coll Cardiol* 1997; **29**: 323–327.

11. Cooper CJ, El-Shiekh RA, Cohen DJ *et al*. Effect of transradial access on quality of life and cost of cardiac catheterization: A randomized comparison. *Am Heart J* 1999; **138**: 430–6.

12. Saito S, Ikei H, Hosokawa G *et al*. The feasibility of using catheters equal or greater than 7 French during transradial coronary intervention. Personal communication.

Chapter 3
Angiographic Views

Thach Nguyen, Ta Tien Phuoc,
Gianluca Rigatelli

The goals of coronary angiographic views
Guidelines for moving the image intensifier
A general overview
    **The game plan
    **How to fully expose the LCX (1)(2)
    **How to fully expose the LAD (1)(2)
    **In order to fully scrutinize the LAD, do we need an LAO cranial view?
    **Angulations to separate the LAD from diagonals
    **Summary of an angiographic sequence
Basic views of the left main
    **How to expose the LM when the heart is horizontal
    **How to expose the LM when the LM is long and has a downward direction
Basic views of the left anterior descending artery
    **Identify the LAD, diagonals and septals
    **Exposure of the high diagonal
    **Best views of ostial and proximal LAD in horizontal heart or short LM
    **Best views of ostial and proximal LAD in patients with long LM
Basic views of the left circumflex artery
Basic views of the right coronary artery
Basic views of the saphenous vein graft
Basic views of the internal mammary arteries
    ***Last resort to visualize the IMA
Trouble-shooting tips
    **How to select the angulation
    CAVEAT: Deceiving angiographic views
    CAVEAT: Missing lesions
    CAVEAT: Magnification artifacts

---

*Basic; **Advanced; ***Rare, exotic, or investigational.

From: Nguyen T, Hu D, Saito S, Grines C, Palacios I (eds), *Practical Handbook of Advanced Interventional Cardiology*, 2nd edn. © 2003 Futura, an imprint of Blackwell Publishing.

THE GOALS OF CORONARY ANGIOGRAPHIC VIEWS

The goal of coronary angiography is to delineate clearly a lesion, so that its morphology can be assessed accurately, the subsequent results of interventions can be compared more objectively, and the changes due to complications can be detected early. Accurate views of the ostial segment of the artery involved, the direction, and course of the segments proximal to the target lesion, are also needed to plan the accurate and timely movement of interventional devices. In order to evaluate difficult eccentric lesions, multiple injections may be needed at slightly different angles. However, when a vessel bends in more than one plane, no single angiographic view can overcome multiple foreshortenings. So one must individualize and select the degree of angulation that best visualizes the problem area.[1] In general, the art of angiography is to expose the most by showing the least foreshortened coronary artery segment at an angulation that causes the lowest radiation to the operators and with the least number of X-ray (XR) pictures.

GUIDELINES FOR MOVING THE IMAGE INTENSIFIER

There are a few rules that govern the visualization of the artery by moving the image intensifier (camera tube) above the patient. The first rule is that the left circumflex (LCX) goes with the image intensifier and the left anterior descending artery (LAD) goes in the opposite direction. In other words, moving the image intensifier leftward to the left anterior oblique view (LAO) will project the LCX to the left on the XR picture and the LAD to the right (rule #1). Cranial angulation will elevate the LCX up and pull the LAD down. It is the reverse with caudal angulation. The same rule is applied to the diaphragm and the spine (Table 3-1).

The second rule is that in order to straighten a tortuous coronary segment, the image intensifier should be moved to an angle with more or less 90° opposite to the present one; the tortuous area would then be seen more straightened (rule #2). The goal of these maneuvers is to view the arterial segment

Table 3-1
Movement of vessels and landmarks according to direction of the camera tube

Same direction	Opposite direction
LCX	LAD
Spine	Diagonals
	Diaphragm

in its most direct (orthogonal) angle, with the least angled projection effect.

A GENERAL OVERVIEW

There are many possible views to start a study of the coronary system. We prefer the neutral AP view because in the first view, we can have a global assessment of the LM, the proximal segment of the LCX and the exact position of the LCX in comparison with the LAD. In this AP view, usually the distal LM, the proximal LAD and LCX would overlap each other so this view would dictate the next area to be elucidated and, practically, the next move of the image intensifier (Figure 3-1).

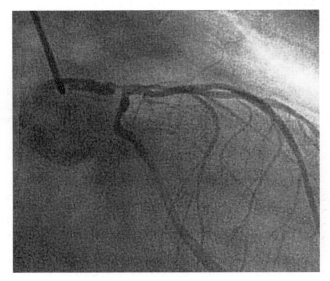

Figure 3-1: The anterior-posterior (AP) view of the left main (LM) artery. This view very clearly showed the severe lesion at the distal LM artery.

TECHNICAL TIPS

**The game plan: In general, there are no exact rules of where to start an angiogram and what to view next. Usually, the operator likes to visualize the area of interest with the culprit lesion quickly. Our personal preference is to get an AP view in order have a global assessment of the LM and to be sure there is no LM disease. Then a severe LCX lesion can be ruled in or out very quickly by only one right anterior oblique (RAO) caudal or anterior-posterior (AP) caudal view. Most of the time, with only two views we can rule out severe LM and LCX disease, and then we like to concentrate on scrutinizing the distal LM and the proximal LAD. Usually, at this stage, the above views would have given enough information regarding the mid and distal segment of the LAD or LCX (Table 3-2).

**How to fully expose the LCX (1): After the first plain AP view, the goal of the next angulation is to see clearly the LM at the same time as the LCX. If the LCX is below or at the same level with the LAD in the plain AP view, then the next view would be any caudal view or maneuver which pulls the LCX down further. Deep inspiration would further elongate the LCX, so there is no foreshortening in the proximal segment or no overlapping by the LAD (Figure 3-2 A,B). These are the two views: RAO caudal and AP caudal. If the proximal segment of the LCX is quite tortuous in the AP view then the RAO caudal view will elongate the LCX and straighten the proximal segment (rule #2). If in the AP view the proximal segment of the LCX is just foreshortened without being too tortuous, then the next view should be the AP caudal view, with deep inspiration to elongate the heart, depress the diaphragm and so pull the LCX straight down further (rule #1). These two views (RAO caudal and AP caudal) will best expose the whole LCX. Most of the time, just after a second XR picture, almost all the segments of the LM and the LCX arteries are completely scrutinized.

Table 3-2
Results of the first anterior-posterior neutral view

Global assessment

1. Ostial LM
2. Distal LAD, LCX
3. Position of the LCX in comparison with the proximal LAD

Overlapped segments needed to be exposed

1. Distal LM
2. Proximal and mid-LAD
3. Proximal and mid-LCX

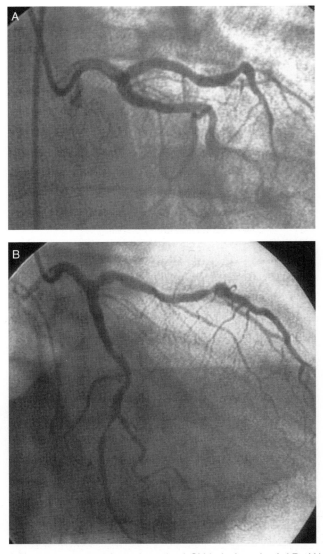

Figure 3-2: Angulation when the LCX is below the LAD. (A) The LCX is below the LAD in this plain AP view. It is also tortuous so the next view would be the RAO caudal view. (B) In this RAO caudal view, the LCX is well elongated and so fully exposed.

**How to fully expose the LCX (2): If the LCX is seen above the LAD on the plain AP view, then the best maneuver is still to try to elongate the LCX by pulling it down further in the RAO caudal or AP caudal view. The reason is that all cranial angulations will project and foreshorten the LCX further above the LAD (Figure 3-3 A,B). Then an LAO cra-

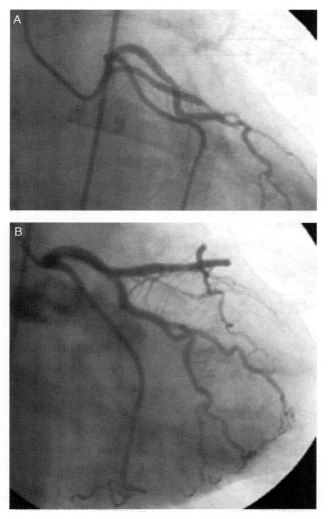

Figure 3-3 A,B: Angulation when the LCX is above the LAD. (A) In this AP view, the LCX is above the LAD, so the next view is to pull the LCX down further to expose it fully. (B) The LCX in the RAO caudal view so it can be elongated more. *(Continued)*

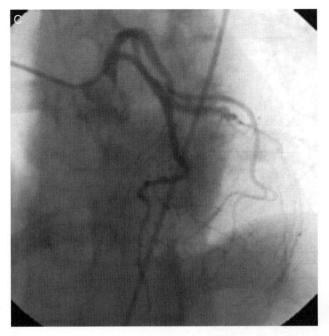

Figure 3-3 C: In this AP cranial view, the LCX is moved further above the LAD so the LAD can be fully seen.

nial or caudal (spider) view will be a good alternative view for the proximal LCX, although it will be seen over the hazy background of the spine. The LAO caudal view is also very helpful for wire entry into the LAD, LCX and the ostium of the first OM (Table 3-3).

**How to fully expose the LAD (1): If in the AP view the LCX is clearly below the LAD, then the next view has to be

Table 3-3
How to expose the LCX

Location of LCX	Best view
If the LCX is below or same level as the LAD in the AP view	RAO or AP caudal
If the LCX is above the LAD in the plain AP view	RAO or AP caudal
	LAO caudal (best alternative view)
	LAO cranial (best alternative view)

any caudal view to pull the LCX down further in order to remove overlapping of the LCX over the proximal LAD (rule #1). This view could have been done to expose the LCX and the LAD at the same time. If the LCX is at the same level with the LAD (Figure 3-4 A), then the next angulation is still any caudal view with deep inspiration to pull the LCX down and to uncover the proximal LAD overlapped by the LCX (Figure 3-4 B,C). Usually the RAO caudal view would expose the LCX and the LAD well and has less interference by the diaphragm than the AP caudal view. However, the main effect of these two RAO and AP caudal views is to remove the

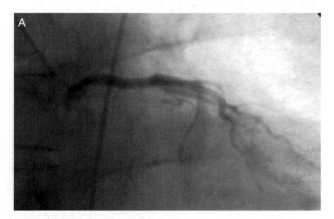

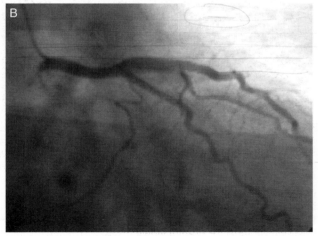

Figure 3-4 A,B: Rationale for selecting angulation of a filming sequence. (A) The LCX at the same level as the LAD in the AP view. (B) The AP caudal view with the LCX being pulled down. *(Continued)*

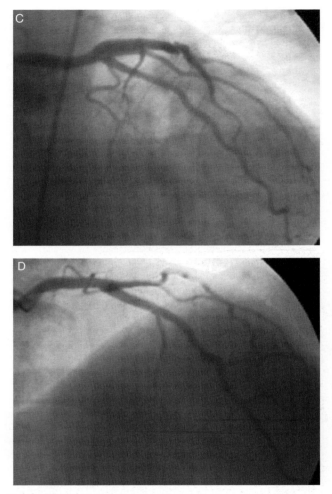

Figure 3-4 C, D: (C) The RAO caudal view with more elongation of the LCX so more exposure of the LCX. (D) Because the LAD was tortuous in the RAO caudal view, the next view is at 90° angle to this RAO caudal view, which is the RAO cranial view. *(Continued)*

LCX away from the LAD and does not purposely expose the LAD. The views that purposely expose the LAD are the RAO cranial and AP cranial views. If the LCX is above the LAD, then the only way to see the LAD is to move the LCX further above the LAD (rule #1) by using the AP cranial view, with deep cranial angulation as possible. It may help if the pillow of the patient can be removed temporarily so

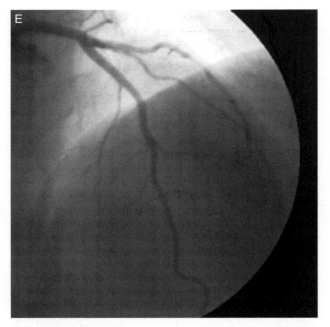

Figure 3-4 E: Because there was overlap of the LCX above the proximal LAD, an AP view with deep cranial angulation is taken and shows the total LAD without overlap.

the camera can be angled more in the cranial direction. An RAO cranial view is also good to lift the LCX up and expose totally the proximal and mid-LAD. However, in these RAO or AP views with extreme cranial angulation, more OMs would overlap the mid- and distal LAD, especially if the LCX is long and dominant (rule #1).

**How to purposely expose the LAD (2): If the LAD is seen tortuous in the RAO caudal view (which is usually the second or third view of the angiographic sequence) (Figure 3-4 C), then the next view to straighten the LAD is the RAO cranial view (rule #2) (Figure 3-4 D). In order to remove the LCX overlapped on the LAD, if the LCX was seen above the LAD, then really deep inspiration will elevate the LCX further above the LAD. If the LCX was seen below the LAD in the AP view, then no deep inspiration is needed, otherwise the LCX would be elevated and overlap the proximal LAD. These maneuvers can be repeated for the AP cranial view. The ostium and the proximal segment of the LAD can be seen well by the LAO cranial view.

**In order to completely scrutinize the LAD, do we need an LAO cranial view? A full exposure of the LAD always requires the LAO cranial view to separate the LAD and the diagonals and expose the lesions at the ostium or bifurcations of the diagonals (Figure 3-5). In patients with prominent abdomen, the AP cranial view with really deep inspiration would move the LCX up high above the LAD (rule #1) and the diaphragm down in order to uncover the whole LAD.

**Angulations to separate the LAD from diagonals: In the RAO view, if the first diagonal is above the LAD and

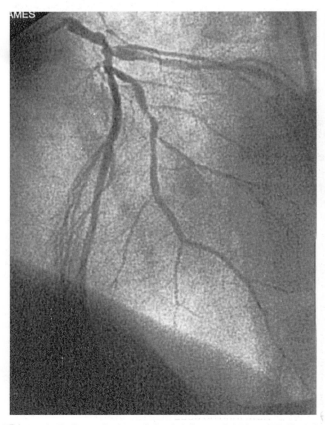

Figure 3-5: Boundaries of the LAO cranial view: a triangle created by the diaphragm, the spine, and the edge of the intensifier. The LAD should be seated at the top of this triangle for adequate visualization. The diagonals are on the right side and the septal arteries on the left side.

overlaps the proximal LAD, a cranial angulation would separate the LAD and its diagonals well. However, the LCX would be moved up and overlap the proximal LAD. If the diagonals are seen below the LAD in the plain RAO view, then a caudal angulation would help to separate the LAD and its diagonal branches (Table 3-4).[2]

**Summary of an angiographic sequence: There are many ways to start a coronary angiogram: the AP view, the RAO view or the LAO view. However, after any first basic XR picture, the second picture should show either a lesion or prove the patency of a major branch. In the left coronary angiogram there are a few areas to be scrutinized: the LM, proximal, mid- and distal LAD, proximal, distal LCX, obtuse marginal (OM) and diagonals. The areas of interest in the right coronary angiogram are: the ostial, proximal, mid- and distal RCA, with the right ventricular (RV), posterior descending artery (PDA), posterior lateral (PLB), and sinus node branches. In Figure 3-4 A–E, all major coronary branches were shown with seven angiograms, with 70 cc

---

Table 3-4
How to expose the LAD and the diagonals

Moving the LCX away from the LAD	
First AP view	Next view with deep inspiration
If the LCX is below the LAD	RAO caudal or AP caudal
If the LCX is the same level	RAO caudal or AP caudal
If the LCX is above the LAD	RAO cranial or AP cranial with deep inspiration

Purposely exposing the LAD	
If the LAD is tortuous in the RAO caudal view	Take a RAO cranial view with deep inspiration to lift the LCX above the LAD
If the proximal LAD is not well seen in the RAO cranial view	Take a steep AP cranial view with deep inspiration in order to lift the LCX higher above the LAD
	The LAO caudal can show best the ostium and the proximal segment of the LAD

Separating the LAD and the diagonal	
First RAO view	Next view
If the first diagonal is above the LAD	RAO cranial view
If the first diagonal is below the LAD	RAO caudal view

of contrast agent used. At first, an AP view was done to see the LM and the location of the LCX compared with the LAD. In Figure 3-4 A, the LCX was at the same level as the LAD. So the next view should be the AP caudal view to pull the LCX down further and expose it (Figure 3-4 B). Because the AP caudal view did not reveal the LCX well, the RAO caudal view was taken and showed the LCX better (Figure 3-4 C). It was a small non-dominant LCX without significant lesion. Because the mid-LAD was seen tortuous in the RAO caudal view, the view that would straighten it was the RAO cranial view (Figure 3-4 D). In order to elevate the LCX high above the LAD so the LAD can be exposed more, the patient was asked to take a deep breath so that the diaphragm is depressed and the LCX elevated further. The LAD was seen fairly well. However, the proximal LAD still had some overlapping. So an AP cranial view was selected; the pillow was taken away so there was more cranial angulation. The AP cranial view showed the whole LAD much better without any overlap by the LCX (Figure 3-4 E). Then to complete the scrutinization of the LM and LAD, an LAO cranial view was done to check the ostial and proximal segments of the diagonals and septals (Figure 3-5). An LAO caudal view was taken to check any lesion in the LM ostium and the proximal segments of the LAD and LCX. In the right coronary angiogram, the LAO caudal was done to check the ostial and proximal RCA. The RAO was done to check the mid-segment and the AP cranial was done to check the patency of the distal RCA and the PDA.

BASIC VIEWS OF THE LEFT MAIN

The left main: The LM has variable length (1–10 mm), no side branches, and bifurcates into the LAD and LCX. Occasionally, there is no functional or very short LM and the LAD and LCX arise from separate ostia. It is an important part of the scrutinization of the coronary artery system, because a lesion on the LM is the main cause of mortality from even diagnostic coronary angiography. The first basic views of the LM are the AP view or the shallow RAO view. If these two views do not show the LM clearly, various views can be taken according to the vertical or horizontal position of the heart and the length of the LM.

TECHNICAL TIPS

**How to expose the LM when the heart is horizontal:
In this case, the LM is short and the proximal LAD has a cephalad orientation; the LAO caudal view is better than the LAO cranial view.[3] The LAO caudal view would help to show the length of the LM, and the direction of bifurcation of

the LAD or LCX where the wire needs to be directed (Figure 3-6). To have the best LAO caudal (or spider) view, the tip of the guide should be positioned at the center of a full half-circle extending from 12 to 6 o'clock formed by the shadow of the cardiac silhouette. However, angulation that is too steep would cause foreshortening of the LM and overlapping by the diaphragm and spine.

**How to expose the LM when the LM is long and has a downward direction: As in vertical hearts, the LAO cranial view will best show the LM and its bifurcation to the LAD and LCX.[3] A LAO cranial angulation that is too steep would further foreshorten the LM and, in conjunction with poor inspiration, would produce a hazy background due to diaphragm overlapping.

If the above views could not clearly delineate the LM lesions, other possible views suggested by a faculty of an interventional cardiology board review course include all the possible combinations of angulation set by an image intensifier (except the AP cranial and lateral views) (Table 3-5).[4]

BASIC VIEWS OF THE LEFT ANTERIOR DESCENDING ARTERY

The proximal LAD is defined as the segment from the ostium to the origin of the first septal. The distal end of the mid-segment is less rigorously defined and is typically the location where the LAD dips downward on a right anterior oblique view.

The RAO cranial view: This is one of the best first views that may delineate the ostial segment, then the mid- and distal segment of the LAD. In patients with long left main, during PCI in the proximal or mid-LAD lesion, this view is very useful to show the course for the wire as it enters the LAD and goes forwards without interference from the septal and diagonal branches. The RAO cranial view can be taken while the patient performs deep inspiration if there is intention to elevate

Table 3-5
Other possible angles to delineate the left main

Vessel segment	Routine views	Adjunctive views
Ostial	LAO caudal	AP caudal
Body	RAO caudal	AP caudal
	RAO cranial	
Distal	LAO caudal	LAO cranial
	RAO caudal	

the LCX above the proximal LAD. If the LCX is way below the LAD, then inspiration is not needed because it will elevate the LCX to overlap the LAD.

The LAO cranial view: This view delineates clearly the course of the LAD, from its origin to the apex, and the correlation with its septals and diagonals. In this view, the LAD is best seen if the tip of the guide is positioned in a triangle made with the spine, the diaphragm, and the edge of the intensifier, over a clear lung background (see Figure 3-5). To move the spine away from the center, just move the tube to the left, then the spine will be moved to the left (rule #1). If the result is suboptimal, better definition of the proximal LAD can be achieved by changing the steepness of the cranial angulation and by having the patient take a deep breath, to lower the diaphragm and thus make the heart more vertical.

This LAO cranial view would help to delineate any lesion on the LAD, especially at the bifurcations with the diagonals and septals. It helps to show the pathway of the wire. However, in this view, the proximal LAD is foreshortened so it does not give an accurate evaluation of the result of angioplasty or stenting in the very proximal LAD.

TECHNICAL TIP

**Identify the LAD, diagonals and septals: The LAO cranial view is the best view to identify and confirm the identity of the LAD. The diagonals will be on the left and the septals will come out from the right of the screen. It is almost unthinkable for there to be no septals. This view would confirm the identity of a compensatory enlarged diagonal because it has no septals (except in very rare cases).[3] The diagonals will point more to the left; however, a long LAD in a very dilated LV could have the apex moved towards the left of the screen, too. Another way to differentiate the septals from the diagonals is that the diagonals move (buckle) during systole while the septals are straighter and move very little with ventricular contraction. The presence of the septals would confirm the identity of the artery that is the LAD.

The AP cranial view: To see clearly the proximal and mid-segment of the LAD with its bifurcation, the AP cranial view could also show very clearly the ostial and the proximal segment of the LAD, if the LCX can be moved entirely above the LAD. The mid- and distal segments of the LAD are well exposed in a single view on the screen so this view is a favorite view during procedures, as the operator can monitor the position of the tip of the guide, the movement of the devices in the proximal segment and of the tip of the wire at the distal segment.

The RAO caudal view: This has much overlapping by the diagonal in the mid-segment. If the LCX is positioned below the LAD, then the proximal LAD is well exposed while being foreshortened.[5] This view best demonstrates the lesions in the mid-LAD in relation to the septals.

The lateral view: To highlight a lesion at the bifurcation of the LAD and the diagonals, the lateral view can help to pinpoint its location and assess its severity. It is more useful for a diagnostic injection rather than for an interventional procedure because a prolonged position of the arm above the head would make any patient tired and uncomfortable.

TECHNICAL TIPS

**Exposure of the high diagonal: Usually the ostium of a high diagonal is not well seen in the RAO cranial view because the area is overlapped by an elevated LCX, so the LAO with steep cranial view (LAO 10, cranial 40) can be tried. However, a good spider view with steep caudal angulation is most likely the best view to expose it (Figure 3-6).

**Best views of ostial and proximal LAD in horizontal heart or short LM: When the heart is horizontal, the LM is short and the proximal LAD has a cephalad orientation; the LAO caudal view is better than the LAO cranial view because of proximal circumflex overlapping.[6] Positioning the proximal end of a stent during PCI of the ostial LAD can be done best in the caudal view. However, the proximal LAD

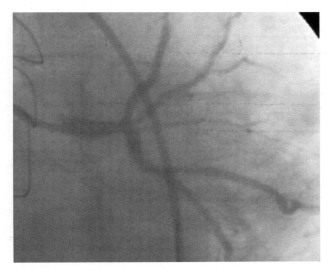

Figure 3-6: The LAO caudal view of the left main. In this (spider) view, the left main is seen very clearly at the bifurcation into the LAD and LCX.[2]

segment is foreshortened so this view is not best for checking the complete deployment at the distal end of a stent or
the appearance of new dissection distal to the stent.

****Best views of ostial and proximal LAD in patients with
long LM:** If the LM is long, then the RAO cranial view should
be the first view, especially if the LCX can be moved above
the LAD. If the LAD cannot be assessed in this view, the
next best view is the LAO cranial, which will best show the
LM and its bifurcation to the LAD and LCX.[3] Thus the best
views for distal LM or ostial LAD can be with either RAO
or LAO cranial angulation.[4] The next try would be the LAO
caudal view. Appropriate views would give the best delineation of the lesion if selected intelligently by the operator.

BASIC VIEWS OF THE LEFT CIRCUMFLEX ARTERY

The proximal segment of the left circumflex artery (LCX)
begins from the ostium up to and including the origin of the first
obtuse marginal (OM). The distal LCX is beyond this point.
When looking at the LCX, a standard RAO caudal view may
provide much-needed information (Figure 3-4 C). However, a
shallow angulation has two limitations: (1) it can foreshorten
the proximal segments of the LCX, so the exact morphology
of a lesion in that segment cannot be optimally assessed or
the direction or its tortuosity is overlooked; and (2) the ostial
segment may be overlapped and not seen clearly. The more
caudal, the better the proximal part is seen. To complement
the limitations of the RAO shallow caudal view, an AP caudal
or an LAO caudal view can help to clarify the problem in that
segment (see Figs 3-4 C and 3-6).

While taking these views, the patient is asked to take
a deep breath, which moves the diaphragm downward and
clears the field for optimal vessel opacification. In the case of
mid- or distal LCX-OM intervention, an RAO caudal view can
foreshorten the proximal LCX and could mask the severity of
the takeoff angle with the LM, and the tortuosity and severity
of any possible obstructive lesions at the proximal segment.
On many occasions, only after unsuccessful advancement
of balloons and stents across the proximal segments, is the
severity of the lesions and tortuosity of the proximal segment
of the LCX appreciated. If properly taken, the AP caudal or
LAO caudal (spider) view would give a sharp delineation of
the ostium and proximal segment of the LCX, so a wire can be
shaped appropriately to enter the artery and the proximal segment without unexpected difficulty.

BASIC VIEWS OF THE RIGHT CORONARY ARTERY

The right coronary artery (RCA): The proximal coronary artery originates at the ostium and ends after the first curve. The mid-segment begins with the first curve and ends at the second curve, and is usually considered the straight segment in the RAO view. The distal segment is the remainder of the artery.

The origin of the RCA is extremely variable, from a straight perpendicular takeoff from the aorta, to a marked caudal direction, to a superior takeoff with the shepherd's crook configuration. A strong hand injection into the low right coronary cusp may help to show the origin of the RCA. If it is not seen, it may originate anteriorly, or from the left sinus of Valsalva, or above the sinotubular ridge.

The LAO view: In the LAO projection, the artery appears like a letter C, while in the RAO position, it appears like a letter L (Figure 3-7). To check the correct alignment of the catheter with the RCA, the best view is the RAO shallow cranial projection. In this location, the tip of the catheter is seen head-on as a

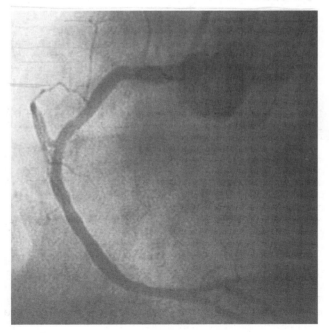

Figure 3-7: The LAO view of the RCA. In this view, the RCA is like a letter C. To focus on the ostial segment, a caudal angulation is needed. A cranial angulation would help to visualize the bifurcation, origin, and course of the PDA.

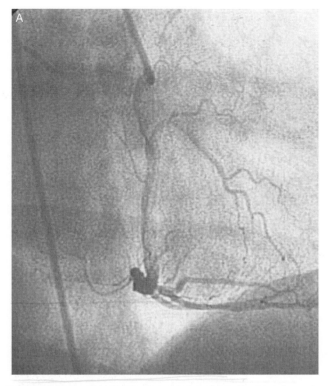

Figure 3-8 A: The RAO view of the RCA. In this view, the guide is truly coaxial, so the tip of the guide will be seen head-on as a circle. *(Continued)*

circle (Figure 3-8 A). If there is an angle formed by the tip of the catheter with the proximal RCA, then there is no coaxial alignment of the catheter (Figure 3-8 B). There would be friction at the angle of transition, which may diminish the forwarding force, the torquing capacity, and obstruct the smooth advancement of interventional hardware across a tight lesion.

When imaging an ostial lesion, it is useful to place the catheter just under the coronary ostium and inject a large volume of contrast to define both the extent of the lesion and its precise position on the aortic wall. This is a particularly important view when contemplating deployment of a stent in the ostial RCA.[7] The exact location of the ostium can often be best seen in an extreme LAO position (more than 50°) or the LAO with caudal angulation.

In order to visualize the ostial segment of the RCA, the best view is the LAO caudal that exposes the ostial and proxi-

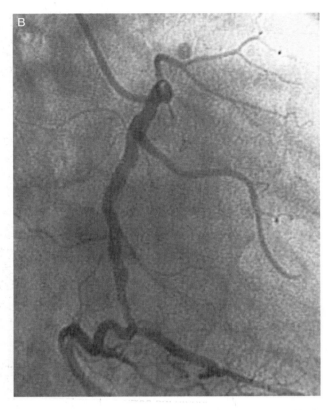

Figure 3-8 B: The RAO view of an RCA anomaly with the ostium in the anterior position. In this view, if the guide is truly coaxial, then the tip of the guide should be seen head-on as a circle. As the location of the ostium in this case is abnormal, so the tip of the guide points to the left.

mal segment of the RCA. In order to view the distal PDA, then the LAO cranial view, coupled with deep inspiration, which moves the diaphragm outside the field, will expose the distal RCA and its bifurcation with the PDA. If there is a need for further exposure of the distal RCA, then an AP cranial view will complement fully the LAO cranial view. Without being overlapped by the diaphragm, the shadow of a previously deployed stent can be visualized more sharply.

   The RAO view: In the LAO view, the mid-segment may not be visualized well because of overlap of the RV branch (see Figure 3-7). The RAO view would separate the mid-segment of the RCA from the RV branches (see Figure 3-8 B). When wiring the RCA, an LAO view would help to direct the

wire from the guide into the proximal segment. It also helps
to appropriately select the different PDAs in the distal segment. However, because of the presence of a few marginal
branches, an RAO view would help to direct the wire at the
mid-segment, avoid the marginal branches, and advance it
easily to the distal segment.

BASIC VIEWS OF THE SAPHENOUS VEIN GRAFT

The best view for the ostium or body of the SVG to the
LAD and diagonals is the LAO view. For the SVG to the LCX,
the best view is the RAO caudal view. The views for the insertion sites and native arteries beyond are the best views of the
distal segments of these native arteries: the AP caudal view
for the OM, the LAO cranial view for the distal PDA, and the
LAO cranial and RAO cranial for the LAD or the diagonals.

BASIC VIEWS OF THE INTERNAL MAMMARY ARTERIES

Usually the left internal mammary artery (LIMA) graft is
inserted into the LAD, so the basic views of the LIMA and its
insertion site should be the LAO cranial or the RAO cranial
views. The insertion site of the LIMA to the LAD can also be
seen well in the lateral view.

Though the LIMA catheter is usually engaged on the AP
view, to check the position of the catheter tip in relation to the
ostium, the best views are the 60° LAO or the RAO 45°. These
angulations would elongate the aortic arch and separate the
subclavian artery to identify clearly the LIMA ostium (Figure
3-9 A–C).

TECHNICAL TIP

***Last resort to visualize the IMA:** In the rare case of
difficulty engaging the left and right internal mammary arteries, a nonselective angiogram with the tip of the catheter
just in the vicinity of the ostia can be done. Complete opacification of the vessel can be achieved with 10 cc manual injection with a blood pressure cuff inflated 10 mm Hg above
the systolic pressure on the ipsilateral arm.[8]

TROUBLE-SHOOTING TIPS

How to select the angulation: There are a few rules
on how to select the angulations mentioned earlier. The
main concerns are how to obtain XR pictures showing the
problematic areas with the least number of XR pictures, the
least amount of contrast agent and with the least radiation

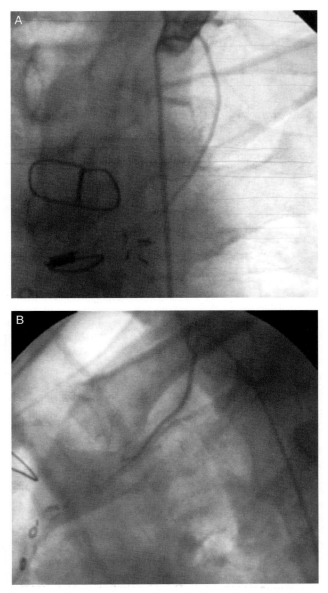

Figure 3-9 A,B: The angulation selection of the LIMA. (A) The LIMA in the AP view without clear exposure of the origin of the LIMA. (B) Because of poor exposure of the origin of the LIMA with the AP view, an LAO 60° was taken and showed exactly the origin and the proximal segment of the LIMA. *(Continued)*

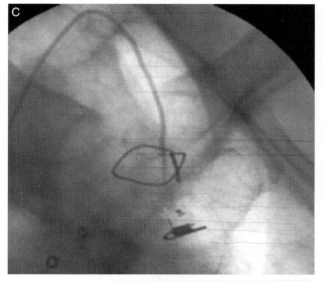

Figure 3-9 C: An RAO 45° showed the origin of the LIMA so the tip of the guide can be advanced.

exposure for the patients, operators and staff. How to angle the camera is summarized in Table 3-6.

Table 3-6
How to select the angle for the camera

Problems	Solutions
The LAD is not central in the LAO cranial view	Move camera tube more LAO
The LAD is too tortuous or foreshortened in the LAO cranial view	Move the camera more or less cranial
If LCX overlaps LAD in the RAO cranial view	Move the camera more cranial and deeper inspiration to lift the LCX more above the LAD or change to AP cranial view
If the LCX is clearly below the LAD in AP view	RAO caudal view with deep inspiration
If the proximal LCX is too tortuous in the AP view	Deep inspiration and take RAO caudal view
If the proximal LCX is foreshortened in the AP	Make view more caudal and deep inspiration
If there is difficulty in cannulating the RCA	Take an RAO view to check co-axial position of the guide

CAVEAT: Deceiving angiographic views: There are angiographic views that minimize the severity of an angulated segment or the severity of a lesion. The most common situation is the RAO caudal view for a lesion in the LCX. This view foreshortens the proximal segment of the LCX so the ostial lesion of the LCX can be missed and the lesions in the proximal segment can be overlooked. In the RAO cranial or LAO cranial views, the lesion in the distal LM can also be missed; if there is a problem advancing the device or thrombus formation after manipulation of interventional hardware, then the severity of the lesion is much more appreciated. In the LAO cranial view, the lesion in the proximal LAD can be missed, because it is foreshortened and a lesion there can be seen better in the RAO cranial view or AP cranial view. During PCI of an RCA lesion, the guide is thought to be coaxial in the LAO view; however, after failing to advance the interventional devices or difficulty in withdrawing them, it is found that the guide is not coaxial in the RAO view (Table 3-7).

CAVEAT: Missing lesions: Coronary angiography or "luminography" is well known to miss severe lesions, especially the short, napkin ring lesion or short aorto-ostial lesions. The reason is that when the lesion is viewed from an angled projection, the lesion is not seen because the adjacent contrast-filled vessel segments are projected over the short and diseased segment and mask it. In the case of an ostial lesion, the tip of a small catheter can be engaged too deeply without causing ventricularization of blood pressure and spill-over of contrast in the aorto-ostial area would mask a short, severe ostial lesion. This is the same problem of PCI in ostial lesion, where it is difficult to position the proximal end of the stent because an angiogram will spill contrast over the ostial area (Figure 3-10).

Table 3-7
Suboptimal and deceiving angiographic views

1. RAO caudal views for the ostial and proximal LCX. **Better view:** AP caudal with deep inspiration (or vice versa)
2. LAO view of the proximal or ostial RCA. **Better view:** LAO caudal to have better delineation of the ostium. RAO view to check coaxial position.
3. LAO view for origin of distal PDA. **Better view:** LAO cranial or AP cranial view with deep inspiration in order to depress the diaphragm further.
4. AP view of the distal LM. **Better view:** LAO caudal (spider view) or cranial angulation.
5. LAO cranial view for the proximal LAD. **Better view:** RAO cranial or AP cranial.

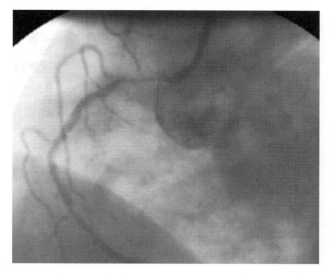

Figure 3-10: During angiogram of the ostial RCA, spill-over of contrast may mask the exact location of the ostium and its abnormality.

Balloon and stent oversizing: In the RAO caudal view, the size of the tip of the guide is projected smaller than the projected size of the LCX, OM or distal RCA because the LCX, OM, distal RCA is more posterior, so it is more enlarged than the tip of the guide on the image intensifier. It is the same problem for measuring the size of the distal LAD in the RAO cranial view. In all circumstances, the image intensifier should be as close to the patient's chest as possible (Table 3-7).

CAVEAT: Magnification artifacts: In many patients undergoing PCI in the LCX, the reference size of the mid-segment of the LCX is measured on the RAO caudal view. In this view, the tip of the guide at the LM ostium is more anterior, while the mid-segment of the LCX is more posterior, at the level of the aorta, so the mid-segment of the LCX (and the shaft of the guide compared with its tip) is projected bigger on the camera screen. This is why the size of LCX as measured by QCA can be quite deceptive (bigger than real life). This is the cause of balloon or stent oversizing in PCI of LCX. The same problem happens with mid- and distal segments of all arteries (Table 3-8) (Figure 3-11 A–D).

   Radiation exposure to the operators: The operator should be cautious in using the views in order to protect himself or herself and the staff against radiation exposure.

Table 3-8
Best views for balloon or stent sizing

Left anterior descending artery

Segment	Best view
Proximal or mid-LAD	RAO or left lateral
Distal LAD	RAO cranial (caution for magnification artifact)

Left circumflex artery

Segment	Best view
Proximal LCX	RAO caudal and LAO
Distal LCX or OM	RAO caudal (caution for magnification artifact)

Right coronary artery

Segment	Best view
Proximal, mid-RCA	RAO, LAO, left lateral
Distal RCA, PDA, PLB	AP, LAO cranial (caution for magnification artifact)

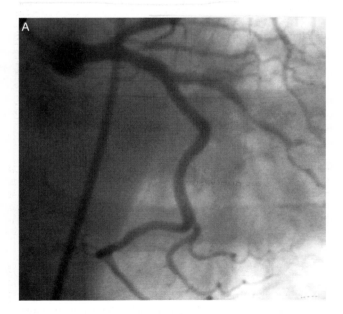

Figure 3-11: False magnification of the LCX. (A) With the size of the guide tip as reference, the OM was measured as 3.8 mm proximally to the lesion and 3.3 mm distally to the lesion, so a 3.25-mm balloon was selected for predilation. *(Continued)*

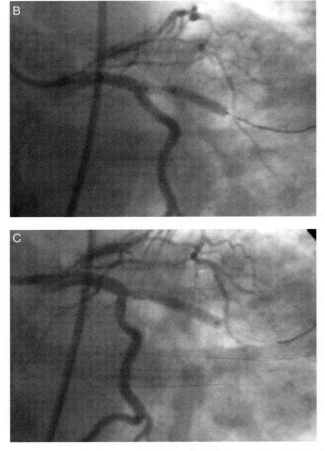

Figure 3-11: (B) During inflation, an angiogram showed total occlusion of the artery, so the balloon fitted well. The body of the guide looked bigger than the tip. (C) Then a 3.0-mm stent was selected and deployed. The angiogram also showed the same size for the proximal segment and the stent. *(Continued)*

TECHNICAL TIPS

**Angulations that cause the most radiation exposure to the operators: The steep caudal angulation is the view that results in the most radiation exposure. It is due to redirection of scatter radiation toward the operator, and the increased scatter produced by the higher kVp level required for hemiaxial angulation.[9]

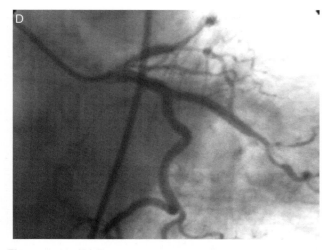

Figure 3-11: (D) The post-stenting angiogram showed there was no discrepancy between the diameter of lumen in the stented area and its proximal segment. The real diameter of the artery was around 3.0 mm, not 3.8 mm, as measured with the tip of the guide as reference.

**Angiographic views and avoidance of radiation over-exposure in obese patients: In order to permit adequate XR penetration, avoid deep angulation, especially caudal angulation. The image magnification is also lower, to reduce patient and operator radiation exposure and limit the amplitude of table panning, thus reducing motion artifacts. In selected suspicious areas, the areas will be re-imaged with higher magnifications.[9]

CORONARY ARTERY ANOMALIES

The most common anomaly is the variation of coronary artery origin from the aorta. Usually, they are of no clinical significance, except in the case of origin of the LM from the right sinus or the RCA from the left sinus that is compressed, resulting in ischemia and sudden death.[10–11] When the LCX originates from the RCA or right sinus, usually it takes the retroaortic course to supply the lateral wall of the ventricle and is benign. The left or right coronary artery can originate from the posterior sinus (very rare) or from the ascending aorta like a bypass graft.[12] Besides an ectopic origin, their anatomic course is usually normal. These anomalies are considered benign.

When the LCA or RCA originate from the opposite sinus, there are four pathways. The rare form is the interarterial course and the most common is the septal course. The other two forms are the retroaortic and the anterior courses. The interarterial course is the most serious one because it can cause ischemia, leading to sudden death.

TECHNICAL TIPS

**The dots and the eyes: The course of an anomalous coronary artery is confirmed by the filming of the pathway in the 30° RAO view. In this visualization, a dot representing the artery seen end-on is noted. The most severe one, the interarterial pathway of an anomalous LM crossing between the aorta and the pulmonary artery, is recognized by the position of the "dot" anterior to the aorta. If the "dot" is behind the aorta, this is the retroaortic benign pathway.[13] The septal pathway is recognized by the fish-hook picture in the RAO view, because the LM goes down to the septum, then comes up to the epicardium, making a picture of a fish-hook. Then the LCX would curve backward and form the "eye", with the LCX as the upper border.[13] In the anterior (pathway) the LM is in front of the pulmonary artery. This pathway is recognized by the "eye", with the LM as the upper border and the LCX as the inferior border (Figure 3-12).

**How to identify and locate the dots and the eyes: In the 30° RAO view, a selective coronary angiogram can show clearly a dot as the artery is filmed end-on. This dot is considered behind the aorta if, during the left ventriculogram, the dot is seen again when the late flow opacifies the aorta and barely both coronary arteries. This ventriculogram locates the dot in front (interarterial pathway) or behind the aorta (retroaortic pathway). The most practical way is to film the coronary artery in the 30° RAO view to show the dot and to do the left ventriculogram with the same angulation. Then the dot can be identified by superimposing (mentally) these two pictures. Another way (for academic purposes) to locate the dot is to do a root aortogram to locate exactly the aorta and the dot.

**How to locate the pathways: In order to clarify the position of an anomalous LM branch in respect of the aorta and pulmonary artery, it may be useful to insert a pulmonary artery (Swan-Ganz) catheter in the main pulmonary artery and to perform a coronary angiogram in the 90° lateral and in the 45° LAO projections. Angiographically, in case of interarterial course, the anomalous LM crosses the pulmonary artery catheter with an almost linear posterior course. If the anomalous vessel is anterior to the pulmonary artery, it crosses the main pulmonary catheter with a circular

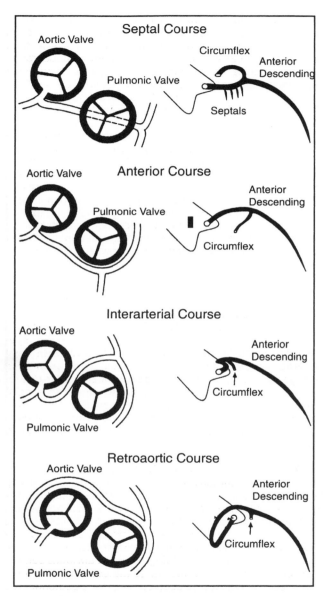

Figure 3-12: General view of coronary anomalies. (Adapted from Serota H, Barth III CW, Seuc CA *et al.* Rapid identification of the course of anomalous coronary arteries in adults: The "dot and eye" method. *Am J Cardiol* 1990; **65:** 891–8.)

anterior course forming the base of a virtual eye. Moreover, in the 45° LAO projection, the presence of a septal branch arising directly from the left main with a parallel course to the pulmonary catheter excludes the interarterial course and identifies the septal type. Another way to locate the anomalous LM (right to left) or the anomalous RCA (left to right) pathway is to insert into the LM or the anomalous RCA only the opaque tip of an angioplasty wire (30 mm long), with the pulmonary artery catheter across the main pulmonary artery. First it is filmed on a plain AP view to see where these two wire-catheters are crossing each other. Then it is filmed on the 45° LAO or LAO caudal view to see whether the first part of the LM is in front or behind the pulmonary artery catheter. If it is in front, then it is the anterior pathway. If it is behind the pulmonary artery, then it is the interarterial pathway. If it is far behind, around the aorta, then it is the retroaortic pathway. In 2003, the best way to definitively identify an anomalous pathway is to do a fast CT scan or MRA. The pathway can be imaged clearly in a static view.

ANGIOGRAPHIC VIEWS

The single coronary artery

The single coronary artery (SCA), defined as an artery that arises from an arterial trunk and nourishes the entire myocardium, is rare. This anomaly, divided into two types, right and left single coronary artery, can be classified in four distinct subtypes depending on the course of the major branch: "anterior" to the pulmonary artery, "posterior" to the aorta, between the aorta and pulmonary artery ("interarterial"), and "septal". The prognosis depends on the pathways as in any anomalous major branch crossing from left to right or vice versa (Figure 3-13).

The left circumflex artery from the right sinus

The most common coronary anomaly is the LCX arising from the proximal RCA. This variant is benign. When the LCX arises from the right coronary cusp or the proximal RCA, it invariably follows a retroactive course, with the LCX passing posteriorly around the aortic root to its normal location. On the LAO, the LCX is seen originated from the proximal RCA. On the selective left coronary angiography, the LM looks surprisingly long and the LAD is seen large without an LCX. In a 30° RAO view, the LCX will be seen curving in the posterior area and is seen head-on, as a dot, posterior to the aorta.[13] When the LCX originates from the proximal RCA, near the ostium, if the catheter tip is engaged too deeply, it can pass the ostium of the anomalous LCX and miss opacifying the LCX (Figure 3-14).

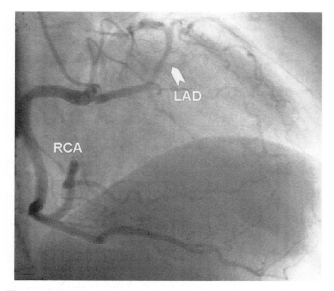

Figure 3-13: The single coronary artery originated from the right sinus. In this RAO view, the left main forms the base of the eye and the LAD curves above it forming the upper part of the eye. The left main had a septal pathway. (Courtesy of the Catheterization Laboratories, Department of Specialistic Medicine, Division of Cardiology, Legnago Teaching Hospital, Verona, Italy.)

The right coronary anomalies
Anterior position of the ostium: If the origin of the RCA is minimally displaced anteriorly, at that time, the tip of the right Judkins catheter may not be directed to the right, but rather looks foreshortened in the familiar LAO view. Directing the tip to the right in the usual fashion using the LAO view permits easy cannulation of the anteriorly directed RCA orifice.[14] In the RAO view, there would be an angle between the catheter tip and the ostium, with the tip pointing toward the left (see Figure 3-8 B).

Anomalous origin of the RCA from the left sinus: When the RCA arises from the left sinus or from the proximal LM, in the RAO view, the RCA will be seen head-on, as a dot anterior to the aorta.[13] The patient in Figure 3-15 is a middle-aged nurse with acute myocardial infarction (AMI). Two years later her son had an angiogram that showed exactly the same anomaly (Figure 3-15).

The left main coronary artery anomalies
The incidence of LMCA originating from the right sinus is very low (1.3%).[15] The artery, seen in the RAO view, may

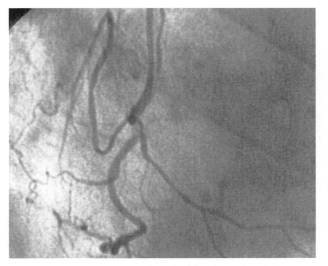

Figure 3-14: In this RAO view, the LCX that is originated from the RCA is seen in a retroaortic pathway as the dot is seen behind the aorta and the artery curves posteriorly.

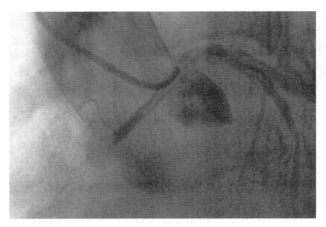

Figure 3-15: In this left coronary injection, an anomalous RCA originated from the left sinus was seen. It was occluded because of AMI. It was then successfully opened.

course in front of the pulmonary artery (anterior course), through the septum (septal course), between the aorta and the pulmonary artery trunk (interarterial course), or behind the aorta (retroaortic course) (see Figure 3-12). Accurate diagnosis is prognostically important because of fatal events associated with the interarterial pathway.[16]

The septal course: The LM runs an intramuscular course through the septum along the floor of the RV outflow tract. It then surfaces at the mid-septum, where it bifurcates into the LAD and LCX. Because the artery divides at the mid-septum, the initial portion of the LCX curves above the LM toward the aorta (the normal position of the LAD) and forms an ellipse with the LM (similar to the shape of an eye, with the LM as the inferior border), seen best on the 30° RAO view. The LAD is relatively short because only the mid- and distal LADs are present. One or more septal vessels can originate from the LM. This type of coronary anomaly is considered benign without ischemia (Figure 3-16).[13]

The anterior free wall course: In the anterior course, the LM crosses the free wall of the right ventricle, in front of the pulmonary artery, and divides into the LAD and LCX at the mid-septum. The LCX would curve back toward the aorta (the position of the normal LAD). On the 30° RAO view, the circumflex forms an ellipse ("eye") with the LM on the superior border. There is no myocardial ischemia associated with this coronary anomaly.[13]

The retroaortic course: In this anomaly, the LM goes around the aortic root to its normal position on the anterior surface of the heart. It divides into the LAD and LCX at its normal point so the LAD and LCX have normal length and course. In the RAO view, the LM is seen head-on, as a circle, posterior to the aorta. This retroaortic dot is diagnostic of a posteriorly coursing artery. There are only rare cases of ischemia reported with this type of anomaly.[13]

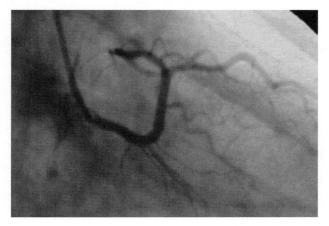

Figure 3-16: The LM from the right sinus by the septal course. The LM forms the inferior border of the eye while the LCX forms the superior border of the eye.

The interarterial course: In this anomaly, the LM courses between the aorta and the pulmonary artery to its normal
position on the anterior surface of the heart. In the RAO view,
the LM is seen head-on, as a dot, on the anterior aspect of
the aorta.[12] The circumflex arises with a caudal orientation.
This type of anomaly is associated with exertional angina,
syncope, and sudden death at young age. Revascularization
in young patients is indicated. However, the surgical indication for asymptomatic elderly patients is not clear because, at
older ages, the arteries are less compressible, unless there is
concomitant obstructive coronary artery disease.[13]

Left main from the posterior sinus

In the AP view, the noncoronary cusp is on the right side
and inferior to the left aortic sinus. However, it is seen best in
the RAO view, in its posterior location, and identified by the
catheter tip in the posterior direction. An injection in the sinus
would outline the artery and the posterior wall of the aorta.[17]

Left main atresia: Left main atresia is rare. Angiographically it should be differentiated from LM occlusion by the fact
that in LM atresia, ipsilateral collaterals are the first portion
of the LAD to be filled, which can be seen best in the RAO
projection.

Anatomic consideration of the ostial segment: Not
every anomaly has a wide ostium that the tip of the guide
can hook onto, or a narrowing at the opening that needs to
be stented. There have been several reports that an anomalous RCA from the left coronary artery can leave the aorta
in oblique fashion, so the ostium has a slit-like configuration
formed by flaps of aortic and coronary tissues. During exercise, the aorta can expand its part of the flap, narrowing farther
the slit-like opening and causing ischemia.[10]

Mechanism of ischemia due to anomalous pathway:
If an anomalous artery has to course between the aorta and
the pulmonary artery, the expansion of the aorta during exercise can cause narrowing of the mid-segment and subsequent
ischemia. If it happens in young patients, there is an indication
for corrective surgery. If the anomaly is found incidentally in
asymptomatic elderly patients, surgery is indicated only if
objective signs of ischemia can be demonstrated (e.g. nuclear
scan). The reason is that the hardened aorta in older patients
does not expand much any more, so it does not cause as much
exercise-induced ischemia as in young patients.[18]

Some anomalous coronary arteries with an intramural
course may adhere to the wall of the aorta, and can even
share a common media with the aorta without intervening
adventitia.[19, 20]

Right coronary artery from the pulmonary trunk

This anomaly is very rare. The RCA is originated from the
pulmonary trunk. Because of the low pulmonary resistance,

the fully oxygenated blood arriving in the anomalous coronary artery, via collaterals from the normal coronary artery, is stolen by the pulmonary trunk, resulting in myocardial ischemia. The treatment includes surgical ligation of the RCA and bypass or re-implantation of the RCA.[21]

REFERENCES

1. King III SB, Douglas JS. New views in coronary arteriography. In: King SB, Douglas JS, eds. *Coronary Arteriography and Angioplasty.* McGraw-Hill, 1985: 274–87.
2. Boucher RA. Coronary angiography and angioplasty. *Cathet Cardiovasc Diagn* 1986; **14**: 269–85.
3. King III SB, Douglas JS. Percutaneous transluminal coronary angioplasty. In: King SB, Douglas JS, eds. *Coronary Arteriography and Angioplasty.* McGraw-Hill, 1985: 443.
4. Vetrovec G. *Cardiac catheterization and interventional cardiology self-assessment program.* American College of Cardiology, 1999.
5. Gershlick AH, Smith LS. Angiography for the interventional cardiologist. In: Grech ED, Ramsdale DR, eds. *Practical Interventional Cardiology.* Martin Dunitz, 1997.
6. Arani DT, Bunnell IL, Greene DG. Lordotic right posterior oblique projection of the left coronary artery: A special view for special anatomy. *Circulation* 1975; **52**: 504.
7. Roubin G. Angiographic views and techniques for coronary interventions. In: Roubin GS, O'Neill WW, Stack RS *et al.*, eds. *Interventional Cardiovascular Medicine: Principles and Practice.* Churchill Livingstone, 1994: 431.
8. Bhatt S, Jorgensen MB, Aharonian VJ *et al.* Nonselective angiography of IMA: A fast, reliable and safe technique. *Cathet Cardiovasc Diagn* 1995; **36**: 194–8.
9. Nissen S. Physical principles of radiographic and digital imaging in the cardiac catheterization laboratories. In: *Interventional Cardiovascular Medicine: Principles and Practice*, 2nd edn. Churchill Livingstone, 2002: 444–64.
10. Cheitlin MD, De Castro CM, McAllister HA. Sudden death as a complication of anomalous left coronary artery origin from the anterior sinus of Valsalva: A not-so-minor congenital anomaly. *Circulation* 1974; **50**: 780–7.
11. Barth CW III, Robert WC. Left main coronary artery originating from the right sinus of Valsalva and coursing between the aorta and pulmonary trunk. *J Am Coll Cardiol* 1986; **7**: 366–73.
12. Santucci P, Bredikis A, Kavinsky C *et al.* Congenital origin of the LMCA from the innominate artery in a 37-year-old man with syncope and right ventricular dysplasia. *Cathet Cardiovasc Interv* 2001; **52**: 378–81.

13. Serota H, Barth III CW, Seuc CA *et al*. Rapid identification of the course of anomalous coronary arteries in adults: The "dot and eye" method. *Am J Cardiol* 1990; **65**: 891–8.

14. Deligonul U, Roth R, Flynn MS. Arterial and venous access. In: Kern M, ed. *Cardiac Catheterization Handbook*, 3rd edn. Mosby, 1999: 51–122.

15. Yamanaka O, Hobbs RE. Coronary artery anomalies in 126,595 patients undergoing coronary arteriography. *Cathet Cardiovasc Diagn* 1990; **21**: 28–40.

16. Wang A, Pulsipher MW, Jaggers J *et al*. Simultaneous biplane coronary and pulmonary artery: A novel technique for defining the course of an anomalous left main coronary artery originating from the sinus of Valsalva. *Cathet Cardiovasc Diagn* 1997; **42**: 73–8.

17. Lawson MA, Dailey SM, Soto B. Selective injection of a left coronary artery arising anomalously from the posterior aortic sinus. *Cathet Cardiovasc Diagn* 1993; **30**: 300–302.

18. Grollman JH, Mao SS, Weinstein SR. Arteriographic demonstration of both kinking at the origin and compression between the great vessels of an anomalous RCA arising in common with the left coronary artery from above the left sinus of Valsalva. *Cathet Cardiovasc Diagn* 1992; **25**: 46–51.

19. Topaz O, Edwards JE. Pathologic features of sudden death in children, adolescents and young adults. *Chest* 1985; **87**: 476–82.

20. Rigatelli G, Docali G, Rossi P *et al*. A new classification of coronary artery anomalies based on the analysis of their clinical significance in an adult Italian population. (In press).

21. Vijitbenjaronk P, Glancy L, Ferguson B. *et al*. RCA arising from the pulmonary trunk in 63-year-old man. *Cathet Cardiovasc Interv* 2002; **57**: 545–547.

Chapter 4

Guides

Thach Nguyen, Nguyen Thuong Nghia, Vijay Dave

General overview
Practical analysis of guide design
    TAKE-HOME MESSAGE: Standard safety techniques
    *Advancement through tortuous iliac artery
    *Dampening of arterial pressure
    *Checking stability and potential of backup capability
    **Simple coaxial position or active support position?
Maneuvering a Judkins guide
    **Selecting the size of Judkins guide
    *Engagement of a Judkins left guide
    **Non-coaxial position of a small Judkins guide
    *Guide that is too large
    *Guide that is too small
    *Engagement of a Judkins right guide
Maneuvering an Amplatz guide
    **Selection of an Amplatz guide
    **Engagement of an Amplatz guide
    **Optimal position of an Amplatz guide
    **Withdrawal of an Amplatz guide
    **Withdrawal of an Amplatz guide after balloon inflation
Maneuvering a Multipurpose guide
Maneuvering an extra-backup guide
Guide selection and manipulation for LM lesions
    *Guide position in suspected LM
    **Dampening pressure
    **Contrast agents
Guide selection and manipulation for LAD lesions
Guide selection and manipulation for LCX lesions
    *Pointing towards the LCX
    **Selection of guides
    ***Rotational Amplatz maneuver
    ***Passive Amplatz maneuver

*Basic; **Advanced; ***Rare, exotic, or investigational.

From: Nguyen T, Hu D, Saito S, Grines C, Palacios I (eds), *Practical Handbook of Advanced Interventional Cardiology*, 2nd edn. © 2003 Futura, an imprint of Blackwell Publishing.

Guide selection and manipulation for RCA lesions
  **Selection of guides for horizontal takeoff angle
  **Selection of guides for superiorly oriented takeoff angle
  **Selection of guides for inferiorly oriented takeoff angle
  **Avoiding selective entry of the conus branch
  **Deep-seating an RCA guide
  ***Rotational Amplatz maneuver for the RCA
Guide selection and manipulation for aortic aneurysm and dissections
  **Is the catheter in the true lumen?
  **Ascending aortogram
  **Engagement of the coronary guides
Selection and manipulation of guides for coronary anomalies
  ***Guides for right aortic arch
  ***Guides for anomalous coronary arteries arising above the sinotubular ridge in the ascending aorta
  ***Guides for anomalous coronary arteries arising from the left sinus
  ***Guides for right coronary artery with anomalous origin
  ***Guides for anomalous coronary arteries arising from the right sinus
  ***Guides for coronary arteries arising from the posterior sinus
  CAVEAT: Guides to locate missing arteries
  Trouble-shooting tips
  **When should a guide with side hole be used?
  **Selection of guides according to inner diameter
  **Deep-seating maneuver
  ***Difficult engagement of a guide while easy engagement with a diagnostic catheter
  **Changing a guide with wire across lesion
  **How to keep the angioplasty wire immobile across the lesion when changing the guide
  **Readvancement of the guide with a wire across the lesion
  **Stabilizing a guide with the "buddy wire" technique
  **Stabilizing a guide with two wires in two branches
  **How to untwist a twisted guide
  ***If the guide is too long
  ***Shortening a guide
  ***Guides for unusually wide ascending aorta

GENERAL OVERVIEW

An optimal guide provides a stable platform for the operator to advance interventional devices to the coronary ostium, through tortuous arterial segments and across tight lesions. It is selected according to the size of the ascending aorta, the location of the ostia to be cannulated, and the orientation of the coronary artery segment proximal to the target lesion. Once engaged in the ostial segment, its soft tip is to be positioned with atraumatic coaxial alignment. In addition to being a conduit for hardware, the guide is also a conduit for delivery of contrast agents, fluids, or medications.

To secure a smooth advancement of interventional devices, measures are taken to lower local friction, to overcome distal resistance, and to reinforce the firm position of the guide.

Lowering the local friction: In order to lower the local friction, there are six corrective measures available:

1. The lumen of the catheter is lined with a lubricious coating to facilitate the smooth movements of interventional devices.
2. A guide with less sharp bends may be selected, so there is less resistance to the movement of devices. The tip of the guide should be positioned in a coaxial alignment in order to create a smooth transition from the guide tip to the ostial segment.
3. The selected interventional device should be more flexible so less friction is generated.
4. The selected interventional device should be short; since it has less contact with the guide lumen and the arterial surface, less friction is generated.
5. The patient is asked to take a deep breath, making the heart more vertical, and thus the artery becomes more elongated and less tortuous. During this short window of opportunity, the device is to be advanced quickly.

Overcoming the resistance: In order to successfully overcome the stiff resistance created by a tight lesion, four options are available:

1. Use a lower profile balloon to dilate the lesion before using the correct size device.
2. Change to the over-the-wire system to increase pushability.
3. Change to the stiffer wire on which the device can slide more easily (increase trackability). The stiffer wire also straightens the proximal segment.
4. Dilate the moderate lesion at the proximal segment. If there is severe superficial calcification in the lesion that obstructs the passage of the device, debulking with rotablation is needed so the device can be advanced across the lesion.

Reinforcing the firm position of the guide: As the interventional device is pushed toward the lesion, any guide with a tip held still, not being displaced, will be the ideal guide for the procedure. In a simple case with easy access, the

Judkins catheter, even in a relaxed position in the aortic sinus, can provide an adequate platform to advance the interventional device. It is also the ideal guide position in aorto-ostial lesion PCI. In complex cases, where more resistance is encountered, any selected guide with its secondary curve well positioned and standing firm against the opposite aortic wall would provide the strong and stable platform needed.

PRACTICAL ANALYSIS OF GUIDE DESIGN

The most commonly used guides are the Judkins, Amplatz, and extra-backup curve guides. The others that have a niche in various situations include the Multipurpose for the RCA bypass or a high LM takeoff, and the LIMA catheter for the superiorly oriented graft and the right and left coronary bypass graft.

Passive and active support: In the literature, there is discussion about guides with passive or active support. Passive support is the strong support of a guide given by the inherent design with good backup against the opposite aortic wall and stiffness from manufactured material. Additional manipulation is generally not required in order to advance interventional devices. Once passive support is insufficient then active support is required. Active support is typically achieved either by manipulation of the guide into a configuration conforming to the aortic root or by subselective intubation with deep engagement of the guide into the coronary vessels.[1]

The Judkins guide

The Judkins left (JL) guide is designed for coronary angiography with its primary (90°), secondary (180°), and tertiary (35°) curves fitting the aortic root anatomy so it can engage the LM ostium without much manipulation. It knows where to go unless thwarted by the operator.[2] Because of the 90° bend at its tip, it does not make perfect coaxial alignment. Furthermore, in inexperienced hands, the LM ostium can still be easily engaged by the guide due to its preshaped configuration. On many occasions, even when the secondary curve does not sit well on the opposite aortic wall or coronary sinus, diagnostic angiography can still be performed satisfactorily while there is no adequate support for advancement of interventional devices during PCI.[1]

The Amplatz guide

The Amplatz left (AL) guide is designed with its secondary curve resting against the noncoronary posterior aortic cusp, while in the Amplatz right (AR) guide, the secondary curve rests against the left aortic cusp.[3] As its tip is well positioned with coaxial alignment, this guide offers a firm platform for advancement of interventional devices. It is best in the case of a short LM, with downgoing LCX or RCA. However, because its tip is pointing downward, there is higher danger of ostial injury causing dissection.

The Multipurpose guide

The technique of manipulation of a Multipurpose guide requires more operator training and experience than the other techniques using preformed guides.[4] With the exception of a few cases of high LM takeoff or downward RCA, which can be cannulated well with this Multipurpose guide, other guides of different designs can provide the same stable platform without much manipulation.

The extra-backup guide

The names of these guides vary (Voda or XB, EB, C, Q, or Geometric curve guides) according to manufacturers. The common design is that their long tip forms a fairly straight line with the LM axis or the proximal ostial RCA, so they can provide a better transition angle with less local friction. They have a long secondary curve resting firmly on the opposite aortic wall, so their tip or body is more difficult to be displaced. As their tip is being held still and coaxial at the ostium, with their shaft firmly positioned, these guides are able to provide a more stable platform.[5]

Standard techniques

Safety measures: In any situation, the basic safety measures should be applied rigorously when manipulating guides. This important take-home message is listed below.[6]

TAKE-HOME MESSAGE

Standard safety techniques:

1. Aspirate the guide vigorously after it is inserted into the ascending aorta for any thrombus or atheromatous debris floating into the guide.
2. Insist on generous bleed back to avoid air embolism.
3. Flush frequently to avoid stagnation of blood and thrombus formation inside the guide.
4. Constantly watch the tip when withdrawing an interventional device from a coronary artery, especially in patients with ostial or proximal plaques.
5. Watch the blood pressure curve for dampening to avoid inadvertent deep engagement of the tip.
6. During injection, keep the tip of the syringe pointed down so any air bubbles will float up and are not injected into the coronary system.

TECHNICAL TIPS

*Advancement through tortuous iliac artery: Because many older patients have a tortuous ascending and descending aorta, sometimes the guide is barely long enough to reach the coronary artery. On other occasions, because of excessive tortuosity of the iliac artery, rotations at the proximal end do not transmit similar motion to the distal tip. If not constantly watched, the guide can twist on itself. Simple gentle movement of the guide in and out, often over a very short distance, transmits torque to the tip.[7] Then, in these situations, a sheath 23 cm long may help to overcome the problem of iliac tortuosity. In the rare case of a patient with AAA, a 40-cm sheath is needed. A more simple technique is by torquing a guide still cannulated inside by a stiff 0.38" wire inserted through a Y adapter. Manipulate the tip near the ostium, remove the stiff wire, flush the guide, and then engage the tip to the ostium.[7]

*Dampening of arterial pressure: The guide can cause a fall in diastolic pressure (ventricularization) or a fall in both systolic and diastolic pressure (dampened pressure). The causes can be: significant lesion in the ostium, coronary spasm, non-coaxial alignment of the guide, or mismatch between the diameter of the guide and of the arterial lumen. When dampening of the aortic pressure is caused by a small coronary artery, the guide can be exchanged for one with side holes, which allows passive blood flow into the distal coronary artery. The drawbacks include suboptimal opacification of the artery because contrast escapes through side holes, and very rarely, decreased backup support due to weakened guide shaft and kinking of the guide at the side holes, if the guide is excessively manipulated. However, the most common cause of ventricularization is ostial lesion.

*Checking stability and potential of backup capability: Under fluoroscopic guidance, forward advancement of the guide should demonstrate a tendency to further intubate the coronary artery rather than prolapse into the aortic root. As the tip slips out, the guide does not provide sufficient backup. It may need to be changed for another with better support. Active intubation of the guide may be tried if the tip is soft, if the artery is large enough to accommodate the guide, and if there are no ostial or proximal lesions. This active support position is needed temporarily in order to advance the device across the lesion.[8] Once the device is positioned, the guide is then withdrawn to outside or at the ostium.

**Simple coaxial position or active support position? Coaxial guide alignment with the ostium is more important than an active support or "power position" to allow the operator to gently advance and retract the guide as needed, ensuring proper device position and contrast opacification. Because almost all interventional devices (stent, cutting balloon, directional, rotational ablative, thrombectomy or distal protection devices, etc.) are rigid and of large profile, a non-coaxial alignment of the guide may lead to injury, endothelial denudation causing thrombus, or dissection of the ostium of the coronary vessel.

Aggressive guide intubation may impair stent deployment at an aorto-ostial lesion.[1]

MANEUVERING A JUDKINS GUIDE

Selection of a Judkins guide

A Judkins guide is selected according to the width of the ascending aorta, the location of the ostia to be cannulated, and the orientation of the coronary artery segment proximal to the target lesion. The segment between the primary and secondary curve of the Judkins guide should fit the width of ascending aorta: 3.5 cm, 4 cm, 4.5 cm or 5 cm, 6 cm, etc. The locations of the ostia can be low, high or more anteriorly oriented or posteriorly oriented. The ostial or proximal segment can be pointed upwards, downwards or horizontally.

TECHNICAL TIPS

**Selecting the size of Judkins guide: For the average American patient, a 4-cm JL guide is often adequate. For Asian patients, a 3.5 JL guide usually fits well. In patients with a very superior direction of the LAD or in those with narrow aortic root, a smaller size guide with a tip more anteriorly pointed will provide a coaxial position of the tip. In patients with horizontal or wide aortic root (e.g. chronic aortic insufficiency or uncontrolled high blood pressure), a Judkins guide with long secondary curve (size 5 or 6) will fit the width of the ascending aorta well.

*Engagement of a Judkins left guide: When the JL guide is advanced into the coronary sinus in the AP view, if it advances straight down, it may enter the noncoronary sinus. Pull it back and re-advance it while torquing the guide counterclockwise so it can be advanced into the left sinus. A small injection may show that the tip is below the LM ostium. Then pull the guide back and torque it counterclockwise so that its tip will point anteriorly and superiorly toward and engage the LM ostium.

**Non-coaxial position of a small Judkins guide: If a small Judkins guide is chosen, with its tip not coaxial to the LM, that tip will point superiorly to the wall. In that position, even though there is no dampening of aortic pressure, an injection of contrast agent in young patients may not cause dissection, but in elderly patients with many unsuspected plaques, it can cause a localized dissection.[9]

*Guide that is too large: The Judkins tip points in a cranial direction, depending on the length between the primary and secondary curves and how far the heel or secondary curve is advanced into the aortic root. As a guide is advanced down the aortic sinuses, if its tip remains in the vertical axis of the ascending aorta and does not curve upward to reach the left ostium, then this catheter is too large. It should be changed for a smaller one.[10]

*Guide that is too small: If the guide is smaller than needed, or the distance between the primary and secondary curves is too short, the guide would be advanced too far into the aortic root. Its primary and secondary curve would double back on itself inside the sinuses of Valsalva.[10]

*Engagement of a Judkins right guide: The basic maneuver for cannulation of the RCA is by advancing the guide into the aortic root, then rotating the shaft clockwise while gently withdrawing it, so its tip can select the RCA ostium.

When the RCA arises more anteriorly or above the right cusp, the tip of the JR guide will not stay coaxial inside the right ostium. The coaxial position can best be appreciated by viewing the tip of the guide as a ring in a head-on position with the RAO 30° view (Figure 3-8 A).

MANEUVERING AN AMPLATZ GUIDE

**Selection of an Amplatz guide: Selection of proper size is essential. Size 1 is for the smallest aortic root, size 2 for normal, and size 3 for large roots. Attempts to force engagement of a preformed guide that does not conform to a particular aorta, aortic root, or aortic sinus will only waste time and increase the risk of complication.[4] If the tip does not reach the ostium and keeps lying below it, the guide is too small. If the tip lies above the ostium, or the loop cannot be opened, the guide is too large. When the RCA ostium is very high, then the AL guide may be used to engage the right ostium. For arteries that lie in the mid-portion of the right sinus or lower, an AR with a much smaller hook must be used. This guide generally is braced against the left aortic cusp and therefore lies directly opposite the RCA orifice.

**Engagement of an Amplatz guide: The guide is advanced into the ascending aorta behind the long soft distal segment of the wire, with the tip pointed toward the patient's left until the guide lies on the posterior or noncoronary sinus. After being flushed well, the guide is then advanced slowly with the tip pointing upward and anteriorly, rotated (more in the counterclockwise), and retracted until the tip engages the left ostium.

**Optimal position of an Amplatz guide: Once the tip of the Amplatz is inside an LM or RCA ostium, the primary and secondary curves of the guide should form a closed loop with the tip coaxial with the ostial segment. This is the appropriate guide position. If the guide is pulled back, its tip would dip farther into the LM. This deep intubation should be avoided, because it increases the probability of LM dissection. Under fluoroscopy, the undesired position of the primary and secondary curves shows a more open loop, with the tip pointing down the inferior wall of the ostial segment.[11]

**Withdrawal of an Amplatz guide: An Amplatz guide should not be engaged more deeply than needed, to avoid tip-induced injury. To withdraw an Amplatz guide, first advance the guide slightly under fluoroscopy to prolapse the tip out of the ostium, then rotate the guide before withdrawing it. If this maneuver fails to dislodge the tip, then the guide is rotated while being retracted slowly under fluoroscopy to avoid deep engagement of the tip.[10]

**Withdrawal of an Amplatz guide after balloon inflation: After angioplasty or deployment of a stent, the balloon is deflated. If it is pulled out, the tip of the Amplatz guide would have the tendency to be sucked in deeper. This is a situation to avoid. The first best technique is to pull the balloon out while simultaneously pushing the guide in to prolapse the guide out. The procedure has to be done under fluoroscopy to monitor the intended movement of the guide tip.

If the above maneuver fails, then the second technique can be used. The deflated balloon should be advanced slowly to back out of the guide. As the guide stops backing out, then the guide is withdrawn slowly, while watching the tip in order to avoid scratching the inferior aspect of the ostial segment. Once the tip is sensed to point unsafely down the ostial segment, then the balloon is advanced again to lift the tip and back out of the guide farther. This maneuver is repeated until the tip of the guide is totally out of the ostium. Then the guide and the interventional device can be retracted as needed. The tip is less likely to cause damage if retracted over the wire or the shaft of a device catheter.

MANEUVERING A MULTIPURPOSE GUIDE

Most operators advocate starting from the posterior sinus or noncoronary cusp in the 30° RAO position. The guide is advanced with the tip pointed toward the spine. When a loop is formed, slight clockwise rotation flips the tip of the left cusp and points it toward the ostium. The tip is then advanced or withdrawn slightly to cannulate the LM ostium. The RCA is approached in the 45° LAO position. From the left cusp, the tip is directed anteriorly and to the patient's right. Then the guide is rotated clockwise, and then slightly withdrawn to engage the right ostium.[4]

MANEUVERING AN EXTRA-BACKUP GUIDE

Most operators advocate the advancement of the tip of the guide with a wire protruding into the ascending aorta, at the aortic valve sinus, below the coronary ostium. Then the wire is removed. The guide is then withdrawn gently while torquing clockwise or counterclockwise until it seats in the left main or right coronary ostium.

GUIDE SELECTION AND MANIPULATION
FOR LEFT MAIN LESIONS

A significant lesion in the LM can be suspected by clinical criteria: (1) typical angina at low level of activity or exercise testing, (2) typical angina at rest, (3) significant diffuse ST-T segment depression at low level of exercise testing, and (4) no increase of blood pressure or decrease of blood pressure upon exercise stress testing.

TECHNICAL TIPS

*Guide position in suspected LM: Once an LM lesion is suspected, a short-tip Judkins left guide should be chosen. The guide is positioned below the LM ostium, beneath the cusp where an injection of 10 cc of contrast may opacify the cusp and help to have a general assessment of the LM segment. Then the tip of the guide is manipulated to slowly engage the LM ostium, avoiding the uncontrolled jump into the artery, due to its preshaped configuration. If there is no dampening or ventricularization of the aortic pressure, then a small amount of 2–3 cc of contrast is injected in the AP, shallow RAO, or shallow LAO views (Figure 3-1).

**Dampening pressure: Dampening of the aortic pressure can be due to an LM lesion and, in rare cases, due to a mismatch between the large-size guide and a small coronary ostium. Gradual repositioning and withdrawal of the guide may eliminate pressure dampening.[12] A few senior angiographers suggest a small injection of contrast with quick removal of the tip of the guide ("hit and run") technique. It is not wise to do so because the tip of the catheter may lie under a plaque and this is the possible cause of dampening of the aortic pressure. An injection of contrast agent, even with a small amount, can farther lift the plaque and really cause a dissection that can become fatal. If the blood pressure is dampened while the tip of the balloon or stent catheter is ready to be inserted into the coronary system, then advancing the device catheters farther will back out the guide and restore the normal blood pressure tracing.

**Contrast agents: Use non-ionic or low osmolar contrast agents because standard ionic contrast may cause rare hypotension and bradycardia, which can be transient in normal patients but can cause lethal complications in patients with LM lesions.

GUIDE SELECTION AND MANIPULATION
FOR LAD LESIONS

The LAD courses in a superior and anterior direction, so any guide with a tip pointing superiorly, such as the Judkins left guide, will provide a stable and coaxial alignment. In patients with a very superior direction of the LAD or in those with narrow aortic root, a smaller size guide will point the tip more anteriorly or the Voda or XB guide would help to provide stronger backup. In the case of high coronary takeoff, a Multipurpose guide or an Amplatz would easily cannulate the left ostium. In patients with horizontal or wide aortic root (e.g. chronic aortic insufficiency or uncontrolled high blood pressure), a Judkins guide with long secondary curve (size 5 or 6), or an Amplatz-type left guide may be needed.[10]

GUIDE SELECTION AND MANIPULATION FOR LCX
LESIONS

Selection of the LCX usually can be achieved with the Judkins left guide. In the case of high coronary takeoff, use a Multipurpose or an Amplatz guide. In patients with horizontal or wide aortic root, a Judkins guide with long secondary curve (size 5 or 6) or an Amplatz-type left guide may be needed. Because the tip of the Judkins guide points superiorly, better axial support for LCX lesions can be obtained using an Amplatz, or extra-backup guides.

TECHNICAL TIPS

*Pointing towards the LCX: In the case of short LM or separate ostium of the LCX, if the tip of the first Judkins guide does not point toward the LCX, slightly withdraw the guide and turn clockwise. The tip will point posteriorly, toward the LCX. If this maneuver does not achieve satisfactory results, change to a larger size or to an Amplatz-type guide with a tip pointing down. If the LM is very short, a size 1.5 Amplatz will allow acceptable access without over-engagement. However, be careful of dissection caused by the tip.

**Selection of guides: If the LM is long and there is no acute angle at the bifurcation with the circumflex, a JL may be the first best choice. If the LM is long and the lesion is quite severe, an extra-backup guide should be chosen because its secondary curve lies on the opposite aortic wall to provide firm backup to cross any tight lesion.

***Rotational Amplatz maneuver: To enhance the support role of a Judkins guide (active support or "power position"), an alternative approach is to advance it farther, well down into the aortic root over the shaft of an interventional device (stent, balloon catheter, IVUS, etc.). This causes the tip to ride superiorly, creating a U-turn between the tip of the guide in the LM and the LCX. If this maneuver is unsuccessful in providing adequate backup, further advancement while applying counterclockwise torque on the Judkins guide may cause the entire tip of the guide to prolapse into the aortic root, turning the primary curve over and pointing downward, simulating the position achieved with the Amplatz guide. This is called the rotational Amplatz maneuver.[10] The operator should not feel any resistance when attempting this maneuver. After the interventional device is advanced and positioned in place, then the guide is withdrawn from the artery by reversing the earlier torquing energy: gentle clockwise rotation so the guide can untwist itself while pulling the guide back slowly. This technique should be performed with soft-tip guide in coronary artery large enough to accommodate the guide. There should not be disease at the ostium or proximal segment. Another alternative is to exchange the Judkins guide for an Amplatz or extra-backup guide that can provide stronger support and safe advancement of interventional hardware (Figure 4-1).[1]

***Passive Amplatz maneuver: In patients with high-positioned LM ostium, instead of torquing with force, if the length of secondary curve of the guide is appropriate (or equal to the height of the left coronary sinus), the guide is torqued clockwise and pushed gently down until the whole curve sits well in the left sinus, with the tip pointing to the LM. Then PCI can be performed accordingly (Figure 4-2).

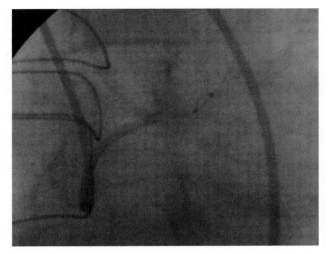

Figure 4-1: Rotational Amplatz maneuver. The Judkins left catheter can be prolapsed into the aortic root, producing a strong backup downward curve of the tip similar to the Amplatz guide.

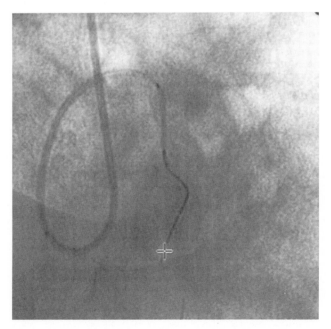

Figure 4-2: Passive Amplatz maneuver. The whole distal part of the Judkins left guide is prolapsed into the aortic root with the tip pointing into the LM ostium.

GUIDE SELECTION AND MANIPULATION FOR RCA LESIONS

The RCA usually arises anterolaterally from the right coronary cusp. In the large majority of cases, its proximal segment has a horizontal configuration and forms a 90° angle with lateral border of the aorta. In the case of an acutely angled takeoff, the "shepherd's crook," the angle is smaller than 90° (Figure 4-3). When the RCA is directed caudally, the downward angle is more than 90° (see Figure 9-3 A). However, there are other minor variations, including the slightly anterior or posterior placed ostium or the one with anomalous origins, that can make cannulation or alignment of guides difficult (see Figure 3-8 B).[13]

TECHNICAL TIPS

**Selection of guides for horizontal takeoff angle: In the majority of cases of RCA with horizontal takeoff, a JR-4 guide can easily engage the ostium. When a JR fails to cannulate the right ostium, an AR would be the next option. If it fails, an AL with backup from the opposite wall of the aorta will usually achieve cannulation of the ostium and provide the required backup.[13]

**Selection of guides for superiorly oriented takeoff angle: When the shepherd's crook or a markedly superior orientation of the RCA is encountered, guides with the

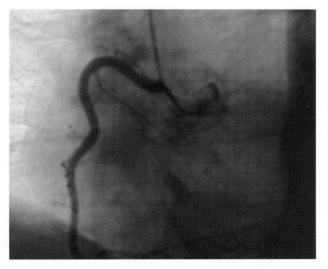

Figure 4-3: The RCA with shepherd's crook configuration.

tip pointing in a cranial direction are necessary. The JR guide, which is effective in diagnostic angiography, does not provide sufficient backup; therefore the AL guide is usually selected. Other guides with a superiorly directed tip, such as the hockey stick, the left venous bypass, and the internal mammary artery guides, can cannulate the vessel, although they offer poor backup support. These preshaped guides may eliminate the need for torquing and are particularly useful in elderly patients or in patients with very tortuous iliac arteries, which sometimes make guide manipulation very difficult.[13]

**Selection of guides for inferiorly oriented takeoff angle: In this orientation of the proximal segment of the RCA, aggressive engagement of the tip from a regular JR tip can abut the lateral wall and cause dissection. The guides with inferiorly directed tips, such as the right venous bypass, Multipurpose, and Amplatz guides, may achieve more effective coaxial alignment with the proximal vessel segment.[13]

**Avoiding selective entry of the conus branch: If the guide keeps entering the conus artery, do one of three things: (1) straighten the tip of the right guide with a heat gun; (2) change the guide for a larger one; or (3) approach the RCA from a posterior direction (counterclockwise rotation of the catheter) entering the main RCA first.[14]

**Deep-seating an RCA guide: In a non-coaxial situation, backup support will not be adequate for advancement of interventional devices. Thus the guide should be better aligned by additional clockwise rotation to allow the tip to engage deeper into the ostium. This maneuver is performed in the LAO view. When the interventional device is advanced into the coronary artery by the right hand, additional pressure should be put on the guide by the left hand placed firmly on the patient's thigh near the femoral sheath so the guide does not back out. While the device catheter is advanced, the assistant should pull the wire back slowly to decrease friction inside the device catheter, thus facilitating its advancement. If the guide needs to be deep-seated then it is advanced over an interventional device (stent, balloon catheter, etc.) while applying clockwise torque. Once the guide is deep-seated, the interventional device is advanced and positioned. After achieving the position needed, the guide is withdrawn with gentle counterclockwise rotation to outside the coronary ostium. This procedure can be done if the artery is large enough to accommodate the guide, if there is no ostial or proximal lesion, and the guide tip is soft.

***Rotational Amplatz maneuver for the RCA:** To en-
hance the support role of a Judkins guide (active support or
"power position"), the guide is torqued counterclockwise,
and simultaneously pushed in such a manner it takes a 90°
bend on its shaft, which then rests on the opposite aortic
wall. The original secondary curve is hence obliterated,
and in fact displaced proximally, to obtain direct support
from the opposite aortic valve. This maneuver is distinct
from deep-seating of the guide where no support is derived
from the opposite aortic wall. This can be done with small
and soft guide (6F). If the guide is stiff, it will tend to prolapse
into the ventricle with the wire projected into the aorta. Such
a catastrophe can be avoided by carefully monitoring the
shape and the position of the guide as the maneuver is carried out. Having rotated the catheter in a counterclockwise
direction, while advancing it, it is essential to have the distal
part of the guide on a plane parallel to the aortic valve. If the
catheter moves downward, toward the aortic valve, further
advancement will result in prolapse of the guide into the
ventricle. At that point, the guide is to be gently pulled back
and rotated further counterclockwise prior to its advancement. If prolapse tends to recur, this maneuver should be
abandoned. It is also very important to avoid excessive
rotation that may lead to kinking of the guide and impede
and/or dislodge stent passage. This maneuver is also useful when a Judkins right cannot engage an RCA because
of ostial lesion. Then an "Amplatzed" Judkins right would
point its tip toward the ostium without direct engagement. In
the rotational Amplatz maneuver, it should be done over the
shaft of an interventional device (stent, balloon catheter,
IVUS, etc.), so there is less trauma to the ostial segment of
the RCA.[15]

GUIDE SELECTION AND MANIPULATION FOR
AORTIC ANEURYSM AND DISSECTIONS

**Guides for ascending or descending aortic aneu-
rysm or dissection:** When performing procedures in patients
with aneurysm in the ascending aorta, the technical problems
could be loss of catheter control or inadequate catheter length
to reach the coronary arteries. In the case of aortic dissection,
the arterial entry route chosen may not allow access to the true
aortic lumen. Other risks include extending a dissection plane
by advancement of the guide or wire, perforation of the aorta
by manipulation or injection in a false lumen, or displacement
of thrombotic material from an aneurysm.[16] For these reasons,
a careful discussion of the goals of angiography should be
carried out with the surgeon. Many surgeons do not require
extensive angiography when CT or MRI confirms the extent of
the pathology and the need for angiography can be avoided.

In cases of aneurysm or dissection limited to the thoracoabdominal aorta, the brachial approach is preferred. When the CT scan showed involvement of the great vessels or carotids, the brachial approach should be avoided. When there is involvement of lower extremities, access from the involved limb is avoided. When extensive ascending and thoracoabdominal aneurysmal disease is present, the femoral approach is chosen because of greater ease of catheter exchange and manipulation.[17]

TECHNICAL TIPS

**Is the catheter in the true lumen? In patients with aortic dissection requiring ascending aortography, at first a pigtail catheter is attempted to enter the left ventricle directly. After pressure measurement is made, the catheter is pulled back and the aortography is performed. In this way, one can be assured of being in the true aortic lumen. It is risky to attempt to cross the aortic valve against resistance. A straight-type catheter with a blunt tip like the Sones or the Multipurpose should be used cautiously in known or suspected aortic dissection due to the possibility of advancing it in the false lumen.[17] Since the majority of the dissection occurs in the lateral wall of the aorta, the pigtail can be positioned in the true lumen by advancing while hugging the medial aspect of the aortic arch in a shallow AP view. In the true lumen, selective cannulation of the coronary artery is possible, as is direct entry into the LV. To be sure it is in the true channel, the pigtail should be able to cross the aortic valve, then go to the LV, then go back easily to the aortic lumen.

**Ascending aortogram: An ascending aortogram in the LAO projection is obtained with 60 cc of contrast with a flow rate 25–40 cc/second. The aortogram is frequently helpful in defining the shape and size of the aorta, showing the position and orientation of the coronary ostia, and in choosing appropriate coronary catheters. Injection is never made if the aortic pressure is damped or there is no brisk blood return through the catheter. If the test injection showed delayed washout or swirling of contrast, it is assumed that the catheter is in the false lumen. It is withdrawn and redirected into the true lumen with a 0.035" high torque floppy wire. When the integrity of the great vessels or aortic arch is in question, a second injection is made with a catheter in a higher position in an LAO projection with approximately 20° caudal angulation.[17]

**Engagement of the coronary guides: When the aortic root is horizontal the JL6 guide is often successful in cannulating the LM. Most often it has to be "pulled into" the LM by a combination of advancement of the catheter below the ostium with simultaneous retraction of the wire, which is curled up into the left sinus. Due to frequent prolapse of the catheter, this maneuver often needs to be repeated many times before successful engagement is achieved. Thus a 0.038" wire is inserted through the Y adapter and left ready in the guide, so the above maneuver can be repeated quickly if needed.

When the aortic root is vertical, the AL4 is more frequently successful in engaging the LM. The guide is engaged by curling the wire well up the left sinus and tracking the guide up just below the LM. The wire is then retracted and the guide is gently advanced up into the LM.[17]

The engagement of the RCA is frequently problematic because its origin is often distorted. Usually it is displaced low in the floor of the right sinus of Valsalva (particularly in an horizontal root), but its origin may occasionally be abnormally high. In many cases, the dissecting plane begins above the RCA. Therefore the aortic diameter may be normal at the level of the right coronary ostium which is usually easily engaged with the standard JR4 or 5 catheters.[17]

In contrast to a patient with aneurysm, the aorta diameter in dissection may be narrower due to systolic compression of the true lumen by the hematoma. One particular problem is a lack of support from the dissecting aortic wall to the Judkins catheter. The Amplatz guides require the support from the aortic valve cups for manipulation and, due to the weakening of the aortic apparatus by the dissection, the guides are more difficult to use, prolapsing frequently into the left ventricle, during attempted engagement.[17]

SELECTION AND MANIPULATION OF GUIDES FOR CORONARY ANOMALIES

Regardless of their rarity, an experienced interventionalist should be aware of all variations of coronary anomalies and systematically search in other aortic sinuses when the vessel in question does not arise from its usual location.[18] Then during intervention, the location of the ostium of the anomalous artery and the geometry of the proximal segment should be the prime determinants dictating selection of a specific guide catheter.[18] An RCA with a long horizontal segment in the LAO view may appear to have an angle of proximal vessel orientation favorable for use of a Judkins curve, but the long segment usually represents an ectopic origin, appreciated more readily in the RAO projection. Coaxial engagement of these arteries may be more difficult and require considerable manipulations. To cannulate the anomalous artery from the right sinus, the best guides are the left, right Amplatz and the Multipurpose guides. For the artery originating from the left sinus, the best guides are the larger left Judkins, left Amplatz, and the Multi-purpose guides.[19] In some very unusual anomalies, "trial and error" guides selection or reshaping guides may be necessary.[19] Approach from the radial artery may offer a better chance of success.

Anatomic consideration of the ostial segment: Not every anomaly has a wide ostium that the tip of the guide can hook onto, or a narrowing at the opening that needs to be stented. There have been several reports that an anomalous RCA from the left coronary artery can leave the aorta in oblique fashion, so the ostium has a slit-like configuration formed by flaps of aortic and coronary tissues. During exercise, the aorta can expand its part of the flap, narrowing farther the slit-like opening and causing ischemia.[20]

TECHNICAL TIPS

***Guides for right aortic arch:** In patients with right aortic arch, dextrocardia, or corrected transposition of situs inversus, a left coronary catheter may be used to cannulate any artery originating from the right aortic sinus. A right coronary catheter will be used for an artery originating from the left sinus. The catheter is torqued in a counterclockwise fashion rather than the usual clockwise one and is based on mirror-image angles.[21]

***Guides for anomalous coronary arteries arising above the sinotubular ridge in the ascending aorta:** Patients can have coronary arteries arising above the sinotubular ridge. In a case report by Yeoh *et al.* because the RCA was not found in its usual location, left ventriculography in the RAO projection showed that the RCA arose from the anterior aspect of the ascending aorta, much like that of a surgically placed vein graft. A Multipurpose guide failed to engage the artery. An AL-1 succeeded in visualizing the artery.[22–23]

***Guides for anomalous coronary arteries arising from the left sinus:** When the right coronary artery arises from the left cusp, usually it is anterior and cephalad to the LM, so in principle, it can also be cannulated by a Judkins left with the secondary curve one size larger than the one for the patient's LAD. This larger Judkins should be pushed deep in the left sinus of Valsalva, causing it to make an anterior and cephalad pointing U-turn. The larger curve will prevent the guide from engaging the patient's LM (see Figure 3-15).[24] By the same principle, an AL-2 with a tip pointed more anteriorly, would help to cannulate the artery.[20] Others reported the use of a JL-4 with an eccentric tip FL4-G (USCI) to cannulate the anomalous RCA from the left sinus. The primary curve of the type G catheter is out of plane to the remainder of the catheter in an anterior orientation, therefore avoiding the normal left coronary ostium.[25]

**Guides for right coronary artery with anomalous origin: This artery usually arises from an anterior and superior location seen in the RAO view. The superb guide for this location is the AL that offers stable seating and great support.[26]

***Guides for anomalous coronary arteries arising from the right sinus: This artery usually arises from the very proximal RCA or from a separate orifice in the right cusp. An AL guide is well suited for cannulating this vessel and will do so selectively rather than entering the RCA. Others have suggested a JR with a posteriorly directed tip or a JR with its tip shortened by 2 mm and smoothed with a sterilized emery board.[25] When the JR cannot provide a stable platform to advance the hardware, then an AR can be cannulated easily.[25]

***Guides for coronary arteries arising from the posterior sinus: The most common anomaly is an anomalous LCX originated from the right sinus. A JR-4 can be cannulated by torquing it clockwise so its tip will point more posteriorly. An AL guide can be cannulated too and its tip should be oriented posteriorly by torquing clockwise in order to successfully engage the ostium.[27]

CAVEAT: Guides to locate missing arteries: On many occasions, when an RCA could not be visualized in the right sinus or an LM could not be detected in the left sinus, a novice angiographer might declare that the patient has congenital omission of that artery. In reality, these arteries may be congenitally mislocated. From accumulated results of prior studies or case reports, the possible abnormal locations of these arteries are tabulated. Then a few suggestions in guide selection may help to pinpoint where the missing arteries can be and how their ostia may be engaged (Table 4-1).

TROUBLE-SHOOTING TIPS

**When should a guide with side hole be used? When there is ventricularization or dampening of aortic pressure, corrective measure by using guide with side holes can give false security because the tip of the guide could be located under a plaque and manipulation or injection of contrast could cause severe dissection. Guide with side holes could be used ideally in PCI of chronic total occlusions of the right coronary artery in case anterograde collaterals are present. This generally guarantees anterograde flow even during deep catheter intubation, which permits distal

Table 4-1
Guides for missing arteries

Missing arteries	Guide selection
Missing LCX due to very short LM	Use larger guide with short tip and turn clockwise to point the tip more posteriorly
Missing LCX originated from RCA	Guide with short tip
No RCA in right sinus	In right sinus: Amplatz left pointing antero-superior of RCA ostium In left sinus: Judkins left one side larger, pointing antero-superior of LM ostium
No LM in left sinus	In right sinus: Amplatz left pointing antero-superior of RCA ostium Check posterior sinus or above the sino-tubular ridge

opacification during contrast injections but avoids possible ischemia.[28]

**Selection of guides according to inner diameter: It is important for the guides to have sufficient inner diameter to accommodate various single or multiple devices while allowing adequate vessel visualization. During intervention with the double balloon technique, the minimal required lumen diameter is calculated by adding 0.006" to the combined diameter of the largest portions of the two balloon catheters. As the lumen size becomes larger due to innovations from manufacturers, the selection of any guide is up to the size of the lumen and its accommodating capacity (Table 4-2).

**Deep-seating maneuver: To provide further support for an interventional device to cross a tight lesion, some operators suggest deeply engaging the tip of the guide into the ostium. For the RCA, the interventional device is retracted as the guide is advanced over the wire and gently rotated clockwise. For the LAD, counterclockwise rotation while advancing the guide provides the best deep-seating. To point the guide toward the LCX, clockwise rotation is suggested (Table 4-3). The operator should not feel any resistance while this maneuver is attempted. The interventional device is then readvanced while maintaining gentle forward pressure on the guide. Extreme care must be taken to maintain distal wire position and avoid proximal vessel trauma or dissection by the deeply engaged tip. Once the lesion is crossed, the guide is pulled back to the free position in the ostium.[29]

Table 4-2
Inner lumen size and accommodating capacity

Size	Accommodating capacity
5F	Diagnostic angiography
5F guide (wide lumen)	Some angioplasty
6F guide	Standard angioplasty and stenting
6F guide (wide lumen)	Some bifurcation angioplasty (including kissing balloons), some IVUS catheters
7F guides (wide lumen)	2.0 mm Rotablator burrs 2 rapid-exchange balloon catheters AngioJet catheter
8F guides	2 over-the-wire balloon catheters 2.25 mm Rotoblator burrs AngioJet catheter, cutting balloon
9F guides	Maximum Rotoblator burr: 2.5 mm Directional coronary atherectomy

Table 4-3
Direction of torquing during deep-seating maneuver

1. Toward the LAD	Counterclockwise rotation
2. Toward the LCX	Clockwise rotation
3. In the RCA	Clockwise rotation

***Difficult engagement of a guide while easy engagement with a diagnostic catheter:** Sometimes a diagnostic catheter can engage easily an artery when it is difficult with an interventional guide. So after the diagnostic catheter engages the artery, a long 0.014" wire is advanced ahead into the artery and the guide is exchanged over. In a similar situation, when there is difficulty in engaging a guide deeply, a 0.014" wire is advanced into the artery and serves as a rail for tracking the guide. Wire with gradual tip transition should be selected to avoid prolapsing at its point of transition and disengagement of the guide.

Changing a guide with wire across lesion: Changing a guide is more difficult if the lesion has already been crossed by a wire. If a wire placement was difficult, it is desirable not to recross the lesion. Techniques have been developed to allow exchange of guides over angioplasty wires. The use of exchange wires with long radiopaque tips facilitates this procedure by minimizing the chance of failing to notice a redundant loop of radiolucent wire in the aortic root.

The other technique is to use a regular length 0.035" wire. Once the guide is disengaged from the coronary ostium and retracted slightly into the aorta, a 0.035" heavy wire is advanced beside the angioplasty wire up the ascending aorta and to the tip. There, the guide is withdrawn with the stiff wire, while the soft angioplasty wire is kept immobile (Figure 4-4).[30] Once the guide is out, the new guide is inserted over the two wires. When the guide is in the ascending aorta, the 0.035" wire is removed. A balloon catheter is inserted and the guide is re-engaged into the ostium over the balloon catheter (Figure 4-5).

**How to keep the angioplasty wire immobile across the lesion when changing the guide: When changing a guide over a wire across the lesion, in order to keep the angioplasty wire immobile, advance the coronary wire so a large loop is created in the aortic root. In this way, any movement over the angioplasty wire is not transmitted

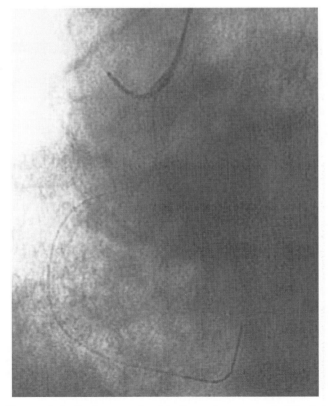

Figure 4-4: Exchange of guide through a second stiff wire while the soft angioplasty wire is still across the lesion.

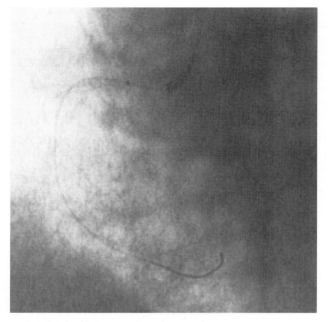

Figure 4-5: The guide is reinserted into the ostium through the angioplasty wire. A balloon is positioned at the ostium as a rail to strengthen the wire so the guide can slide on.

and the wire will stay immobile inside the coronary artery and across the lesion. However, there is a need to use the fluoroscope all the time to be sure that the wire is not moving. When reinserting the guide, the guide should be reinserted over two wires, the soft angioplasty and the stiff 0.035". Once at the ascending aorta level, the 0.035" wire is removed and a balloon catheter is inserted. The new guide is then to be engaged into the coronary ostium not only over the soft angioplasty wire but also over the stronger balloon catheter shaft. Once the balloon is at the ostium of the coronary artery, the stiffer shaft of the balloon catheter will provide a better rail for the guide than the wire alone would, to engage the ostium (Table 4-4).

**Readvancement of the guide with a wire across the lesion: After a balloon or stent is positioned at an intended location, a guide has to be repositioned in order to have an angiogram to check the exact location of the device. The wire should be withdrawn slowly in order for the tip of the guide to advance farther inside the ostium, rather than the guide being pushed in. Be sure the balloon or stent does not move.

Table 4-4
Different techniques for changing guide

---

1. Remove the whole system, change the guide, and recross the lesion.
2. Change the guide through the extension of the existing angioplasty wire.
3. Change the guide through a second regular length 0.035" wire while the angioplasty wire is kept immobile across the lesion.[31]
4. Reinsert the guide through a balloon catheter.

**Stabilizing a guide with the "buddy wire" technique: When working with an unstable guide, after unsuccessful advancement of interventional hardware, a second angioplasty wire can be advanced parallel to the first one. It straightens the tortuous vessel and provides better support for device tracking.

**Stabilizing a guide with two wires in two branches: When working with an unstable guide, especially the small 6F from the radial approach, a stiff 0.014" steerable wire may provide support and a second stiff wire in a side branch can be very useful in "anchoring" the guide (e.g. second wire in LCX when dilating LAD lesion). This provides for better "backup" and allows retraction of the guide catheter without loss of position when necessary (see Figure 5-7). It also prevents the guide from being "sucked in" beyond the LM when pulling back high-profile, poorly rewrapped balloon catheters following stent deployments or post-stent dilations. However, a second wire in a non-diseased branch would cause unnecessary denudation of endothelium in that vessel. Risks and benefits should be evaluated before this maneuver is attempted.

**How to untwist a twisted guide: When the iliac artery is very tortuous, torquing maneuver can twist the guide at its proximal segment. Usually the pressure curve would disappear on the screen. The patient can complain of pain in the lower quadrant area because when the guide becomes twisted, it forms a sharp bend pointing laterally and can cause perforation. When seeing a twisted guide, the first thing to do is to move the twisted segment to a large area by advancing it into the aorta rather than leaving it in the iliac artery. Then cannulate the guide with a 0.035" wire, moving its tip to the twisted area. Then try to untwist the guide by torquing it in the opposite direction you did before. If you torque clockwise more in the last few minutes, then try counterclockwise (or vice versa). Work on a trial and error basis. However, as you torque, slowly advance the wire to secure the segment you just untwisted. If you see on the fluoroscope that the guide is becoming more tortuous, this means you are making the situation worse. Try the opposite way. Advance the wire gently as you torque. In a matter of less than one minute, the guide should be untwisted, straightened and removed.

***If the guide is too long:** In cases of interventions through long SVG or IMA grafts, care must be taken to ensure that there is sufficient catheter length to reach distal sites with extra-long (145 cm) balloon catheters or short guides (80 cm) or the guide can be shortened and capped with a flared, short sheath one size smaller.[32]

***Shortening a guide:** In many circumstances, when the balloon catheter does not reach the lesion through the guide, the whole system has to be changed and the lesion recrossed with a wire. To avoid removing or exchanging the guide or wire, there is a technique of shortening the guide so a balloon can reach the lesion.[32]

TECHNIQUE

First cut the guide with a scalpel. While the guide is still engaging the artery with a wire across the lesion, the guide should be clamped by a hemostat to prevent bleeding during the shortening procedure. Care must be taken so the scalpel does not damage the wire.

Next, a standard introducer that is 1 French size smaller than the guide is cut with 2 cm of sheath attached to the hub. The newly shortened sheath tip is then "flared" with a vessel dilator that is 1 French size larger than the sheath. This is accomplished by inserting the tapered end of the dilator retrograde into the sheath tip.

Insert a dilator into the shortened sheath and then thread the sheath on the indwelling wire through the dilator. Remove the dilator.

Finally, the flared end of the sheath stub is advanced over the cut end of the guide catheter with a firm friction fit. The hemostatic clamp is removed and the side port is attached to the manifold. The newly assembled system is carefully aspirated through the manifold to assure there is no air trapped within it.[32]

***Guides for unusually wide ascending aorta:** In extremely enlarged aortas due to long-standing aortic insufficiency or hypertension, the usual guides do not fit the large size of the aorta to cannulate the ostium. If the guide has a Judkins shape, the primary curve is lengthened to 7, 8, or 9 cm. For the Amplatz catheter, it is like the AL-5 or AL-6. However, the radius of the curvature is increased so the tip remains lower. For the guide with the Voda curve, the distal tip is lengthened to fit the extra-wide aortic sinus.[33]

TECHNIQUE

Shaping the guide: Stainless steel wires (0.035") are mounted into the desired shapes and kept in sterile condition. 6F Multipurpose guides are mounted on the preformed wires and heated using an industrial warm air blower. Then the guides are immersed in cold saline and the wire removed.[33]

REFERENCES

1. Tenaglia A, Tcheng J, Phillips III HR. Coronary angioplasty: Femoral approach. In: Stack R, Roubin G, O'Neill W, eds. *Interventional Cardiovascular Medicine, Principles and Practice*, 2nd edn. Churchill Livingstone, 2002: 477–89.
2. Judkins M, Judkins E. The Judkins techniques of coronary arteriography. In: King III SB, Douglas JS, eds. *Coronary Arteriography and Angioplasty.* McGraw-Hill, 1985: 182–238.
3. Deligonul U, Roth R, Flynn MS. Arterial and venous access. In: Kern M, ed. *The Cardiac Catheterization Handbook*, 3rd edn. Mosby, 1999: 51–122.
4. Pepine C, Lambert CR, Hill JA. Coronary angiography. In: Pepine C, ed. Diagnostic and Therapeutic Cardiac Catheterization, 3rd edition. Williams and Wilkins, 1998.
5. Voda J. Long tip catheter: Successful and safe for left coronary angioplasty. *Cathet Cardiovasc Diagn* 1992; **27**: 234–242.
6. Douglas J. *Cardiac Catheterization and Interventional Cardiology Review Course.* American College of Cardiology, 1999.
7. Hill JA, Lambert CR, Vlietstra RE *et al*. Review of techniques. In: Pepine CJ, ed. *Diagnostic and Therapeutic Cardiac Catheterization.* Williams and Wilkins, 1998.
8. Sweeney J, Schatz R. The Palmaz-Schatz stent. In: Stack R, Roubin G, O'Neill W, eds. *Interventional Cardiovascular Medicine, Principles and Practice*, 2nd edn. Churchill Livingstone, 2002: 793–808.
9. Ellis S. Elective coronary angioplasty. In: Topol E, ed. *Textbook of Interventional Cardiology.* WB Saunders, 1999.
10. King SB, Douglas JS. *Atlas of Heart Diseases: Interventional Cardiology.* Mosby, 1997.
11. Ghazzal Z. Balloon angioplasty. In: *Cardiac Catheterization and Interventional Cardiology Self-Assessment Program.* American College of Cardiology, 1999.
12. Deligonul U, Kern M, Roth R. Angiographic data. In: Kern M, ed. *The Cardiac Catheterization Handbook*, 3rd edn. Mosby, 199: 278–390.

13. Myler RK, Boucher RA, Cumberland DC, Stertzer SH. Guiding catheter selection for RCA angioplasty. *Cathet Cardiovasc Diagn* 1990; **19**: 58–67.

14. King SB. Approaches to specific sites. In: King SB, Douglas JS, eds. *Atlas of Heart Diseases: Interventional Cardiology.* Mosby, 1997: 10-1–10-17.

15. Abhaichand RK, Lefevre T, Louvard D *et al.* Amplatzing a 6 Fr JR guiding catheter for increased success in complex RCA anatomy. *Cathet Cardiovasc Interv* 2001; **53**: 405–9.

16. Hart WL, Berman EJ, LaCom RJ. Hazard of retrograde aortography in dissecting aortic aneurysm. *Circulation* 1963; **27**: 1140–2.

17. Israel DH, Sharma SK, Ambrose JA *et al.* Cardiac catheterization and selective coronary angiography in ascending aortic aneurysm or dissection. *Cathet Cardiovasc Diagn* 1994; **32**: 232–7.

18. Tenaglia A, Tcheng JE, Phillips HR. Coronary angioplasty: Femoral approach. In: Roubin GS, O'Neill WW, Stack RS *et al.*, eds. *Interventional Cardiovascular Medicine, Principles and Practice.* Churchill Livingstone, 1994: 447.

19. Topaz O, DiSciascio G, Goudreau E *et al.* Coronary angioplasty of anomalous coronary arteries: Notes on technical aspects. *Cathet Cardiovasc Diagn* 1990; **21**: 106–11.

20. Cheitlin MD, DeCastro CM, McAllister HA. Sudden death as a complication of anomalous left coronary origin from the anterior sinus of Valsalva: A not-so-minor congenital anomaly. *Circulation* 1974; **50**: 780–787.

21. DiSciascio G, Lewis SA, Cowley MJ. Coronary angioplasty of multiple vessels in corrected transposition with situs inversus. *Am Heart J* 1988; **115**: 892–4.

22. Yeoh JK, Ling LH, Maurice C. PTCA of anomalous RCA arising from the ascending thoracic aorta. *Cathet Cardiovasc Diagn* 1994; **32**: 254–6.

23. Chen HL, Lo PH, Wu CJ *et al.* Coronary angioplasty of a single coronary artery with an anomalous origin in the ascending aorta. *J Invasive Cardiol* 1997; **9**: 188–191.

24. Cohen M, Tolleson T, Peter R *et al.* Successful PCI with stent implantation of anomalous RCA arising from left sinus of Valsalva: A report of 2 cases. *Cathet Cardiovasc Interv* 2002; **55**: 105–8.

25. Kimbiris D, Lo E, Iskandrian A. Percutaneous transluminal coronary angioplasty of anomalous LCX artery. *Cathet Cardiovasc Diagn* 1987; **13**: 407–10.

26. Yip H, Chen M, Wu C *et al.* Primary angioplasty in acute inferior myocardial infarction with anomalous-origin RCA as infarct-related arteries: Focus on anatomic and clinical features, outcomes, selection of guiding catheters and management. *J Invasive Cardiol* 2001; **13**: 290–7.

27. Lawson MA, Dailey SM, Soto B. Selective injection of a left coronary artery arising anomalously from the posterior aortic sinus. *Cathet Cardiovasc Diagn* 1993; **30**: 300–302.

28. Fajadet J, Hayerizadeh B, Ali H *et al*. Transradial approach for interventional procedures. In: Fajadet J, ed. *Syllabus for EuroPCR*, 2001: 11–28.

29. Bartorelli A, Lavarra F, Trabattoni D *et al*. Successful stent delivery with deep seating of 6F guiding catheters in difficult coronary anatomy. *Cathet Cardiovasc Interv* 1999; **48**: 279–84.

30. Newton CM, Lewis SA, Vetrovec GW. Technique for guiding catheter exchange during coronary angioplasty while maintaining guide wire access across a coronary stenosis. *Cathet Cardiovasc Diagn* 1988; **15**: 173.

31. Azrin MA, Fram DB, Hirst JA. Maintenance of coronary wire position during guide catheter exchange. *Cathet Cardiovasc Diagn* 1996; **37**: 453–4.

32. Stratienko AA, Ginsberg R, Schatz RA *et al*. Technique of shortening angioplasty guide catheter length when therapeutic catheter fails to reach target stenosis. *Cathet Cardiovasc Diagn* 1993; **30**: 331–3.

33. Abhyankar AD. Modified catheter shapes for engaging left coronary ostium in unusually wide ascending aorta. *Cathet Cardiovasc Diagn* 1996; **39**: 327.

Chapter 5
Wires

Thach Nguyen, Lihua Shang

Basic designs and maneuvers
Advancing a wire
    **Direction and movement of wire when trying to enter the LAD
    *Better torque control
    *Wire prolapsing
    BEST METHOD: Increase the chance of entering the LCX
    **Directing the tip of the wire with a transport catheter
    **Avoiding the unwanted lumen by deflection with a previously unsuccessful wire
    ***Deflecting the tip of a wire by a distal inflated balloon
    **Advancing a wire through a severely angulated segment by pulling it back
    **Soft wire or stiffer wire
    **Directing the wire when navigating the LAD
    **Crossing a stent
    **Prevention of dissection by a wire
    **Measure the length of a lesion with a wire
    **Confirmation of the intraluminal position
Wiring in chronic total occlusion
    **Failure to cross a lesion
    **Bending the wire to increase device trackability
    **To advance a device with the "buddy wire" technique
    ***Double wire to position ostial stent
    ***Withdrawal of an uncoiling ribbon of a wire
    ***Entangled wires with the IVUS catheter
    ***Avoiding entangled IVUS catheter and wire
The techniques of exchanging catheters
    ***Advancement of an over-the-wire balloon catheter over a regular length wire
    ***Exchanging the balloon catheter over a regular-length wire without sacrificing the wire position

*Basic; **Advanced; ***Rare, exotic, or investigational.

From: Nguyen T, Hu D, Saito S, Grines C, Palacios I (eds), *Practical Handbook of Advanced Interventional Cardiology*, 2nd edn. © 2003 Futura, an imprint of Blackwell Publishing.

BASIC DESIGNS AND MANEUVERS

A wire consists of two main components: (1) a central shaft of stainless steel or Nitinol, and (2) a distal flexible tip shaped as a spring coil made with platinum or tungsten. Wires with a Nitinol core are kink-resistant while those with stainless steel are more susceptible to kinking. The usual wire is the flexible tip 0.014" diameter lightweight wire, while the larger size wires (0.16–0.18") or the much stiffer 0.014" wire (e.g. Ironman, ACS, Temecula CA or Platinum-Plus, Boston Scientific, Quincy MA) are used to straighten tortuous coronary segments and to provide more support for device tracking and when the support offered by 6F guide needs bolstering. In general, the flexible wires are less steerable and the stiffer wire offers more torque control.[1] However, since the wires are stiff, they can straighten the curved segment, change the vessel shape and cause wrinkles or pseudolesions. Removing the stiff part of the wire while leaving the radiopaque flexible end across the pseudolesions, exchanging for a more flexible wire or pulling the wire completely out, would abolish these pseudolesions. Other disadvantages of stiff wire include difficulty of tracking stents because of the wire bias inducing coronary spasm, even obstruction of flow induced by vessel kinking, and wire buckling due to sharp transitions. Sometimes, stiff wires can act as a "cheese cutter" when the wire is so straight and stiff that it cuts through the curve of a vessel. In these situations, the wire should be exchanged and use of atherectomy devices avoided because of excessive wire bias.

A wire is advanced gently and should pass smoothly through the stenosis. Withdrawal and reorientation of the wire is required when buckling occurs. It should not be forcefully jammed, because it can disrupt the plaque, cause thrombus formation and ultimately acute occlusion. Repeated rotation of 180° in clockwise and counterclockwise directions also seems to aid wire advancement and reduces subselection of unwanted small branches.[1] Never rotate the wires 360°. This may result in entanglement with a second wire or tip fracture if it is caught in a small branch. In any case, the tip of the wire has to be placed as distally as possible, so the stiff part of the wire is across the lesion where the stent or other interventional devices are to be tracked.

When side branch selection is desired, it is important to make the radius of the curve on the tip of the wire match the diameter of the main vessel proximal to the origin of that branch. A double bend can be useful if there are two different angulated segments to cross.[1]

Wiring the LAD: The LAD typically has little tortuosity; therefore, the wire transition point between the flexible tip and the more rigid body is usually not a major problem.

Wiring the LCX: For LCX interventions, the wire needs to pass the LM, turn into the LCX, then move forward to cross the lesion. Sometimes it requires a broad curve to successfully enter the LCX and a shorter curve to cross the lesion. Wires with gradual transition from the body to the spring tip are preferred to avoid continuous prolapsing into the LAD.[1]

Wiring the RCA: When the origin of the RCA is relatively normal, a conventional soft wire with good steerability to avoid side branches is usually chosen first. When the RCA arises anteriorly, the wire sometimes may be required as an aid to guide engagement. In this situation, wires with improved tip transition are selected to avoid prolapsing at the point of transition and disengagement of the guide.[1]

ADVANCING A WIRE

TECHNICAL TIPS

**Direction and movement of wire when trying to enter the LAD: Usually in the RAO cranial position, when the wire is being manipulated to enter the LAD, if the wire is pointing too much downward or upward, most likely it enters the LCX (in the AP view, the LCX points downward, however, in the cranial angulation, the LCX is lifted upward). If the wire swings widely, then it may enter the ramus intermedius which buckles with contraction of the LV like the diagonals.[1]

If there is too much difficulty entering the LAD by the RAO view, then the wire should enter the LAD by the LAO caudal view (spider view) and, once it is in far enough, the angle is changed to the RAO cranial view so the wire can be moved to the mid- and then tip of the LAD.

*Better torque control: When a wire is harder to manipulate after it has passed through too many curves, advancement of a balloon catheter near the wire tip will improve wire support, torque control, and steerability. Other options include use of stiffer wire or hydrophilic wires, which are very sleek and kink-resistant. However, since they are so smooth, the operator has little tactile feedback, and they can easily go subintimally or cause distal perforation if inadvertently advanced into a small and short branch. These small wire perforations will not seal themselves when glycoprotein 2b3a inhibitors are on board. When manipulating a hydrophylic wire, always watch the distal tip, to avoid inadvertent migration and perforation.

*Wire prolapsing: When navigating a curve in order to enter an artery (e.g. from the LM into the LCX), a floppy wire may keep prolapsing into an unintended artery (e.g. LAD). The cause is the abrupt transition between the short tip and the main shaft. The way to resolve this is to change to a wire with a gradually tapered core so that, as the tip is deeply advanced, it stabilizes the wire and the stiffer shaft can negotiate the angle better, without prolapsing into an unintended area (or LAD).[1]

BEST METHOD

Increase the chance of entering the LCX: When navigating the LM in order to enter a sharp bifurcation of the LCX, there are two best maneuvers manipulating a wire into the LCX.

1. **First maneuver:** Torque the guide clockwise so its tip will point toward the LCX ostium, especially if the LM is short.
2. **Second maneuver:** Park the flexible tip of the wire around the bend with the LCX, then ask the patient to take a deep breath that elongates the heart and straightens the angle between the LM and LCX. In this window of opportunity, advance the wire further into the LCX.
3. **Third maneuver:** If these two above maneuvers are unsuccessful, then remove the wire. Shape the tip to conform with the entry angle of the LM and LCX.
4. **Change one device:** If all of the above fail to advance the wire, then the wire needs to be changed for a better wire with smoother transition between the soft tip and the stiff shaft.
5. **One more device needed:** If the artery is calcified and the angle is rigid, then park the wire around the bend of the LM-LCX angle. Advance a balloon very slowly around the bend. Once the balloon is curved around the bend, advance the wire gently.

**Directing the tip of the wire with a transport catheter: Sometimes, it is difficult to curve a wire into a branch of a large artery because of the short stem of the branch, so a transport catheter may help to stabilize the wire at the stump. In a case report by Violaris *et al.*, a patient presented with complete occlusion of the proximal LCX 5 months after the first angioplasty. At the second intervention, despite persistent manipulation, the 0.014" wire kept buckling under pressure and prolapsing into the LAD. A small transport catheter was inserted through the wire into the proximal LCX. The new catheter prevented buckling of the wire and helped the wire cross the tight lesion.[2]

**Avoiding the unwanted lumen by deflection with a previously unsuccesful wire: Sometimes, a wire keeps persistently entering an unwanted branch or area. Keep the wire stuck in that location and insert a new wire. This new

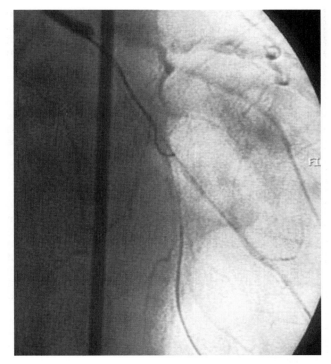

Figure 5-1: The old wire is stuck in the unwanted lumen and the new wire is deflected to the new channel and enters it successfully.

wire will be better at seeking another channel and avoiding the unwanted area, thus entering the desired lumen (Figure 5-1).

***Deflecting the tip of a wire by a distal inflated balloon:** Sometimes, it is difficult to curve a wire into a side branch with extreme angle takeoff. In a case report by Gershony *et al.*, a 74-year-old patient with unstable angina underwent a coronary angiogram, which showed severe ostial lesion of an obtuse marginal (OM). This OM originated from the LCX at an extreme angle. Multiple attempts to wire the OM were unsuccessful because of repeated prolapse of the wire in the main LCX. A perfusion catheter was then advanced to the distal LCX and inflated with its proximal end right beyond the ostium of the diseased OM. A new wire was inserted and successfully entered the ostium of the OM, steering it towards the opening of the side branch with extreme angle takeoff. In this case, the inflated perfusion balloon prevented the continuing prolapse of the wire and deflected the tip to the desired retrograde direction.[3]

Advancing a wire through a severely angulated segment by pulling it back: In rare instances, a wire has to enter a very severely angulated segment. The tip of the wire should be curved to form a large diameter curve. Once the tip enters the branch, the wire is withdrawn to prolapse the tip into the intended branch. Then rotate the wire towards the main lumen, clockwise if the tip was pointing towards the left and counterclockwise if the tip was pointing towards the right. If there is enough stiff segment inside the side branch (not just the soft tip), then the wire will advance further, without prolapsing back (Figure 5-2).

**Soft wire or stiffer wire: If a wire to enter a very short and small stump, a soft wire fails to anchor the wire. However, a stiffer wire will stay put inside the stump and an over-the-wire balloon can be advanced near the tip and locked in the stump to support the advance of the wire and serve as a channel so wires can be exchanged or advanced (Figure 5-3).

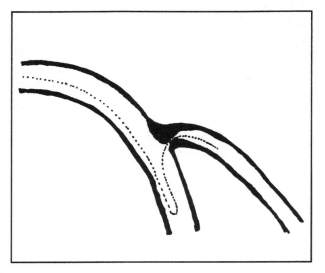

Figure 5-2: Pulling the wire to advance it. A wire is inserted and manipulated to enter an angulated tortuous branch. In order to advance the tip further, the technique is to pull the wire back to prolapse the tip deeper into the branch. (Adapted from Angelini P. Chapter 3: The Procedure. In: Angelini P, ed. *Balloon Catheter Coronary Angioplasty.* Futura Publishing Co, 1987.)

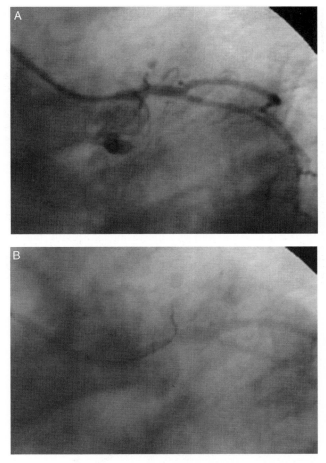

Figure 5-3 A,B: (A) The LAD is only a tiny stump in the upper part of the LM in this LAO caudal view. (B) A soft wire was able to enter the stump. However, its tip was so soft that it could not hold still and be tracked by a balloon. *(Continued)*

**Directing the wire when navigating the LAD: In case of navigating the LAD, at first at the LAO caudal view, the wire should point to right of the patient. The left is toward the diagonal. Once inside the proximal segment, the better view is the LAO cranial view. Here the wire should move downward. Any straying to the left will point to the diagonal and to the right will point to the septals (Figure 5-4 A–C).

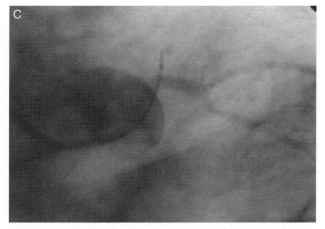

Figure 5-3 C: A stiff wire was able to enter the stump, held on and had an over-the-wire balloon tracked to the tip. The over-the-wire balloon became a channel for exchanging wire and provided a strong platform so the wire could cross this chronic total occlusion (Figure 5-4 A–C).

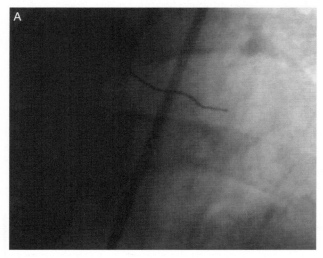

Figure 5-4 A: In the AP cranial view, the wire pointed too much to the left, so it entered the diagonal instead the LAD. It should point more downward and to the right of the patient. *(Continued)*

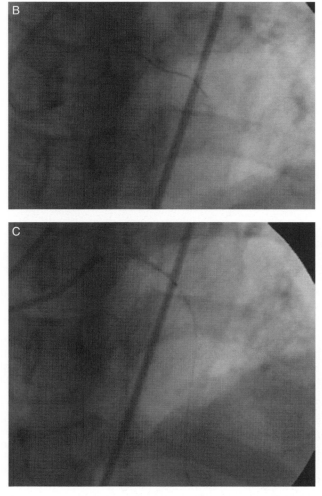

Figure 5-4 B,C: (B) In the LAO cranial view, the tip was re-shaped to point more downward. (C) The wire successfully entered the LAD.

**Crossing a stent: If a stent needs to be recrossed, the tip of the wire should be curved well into a wide J and the whole wire can be advanced while being rotated. This maneuver will help to avoid the inadvertent migration of the tip of the catheter under a strut, changing the direction of the whole wire to outside the stent. If there is subtle resistance, wire exit through or behind the struts is suspected. If the stented area has sudden acute thrombosis, and a curved tip fails

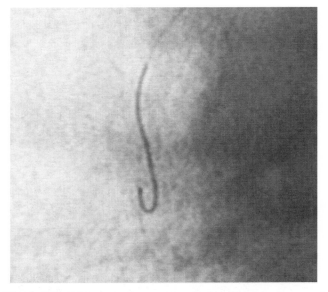

Figure 5-5: When crossing a stent, the tip of the wire is curved so there is no migration through the side struts.

to cross the stent, then an intermediate wire with a mildly bent tip can be manipulated to cross the stent (Figure 5-5). Try to have the pictures of the segments in two orthogonal views so the wire can be advanced inside the lumen as well as possible.

**Prevention of dissection by a wire: A wire should be advanced smoothly without any resistance and tip buckling. Otherwise, it can go through soft plaque, under the intima, and cause dissection. In case of a perfusion balloon, a wire can exit through a proximal side hole. When the perfusion catheter is readvanced, with the sharp metallic wire entangled on its side, the balloon can break the plaque and dissect the artery. Therefore it is important to advance the wire while the perfusion balloon remains inflated and to watch its course under fluoroscopy.[4]

**Measure the length of a lesion with a wire: It is not easy to guess accurately the length of a lesion if some segments are foreshortened because of tortuosity. When a vessel bends in more than one plane, no single angiographic view can overcome multiple foreshortening. Most radiolucent wires have a 20 to 30 mm radiopaque distal end. Position

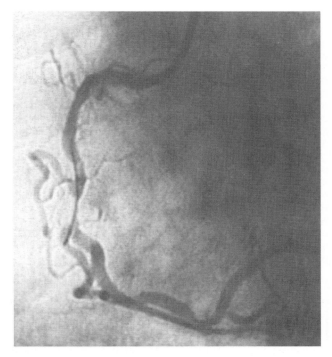

Figure 5-6: Measuring the length of a lesion with a wire. Usually the opaque tip of the wire measures 30 mm. In a tortuous lesion, the tip of the wire can give an estimated length of the lesion better than the angiogram.

this radiopaque segment across the lesion so the length of the lesion can be estimated. Another way is to measure the lesion length with a balloon that has markers at its two ends (Figure 5-6).[5]

**Confirmation of the intraluminal position: After crossing a total occlusion, a wire is advanced distally. Balloon dilation can cause perforation if the wire is inadvertently positioned outside the true lumen. To avoid this complication, it is wise to perform an injection through the guide to see if the contrast tracks along the wire. Then advance an over-the-wire balloon catheter or a transport catheter distally to perform a distal dye injection to confirm the intraluminal position of the wire prior to any dilation. Full-strength contrast enables less volume to be injected, thus reducing the risk and the extent of dissection, if it happens.

WIRING IN CHRONIC TOTAL OCCLUSION

Wire selection is based on a detailed angiographic assessment: the presence of tapering versus abrupt occlusion; the length of the occlusion; the presence of recanalized channel versus bridging collaterals; the size, location, and condition of the distal vessel. In case of recent occlusion (1–2 months), it can be crossed with a 0.014" high-torque floppy (or comparable) wire which can be stiffened by advancing a balloon near the tip. If the duration of the occlusion is longer than 3 months, then the choice of the wire is determined by the angiographic features of the lesion. Tapered occlusions are approached with a 0.014" soft high-torque floppy wire. However, in some cases, a stiff 0.010" standard wire is needed. In cases of an occlusion that does not taper, soft wire is usually ineffective. Then, with firm and steady pressure a hydrophilic-coated wire may slowly "glide" through. Also in these non-tapered old occlusions, a Magnum wire (Schneider, Switzerland) can be used to cross the chronic total occlusion. It requires very firm push and excellent guide backup support.[6]

TROUBLE-SHOOTING TIPS

**Failure to cross a lesion: When a wire does not seem to be able to cross a lesion, the most appropriate step is to check the wire position in a second orthogonal view. Maybe the tip of the wire is in a side branch or has migrated outside the true lumen. Once the wire is sure to be inside the true lumen, other strategies include changing to a stiffer wire, smaller wire or a hydrophilic wire, or passing a balloon to near the tip to increase support to the wire.

**Bending the wire to increase device trackability: When any interventional device (stent or balloon, etc.) needs to be advanced through many angulated segments, bending the wire in strategic locations facilitates the forward movement of the device. This helps relieve the tendency of the wire to hug the outer curve of the vessel (wire bias). This will also decrease the tendency of the device to be forced against the outer wall of the vessel, where resistance to its passage is increased.[7]

**To advance a device with the "buddy wire" technique: When it is difficult to advance a device over a wire, changing to a stiffer wire or advancing a second wire along the first one may help to advance the device.

***Double wire to position ostial stent: Difficulty in positioning the guide during stenting of an ostial RCA lesion is sometimes made easier by use of a second steerable wire placed in the aorta just above the coronary sinus or in an

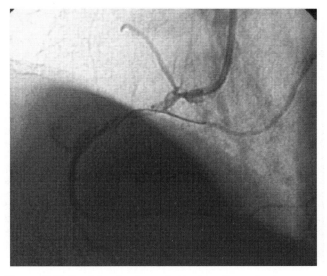

Figure 5-7: Double wire for ostial lesion. One wire is seen at the distal RCA. One wire is seen in the anomalous LCX originated from the proximal RCA.

anomalous LCX (Figure 5-7). This second wire stabilizes the guide outside the coronary artery and also defines the junction of the coronary artery and aorta, an important landmark for stent placement. The position of this landmark is frequently difficult to identify with certainty (see Figure 3-10).

***Withdrawal of an uncoiling ribbon of a wire:** After excessive manipulation of a wire (more than 180° turns), its distal segment can become uncoiled. This is detected as the distal tip shows a radiolucent segment. Instead of pulling the wire in an effort to remove it out of the coronary system, the best technique involves proper seating of the guide, then advancing an over-the-wire balloon or a transport catheter over the whole wire including the uncoiled segment, if it tracks easily. After the radiolucent segment is advanced over by the balloon or a transport catheter, the whole system, guide, catheter, and wire, is removed as a unit.[8] If the balloon catheter does not track easily over the floppy tip, it may dissect the artery. In this case, it may be better to simply pull the wire and all the devices as a unit.

***Entangled wires with the IVUS catheter:** In complex PCI with advanced physiologic or imaging studies by pressure flow wire (PW) and IVUS, there is a possibility of entanglement of wires. In a caseload of 704 patients who had

IVUS, 0.5% had entanglement with angioplasty wire while it happened in 13% with the PW (Radi Medical System, Upsala, Sweden). Besides some minor difficulties in advancement of either wire, the problem began to unravel when the IVUS catheter was withdrawn. Under fluoroscopy, the IVUS catheter was seen entangled with the PW, stuck on the PW, or found retrieving on the PW. So after multiple unsuccessful attempts to pull the IVUS catheter, all wires and guides were removed as a unit. Once outside, direct inspection showed: (1) unraveling coils in the distal segment of the PW, (2) the IVUS catheter was stuck into an acute bend of the PW, or (3) a kinked PW stuck to the distal tip of the IVUS catheter and looped around it.[9] The predisposing factor for these entanglements is most likely the short monorail segment of the IVUS catheter. In order to avoid entanglement of the wires, it is wise to ensure that the short monorail segment of the IVUS seats near the stiff segment of the PW or angioplasty wire. If entanglement is noticed, attempt to advance the PW or the PTCA wire farther in order to separate its kinked part from the corresponding tip of the IVUS catheter. Another option is to slide the IVUS catheter distally over the kinked wire. However, overmanipulation may be hazardous and predispose to generate loops and further kinking of the PW. Removal of the complete system as a single unit may be a last resort and a pragmatic option.[9]

***Avoiding entangled IVUS catheter and wire:** When the proximal segment to be crossed is too tortuous and calcified, the advancement of the IVUS catheter is less than smooth. If too much force is inadvertently applied to advance the IVUS catheter, displacement of the catheter away from the wire could be induced and the wire could be kinked.[10] If the problem is not recognized early, advancing a kinked wire can cause perforation or dissection. Because the IVUS catheter slides on a short monorail distal segment, torquing movement is not transmitted well to the tip. This hampers its capacity to negotiate distal tortuous segments or cross tight curves, lesions or acute angles.

THE TECHNIQUES OF EXCHANGING CATHETERS

***Advancement of an over-the-wire balloon catheter over a regular length wire:** A regular-length angioplasty wire is inserted and manipulated to cross the lesion. Be sure that the wire tip is positioned at the most distal segment of the artery. An over-the-wire balloon catheter is then advanced over the wire without manual control of the wire. This is performed with fluoroscopic guidance until the proximal end of the wire reappears through the wire port of the balloon catheter. During the passage of the balloon catheter, extreme care is taken to make the movement as smooth as possible with no tactile evidence of any hindrance. An absolute requirement is to refrain from any forceful forward motion of the balloon catheter over the wire, if any resistance is felt. This precaution would limit any forward migration of the wire. Any resistance or evidence of ventricular ectopy should prompt immediate reassessment of the wire, balloon catheter, and guide positions under fluoroscopy. There was no reported damage to the coronary artery due to inadvertent advancement of the wire. With forward motion of the balloon catheter, increased tension in the wire can back out the guide, so the tip of the guide needs to be watched.[11]

This technique is cost-effective as only one wire is used, saving the cost of an extension. It is also advantageous when the proximal end of the wire is damaged and therefore cannot be extended, or if the wire is not constructed to be extended, or there is no extension wire available.

***Exchanging the balloon over a regular-length wire without sacrificing the wire position: There are many ways to exchange over-the-wire balloons without sacrificing the wire position across the lesion (Table 5-1).

TECHNIQUE

Exchanging over a regular length wire: The over-the-wire balloon is pulled back over the wire until the stiff end of this wire remains just within the hub of the balloon catheter. The stiff end of a second wire is then introduced into the catheter hub in end-to-end apposition to the first wire inside the catheter. This introduction can be facilitated by the use of a 20-gauge IV cannula with the tip placed inside the hub. The balloon catheter is then gradually pulled back over this combination while maintaining a forward push on the second wire. Be sure that this wire is compatible with the lumen size of the balloon catheter.[14]

Table 5-1
Exchanging balloon catheter over a regular-length wire

---

1. Cutting the balloon catheter to be removed whenever it arrives at the end of the wire (2 cuts required)[12]
2. Injecting contrast agent through the central lumen during withdrawal of catheter[13]
3. Using extension device
4. Using the back end of a regular wire[14]

REFERENCES

1. King SB, Warren RJ. Equipment selection and techniques of balloon angioplasty. In: King SB, Douglas JS, eds. *Atlas of Heart Diseases: Interventional Cardiology.* Mosby, 1997: 3.1–3.15.

2. Violaris AG, Tsikaderis D. Tracker tricks: Applications of a novel infusion catheter in coronary intervention. *Cathet Cardiovasc Diagn* 1993; **28**: 250–1.

3. Gershony G, Hussain H, Rowan W. Coronary angioplasty of branch vessels associated with an extreme angle take-off. *Cathet Cardiovasc Diagn* 1995; **36**: 356–9.

4. Werns S, Bates E. Coronary artery dissection caused by exit of the wire through the distal perfusion sidehole of an auto-perfusion angioplasty balloon catheter. *Cathet Cardiovasc Diagn* 1994; **33**: 32–5.

5. Dixon SR, Ormiston JA, Webster MW. Long lesion length assessment. *Cathet Cardiovasc Diagn* 1998; **45**: 299–300.

6. Douglas JS. Percutaneous interventional approaches to specific coronary lesions. In: King SB, Douglas JS, eds. *Atlas of Heart Diseases: Interventional Cardiology.* Mosby, 1997.

7. Feldman T. Bent stents: A crooked stick to walk a crooked mile. *Cathet Cardiovasc Diagn* 1999; **44**: 345.

8. Iyer SS, Roubin GS. Nonsurgical management of retained intracoronary products following coronary interventions. In: Roubin GS, Califf RM, O'Neill WW, Phillips HR, Stack RS, eds. *Interventional Cardiovascular Medicine: Principles and Practice.* Churchill Livingstone, 1994.

9. Alfonso F, Flores A, Escanend J *et al.* Pressure wire kinking, entanglement, and entrapment during IVUS ultrasound studies: A potential dangerous complication. *Cathet Cardiovasc Interv* 2000; **50**: 221–5.

10. Alfonso F, Goncalves M, Goicolea *et al.* Feasibilies of IVUS studies: Predictors of imaging success before PCI. *Clinical Cardiol* 1997; **20**: 1010–16.

11. Ahmad T, Webb JG, Carere RG *et al.* Guide wire extension may not be essential to pass an over-the-wire balloon catheter. *Cathet Cardiovasc Diagn* 1995; **36**: 59–60.

12. Meier B. Chronic total occlusion. In: Topol EJ, ed. *Textbook of Interventional Cardiology.* WB Saunders, 1990: 300–326.

13. Hoorntjie JCA. How to change an over-the-wire PTCA balloon over a normal short guide. *Cathet Cardiovasc Diagn* 1989; **18**: 284.

14. Agarwal R, Shah D, Matthew KS. New technique of exchanging an over-the-wire balloon dilation catheter. *Cathet Cardiovasc Diagn* 1995; **36**: 350–1.

Chapter 6
Balloon Angioplasty

Thach Nguyen, Nguyen Ngoc Quang, Huan Quang Do, Meilin Liu, Rijie Li

Design and maneuvers
    **Length of the balloon
    **Compliant balloons
    **Non-compliant balloons
    **Where the markers should be
    **Positioning a balloon when the blood flow is cut off by an undeployed balloon
    **Advancement of balloon
    **Speed of inflation pressure
    **Checking the appropriate size of the balloon or stent
    **Looking for collaterals
    **Exchanging a balloon catheter over a regular-length wire
    **Balloon angioplasty of large vessels
Trouble-shooting tips
    *How to cross a lesion
    **Failure to cross a lesion
BEST METHOD: Advancing a balloon across a tight lesion
BEST METHOD: When a balloon fails to dilate a lesion
    ***Force-focused angioplasty
    **Manipulating the cutting balloon
    ***Extraction of stent by cutting balloon
    **Failure to deflate the balloon
    ***Impending rupture due to material fatigue
    **Entrapment of deflated balloon during withdrawal
    ***Using a commercial snare to remove a balloon
    ***Management of repeated rupture
    ***Damage control for balloon rupture
Conclusion

---

*Basic; **Advanced; ***Rare, exotic, or investigational.

From: Nguyen T, Hu D, Saito S, Grines C, Palacios I (eds), *Practical Handbook of Advanced Interventional Cardiology*, 2nd edn. © 2003 Futura, an imprint of Blackwell Publishing.

DESIGNS AND MANEUVERS

Angioplasty balloons come in different diameters and are made from diverse materials [polyethylene (PE), polyethylene terephthalate (PET), etc.] to give an exact or oversized diameter with various inflation pressures and a degree of balloon hardness dependent on material characteristics (compliant or non-compliant). The catheter can be advanced over a wire that passes through the lumen inside the whole length of the shaft (over-the-wire system) or only inside the distal segment (monorail system) or without an indwelling wire at all (fixed wire). A perfusion balloon has extra lumen with antegrade flow while the balloon is in inflation. A cutting balloon has micro-blades arranged lengthwise along the sides of the balloon. Once inflated, the mechanism of acute lumen gain after PTCA in calcified lesions is dissection while it is plaque compression and vessel expansion in fibrotic lesions.

Ideally, a balloon has a very low profile in its undeployed state. However, low profile is less important for most lesions than trackability and pushability. Trackability is the ease of advancing a balloon over a wire through an angulated coronary artery segment. Pushability is defined as the ability to push a balloon through tortuous segments or across a lesion. In the monorail system, smaller guides can be used with better opacification and reduced fluoroscopy time. However, the wire is unable to be exchanged or reshaped without being removed, giving up position or use of a transport catheter. The over-the-wire balloon may be more trackable and the fixed-wire balloon has a much lower profile and can be useful in tortuous arteries and extremely tight lesions. Because of the excellent result of stents in sealing off dissections, the use of perfusion balloon catheters has disappeared, except in the case of perforation, which requires prolonged inflation or in the case of poor results of initial balloon but inability to stent.

The choice of the exact balloon and wire system is less important than the operator's overall approach to the technique of dilation, the familiarity with the system chosen, the balloon size, and the capacity to treat possible complications.[1]

Size of balloon: The ratio of balloon to artery size should be approximately 1:1. A higher balloon:artery ratio has been shown to be associated with dissection and acute closure.

TECHNICAL TIPS

**Length of the balloon: In a long lesion with diffuse disease, long balloons can distribute inflation pressure more evenly across the diseased segment, without the inconvenience of multiple short and overlapped inflations, or the danger of untreated plaques protruding into the lumen. The probability of dissection with a long balloon is thought by some operators to be lower because a short balloon can partially disrupt an atherosclerotic plaque and allow the blood to enter the channel created behind the broken plaque. The longer balloon also exerts less straightening force on the vessel, tending to maintain the curved configuration during balloon inflation.[2] When dilating a long lesion in an artery that tapers, the disadvantage of a long balloon is that it may underdilate the proximal segment and overdilate the distal segment.

**Compliant balloons: Compliant balloons are used routinely because of their low profile and good "re-wrapping" after deflation. They are also useful when vessel size is uncertain, such as an undersized vessel due to chronic low flow or total occlusion. Once the lesion is open and nitroglycerin is given, the vessel may show a larger lumen; then a second dilation at higher pressure further expands a compliant balloon. Similarly, when multiple lesions are targeted in different size vessels, use of a compliant balloon may be more cost-effective. At first, the balloon is to dilate a lesion in a small diameter vessel, then it is moved to a larger vessel where the balloon can be inflated with higher pressure in order to achieve a higher diameter. However, if a stent is hand-mounted on a compliant balloon, then because of unexpected calcification at the index lesion, the balloon needs to be inflated with higher pressure in order to fully dilate the stent, and the final diameter of the balloon could be higher than the reference diameter of the distal segment. There is then a potential risk of over-expansion causing dissection of the distal part of the lesion.[1]

**Non-compliant balloons: Non-compliant balloons are needed in different situations. When post-dilating a stent, a short non-compliant balloon may be needed to maximize the stent size without overstretching the vessel at the stent edges. In a long lesion, a non-compliant balloon will not overstretch the distal segment, which is frequently smaller than the proximal segment. In hard and calcified lesions, compliant balloons may preferentially overdilate the soft segments while being unable to break the plaque in the hard and calcified segment. The artery still looks bigger, thanks to the overstretched normal segment, which may recoil with time. In the same lesion, a non-compliant balloon would concentrate its dilating force more directly on the hard and calcified segment without stretching the adjacent normal segment. With high pressure, it would break the plaque and shift the atherosclerotic burden equally along the longitudinal axis, and reconstruct a bigger and more stable lumen.[1]

**Where the markers should be: A balloon with a marker in the middle should be chosen if the lesion is very tight.

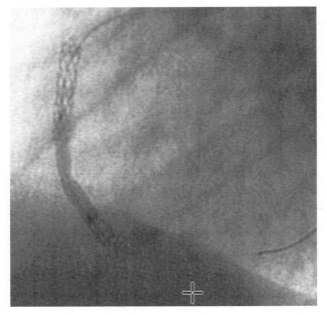

Figure 6-1: When the operator sees the marker at the middle of the lesion, he or she will know that the balloon is succeeding in crossing the lesion and inflation can be started. A balloon with markers at both ends will be needed to ensure that the lesion is covered in its whole length.

When the operator sees the marker at the middle of the lesion, then inflation can be started (Figure 6-1). When doing PCI for a long lesion, then a balloon with markers at two ends will be needed in order to be sure that the whole length of the lesion is covered.

**Positioning a balloon when the blood flow is cut off by an undeployed balloon: In many cases, just advancing across a severe lesion cuts off the coronary flow. Once the balloon is in place, there is no way to check the location of the balloon before inflation. Then select a balloon long enough to cover the lesion well. Inject the contrast agent while advancing the balloon. The balloon will trap the contrast that stops exactly at the critical point of the lesion. If the balloon totally covers the lesion, then it can be inflated (Figure 6-2).

**Advancement of balloon: The left hand of the operator may advance the balloon while the right hand or another operator keeps a gentle traction on the wire. The balloon

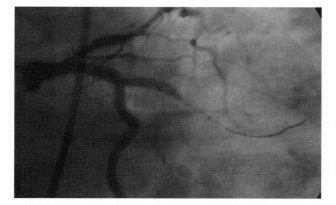

Figure 6-2: There was a tight lesion at the OM. When the balloon was across the lesion, it obstructed the flow so a coronary angiogram could not be done to check the exact location of the balloon. Injecting the contrast while advancing the balloon will trap the contrast exactly at the center of the lesion.

should be advanced by constant pressure rather than by jerky movements. While the balloon is advanced, carefully watch the tip of the guide. Too deep or aggressive intubation may cause proximal injury or dissection. As the balloon is being pushed harder, an unstable guide may back out and even become completely disengaged, forfeiting the wire position. If resistance is encountered at the lesion, gentle forward pressure on the balloon catheter, while pulling back on the wire and deeply but gently seating the guide, will often cause the balloon to cross.

**Speed of inflation pressure: Most operators inflate the balloon slowly until its waist disappears. This gradual inflation will slowly rearrange the atheromatous material within the plaque along the longitudinal and radial axis. In this way, the vessel is being stretched and deformed in a more predictable fashion than with sudden inflations that are more likely to cause extensive tearing (dissection) of the vessel wall. However, no studies have defined an optimal inflation strategy.

**Checking the appropriate size of the balloon or stent: After successful inflation of the balloon, 5 seconds before deflating it, a small injection of contrast agent will verify the correct fitting of the balloon with the proximal segment of the dilated lesion. The same maneuver after deploying a stent will verify the correct size of the stent with the proximal segment of the dilated area. If contrast agent is seen flowing around the proximal segment of the inflated stent-balloon complex, the balloon needs to be inflated at higher pressure in order to upsize the stent or larger size balloons should be used (Figure 6-3). This is only a rough assessment for the appropriate size of a balloon or stent, when IVUS is not available. It can check only whether the balloon is undersized and not if the balloon is oversized. If the balloon is inflated in a proximal segment without a side branch, there may not be enough flow to opacify the artery, so in this situation it is not possible to evaluate the balloon size with the above technique.

**Looking for collaterals: Collaterals seen during the diagnostic study or appearing with a contrast medium during balloon occlusion project a low-risk profile for the patient and reduce the stress for the operator. They can be looked for by injecting contrast medium while the balloon is about to be inflated. If the contrast medium caught in the distal vasculature the moment the balloon is fully inflated is washed out promptly, good collaterals are documented. If it

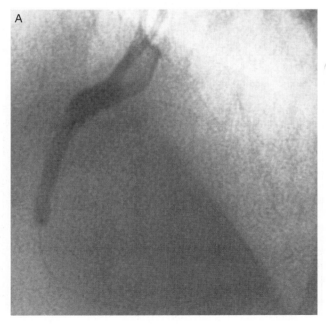

Figure 6-3: Assuring the adequate the size of the balloon and stent: (A) A balloon is inflated. Five seconds before deflation, inject contrast agent. Compare the size of the balloon and the proximal segment. In this case, the size of the balloon is clearly smaller than the proximal arterial segment. *(Continued)*

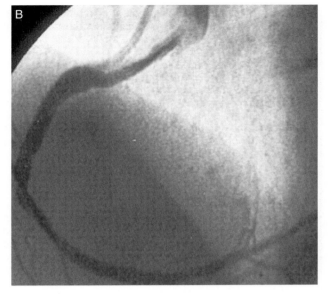

Figure 6-3: (B) A larger stent is selected and deployed. A post-stenting angiogram shows larger luminal diameter in the stented area, with a smooth transition from the non-stented proximal arterial segment to the stented segment.

stays put, the territory is devoid of collateral blood flow in the event of a later vessel occlusion.[3]

**Exchanging a balloon catheter over a regular-length wire: It is simple to exchange a balloon catheter over the monorail system, and fluoroscopic monitoring is not necessary. When exchanging a balloon on the over-the-wire system, the indwelling wire must be extended (docked) to a 300-cm wire, or a long exchange wire is needed. However, an over-the-wire balloon catheter can be exchanged without the need for a longer wire. With the indwelling wire held still, the balloon catheter is removed slowly until its proximal hub meets the proximal tip of the wire.

In another method, the wire is still across the lesion but its proximal segment is no longer extending out of the hub of the catheter. Attach a 5 cc syringe of contrast to the central lumen of the balloon catheter. Persistently inject the contrast while simultaneously withdrawing the balloon. This persistent injection will move the wire forward while the balloon is removed slowly. To successfully accomplish this exchange, there must be no friction at the Y-connector and no traction on the catheter. The wire should not be bent and the catheter should be well flushed before starting the procedure. The catheter should be positioned on a straight line, to minimize any friction with the wire.[4]

**Balloon angioplasty of large vessels: Current maximal balloon size is 4 mm in diameter, so when the coronary artery or the SVG is larger than 4 mm, the hugging balloon technique or use of a peripheral balloon is suggested. The two balloons are positioned side by side and inflated simultaneously. The combined diameter will be 70% of the sum of each balloon alone and the cross-section area will be oval rather than round.[5,6]

TROUBLE-SHOOTING TIPS

*How to cross a lesion: The standard maneuver is to advance a balloon with the left hand while pulling the wire taut with the right hand (or with the help of an assistant). This technique is to decrease the friction between the wire and the lumen of the balloon catheter. It also helps to keep the wire straight and taut so the balloon catheter can slide more easily on it.

**Failure to cross a lesion: The causes of failure to advance a balloon across a tortuous segment in order to reach a lesion are multiple. If the lesion is too severe, the balloon tip will not cross, and the guide will back out; then the guide should be held steady, engaged deeper or be replaced. If there is excessive tortuosity of the arterial segment proximal to the lesion, the solutions are (1) to secure a more stable position of the guide, or (2) to use a stiffer wire for the balloon to be tracked on, or (3) to straighten the artery by asking the patient to take a deep breath, or (4) using a "buddy wire", placed adjacent to the primary wire. A "wiggle" wire is useful at deflecting the tip of the balloon of plaques and stent struts, better allowing lesions to be crossed. A smaller balloon with a lower profile or length may also succeed in crossing a tight lesion. Once inflated, it creates a channel sufficient for the optimal size balloon to enter. The different methods for advancing a balloon across a tight lesion are listed below.

BEST METHOD

Advancing a balloon across a tight lesion:

1. **First maneuver:** Check the guide position, optimize coaxial alignment, deep-seat the guide if needed, so the guide can provide sufficient support for advancing the balloon.

2. **Second maneuver:** Ask patient to take a deep breath in order to elongate the heart and make the artery less tortuous. During this short window of opportunity, advance the balloon. This maneuver works best in the RCA.
3. **Add a second device:** If the balloon could not be advanced because of tortuous proximal segments and if the first two maneuvers fail to advance the balloon, then insert a second (moderately stiff) wire to straighten the proximal segment and most likely it will help to advance the balloon.
4. **Change one device:** Use a stiffer wire so the arterial segments are straightened and the balloon can be tracked on more easily. The disadvantage of this tactic compared to adding a second wire is the need to remove the first wire and exchange for a second wire. Tactic (3) above just involves inserting a new wire, so it is simpler and faster. However, if tactic (3) fails to advance the balloon, then the balloon may slide better on the second, stiffer wire.
5. **Change to an expensive device:** Use a lower profile balloon (monorail, compliant balloon material, center marker).

**Failure to dilate a lesion: A rigid lesion with heavy calcification may prevent the full expansion of a balloon. The first choice is high pressure inflations with a non-compliant balloon. It may be successful but it exposes the patient to the risk of dissection or balloon rupture. The second choice is to use a cutting balloon (CB). If the CB is not available then force-focused angioplasty with an extra wire besides the inflated balloon can be used. In lesions with heavy superficial calcium, the problem can be resolved with debulking by rotational atherectomy, followed by low-pressure angioplasty. The cutting balloon is the best option in PCI of the undilatable lesion, because the use of rotational atherectomy has become uncommon due to concerns over excessive debris embolization. The different options are listed below.

BEST METHOD

When a balloon fails to dilate a lesion:

1. **First maneuver:** High pressure inflation of non-compliant balloon. This balloon should be selected right from the start of the procedure. Now just inflate the balloon to its maximal pressure possible.
2. **Add one device – force-focused angioplasty:** Insert a second wire across the lesion and inflate the non-compliant balloon. The pressure will focus on the second wire and break the plaque. This tactic is better than

angioplasty with a cutting balloon because it is cheaper (one extra wire) and may be the only possible choice (it is difficult or impossible to advance a stiff cutting balloon across a tortuous segment).

3. **Change one device:** If the non-compliant balloon fails to dilate the lesion at high pressure then cutting balloon angioplasty is the next best choice if it can be advanced across the lesion.

4. **Add a new device – rotational atherectomy:** Although rotablation is excellent in shaving the superficial calcium from the plaque and making it susceptible to dilation by balloon angioplasty or stent, this technique is out of favor because of excessive debris embolization causing release of cardiac enzymes.

**Force-focused angioplasty: If the balloon fails to break a plaque, it is withdrawn into the guide. A second wire is advanced beyond the lesion. The balloon is readvanced, positioned across the lesion, and inflated as usual. With the wire across the lesion, the pressure is then focused on the wire, which then acts as a cutting wire to selectively put pressure and crack the plaque. Complications include dissection, which can be treated by stenting.[7] It is best done with an undersized non-compliant balloon that allows the operator to go to high pressures without concerns of balloon oversize relative to vessel size or balloon rupture.

**Manipulating the cutting balloon: Because of the presence of the microblades at its side, the cutting balloon is quite stiff, and is difficult to curve around sharp bends. To overcome this problem, the cutting balloon is designed with very short length (10 mm). While dilating the cutting balloon, a slow inflation strategy is used. There should be 3–5 seconds interval between each atmosphere increase, to ensure that the peripheral balloon wings unfold slowly, first around the blades, before inflation of the central core of the balloon. Rapid inflation could result in the blades puncturing the balloon. The cutting balloon is effective in PCI of patients listed in Table 6-1.

***Extraction of stent by cutting balloon: The CB has its blades mounted along its length. During inflation, the

Table 6-1
Indications for use of cutting balloon

1. Aorto-ostial lesion
2. Bifurcation lesion
3. Restenotic lesion
4. Highly resistant lesions

blades are protruded outwards and exposed. Then, during deflation, there is a mechanism for rewrapping the balloons with multiple wings. During this process of rewrapping, there is possibility of the creation of an anchor formed by the balloon and the blades or just because the higher profile balloon is strengthened with the blades. This recess can get stuck into the stent struts and prevent withdrawal of the CB. If the CB is pulled strongly enough it could pull with it the stent or part of the stent. Because the lumen of the artery is removed with the stent, the lumen can become avulsed and have acute occlusion.[8,9]

**Failure to deflate the balloon: Inability to deflate the balloon is a rare occurrence. Possible causes are excessive twisting (more than 360°) in order to cross a distal lesion[10] or entrapment in the distal portion by a tight lesion. Usual maneuvers to deflate the balloon are listed in Table 6-2.

After exhausting all maneuvers without success, one rarely used measure is to bring a new over-the-wire balloon immediately next to the entrapped and inflated balloon. Reverse the wire by reinserting the back end first. Inflate the new balloon at low pressure to position the sharp tip of the wire at the center of the vessel lumen. Try to puncture the inflated balloon with the back end. A 190-cm wire which has a tapered back end to allow extending may be most effective in puncturing. Although there is a risk of coronary perforation, the hole would be quite small and unlikely to cause any significant complication. In addition, vessel trauma from balloon rupture can be much more extensive and more uncontrolled than a single pinhole puncture.[12]

***Impending rupture due to material fatigue: Besides rupture due to excessive inflation or calcified plaque, another cause of rupture is material fatigue.[11] Balloon fatigue generally occurs after numerous inflations and deflations of a re-used balloon – seen frequently outside the US. As the balloon material undergoes fatigue, a focal bulging in the balloon during inflation may be observed. It is sug-

Table 6-2
Technical options when the balloon fails to deflate

1. Deflate the balloon with the inflation device.
2. Deflate the balloon with a 50 cc syringe directly at the inflation port.
3. As a last resort, inflate the balloon to rupture it. Prepare for damage control from dissection or coronary perforation.[11]
4. Surgical removal of balloon.
5. Investigational: puncture the balloon with the back end of a wire.

gested that when faced with an unyielding stenosis, inflation pressure sufficient to cause balloon rupture should be
avoided.[13]

***Entrapment of deflated balloon during withdrawal:**
Even though the incidence of entrapment of a deflated
balloon is low, once it happens, it is quite traumatic to the
patient, operator, and the interventional team. The entrapment can happen in an unpredicted way. Different options
for management are listed in Table 6-3. There are no best
options. Different modalities of treatment can be attempted
on a trial-and-error basis.

***Using a commercial snare to remove a balloon:** Cut
the proximal end of the balloon catheter. Advance the snare
using the balloon catheter as a wire. Once arriving at the
entrapped balloon site, loop the snare around the balloon,
tighten the loop by advancing the transport catheter, and
pull the snare and the catheter end to free the balloon.[16] Be
prepared to unwrap the snare and pull it back alone if it is not
able to remove the trapped balloon.

***Management of repeated rupture:** Balloon rupture
can happen repeatedly as in a case reported by Gilutz *et al.*
In a patient with ISR, three balloons were ruptured during

Table 6-3
Management of entrapment of balloon after inflation

---

1. Pull the balloon back more forcefully.[14]
2. Push the balloon forward then pull it back.
3. Twist the balloon in an attempt to rewrap the balloon
   before pulling back.
4. Insert a stiffer wire alongside the entrapped balloon
   before pulling the balloon back so the artery can be more
   straightened.
5. Advance and inflate any new balloon alongside the
   entrapped balloon, or at least in the proximal vicinity,
   to prepare a pathway so the entrapped balloon can be
   withdrawn.[15]
6. Advance a second wire distally, then insert an over-the-
   wire balloon alongside the entrapped balloon, and inflate
   the new balloon at low pressure to free the entrapped
   balloon.
7. If the over-the-wire balloon cannot be advanced, then
   advance a balloon-on-a-wire alongside the entrapped balloon and inflate it to free the entrapped balloon.
8. Advance a commercial microsnare, and tighten the loop
   near the balloon as much as possible, then pull the balloon back as any embolized material.[16]

inflation. IVUS study showed a ridge of calcium protruding into the lumen. Management of this problem includes use of stronger balloon, rotational atherectomy, which can be problematic because it can ablate the metallic stent struts, or, as in this case report, CABG.[17]

***Damage control for balloon rupture:** Balloon rupture is seen under the fluoroscope as a quick dispersion of contrast agent from the balloon, with short contrast opacification of the vessel or decrease in the inflation pressure. When this occurs, slowly withdraw the balloon proximal to the lesion and inject some contrast to detect whether there is perforation. The balloon is then removed if not entrapped in the lesion. Stenting should be performed if there is dissection.

CONCLUSION

Balloon angioplasty is the basic technique of coronary intervention. In many situations it is the only one available, for example, in intervention in small vessels, very tortuous arteries, ISR, bifurcation, and AMI. It is still the only procedure available in many developing countries because of the high cost of stent. Manipulation of a balloon and opening an artery without causing complications requires more than technical skill. Balloon angioplasty is an art: how to unblock diseased arteries in a cost- and time-effective manner.

REFERENCES

1. Ellis S. Elective coronary angioplasty: Techniques and complications. In: Topol E, ed. *Textbook of Interventional Cardiology,* 3rd edition. WB Saunders, 1999.
2. King SB. Complications of angioplasty. In: King SB, Douglas JS, eds. *Atlas of Heart Diseases: Interventional Cardiology.* Mosby, 1997: 12.1–12.15.
3. Meier B. Balloon angioplasty. In: Topol E, ed. *Textbook of Cardiovascular Medicine.* Lippincott-Raven Publishers, 1998: 1983.
4. Nanto S, Ohara T, Shimonagata T *et al.* A technique for changing a PTCA balloon catheter over regular length guidewire. *Cathet Cardiovasc Diagn* 1994; **32**: 274–7.
5. Krucoff MW, Smith JE, Jackman JD *et al.* "Hugging balloons" through a single 8F guide: Salvage angioplasty with lytic therapy in the IRA of a 40-year-old man. *Cathet Cardiovasc Diagn* 1991; **24**: 45–50.
6. Feld H, Valerio L, Shani J. Two hugging balloons at high pressures successfully dilated a lesion refractory to routine

coronary angioplasty. *Cathet Cardiovasc Diagn* 1991; **24**: 105–7.

7. Yazdanfar S, Ledley GS, Alfieri A *et al*. Parallel angioplasty dilation catheter and guide wire: A new technique for the dilation of calcified coronary arteries. *Cathet Cardiovasc Diagn* 1993; **28**: 72–5.

8. Kawamura A, Asakura Y, Ishikawa S *et al*. Extraction of previously deployed stent by an entrapped CB due to blade fracture. *Cathet Cardiovasc Interv* 2002; **57**: 239–43.

9. Harb T, Ling F. Inadvertent stent extraction six months after implantation by an entrapped cutting balloon. *Cathet Cardiovasc Interv* 2001; **53**: 415–19.

10. Hamada Y, Matsuda Y, Takashiba K *et al*. Difficult deflation of Probe balloon due to twisting of the system stenosis. *Cathet Cardiovasc Diagn* 1989; **18**: 12–14.

11. Breisblatt WM. Inflated balloon entrapped in calcified coronary stenosis. *Cathet Cardiovasc Diagn* 1993; **29**: 224–8.

12. Personal communication with Khoi Le MD, Palm Spring CA.

13. Kussmaul III WG, Marzo K, Tomaszewski J *et al*. Rupture and entrapment of a balloon catheter in the LAD: Fluoroscopy of impending balloon rupture. *Cathet Cardiovasc Diagn* 1993; **19**: 256–9.

14. Rizzo TF, Werres R, Ciccone J *et al*. Entrapment of an angioplasty balloon catheter: A case report. *Cathet Cardiovasc Diagn* 1988; **14**: 255–7.

15. Colombo A, Skinner JM. Balloon entrapment in a coronary artery: Potential serious complications of balloon rupture. *Cathet Cardiovasc Diagn* 1990; **19**: 23–5.

16. Watson LE. Snare loop technique for removal of broken steerable PTCA wire. *Cathet Cardiovasc Diagn* 1987; **13**: 44–9.

17. Gilutz H, Weistein J. Repeated balloon rupture during coronary stenting due to a calcified lesion: An IVUS study. *Cathet Cardiovasc Interv* 2000; **50**: 212–14.

Chapter 7
Stenting

Thach Nguyen, Jia Sanqing,
Wang Lei, Yan Songbiao

---

*Basic; **Advanced; ***Rare, exotic, or investigational.

From: Nguyen T, Hu D, Saito S, Grines C, Palacios I (eds), *Practical Handbook of Advanced Interventional Cardiology*, 2nd edn. © 2003 Futura, an imprint of Blackwell Publishing.

BEST METHOD: Redeploy a stent after failed expansion by balloon

BEST METHOD: Redeploy a stent after failure of stent expansion

Recrossing a stent

BEST METHOD: Recrossing a stented area by a balloon or stent

**Dottering for recrossing a newly stented area

***Other exotic techniques

***First balloon deflecting second balloon from problematic area

***Recrossing a stent with a bent stiff wire

CAVEAT: Manipulation near a previously deployed stent

Side branch dilation

***Opening of a stent at its side by balloon inflation

***Mechanisms of side opening following dilation

***Main lumen distortion and restoration following dilations

CAVEAT: Entrapment of a balloon during side branch dilation

***Entrapment of the distal tip of an IVUS catheter

Stent deformations

TAKE-HOME MESSAGE: Perfect stenting in the era of drug-eluting stents

STRUCTURAL DESIGNS AND FUNCTIONAL EXPECTATIONS

As a clinical cardiologist must know the pharmacologic properties of a new cardiovascular drug or the mechanism of a new therapeutic device, interventional cardiologists must understand the basic physical or bioengineering principles of stenting so that the most suitable stent for a given lesion can be selected.

Easy delivery = high longitudinal flexibility + low profile: A stent mounted on a delivery balloon should be able to negotiate easily the tortuous segments proximal to the target site, without injuring the intima or eliciting spasm. This smooth delivery is termed high trackability as a stent is passed easily over a wire. The two properties, high longitudinal flexibility and low profile, help to bring the stent to the target site within an allotted time frame and with minimal manipulation.

A stent can easily cross an angulated segment if its length can fit in the widest interval at the curve. If it is longer, it can be advanced as long as it can be bent or curved, or the arterial segment is not too calcified to relax and compliantly accommodate the stent.

Perfect deployment = great radial strength and curve conformity: Once deployed, a stent must have sufficient radial strength to resist the elastic recoil of the media and of the shifting plaque. In an emergency situation, it has to be strong to seal the entry of a dissection, patch a dissecting flap, or brace against the persistent compression of a growing intramural hematoma. In addition, an adaptively deployed stent would mold its shape along the contour of a curved segment rather than straighten it and still provide a large desired lumen. These two properties of a deployed stent, great radial strength and curve conformity, would give an instant perfect angiographic result. Following deployment, the struts should be well imbedded into the arterial wall and stop any systolic contraction or diastolic relaxation. Therefore, they effectively immobilize the stented arterial segment and prevent any ongoing injury to the intima, which is the nidus for any endothelial thrombotic formation. Excellent apposition of the struts on the vessel wall will guarantee the delivery of the cytostatic drug preventing intimal hyperplasia.

No subacute thrombosis = high acute gain: While restenosis following angioplasty typically is caused by a combination of early elastic recoil, intimal hyperplasia (IH), and late vessel remodeling, the primary cause of restenosis following stenting is excessive IH and late negative remodeling. By serving as a rigid metallic frame, stents prevent early elastic recoil and late remodeling. Therefore, the largest achievable lumen diameter at the acute phase may help to avoid subacute thrombosis, and overcome late lumen loss. With the advent of DES, late restenosis is effectively prevented by cytostatic drugs coated on the stent struts.

ENGINEERING CRITERIA FOR STENT EVALUATION

Longitudinal flexibility: In the coil design, a single wire is coiled in different curves and crimped tightly around a deflated balloon. It has no longitudinal strut so it uses the delivery balloon as a platform for its struts to be positioned on the longitudinal plane. Without stiff longitudinal shafts, the coil stent is very flexible. In the tubular design, the primary mechanism for flexibility is that the longitudinal struts should be rather short and interrupted while the circular struts should be bent or folded and positioned sideways along the longitudinal axis, before deployment. This arrangement of struts makes a stent highly flexible during delivery.

Radial strength: At the target site, the balloon is inflated to deploy the stent. In the tubular design, the struts that were previously longitudinal or folded along the length of the stent rotate outward away from the long axis, and become the circumferential struts. In the coil design, the circumferential loops are just stretched wider to attain the desired diameter. Because they are incomplete loops, their radial strength is lower, as evidenced by 15%–20% loss of achieved diameter due to intrinsic recoil.

In general, a stent has higher radial strength if its longitudinal struts rotate more circumferentially during deployment and it has more struts that are thicker and wider. Thus, the majority of coil stents have thicker struts (0.12–0.20 mm) to increase radial strength while the other design stents have thinner struts (0.05–0.12 mm) to increase longitudinal flexibility.

PRACTICAL CLINICAL EVALUATION OF A STENT

Is this stent flexible?
In general, if a stent has no stiff longitudinal shaft along its length, it will be quite flexible. This is well evidenced in any coil stent design. With better supportive equipment to advance a stent (stiffer wire, more stable guide), or in the case of minimal tortuosity, the flexibility of a stent is not a major concern in today's busy cardiac catheterization laboratories.

How is the radial strength?
Most currently available stents have adequate radial strength. However, the most important concern is the even and reliable distribution of their struts or radial strength.

In the left main trunk, at the anastomotic site of a saphenous vein graft, or in the lesions of elderly patients, the lesions are composed of extensive fibrotic tissue and have significant recoil pressure. In these situations, stents with high radial strength are particularly needed. They are also required for the long-term success in stenting of the carotid, femoral, popliteal, or tibial arteries, which may be subjected to external compression.

Does this stent brace itself against the wall with a strong strut network?
IVUS has demonstrated that stenting a lesion shifts the mass of atheromatous material along the longitudinal and radial axes. To achieve the best luminal diameter, a newly deployed stent has to provide a strong network of struts to fence off the recoiling atheromatous mass and provide a controlled shifting of the plaque burden along the longitudinal axis. It has to be able to prevent any intraluminal herniation of the plaque through its struts and any possible distal embolization. The strong apposition of the struts into the vessel wall will guarantee the delivery of cytostatic drugs which will prevent intimal hyperplasia and restenosis.

Is the stent user-friendly?
In general, an elective stenting procedure should not require more than 30 minutes if the equipment is reliable and user-friendly. Every step of the procedure should be achieved on the first try. Besides a strong guide support, the success of delivery depends on the size, flexibility of the stent-balloon

complex, and the compliance of the arterial segments proximal to the target site.

A flexible and small stent can slide on a floppy wire while a stiffer wire is needed to track a bulky, stiffer stent. A short stent can easily negotiate a sharp bend, while some longer stents cannot. During delivery, a stent should hold well to the balloon, thus avoiding the risk of inadvertent embolization. In case of failure of delivery, while attempting to withdraw an undeployed stent into the guide, there should be no feeling of resistance and the stent should be watched carefully to ensure it does not slip off the balloon. If this occurs, the guide, stent, and wire should be withdrawn together *en bloc*. In all situations, the choice of a stent depends on the operator's preference, experience with a particular design, and critical evaluation of different structural features to maximize benefits.

ADVANCING A STENT

When a stent fails to move forward, it is imperative to assess the stability of the guide position, the sufficient stiffness of the wire, and the tortuosity of the vessel. If the guide position is fairly stable but the artery is more or less tortuous, then an extra support wire may compensate enough for this mildly deficient guide backup. However, if the guide is also unstable, then an extra wire is not enough to correct the problem. If the problem is not from the guide, then possibly, a firm wire passed through a heavily calcified and angulated lesion may occasionally "force" the stent against the wall of the lesion and make stent passage difficult. To avoid the above wire bias, a floppy or moderately balanced wire should be used. If there are no problems with guide support or wire bias, then the balloon may be too stiff to make the turn around the lesion. The best options in advancing the stent are listed below and in Table 7-1.[1]

BEST METHOD

When a stent fails to advance:

1. **First maneuver:** Secure a more stable guide position or, if possible, the guide can be deep-seated safely (Figure 7-1).
2. **Second maneuver:** Constant forward pressure on the stent catheter while pulling the wire back to decrease friction inside the stent catheter lumen and to straighten the stent catheter while asking the patient to take a deep breath in order to elongate and straighten the artery.
3. **Add a device:** Advance a second stiffer wire to straighten the artery (the "buddy wire" technique).

Table 7-1
Other options when a stent fails to advance

Wire manipulations

1. Shape the wire along the curve of the artery in order to lessen wire bias, so there is less friction or resistance at the outer curve of the vessel and the path of the wire is more coaxial with the path of the vessel. (rare)

Stent manipulations

2. Partial stent-balloon inflation. (rare)
3. Inflate tip slightly. (bubble stent)
4. Change the stent to a shorter one, if the problem is due to tortuosity of the proximal segment.
5. Select a different type of stent with better flexibility.
6. Bend the stent to conform the stent along the curve of the artery.

Guide manipulations

7. Different curve to achieve better backup and less friction at the ostium.
8. Larger or smaller guide to achieve better backup.

Balloon manipulation

9. The buddy balloon technique: Advance a second balloon beyond the deployment area, inflate the balloon to hold the first wire steady, pull the first wire to keep tension on it, and slide the stent on this taut wire.

---

4. If the stent could not be advanced on the first soft wire, then advance the stent on the second, stiffer buddy wire.
5. Additional proximal segment dilation or plaque removal to facilitate stent advancement

TECHNICAL TIPS

**To secure a stent on a balloon: Most of the hand-crimping should be applied to the middle of the stent and not to the ends, to make sure the balloon material is not damaged. Always inflate the balloon first before mounting the stent, since the winged balloon material tends to hold the crimped stent in position more reliably than an uninflated balloon.[2]

***Hand-crimp a stent on a balloon with the tip partially inflated: After the stent is securely hand-crimped, the balloon is inflated to half an ATM, or until a small bubble is visible at the distal end of the stent. If a proximal bubble appears, the operator should squeeze the bubble between the fingers to induce the formation of a distal bubble. This

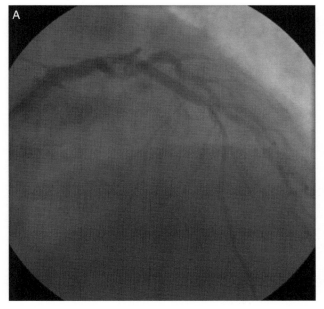

Figure 7-1: Deep-seat a guide in order to advance a stent across another stent. (A) A patient came with AMI in the LAD. A stent was deployed. There was dissection at the distal end of newly deployed stent at the mid-LAD. *(Continued)*

bubble would direct the stent to the center of the stented lumen and would facilitate the crossing of the stented area. The only word of caution when using this technique with 6F guides is to carefully flush the system during advancement of the balloon catheter inside the guide, in order to prevent air suction by the vacuum and subsequent coronary air embolism.[3]

**Partial inflation of a stent in order to cross tortuous segments: In a case report by Fernandes *et al.*, a stent failed to cross a sharp bend despite all manipulations. Then the authors inflated the balloon-stent with 2–3 ATM and all stents were successfully delivered and deployed. The technique of partial balloon inflation is described in the previous paragraph for the purpose of stabilizing a stent and preventing its embolization. Partial balloon inflation also makes the balloon stent complex stiffer, straighter and more coaxial with the lumen thereby eliminating local wire-bias. This makes the stent more able to go along and around a bend rather keep pointing straight toward the wall and getting stuck under a plaque. Of the angiograms illustrated in the

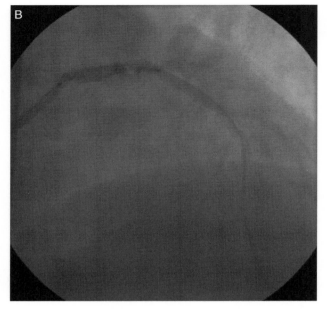

Figure 7-1: (B) The second stent could not be advanced across the first stent. The two markers of the second stent were seen at the LM. *(Continued)*

case report, there is one common factor: the angle at the bend is very acute and a sharp straight stent would point towards the wall and can get stuck there. A further push could have perforated the wall. So a round tip of a partially inflated balloon will smoothen the tip and make it less sharp to be able to curve (or to float) along and around the bend. In this report, the authors were successful in delivering the stents with a partially inflated balloon. However, if this trick is not able to advance the stent, then the stent has to be withdrawn. In theory, it is not able to be withdrawn back into the guide because the balloon is inflated, however, in a recent case of mine, the balloon could be withdrawn as I made sure that the stent was coaxial with the opening of the guide (TNN). Otherwise, the only way is to withdraw the whole system (wire, balloon-stent complex and guide) as a unit. Then the procedure has to be started over again.[4]

**Testing the road: After the lesion is predilated with a balloon, a stent is prepared to be advanced for deployment. If the proximal segment is tortuous, there is a question as to whether the stent can succeed in arriving at the lesion area. One way to test the possibility is to advance the predilating

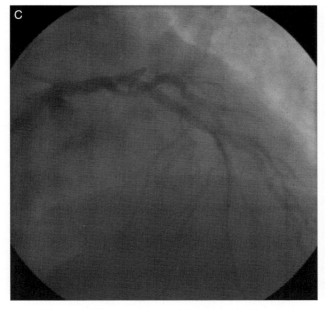

Figure 7-1: (C) With deeper guide intubation, the second stent succeeded in crossing the first stent and was deployed at the dissected are. (Courtesy of the Cardiac Catherization Laboratories of The Heart Institute, National University Hospital, Singapore.)

balloon, now deflated, with its wings still out, to recross the lesion. If the balloon can recross the tortuous segment and lesion, then there is higher chance (>50%) a stent can do so too.

**The "buddy wire" technique: The "buddy wire" approach requires one extra-support or heavy-duty wire to straighten the artery. Advance a heavy wire across the lesion, then advance the stent as usual. Once the stent is positioned across the lesion, the buddy wire is removed and the stent deployed.[5]

***Bend the wire: To advance a stent across some angulated segments, a wire can be bent to direct the wire more coaxially, by relieving the tendency of the wire to hug the outer curve of the vessel (wire bias). When a stent is tracked on the bent wire, the stent will have less tendency to be forced against the outer wall of the vessel, where resistance to its passage is increased. A wire with a deformable, non-

Nitinol shaft must be used. Care must be taken to avoid stripping the coating off the wire.[6]

**How to calculate the location of the bend: The spring coil of the wire is used as a measuring device to place the location of the bends. Usually it is 20–30 mm long and it is marked on the label cover. After the vessel is wired, the approximate location of the bends can be estimated, as a multiple of the length of the spring coil. A transport catheter is placed over the wire and the wire is removed. After the bends are strategically placed, the wire is replaced into the transport catheter, which is then itself removed. Once the curves have "locked" into place, the stability of the wire is remarkable.[6]

***The buddy balloon technique: On many occasions, because of poor support from the guide, a stent cannot be advanced to the intended area. After exhausting all the technical tricks (the buddy wire, bubble stent, bending the stent), an operator advances an ACE balloon beyond the target lesion in the distal segment. There he inflates the balloon to entrap the wire. While pulling the entrapped wire to keep tension on it, the stent is advanced successfully on this taut wire. The mechanism of this technique is highlighted in Table 7-2.[7] The negative sides of the trick are: (1) need for an extra balloon, (2) inflation of a distal balloon, which can cause endothelial denudation, the initial lesion of the restenosis process, and (3) rupture of a new plaque, causing thrombosis or acute occlusion. If the benefits outweigh the risks then this technical tip can be used.

DEPLOYING A STENT

As more percutaneous coronary interventions are done without formal surgical backup, many lesions are strategically underpredilated to be stented immediately at standard size and higher pressure. Other operators suggest direct stenting without prior balloon inflation.

Direct stenting: Direct stenting is a feasible and safe technique when used in selected coronary lesions, without significant calcifications and/or angulation. The degree of

---

Table 7-2
Mechanisms of the buddy balloon technique

1. Pulling on the wire will seat the guide more deeply and firmly.
2. Providing a stiff rail over which the stent is easily tracked.
3. Straightening the proximal segment of the vessel.

stenosis is not an important limitation, particularly in unstable angina where thrombus plays an important role. In the case of a type A lesion, there is not much difficulty involved in measuring the reference diameter for accurately sizing a stent. In a lesion with chronic distal vasoconstriction due to low flow, the angiographic distal reference diameter may be smaller. Sometimes the strategy of direct stenting backfires because of the potential for only partial stent deployment (e.g. due to lesion fibrosis, calcification, or balloon rupture), the risk of stent loss and difficult stent retrieval, and inaccurate stent placement if there is poor distal vessel opacification. Therefore it is important to check the presence of heavy calcium at the lesion and in other branches prior to angioplasty and stenting for possible rotational debulking. Fluoroscopy alone is not sensitive enough to detect superficial calcium. The important take-home message is summarized below. The factors favoring successful direct stenting and its contraindications are listed in Tables 7-3 and 7-4.[8]

TAKE-HOME MESSAGE

Direct stenting: [9]

1. Do not attempt direct stenting in patients older than 75 years old with chronic angina because unexpected calcified or fibrotic lesion can prevent full deployment of a stent. Suboptimal stent deployment predisposes to subacute stent thrombosis.
2. Do not attempt direct stenting before establishing control and good coaxial alignment of the guide

---

Table 7-3
Factors favoring successful direct stenting

1. Young age <70
2. No calcium at the target and other coronary vessels
3. No severe proximal tortuosity
4. Not an LCX lesion
5. Not too distal location

Table 7-4
Lesions unsuitable for direct stenting

1. Total occlusion
2. Bifurcation lesions
3. Important side branch
4. Long lesions
5. Proximal tortuosity

3. Do use a moderate push to attempt the passage of the stent to the desired position at the lesion site. Avoid prolonged or forceful manipulation to cross the lesion because the stent can be stripped off the balloon and embolized distally.
4. If the lesion cannot be easily crossed, try a deeper intubation of the guide but without aggressive manipulation because it can cause ostial trauma.

TECHNICAL TIPS

**Predilating balloon angioplasty in the DES era: The goal of predilation is not to achieve a perfect result, but it is to facilitate the positioning of the stent. Perfect angioplasty may eliminate the angiographic landmark of the lesion and make the location of stent deployment uncertain and full coverage of the injured segment doubtful.

***Deploying a stent from the radial approach: When using radial approach, breath movement may induce greater guide movement compared to the femoral approach, so it is critical to ask the patient to stop breathing for a few seconds during stent positioning and deployment.[9]

***Redeploying an embolized stent: In case of inadvertent embolization of an undeployed or partially deployed stent, the best way to resolve the problem is to insert a new non-compliant balloon into the stent. Then deploy the stent with prolonged high pressure. However, it is not easy and it may take a lot of time, patience, and skill to advance a new balloon across a partially deployed stent. If not successful, the stent has to be removed.

***Balloon rupture: Not infrequently after deployment of a stent, especially if it is a reused balloon, the balloon can rupture. Rarely, as proved by IVUS, an irregular jagged-appearing calcified lesion can penetrate into the lumen of the stented lesion and can cause repeated perforation of the balloon. While the PET material of a balloon ruptured twice, the nylon material of a balloon was able to withstand high pressure without being punctured. If the heavy calcification had been detected earlier, rotablational atherectomy would have been helpful. However, once the lesion is stented, ablation with the burr is not an option as the stent abuts the calcified plaque.[10]

**Avoid high-pressure post-dilation in the DES era: As a bigger lumen is found to have a better restenosis rate, there was a trend of post-dilating the stent with high pressure in order to achieve the largest lumen possible. A shorter non-compliant balloon is used so there is no stent edge dissection. However, with high-pressure post-dilation, there was more plaque extrusion on the longitudinal axis, even exceeding the stent margins.[11] This observation explains the minimal haziness on the proximal or distal stent edges after deployment or the transient worsening of the ostial size of a side branch in the vicinity of the stented area and more distal embolization causing distal low flow.

Because of the new appearance of atheromatous material at the proximal or distal edge of the newly stented area (step up, step down), there is more turbulent flow in these areas. This increased shear stress is the most likely cause of proximal edge restenosis after DES in the SIRolImUS-Eluting Stent in De Novo Native Coronary Lesions (SIRIUS) trial. Therefore, when deploying a DES, the operator should avoid causing endothelial denudation in the proximal segment while advancing the stent towards the index lesion, avoid having different flow patterns at the entry and exit of the stented area (no step up, step down) and try to cover the DES on all instrumented (possibly future restenotic) areas.

**Deployment of a stent in a tortuous artery: When a stent is deployed in a very tortuous arterial segment, the vessel wall forms many invaginations beyond the struts rather than being well stretched. To maximize the length of the stented segment along the natural curve of the tortuous artery and to ensure that the struts are well apposed to the vessel wall, the stent is deployed while the patient takes a deep breath. Deep inspiration will make the heart more vertical, elongate the artery, and in that short window of opportunity, the stent is deployed (Figure 7-2 A,B).

When deploying a stent in a tortuous segment, do not position the proximal or distal end of the stent at a curved or angled segment. The sharp angulation formed by the stent and the wall will make recrossing the stent difficult for the redilation balloon, a newer distal stent, or an embolic protection device.

***Stent deployment after balloon rupture: When a balloon ruptures during stent deployment, withdrawal of a partially inflated balloon can dislodge the stent into the proximal segment. In order to deploy the stent, some experienced senior operators suggest using a 20 cc syringe filled with contrast and injecting 2–3 cc very quickly to inflate the balloon and deploy the stent. Keelan *et al.* were able to partly deploy the stent using an automatic power injector. Using 50% diluted contrast at a rate of 20 cc/sec over 0.25 sec and a pressure limit of 200–400 psi, they found that 1 cc was injected before the pressure maximum was exceeded. The stent was sufficiently deployed with the damaged balloon to allow its removal.[12] Many times, the balloon ruptures because of a tiny pinhole, so these quick injections can

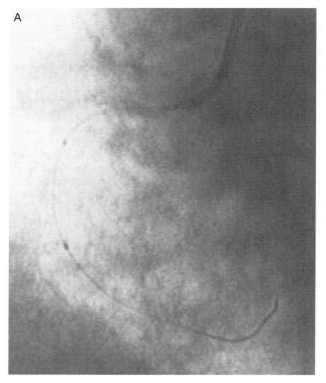

Figure 7-2: Deploying stent in a tortuous artery. (A) The short curve of the RCA prior to stenting. *(Continued)*

sufficiently inflate a balloon and partially deploy a stent; however, these injections can cause a jet injury at the arterial wall and may cause perforation.

***How to prevent damage from balloon rupture:** After deployment of a stent, the post-dilation high-pressure balloon should be short and non-compliant. The balloon should be short so it can fit entirely inside the length of the stent, without causing any tear at the two edges. If the balloon is longer than the stent, then the segment of the balloon exceeding the length of the stent is positioned at the proximal end. This position will help to avoid the need to recross the stent if there is a rupture-induced dissection in the proximal end rather than at the distal end. This position also helps to avoid overdilating the adjacent distal segment that is often smaller than the proximal reference segment. Moreover, placing excess balloon length proximal to the stent should decrease the chance

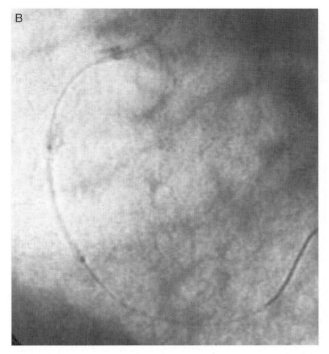

Figure 7-2: (B) The stent is deployed while the patient takes a deep breath to make the heart more vertical and the artery elongated. The curve is longer so the stent can be deployed at its maximal potential to reconstruct the best lumen possible (with less arterial wall invagination).

of entrapment and tethering of the ruptured balloon on the distal end of the stent, which could make the retrieval of the balloon extremely difficult or impossible.

If the balloon cannot be removed easily, the lumen of the balloon should be flushed with saline, aspirated with a 50-cc syringe, and the balloon should be pushed gently forward before being pulled back.[13]

CAVEAT: Check the integrity of a balloon before deployment: To avoid crimping a stent on a ruptured balloon, three observations to confirm the integrity of the balloon should be checked prior to advancement (Table 7-5). In the case of a hand-crimped stent, the balloon-stent complex can be checked again when the stent is at the tip of the guide, before engaging the coronary artery, so there is still time to retrieve it if needed.[14]

Table 7-5
Checking the integrity of a balloon before advancing it into the coronary artery

1. No air bubble in the fluid inside the inflation device.
2. No blood back inside the shaft of the balloon catheter lumen after the catheter is inserted into the guide.
3. While the plunger of the inflation device is in the aspiration position, it does not return rapidly to the neutral position as it is released.

**Appropriate sizing for tapering artery: After successful inflation of the balloon, 5 seconds before deflating it, a small injection of contrast agent will verify the correct size of the balloon with the proximal segment of the dilated lesion. The same maneuver after deploying a stent will verify the correct size of the stent with the proximal segment of the dilated area. If contrast agent is seen flowing around the proximal segment of the inflated stent-balloon complex, the stent needs to be inflated at higher pressure and/or larger balloons are needed. If the stent is underdilated, the now deflated balloon is pulled back a few millimeters in order to avoid overdilating the distal end, and is inflated again with higher pressure to achieve higher size. This is only a rough assessment of the appropriate size of the balloon or stent, when IVUS is not available (see Figure 6-3 A,B).

**Overlapping stent in the DES era: With bare stent, there was a concern of overlapping stent that caused increased metal density triggering restenosis. In the SIRIUS trial, the rate of restenosis in lesions with overlapped stent was double (8.8% with DES) that for the whole group (4.1%). Among the eight cases of restenosis in patients with overlapped stents, five occurred in the overlapped region.[29]

REDEPLOYING A STENT

With the trend of primary stenting or lower pressure balloon predilation, in many occasions, a stent cannot be fully expanded, due to an unexpected severely calcified vessel wall. In other cases, a stent was crushed by inadvertent insertion of the dilation balloon through a strut (Figure 7-3 A). How can the stent be redeployed?

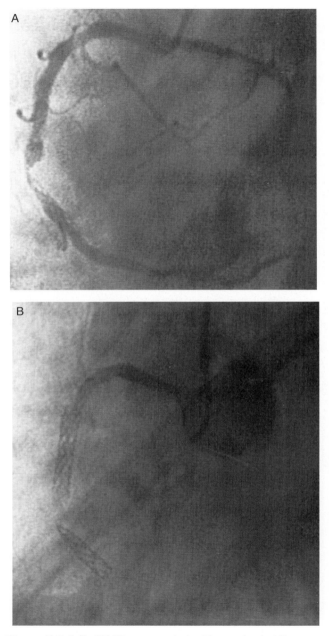

Figure 7-3 A,B: (A) The second stent is crushed at its opening. (B) The RCA in the LAO view. *(Continued)*

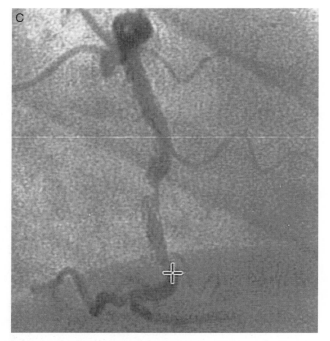

Figure 7-3 C: Because the wire was unable to enter the stent ostium, another angiogram was done in the RAO view (90° opposite) in order to locate the exact location of the true opening. *(Continued)*

BEST METHOD

How to cross a crushed stent:

1.   **The one and only maneuver:** After failure to advance a wire across a crushed stent, the *only* next step is to take another picture from another orthogonal angle (90° opposite to the first angle) in order to locate the exact location of the possible opening.

Then advance a balloon with marker in the middle of the balloon. As soon as the marker is seen in the middle of the lesion, it is assured that the lesion is crossed. From there the stent is redilated successfully (Figure 7-3 B–E).

**Redeploy a stent after failed expansion by balloon: In order to redeploy a stent, usually the operator would insert and inflate a non-compliant, high-pressure balloon. Even so, on occasion, very high-pressure balloon inflation fails to expand the stent. Then the next step is to use a cutting

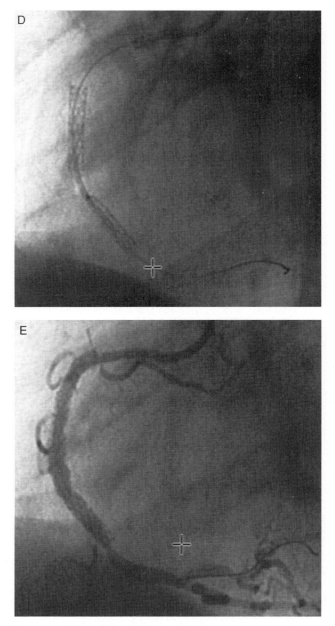

Figure 7-3 D,E: (D) A balloon with marker in the middle of the balloon was advanced across the stent. (E) The stent was redilated successfully.

balloon to try to open the undeployed segment.[2] If there is laser angioplasty equipment available (rare), conventional laser angioplasty in a blood medium would provoke local dissection behind the stent struts. The theory is that excimer laser irradiation of blood results in vapor bubble formation and acousto-mechanical trauma to the vessel wall, causing localized dissection. Usually, during regular laser angioplasty, intracoronary infusion of normal saline is required to displace the blood, and minimize the blood irradiation and consequent arterial wall damage. In case of failure deploying a stent due to unexpected heavy calcification, excimer laser irradiation would provoke local dissection, and weaken the vessel wall and allow full expansion of the stent.[15] The different methods of redeploying a stent are featured below.

BEST METHOD

Redeploy a stent after failure of stent expansion:

1. **First maneuver:** Increase inflation pressure to maximum.
2. **Change a device:** Change current balloon to a high-pressure and non-compliant balloon. Inflate it with maximal high pressure possible so at least the proximal end is opened as much as possible in order to facilitate the reinsertion of a new balloon. It is not always easy to reinsert a new balloon into an underdeployed stent.
3. **Change to a more expensive device:** Cutting balloon is the best bet.
4. **Change to a more expensive (and may not be available) device:** Laser angioplasty in a blood medium to cause local dissection behind the stent struts, then reinflate the balloon to redeploy the stent.

RECROSSING A STENT

When there is a need to cross a stented segment, any suboptimal deployment of the first stent predisposes the second stent to be caught in the first one, with potentially catastrophic outcome.[16] If the first stent is well dilated and deployed, then the best technique to advance the stent is by gently dottering it.

BEST METHOD

Recrossing a stented area by a balloon or stent:

1. **First maneuver:** The technique is to gently bounce the balloon-wire (or device-wire) forwards and backwards

and, because these movements are limited, the wire will bounce up and down (more wire-centering) and create a chance for the balloon-wire (or device-wire) to enter the lumen.

2. **Second maneuver:** Engage the guide in a more stable position or deep-seat the guide to change the entry direction of the wire, and hopefully lessen wire bias.

3. **Third maneuver:** Steer the wire into a different direction, or to a different branch or side branch, in order to lessen wire bias and increase wire centering; hopefully, it will help to advance the stent.

4. **Add a device:** Park a balloon at the resistance site; advance a second balloon as the working balloon. The first balloon should deflect the second balloon away from the problematic area and hopefully the second device can enter the lumen.

TECHNICAL TIPS

**Dottering for recrossing a newly stented area: Hold the interventional device (stent, balloon, cutting balloon, IVUS catheter, etc.) and advance it by gently dottering it. By moving the device gently forward and backward, the indwelling wire is also bounced forwards and backwards gently. Because the tip of the wire cannot go farther, the forward energy will be changed to the up and down direction that bounces the wire up and down the whole diameter of the lumen. This should enable more wire-centering and create a chance for the interventional device to enter the newly stented area. If the wire cannot be bounced up and down, because of small vessel diameter or because the wire is well encased in a tight area or because the monorail segment of the device (e.g. the IVUS catheter) is so short and does not transmit the dottering movement, then this technique does not work (Table 7-6).

***Other exotic techniques: When crossing a stented segment of a vessel, a short stent can cross more easily than a longer one. If the stent fails to cross a stented segment while being tracked on a soft wire, a stiffer wire with less wire bias can direct the balloon-stent complex more to the center of the stented segment and help the stent

---

Table 7-6
Unfavorable factors for the dottering technique

---

1. Small vessel diameter
2. Wire encased in a tight area
3. Too short monorail segment
4. Suboptimal opening of stent

to cross. If the stent fails to pass with a stiff wire in place, changing to a softer one may help. If a balloon cannot cross a stent, the balloon-on-a-wire type can have a higher chance of crossing the stent, because there is no "step up" from the wire to the balloon, and therefore no "lip" on the balloon's nose to get caught inside a stent strut. Unfortunately, these balloons cannot be inflated at high pressure to fully dilate a stent.[17] A new wire with a stiffer distal tip that is flexible as a whole in its radial axis (the wiggle wire) can move up and down the tip of the stent-balloon complex as it is advanced. Recrossing a stented area that was deployed a long time before can be easier, probably due to endo-thelial coverage of the struts and any small gaps between them. Various options in the technique of recrossing a stent are suggested in Table 7-7.

***First balloon deflecting second balloon away from problematic area: In a case report, Abernethy *et al.* suggested positioning a balloon at the resistance site where the balloon could not enter the stented area, then advancing a second balloon as the working balloon. The first balloon would deflect the second balloon away from the problem-atic area and allow the second balloon to enter the intended lumen of the stented area.[18]

Table 7-7
Exotic options to advance a device across a stented area

1. Rotate the balloon catheter while advancing it and let the catheter enter the stent by itself through its rotational energy (like torquing the JR catheter to engage the RCA ostium).
2. Bend the wire and place the bent segment near the ostium of the stent to be crossed in order to position the wire more at the center of the entrance of the stented segment and to decrease wire bias.
3. Use a newly designed wire that wiggles its long tip up and down along the radial axis so the balloon-stent com-plex enters the lumen at the center. (wiggle wire)
4. Insert a second, stiffer wire to straighten the vessel.
5. Change the current wire to a stiffer one.
6. Use a shorter balloon or stent.
7. Use a more flexible balloon or stent.
8. Use a fixed-wire balloon to cross the stent.
9. Use a fixed-wire balloon to track alongside a buddy wire.
10. Mount a stent on a balloon with the tip partially inflated.
11. If only the balloon needs to enter the stented segment, inflate the balloon with 1–2 ATM so the balloon will center the wire at the lumen and facilitate the crossing of the wire and balloon.

***Recrossing a stent with a bent stiff wire:** Often there is a need to cross a stent with a balloon for high-pressure post-dilation, to do angioplasty in the distal area, or to patch a distal edge dissection or perform stenting in the distal segment. If a balloon fails to recross a stent, it is usually due to the nose of the balloon engaging the stented arterial segment eccentrically or nonaxially. In order to facilitate coaxial entry of the balloon within the deployed stent, a stiff guidewire may be shaped so that a bend on the wire directs the balloon tip into the center of the stented lumen, thus facilitating passage.[1]

CAVEAT: Manipulation near a previously deployed stent: Often during PCI near a previously stented area, there is a risk of dislodging or removing the stent by any interventional hardware (balloon, rotablation, cutting balloon, IVUS, DCA, AngioJet catheters, etc.).[19] The first event in a chain leading to later catastrophe is that a wire exits through stent struts. So inability to pass balloons, stents, etc. over the wire must be taken seriously as a clue to this possibility of wrong wire exit. The wire should be advanced with a wide J curve, or repositioned, avoiding the previously stented area. Angiographic views can be deceiving and misleading. Sometimes there is no resistance when the wire exits through the struts.[19] Some caveats for PCI near a previously stented area are listed in Table 7-8.[20]

SIDE BRANCH DILATION

In complex interventions, a stent has to be crossed on its side for side branch dilation. Inflation through the stent struts

Table 7-8
Caveats during PCI near a previously deployed stent

1. Review prior angiogram for stent position and type.
2. Resistance to crossing device suggests passage between or behind struts.
3. Use two orthogonal views in order to assess access, avoiding damage to ostial stents by diagnostic catheter or guide that can cause thrombotic formation.
4. Advance the wire easily with the tip in a wide J curve. The tip should move freely.
5. Use low-profile balloon with good rewrap while crossing side branch. Keep the balloon saddle at the ostium of the side branch with proximal half in main vessel in order to avoid being trapped.
6. IVUS of parent vessel only. Avoid inserting the IVUS catheter through struts.

causes stent deformity that decreases the diameter of the main lumen.[21] Different problems related to the side opening, side struts, and the stent itself are discussed below.

***Opening of a stent at its side by balloon inflation: The average profile of a balloon lies in the range 0.024–0.028" while the profile of a cutting balloon is 0.041–0.046". The mean diameter of the side opening created by inflation of a 2.5-mm balloon ranged from 1.9 mm (NIR stent) to 2.7 mm (AVE, GFX, beStent, Multilink). This diameter increased in proportion with the size of the balloon in use, except it did not change much in the case of a beStent and NIR stent until a 4-mm balloon was used to rupture the struts. The maximum side opening diameter ranged from 3.6 mm (Crown) to 4.1 mm (AVE GFX).[21,22]

***Mechanisms of side opening following dilation: In the stents of slotted tube designs, the side lumen is opened due to straightening and displacement of the stent struts. This mechanism is responsible in part for opening the side lumen in the stent of multicell design. For the AVE GFX, the mechanism was displacement and separation of the zigzag rings. When a 4.0-mm balloon was used, it caused rupture of the struts and marked distortion of the cell shape in the beStent and NIR stent. The reason is that the cells of these stents are of smaller size compared with other stent designs.[21]

***Main lumen distortion and restoration following dilations: In all stents, side dilation produces narrowing of the main lumen immediately distal to the dilation site. The severity increases with larger balloon size, especially after inflation of the 4.0-mm balloon. These changes are mostly reversed after the stent is redilated through its main lumen, especially after the inflation of the balloons in the kissing balloon techniques. The marked distortion of a stent may not be recognized by angiography.[21]

CAVEAT: Entrapment of a balloon during side branch dilation: In a case report by Hongo *et al.*, in order to dilate a side branch, a balloon was advanced through the side struts of a stent. Only the distal tip of the balloon would pass through the stent. Following inflation, the balloon was able to be neither advanced nor withdrawn farther. After an unsuccessful trial with various retrieval devices, the balloon was then removed by alligator forceps.[22] Entrapment may occur due to "wedging" of the catheter between acutely angulated stent struts, strut fracture, or balloon "winging" beyond the confines of a stent. To avoid the entrapment of the balloon across the struts, a few measures are recommended and listed in Table 7-9.[23]

Table 7-9
Recommendations for dilation of a stent on its side

1. Ensure placement of only the distal tip through the stent struts.
2. Use a low-profile, nonwinged, undersized, high-pressure balloon.
3. Avoid excessively high pressure.
4. Expand knowledge of stent design and engineering characteristics so appropriate balloon size can be selected and opening diameter can be achieved.

***Entrapment of the distal tip of an IVUS catheter:** In a case report by Sasseen *et al.*, an IVUS catheter got stuck at the distal edge of a stent after multiple runs. After many manipulations and pulls, the IVUS catheter was finally removed minus the distal 2 cm trapped by the stent.[24]

STENT DEFORMATIONS

During procedures for ostial lesions, the tip of the guide can cause longitudinal collapse or elongation of a coil stent like an accordion, or unravel the stent to become a metallic string. While recrossing a stent, a wire may inadvertently enter the center of the stent through a proximal strut or may exit subintimally through a distal strut. It can also cross the stent purposely to enter a side branch which needs to be dilated later with a balloon straddling the struts. All of these dilations that may deform the stent can go unrecognized, with a perfectly conventional angiographic result, and can be identified only by IVUS (Table 7-10).[25,26] The collapsed segment of the coil stent is seen as a metallic mass by IVUS, while in the PS

Table 7-10
Patterns of deformation of stents

1. Free ends of struts sticking out toward the lumen of other bifurcating branch.
2. Free ends of struts sticking out toward the vessel wall causing perforation.
3. Main lumen diameter decrease due to side cell dilation for bifurcation lesion.
4. Collapse of proximal or distal stent segment seen as continuous half-circle by IVUS.
5. Collapse of the stent seen as a metallic mass by IVUS.
6. Longitudinal stent collapse or elongation like an accordion.
7. Unraveling of a coil stent to become a metallic string.

stent, it looks like a metallic half-circle without signs of struts on the opposite side. A stent can be deformed after a patient has received cardio-pulmonary resuscitation (CPR) due to direct force from chest compression. Once the patient survives a cardiac arrest, the integrity of a stent should be checked.[27]

PERFECT STENTING IN THE ERA OF DRUG-ELUTING STENTS

With more improvements in technology and more operator experience, procedural success has been achieved in more than 99% of patients undergoing more complex PCI, with a low complication rate (less than 1–2%). To achieve these results, the important take-home message is summarized below.

TAKE-HOME MESSAGE

Basic preparations:

1. Perfect the first try anterior wall puncture of the femoral artery so there is no posterior hematoma and no retroperitoneal hemorrhage. Perfect the first try puncture of the radial artery.
2. Optimal anticoagulation with ACT of 250 to decrease bleeding complications.
3. Prior administration of oral or intravenous antiplatelet agents to prevent thrombotic complications in the coronary artery system.
4. Generous blood return after insertion of the guide to remove any atherosclerotic debris or thrombus in order to avoid any emboli-related complications.
5. Gentle and coaxial intubation of the coronary ostium, especially the left main, to avoid any ostial dissection.

Coronary interventions:

6. Gentle advancement of interventional hardware to avoid provoking any spasm or intimal injury, which are the nidus for thrombotic formation.
7. Underdilate the lesion and stent it with optimal pressure and dimension so there is no direct stenting due to concerns of mechanical stress and prolonged blood exposure during excessive manipulation for a perfect position.[28]
8. Handle the stent gently in order to avoid cracking and flaking of the coating layer caused by mechanical stress on the stent during unpacking and delivery. Furthermore, the stent should be placed rapidly in the coronary system. Losses to the blood lipids may occur

during the brief (30 seconds) exposure to the coronary circulation before deployment.[28]

9. The DES should encompass the lesion, the two ends of plaque shifting, and the area injured by the predilating balloon.
10. The stent struts should be apposed well into the vessel wall so the drug can be absorbed and so inhibits the intimal hyperplasia.
11. Avoid causing damage to the endothelium in the proximal segment by interventional hardware during transit.
12. Avoid causing dissection and have all the equipment available if dissection happens. Ensure prompt redilation with the balloon or sealing the entry and exit of the dissecting segment with stent.
13. Achieve an optimal lumen reconstruction by QCA with a good TIMI-3 flow to have the lowest rate of restenosis.

Post-procedure care and follow-up:

14. Femoral or radial sheath to be removed as soon as possible.
15. Good groin compression and follow-up to prevent any hematoma.
16. Watch for late (24–48 hours) renal failure in elderly patients.

REFERENCES

1. Feldman T. Tricks to overcome difficult stent delivery. *Cathet Cardiovasc Interv* 1999; **48**: 285–6.
2. Colombo A, Stankovic G. Cutting balloon angioplasty: Areas of application. In: Colombo A, Stankovic G, eds *Colombo's Tips and Tricks in Interventional Cardiology.* Martin Dunitz, 2002: 29.
3. Fujise K, Ganim M, Floyd D *et al.* Bubble at the tip of the stent delivery system of the PS stent improves trackability to the target site. *Cathet Cardiovasc Diagn* 1998; **43**: 108–10.
4. Fernandez V, Kaluza G, Godlewski B *et al.* Novel technique for stent delivery in tortuous coronary arteries: Report of 3 cases. *Cathet Cardiovasc Interv* 2002; **55**: 485–90.
5. Saucedo JF, Muller DW, Moscucci M. Facilitated advancement of the PS stent delivery system with the use of an adjacent 0.01 stiff wire. *Cathet Cardiovasc Diagn* 1996; **39**: 106–10.
6. Feldman T. Bent stents: A crooked stick to walk a crooked mile. *Cathet Cardiovasc Diagn* 1998; **44**: 345.

7. Lowell BH. Push-pull angioplasty: ACE balloon-facilitated stent passage technique. *Cathet Cardiovasc Interv* 1999; **48**: 93–5.

8. Chevalier B, Royer T, Guyon P *et al*. Predictive factors of direct stenting failure in a single center of 1500 patients. *J Am Coll Cardiol* 2000; **2** (Suppl A): 89A.

9. Marco J, Touati C, Chevalier B. Direct stenting. In: Fajadet J, ed. *Syllabus for EuroPCR*, 2001.

10. Zellner C, Sweeney JP, Ko E *et al*. Use of balloon ultrasound in evaluating repeated balloon rupture during coronary stenting. *Cathet Cardiovasc Diagn* 1997; **40**: 52–4.

11. Honda Y, Yock CA, Fitzgerald PJ. Impact of residual plaque burden on clinical outcomes of coronary interventions. *Cathet Cardiovasc Interv* 1999; **46**: 265–76.

12. Keelan ET, Nunez BD, Berger P *et al*. Management of balloon rupture during rigid stent deployment. *Cathet Cardiovasc Diagn* 1995; **35**: 211–15.

13. Esente P, Giambartolemei A, Reger MJ *et al*. Extensive coronary dissection caused by balloon rupture at high pressure during stent deployment. *Cathet Cardiovasc Diagn* 1996; **38**: 263–5.

14. Antonnellis J. How to avoid having a stent mounted on a ruptured balloon in a coronary artery. Letter to the editor. *Cathet Cardiovasc Diagn* 1996; **38**: 102–3.

15. Sunew J, Chandwaney R, Stein D *et al*. Excimer laser facilitated PCI of a non-dilatable coronary stent. *Cathet Cardiovasc Interv* 2001; **53**: 513–17.

16. Mendzelevski B, Sigwart U. Rupture of coronary artery and cardiac tamponade complicating Wallstent implantation. *Cathet Cardiovasc Diagn* 1997; **40**: 368–71.

17. Philips PS, Kern M, Serruys PW. *The Stenter's Notebook*. Physicians Press, 1998: 171.

18. Abernethy W, Choo JK, Oesterle S *et al*. Balloon deflection technique: A method to facilitate entry of balloon catheter into a deployed stent. *Cathet Cardiovasc Interv* 2000; **51**: 312–19.

19. Grantham J, Tiede D, Holmes D. Technical considerations when intervening with coronary devices in the vicinity of previously deployed stents. *Cathet Cardiovasc Interv* 2001; **52**: 214–7.

20. Sattler L, Pichard A, Kent K. Guidelines for repeat PCI in patients with previously deployed stents. *Cathet Cardiovasc Interv* 2001; **52**: 218–19.

21. Ormiston JA, Webster MW, Ruygrok PN *et al*. Stent deformation following simulated side-branch dilatation: A comparison of five stent designs. *Cathet Cardiovasc Interv* 1999; **47**: 258–64.

22. Hongo R, Brent B. Cutting balloon angioplasty through the stents struts of a "jailed" sidebranch ostial lesion. *J Invasive Cardiol* 2002; **14**: 558–60.

23. Chan AW, Lohavanichbutr K, Carere RG *et al*. Balloon entrapment during side-branch angioplasty through a stent. *Cathet Cardiovasc Interv* 1999; **46**: 202–4.

24. Sasseen B, Burke J, Shah R. *et al*. IVUS catheter entrapment after coronary stenting. *Cathet Cardiovasc Interv* 2002; **57**: 229–33.

25. Hiro T, Leung CY, Russo RJ *et al*. Intravascular ultrasound identification of stent entrapment *in vivo* and *in vitro* confirmation. *Cathet Cardiovasc Diagn* 1997; **40**: 40–45.

26. Pomerantz RM, Ling F. Distortion of PS stent geometry following side-branch balloon dilation through the stent in a rabbit model. *Cathet Cardiovasc Diagn* 1997; **40**: 422–26.

27. Windecker S, Maier W, Eberli F *et al*. Mechanical compression of coronary stents: Potential hazard for patients undergoing cardiopulmonary resuscitation. *Cathet Cardiovasc Interv* 2000; **51**: 464–7.

28. Regar E, Degertekin M, Tanabe K *et al*. Drug Eluting Stent. In: Marco J, Serruys P, Biamino G *et al*., eds. *Syllabus of The Paris Course on Revascularization* 2003: 265–82.

29. Weisz G, Moses J, Popma J *et al*. Do overlapping multiple sirolimus-eluting stent impact angiographic and clinical outcomes? Insight from the SIRIUS trial. *J Am Coll Cardiol* 2003; **6**: 33A.

Chapter 8
High-risk Patients

Thach Nguyen, Nithi Mahanonda, Sarana Boonbaichaiyapruck

From: Nguyen T, Hu D, Saito S, Grines C, Palacios I (eds), *Practical Handbook of Advanced Interventional Cardiology*, 2nd edn. © 2003 Futura, an imprint of Blackwell Publishing.

EVALUATION OF HIGH-RISK PATIENTS

High risk is defined as the probability and, more importantly, the consequence of abrupt closure of the dilated site, occlusion of large side or distal branches or widespread microvascular obstruction with spasm.

Abrupt closure of a large epicardial artery or of a side or distal branch is recognized by standard angiogram while occlusion at the microvascular level is seen as slow flow or no-reflow secondary to showers of atheromatous material from ruptured plaques. Their immediate clinical presentation and long-term outcome is determined by the amount of myocardium in jeopardy and the degree of myocardial reserve. The treatment for abrupt closure at the epicardial artery is mainly by prompt stenting. However, the preventive measures of occlusion at the distal branches and at the microvascular level may require deployment of embolic protection devices. The ultimate goals are to preserve the patency of the coronary arteries and the systolic function of both right and left ventricle, and to prevent negative localized or global ventricular remodeling.

In general, as the patients undergoing percutaneous coronary interventions (PCI) are older and present to the hospital sicker, they are more vulnerable even with short episodes of ischemia or worse when there is irreversible acute closure due to extensive dissection or refractory thrombus. To facilitate short- and long-term success of PCI in complex lesions, the rationale to justify the procedure and strategies to achieve clinical and procedural goals includes:

1. identify clinical and angiographic features of complex PCI
2. determine the appropriateness of complex PCI compared to alternative therapies such as open heart surgery (CABG) and
3. formulate a strategy that maximizes immediate and long-term success.[1]

The clinical risk factors predicting in-hospital mortality and morbidity are listed in Table 8-1.[2] The most important factor is severe left ventricular (LV) dysfunction. However, the risk of acute periprocedural closure depends on the high complexity of lesion morphology (left main disease, angulation >45°, lesions with thrombus, long lesion, bifurcation lesion, multiple vessel with multiple lesions) and the suboptimal results of PCI.

As a result of acute closure of the dilated artery, the most common presentation prior to fatality is profound cardiogenic shock. The predisposing risk factors for shock are listed in Table 8-2. The factors associated with abrupt closure are mostly lesion-based. In contrast, the factors associated with

Table 8-1
Clinical and anatomical predictors of mortality and morbidity following acute closure

1. Left ventricular ejection fraction <40%
2. Creatinine >1.5
3. Diabetes mellitus
4. Triple vessel disease
5. Age >70
6. Acute coronary syndrome
7. Female gender

Table 8-2
High risk of shock if acute occlusion of target vessel

1. Left ventricular dysfunction (ejection fraction <30%)
2. Target vessel supplying more than 50% viable myocardium
3. Circulation to both papillary muscles compromised
4. High jeopardy score (>3)

shock and/or mortality are mostly patient-based, reflecting the poor ventricular function and greater extent of coronary artery disease.

The jeopardy scoring system is used to assess the hemodynamic importance of the culprit lesion occlusion. The coronary tree is divided into six segments of myocardial perfusion. Half a point is given for each myocardial region with baseline hypokinesis and not supplied by a vessel with significant lesion. One point is given for each myocardial region supplied by the artery with lesion of >70% diameter stenosis. One point is also given to the target vessel area. The jeopardy score is the total of all the scores from the six areas, with a maximum of six. The risk of procedure mortality begins with a score above 2.5 and increases as the total score rises.[3]

When performing interventions in complex lesions, more complications must be anticipated. Should disaster occur, the management approach should already be identified and all the mechanisms set in place and put in motion as planned.[4] In the case of acute closure, a stable blood pressure is very important to secure survival. Lower blood pressure correlates with higher risk of death.[5] Thus, every attempt has to be made to keep a decent blood pressure while the patient undergoes cardiopulmonary resuscitation (CPR) or emergent measures to reopen the artery with a perfusion balloon or stent are taken. An important take-home message for PCI of complex lesions in high-risk patients is summarized below.[4]

TAKE-HOME MESSAGE

Strategies for complex and high-risk lesion PCI:

1. Over-prepare for the possibility of a complication. Rehearse the scripted case strategy
2. Attention to the general factors: controlled diabetes, enough hydration to optimize renal function, lower use of contrast, etc.
3. Early and appropriate use of antiplatelet agents
4. Hemodynamic support (IABP) for hypotension or LV dysfunction
5. Meticulous access site management
6. Necessary and adequate sedation and anesthesia
7. Conservative equipment selection (larger guide, rotational atherectomy only if necessary)
8. Short procedure
9. Accept less than perfect results when benefits/risk unfavorable
10. Stop when appropriate before disaster, always favor safety over completion of procedure
11. Obsessive post-procedural care
12. Early follow-up angiography for selected group of patients (e.g. LM disease)

MODIFYING THE RISK FACTORS

LV dysfunction is the most important predictor of immediate and long-term survival in patients with CAD. Ejection fraction less than 30% and a target vessel supplying more than 50% of the remaining viable myocardium are considered high-risk factors for mortality and severe morbidity if there is acute occlusion of the target vessel.[6] The mortality of these patients ranges between 12% and 33%. Therefore, optimal medical management and fluid status, stabilization of decompensated congestive heart failure and unstable angina symptoms plus surgical consultation prior to PCI are needed. There is an absolute need to minimize the impact of peri-procedural ischemia by using short inflation time, or using a perfusion balloon. PCI in lesion of an artery providing collaterals should be efficient, thus avoiding ischemia in far-away areas. A cautious approach should be exercised in PCI of lesions that can cause slow flow or no-reflow (lesion with thrombus, large bulky atheromatous lesion, degenerated vein graft, etc.). In patients with significant baseline LV dysfunction, liberal use of right heart pressure monitoring, inotropic support, and IABP are suggested.

LEFT VENTRICULAR DYSFUNCTION

Right heart pressure evaluation and monitoring: While undergoing complex coronary interventions, all patients, especially those with LV dysfunction and renal insufficiency, need adequate hydration to sustain a stable coronary and renal perfusion pressure. Monitoring the pulmonary capillary wedge pressure (PCWP) prior to intervention helps to optimize fluid management without provoking congestive heart failure and pulmonary edema, and is also a powerful adjunct for procedure planning. In some cases, with an elevated PCWP, the procedure may be deferred to allow time for clinical optimization by medical therapy. These patients may benefit from IABP support. Those with low cardiac output should be treated with afterload reduction or inotropic support during intervention.

Intra-aortic balloon pump: The most common strategy to support LV dysfunction during complex coronary intervention is diastolic counterpulsation by IABP. Its mechanism is to increase the diastolic pressure and, hence, the diastolic coronary perfusion. With inflation of a 40-cc balloon to coincide with the closure of the aortic valve, IABP increases the cardiac output by roughly 30%. The indications for insertion of IABP prior to PCI are listed in Table 8-3. In patients with LVEF <25% with stable BP >100 mmHg and PCWP <20 mmHg, IABP standby is suggested.[7] After the patients successfully undergo the complex procedures, IABP can be removed. In some cases it is useful to continue IABP support on the day after the procedure. This strategy can be followed if the ventricular function is severely depressed, filling pressure is elevated, or PCI results are suboptimal. When the PCWPs are adequate after the procedure, and the PCI results are good, balloon pump support may be discontinued prior to transfer out of the catheterization laboratory. Femoral closure with an arteriotomy closure device makes this approach very practical.

Options for extremely high-risk patients: In general, there are many patients with complex lesions on top of severe LV dysfunction, for whom the temptation of PCI should be resisted under normal circumstances (Table 8-4). However, as the left ventricular assist device (LVAD) is more available and

---

Table 8-3
Indications for insertion of IABP prior to PCI: EF <25% and

---

1. Target vessel supplying the majority of viable myocardium
2. Jeopardy score >3
3. Abnormal resting hemodynamics (low BP <100 mmHg with high PCWP >20 mmHg)
4. Cardiogenic shock and multivessel disease

Table 8-4
PCI should be refused: EF <20% and:[10]

1. PCI to the only patent vessel (especially SVG)
2. Use of rotational atherectomy
3. Complex lesion morphology (e.g. in no-option patients, in degenerated SVG, thrombus contained lesion, etc.)
4. Unstable hemodynamics with decompensated CHF, severe pulmonary hypertension
5. Not an ideal anatomy for stenting

refined, some patients could have PCI while under support of the LVAD and, after successful PCI, could be weaned off the LVAD.[8] Other patients could undergo PCI while having retrograde perfusion via a new investigational device, selective coronary sinus retroinfusion and suction by the Myoprotect SSR device (PTC, Moeling , Austria).[9]

ACUTE CORONARY SYNDROMES

In general, patients with ACS having continued, recurrent, or refractory angina should be referred for coronary angiography PCI because 1–5% will die and 2–10% will progress to MI if PCI is not offered before hospital discharge.[11] In the past, compared with medical treatment, PCIs in these patients were laden with complications. Many of these problems were related to the presence of intracoronary thrombus, the hypercoagulable state triggered by ruptured complex plaque. Complications used to be 3–5% for Q-wave myocardial infarction, 2–3% for emergency bypass surgery, and 5–10% for abrupt closure. At this present time, prompt stenting effectively reversed the problem with abrupt closure. Effective antiplatelet drugs have had a dramatic effect in stabilizing patients prior to intervention and diminishing peri-procedural events. The Evaluation of 7E3 for the Prevention of Ischemic Complication (EPIC) and the Evaluation in PTCA to Improve Long-term Outcome with abciximab GP 2b3a blockade (EPILOG) trials confirmed the clinical benefit of platelet inhibition in acute coronary syndromes.[12]

EVIDENCE-BASED MEDICINE APPLICATIONS

The EPIC trial: This trial was designed to examine the safety and efficacy of abciximab in high-risk patients undergoing balloon angioplasty (PTCA) or directional coronary atherectomy (DCA). The patients were defined as high-risk if they were undergoing primary or rescue angioplasty for acute myocardial infarction (MI), had unstable or post-infarction angina, or had other high-risk clinical and/or morphologic characteristics. The most important 30-day finding was the statistically significant 35% primary end-point reduction in the bolus and infusion group compared with placebo group (8.3% vs 12.8%, P=0.008). The benefits were largely manifested in prevention of MI and the need for urgent intervention. The major drawback of this regimen (bolus + infusion) was a doubling in the rate of major bleeding in the vascular access site (14% vs 7%, P=0.001) and transfusions (15% vs 7%, P= <0.001).

At the 3-year follow-up, the benefit still persisted, with 13% reduction in the composite end-points of MI, death, and TLR (41% vs 47%, P= 0.009).[13] The difference was driven by a 21% reduction in MI, and 13% reduction in revascularization. Compared with placebo, a significant 60% mortality benefit was noted in the subgroup presenting with evolving MI or unstable angina (5.1% vs 12.7%), while no mortality difference was seen in the remainder of the group (7.4% vs 7.2%, P=0.91).[13]

The EPILOG trial: In this trial, the goal was to evaluate the efficacy and safety of abciximab in low- and high-risk patients. In addition, to decrease the bleeding complication, heparin was used with standard dose for an activated clotting time (ACT) >300 seconds or lower dose of heparin (70 units/kg) to achieve an ACT of >200 seconds. At 30 days, the treatment resulted in a 56% reduction of combined end-points MI, death, and target vessel revascularization when compared with placebo (5% vs 11%, P=0.001). This low event rate of 5% was previously observed only after interventions for patients with stable angina.[14] The reduced dose of heparin did not compromise the clinical efficacy but, combined with earlier sheath removal, did result in elimination of excess bleeding. The lower heparin dose (70 units/kg) becomes the standard dose in today's PCI.

The majority of the benefit of glycoprotein 2b3a inhibitors is due to the reduction of MI, especially the non-Q wave MI (3.8%), (defined as CK-MB >5 × normal) and urgent coronary artery bypass surgery (CABG) (0%).[13] While the late mortality correlated with the level of peri-procedural CK elevation, the EPIC trial is the first trial to demonstrate that a pharmacologic intervention that reduced peri-procedural MI could translate into improved late survival.[14] However, glycoprotein 2b3a inhibitors are beneficial when given prior to the procedure in patients with high risk of ischemia caused by thrombus formation. They did not improve the outcomes in low-risk patients (type A lesions), or in procedures with mechanical difficulty (chronic total obstruction), or heavy atheromatous burden with high possibility of distal debris embolization (degenerated saphenous vein graft (SVG).[15]

RENAL INSUFFICIENCY

Acute renal failure (ARF) after PCI is defined as an increase of creatinine level of >0.5 mg/dL or 25% from baseline. The incidence was 3.3%. Among patients with creatinine level <2 mg/dL, the risk of ARF was higher in diabetic than in non-diabetic patients whereas all patients with baseline creatinine level >2.0 mg/dL had significant risk of ARF. Twenty percent of patients with ARF died during the index hospitalization compared with 1.5% without ARF. The risk factors for contrast-induced ARF are listed in Table 8-5.[16]

Risk factor modification: These patients should be hydrated before and after the interventional procedure with normal saline for 12 hours (100 mL/hour) to maintain a urine output of 40–60 cc/hr. The diabetic patients with borderline renal insufficiency (creatinine above 1.7–2.0 mg/dL) would benefit well from this strategy. In unstable patients, it is helpful to use the pulmonary capillary wedge pressure to guide hydration, thus avoiding precipitation of pulmonary edema, because many patients with renal insufficiency have concurrent LV dysfunction. Supplemental loop diuretics are used to prevent pulmonary congestion and facilitate the excretion of contrast agent, even if they do not prevent worsening of renal function,[17] so judicious use of the smallest amount possible of contrast media is critical. A low dose of contrast agent has been variably defined as <70 mL, <125 mL or <5 mL/kg (to a maximum of 300 mL), divided by the plasma creatinine concentration.[18] No patient who received <100 mL of contrast was found to develop renal failure.[19] The average amount of contrast agent for a coronary angiography was 130 mL and it was 191 mL for a PCI.[20] A volume of 140 mL was identified is

---

Table 8-5
Risk factors for contrast-induced nephropathy

---

1. Confirmed factors:

a. Creatinine level >1.5 mg%
b. Diabetic nephropathy
c. Class III or IV congestive heart failure
d. Multiple myeloma
e. Contrast media
f. Repeat contrast injection in <48 hours

---

2. Suspected factors

a. Hypertension
b. Abnormal liver function test
c. Increased age
d. Gender
e. Concomitant use of loop diuretics

---

the cut-off value predicting the occurrence of contrast-media associated nephropathy.[21] There are no convincing data that low-osmolarity contrast agents are less nephrotoxic.[22] These patients should avoid the nonsteroidal anti-inflammatory drugs. Angiotensin-converting enzyme (ACE) inhibitors must be used cautiously since coexistent renal artery stenosis is common in these patients. In a small, single-center, random-ized trial, oral acetylcysteine was given 600 mg BID for 2 days prior to CT scanning with 75 cc of bolus contrast. It was com-pared with plain intravenous hydration. The results showed a 21% incidence of ARF in the hydration group compared with 2% in the acetylcysteine group.[23] However, there was only a small but significant decrease of serum creatinine level at 48 hours. Other subsequent trials did not show consistent incre-mental benefits of acetylcysteine.[21] Further analysis showed a trend of worse outcomes in patients receiving more than 140 cc of contrast compared with patients receiving a lesser amount. It would be anticipated that if an effective agent were identified to prevent ARF, its effect would be amplified with higher risk states – including exposure to higher doses of contrast – rather than the opposite effect.[24] Fenoldopam is a selective dopamine-1 (DA1) receptor agonist that acts to increase renal blood flow and prevent shunting of blood flow from the medulla to the cortex. It was tried on animal models and in small, single-center retrospective human studies or prospective studies with comparison to historical controls.[25] The data are promising but unproven as yet. The strategies to reduce contrast-induced nephropathy are listed in Table 8-6.

About 0.4% of patients will need acute hemodialysis due to ARF after PCI. Although the likelihood of ARF that requires emergency hemodialysis after PCI is low, it is associated with high in-hospital and one-year mortality, and 23% of these patients will require permanent dialysis.[26]

Table 8-6
Strategies for reducing contrast-induced nephropathy

1. Confirmed

a. Minimal contrast (use 5 cc syringe to inject)
b. Saline infusion

2. Investigative

a. Mucomyst (acetyl cysteine) (not working)
b. Fenoldopam

3. Not effective

a. Dopamine
b. Mannitol
c. Loop diuretic

Stents should be used liberally to shorten procedural time and achieve stable acute results. Intravascular ultrasound (IVUS) can be used to monitor the procedure. A variety of adjuncts such as the guidewire with interval markers with digital road-mapping can help in positioning stents or balloons. All of these efforts are to minimize the amount of contrast agent used during the procedure. There is of course no risk of nephrotoxicity in patients already on dialysis, though volume overload should not be overlooked. While patients with chronic renal failure could have high acute procedural success, their long-term outcome is still poor compared with patients without renal failure.[27]

MULTIVESSEL DISEASE: DILATION STRATEGY

Not every lesion needs revascularization because it is too distal, located in a small branch or in completed infarct areas. For patients with significant multivessel disease, there are safety concerns, rationale for indications, principles and strategies guiding the performance of their PCI. They are listed in Table 8-7.

The main strategy: The main strategy of performing high-risk PCI in patients with MVD is to identify, between all the arteries, with or without lesions, which one is essential

---

Table 8-7
Principles and strategies guiding the performance of PCI in MVD

1. Pre-procedure evaluation

a. Solid indications
b. Comprehensive evaluation of risks
c. Practical assessment of chance of success

2. Strategy for safe and successful procedures

a. Stratify the significance of contribution of each lesion in the maintenance of blood pressure
b. Perform PCI *first* on the artery that is not *essential* in maintaining a decent blood pressure

3. Procedural tactics for safety and success

a. Setting up with good rationale the sequential order of lesions to be dilated
b. Constant monitoring of the progress and safety of the procedure
c. Detecting early signs of hemodynamic instability
d. Dilating the first lesion: the challenging first minute
e. Transforming high-risk MVD PCI into simpler PCI

or non-essential in preserving adequate LV contractility and decent blood pressure – in other words, which one is sustaining life. Performing PCI first on the lesion of the artery that is not vital in maintaining decent blood pressure would offer a safe and *best* strategy. The reason is that during PCI of an artery with severe lesion which *does not* contribute to the maintenance of a decent BP, in the case of acute occlusion of that dilated artery, a decent blood pressure is still maintained. Looking at the other side of this coin (the main strategy), there are lesions to watch for that are located in strategic locations where occlusion of these lesions could bring persistent hypotension, shock and mortality. Different tactics in evaluation of lesions and patients by clinical, non-invasive and invasive methods will be discussed and case reports to illustrate this strategy will be presented.

TECHNICAL TIPS

CAVEAT: The lesions that bring catastrophe: During PCI, if there is acute occlusion of the target lesion, the worst catastrophe is persistent shock leading to mortality. The cause of shock is refractory right and left heart failure, aggravated by the infarction of the papillary muscles, triggering acute mitral regurgitation. Other mishaps include persistent complete heart block or right ventricular infarction. Certainly, these complications can happen and are non-lethal in patients with good LV function. However, nowadays, many high-risk patients undergoing PCI have poor LV function. They are more vulnerable to any ischemic challenge and any mildly prolonged low diastolic blood pressure that decreases coronary perfusion. So during PCI of these lesions, the operators should be aware of these possible complications in order to prevent them, suspect their appearance at the earliest opportunity, and reverse their course before they become severe. The list of these lesions in strategic locations can be found in Table 8-8.

**Lesions that are possibly safe to be dilated first: There are many situations where the main strategy of dilating first the lesions that are non-essential for maintaining a decent blood pressure can be applied. In patients with arteries connected by collaterals, it is best to perform PCI on the lesion of the recipient artery, unless the collaterals are minimal. The reason is that acute occlusion of the artery that supplies the collateral can cause remote ischemia and infarction in the recipient artery.[28] PCI of the stenosis on the supplying artery can be done only if the first PCI was successful, with disappearance or reversal of collaterals. In patients with ACS, it is rationally sound to perform PCI first on the culprit lesion. In patients with AMI, it is now accepted to dilate the acute occlusion lesion, even without surgical

Table 8-8
Lesions in strategic locations with possible catastrophic complications

1	Proximal RCA	Large amount of myocardium in jeopardy
		Closure of sinus node artery causing complete heart block
		Closure of PDA causing acute mitral regurgitation
		Persistent right ventricular infarction
2	Proximal LAD	Large amount of myocardium in jeopardy
		Closure of diagonal causing acute mitral regurgitation
3	Sinus node artery	Complete heart block
4	First diagonal	Acute mitral regurgitation due to ischemia or infarction of the antero-lateral papillary muscle
5	First OM (left dominant)	Acute mitral regurgitation due to ischemia or infarction of the postero-medial papillary muscle
6	Left ventricular branch (right dominance)	Acute mitral regurgitation due to ischemia or infarction of the postero-medial papillary muscle
7	PDA of RCA and postero-lateral branch of the LCX (dual dominance)	Acute mitral regurgitation due to ischemia or infarction of the postero-medial papillary muscle

stand-by. In patients with stable angina, performing PCI first on the lesion of the artery that is not vital in maintaining decent blood pressure is the best and safest strategy. In patients with subtotal ostial RCA, if cannulation of the RCA by a diagnostic catheter is causing ventricularization of the pressure, then PCI of the RCA seems to be safe because the RCA may not contribute much to the maintenance of blood pressure (Table 8-9). In the patients with equally significant lesions in large arteries of equal size, without prior infarct, without any non-invasive imaging available, then there is no convincing rationale on a clinical basis for which lesion should be dilated first, except the one that is easier to be opened can be opened first ("hit and run" approach).

**Why these lesions are possibly benign, while others are unpredictable: In patients with an artery receiving collaterals, PCI of the recipient artery may not cause any

Table 8-9
The possible benign lesions to be dilated first

1. The lesion of artery receiving collaterals
2. The culprit lesion of non-Q AMI
3. The acute occlusion lesion in AMI
4. The lesion of old MI
5. The chronic total occlusion (CTO)
6. The subtotal ostial RCA
7. The lesions of small arteries

hemodynamic instability unless there is distal embolization cutting off the contralateral retrograde collateral flow. In patients with AMI, opening the acute occlusion may not cause any hemodynamic disturbance, unless there is transient vaso-vagal symptom, no-reflow or large distal embolization. The reason is that the patient did tolerate the acute occlusion and survive, so the transient occlusion of a balloon should not cause hypotension of catastrophic extent. It is the same rationale for ACS patients with elevated level of troponin, for patients with previous MI, CTO, or subtotal ostial RCA. Patients with stable angina (no previous MI) or unstable angina (without elevation of cardiac enzyme), have never experienced any transient acute occlusion, and the clinical reaction to any acute occlusion has not been tested. These patients also do not have ischemic preconditioning so their reactions are also unpredictable.

CAVEAT: The challenging first minute: When the balloon is inflated for the first time, during balloon occlusion, observe carefully the ECG and the symptomatic reaction of the patient. Marked ST-segment elevation, severe pain, malignant ectopy, hypotension, marked decrease of wire tip movement (distal hypokinesis) all portend a major adverse clinical event in case of acute vessel closure.[29] This is why the first inflation should be short, of lower pressure and the speed of inflation slow and gradual. The second inflation may bring fewer symptomatic reactions because of collateral recruitment and ischemic preconditioning. If the patient is symptomatic with the inflation, keep the inflation time short. The interval between the first and second inflation should be more than 2 minutes in order to trigger ischemic preconditioning.[30]

**How to identify the culprit lesion by ECG and angiographic findings: In any situation, a comprehensive evaluation should be done. The interventional cardiologists come to the bedside, examine the patient, review the history, assess the problems, discuss the risks and benefits. Usually the ECG would show some hints on the location of the lesion and the angiogram would pinpoint the culprit lesion that is subtotal and has haziness due to thrombus. The following case report illustrates this strategy.

Case report

Sequential dilation strategy guided by history, ECG and angiographic findings: A 73-year-old nurse with recurrent typical angina at rest had a coronary angiogram that showed severe lesion in the proximal and mid-LAD and proximal RCA. Both arteries were large, not tortuous, not too close to the ostium, and had no side branch involvement. Which one should be dilated first? There is a need to identify the culprit lesion and rationalize the sequential order of dilation. The ECG showed mild ST depression in 2,3,AVF so most likely the culprit lesion was in the RCA. The lesion in the RCA was subtotal with haziness suggestive of thrombus, a hallmark of unstable, fractured plaque. Even the lesion in the mid-LAD was tight, its borders were sharp, it was most likely a stable lesion. The patient underwent successfully PCI of the RCA first by direct stenting, followed without complication by POBA and stenting of the LAD lesions (Figure 8-1 A–D).

**How to assess the lesion by history and ECG – rationale for the dilation sequence: One way to guess the significance and severity of two lesions is to reconstruct

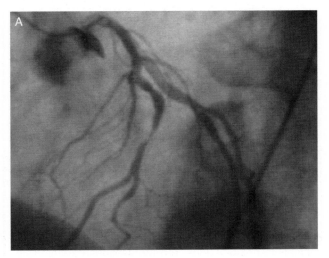

Figure 8-1: Rationale for dilating sequence in PCI of patient with two vessels disease. (A) The patient had a severe LAD lesion in this LAO cranial view. *(Continued)*

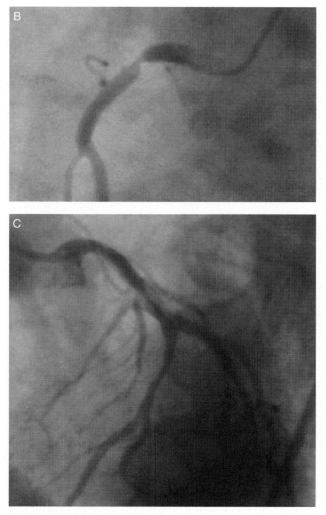

Figure 8-1 B,C: (B) The RCA had a subtotal lesion in its proximal segment. (C) After successful direct stenting of the RCA, the LAD lesion was predilated with undersized balloon. *(Continued)*

the historical sequence of symptoms which show the clinical stability of a significant older lesion (while patient had stable angina after an AMI) and the clinical destabilization by the appearance of a new lesion (patient now has unstable angina). If the first lesion was caused by myocardial

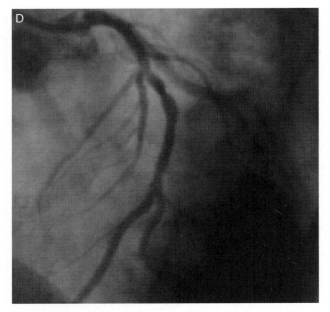

Figure 8-1 D: Successful stenting of the LAD.

infarction, then the artery containing the first lesion was not vital in maintaining a stable clinical condition and indirectly not responsible for the preservation of blood pressure. PCI of the first lesion is most likely safe. The following case report illustrates this strategy.

Case report

Sequential dilation of multiple lesions guided by history of old MI and ECG: An 80-year-old woman with unstable angina had a coronary angiogram that showed severe lesions in the proximal LAD and mid-RCA. Both were of type A. PCI should be technically easy and smooth for both lesions. Which one should be dilated first? In order to evaluate the contribution of each lesion to symptoms and the maintenance of blood pressure, a resting ECG was ordered and a detailed history was taken. The patient had an AMI 7 years ago, which was confirmed by Q wave in V leads. She had had stable angina since then, which means that the LAD lesion caused only stable angina, without much interference to the preservation of LV contraction or blood pressure. About 6 months prior to this hospitalization, she began to have symptoms of unstable angina with chest pain at low level of activities, chest pain at rest, more shortness of breath and more dizziness. Most likely the symptoms were caused by worsening of the lesion in the RCA that (without a lesion) most likely contributed the most to a stable clinical condition in the last 7 years and indirectly to the preservation of blood pressure. By this rationale, PCI was performed on the LAD lesion without causing any hypotension. Once it was successful, PCI of the RCA was done without technical difficulty. However, the patient developed chest pain, hypotension, elevation of ST segment in leads 2,3,AVF due to slow flow in the distal RCA. Coronary angiogram showed persistent patency of the newly stented segment with distal no-reflow. The patient recovered later with intracoronary vasodilators. In this case, clearly the RCA was the vessel that maintained a decent blood pressure. The rationale for PCI first in the LAD lesion was justified. If PCI had been performed in the RCA first, in the case of no-reflow without adequate blood supply from the left system, then severe low blood pressure with cardiogenic shock could have resulted, with possible fatality.

Non-invasive evaluation of lesions: In general, besides a comprehensive history in order to identify the culprit lesion and its contribution in maintaining a decent blood pressure, non-invasive studies (ECG, exercise stress testing, stress echocardiography, nuclear stress testing) can be done in order to identify objectively the culprit lesion, its compromised area and its extent of reversible ischemia, wall motion abnormality or ST segment change. Nuclear scan can also easily identify other areas with adequate perfusion at rest and under stress. Following this, PCI should be performed *first* in the area of ischemia, while adequate blood supply at rest to the other areas that maintain a decent blood pressure is assured by other patent arteries (Table 8-10).

Table 8-10
Identification of essential and non-essential arteries

---

1. Historical reconstruction of symptoms in order to identify the old stable diseased lesion versus the new clinically destabilizing lesion
2. Resting ECG for extent of Q wave or ST-T change
3. Nuclear scan for reversible ischemic change and extent of abnormal and normal areas
4. Cardiac enzyme measurements (CK-MB and troponin level)
5. Wall motion abnormality and its extent in stress echocardiography
6. Extent of ST segment depression during exercise stress testing
7. Pressure tracing showing ventricularization during cannulation of RCA ostial lesion by a diagnostic catheter

TECHNICAL TIP

CAVEAT: Deceiving nuclear scan: The main mechanism of a nuclear scan is to show a difference of isotope uptake between territories. If there is a dramatic change in one area, subtle changes in other areas may be missed. If there is diffuse disease, then there is not much difference between territories even where there are significant lesions. It is well known that a nuclear scan can look normal in patients with three-vessel disease because there is homogenous, diffuse and widespread decrease of blood flow at stress and at rest.

**Important meaning of ventricularization of pressure during diagnostic cannulation of the RCA ostial lesion: The combination of a subtotal ostial lesion and ventricularization of pressure by a diagnostic catheter might suggest the irrelevant contribution of that artery in maintaining blood pressure. The case report below illustrates that notion and the safety of performing PCI in this kind of subtotal ostial lesion.

Case report

Tactic during PCI of patient with subtotal ostial RCA and LM disease: A patient came to the emergency room with recurrent angina at rest. A coronary angiogram showed subtotal ostial lesion in the RCA and 50% lesion in the mid- and distal LM. Could the patient undergo safely PCI of the ostial RCA? The cardiac surgeon refused to do CABG surgery because the LM lesion seemed not severe enough to warrant surgery. During the diagnostic angiogram, cannulation of the RCA with severe ostial lesion by a 4F Judkins Right persistently caused decrease of systolic and diastolic blood pressure without any symptom. Because the patient was asymptomatic with occlusion of the RCA by a JR catheter, it seemed likely that PCI of the RCA would not cause any major hemodynamic and symptomatic disturbance. Convinced by this rationale, a long and complex PCI of the ostial lesion was successfully carried out without any decrease of blood pressure. Following the same strategy, recently another patient with severe ostial RCA and proximal LAD underwent successfully PCI of two vessels. Because the RCA seemed not to contribute much in maintaining blood pressure, the RCA lesion was dilated successfully and without problem; the lesion of the LAD was dilated next. This observation needs to be verified and confirmed in a larger number of cases (Figure 8-2 A–C).

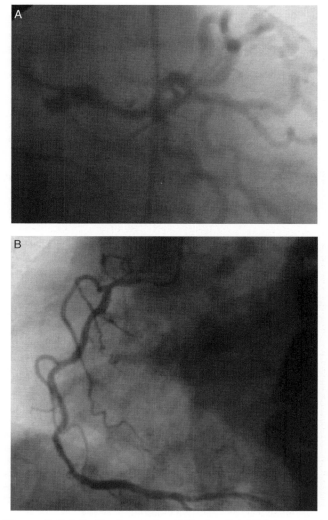

Figure 8-2 A,B: Tactics during PCI of ostial RCA in patient with LM disease. A patient presented with recurrent resting angina. The right angiogram showed subtotal ostial lesion. There was ventricularization of pressure every time the RCA was cannulated with a diagnostic 5F catheter. (A) There was a 50% lesion in the mid- and distal LM. (B) The RCA had a subtotal lesion in its ostium. *(Continued)*

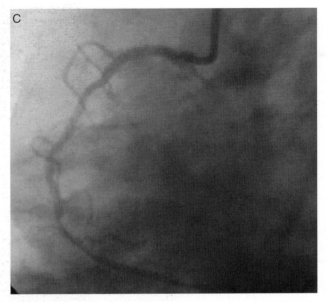

Figure 8-2 C: The patient underwent successful PCI of the ostial RCA without any hemodynamic disturbance.

**How to perform PCI in patients with ACS or AMI: In patients with non-Q AMI, opening the subtotal occlusion may not cause any hemodynamic disturbance, unless there is transient vaso-vagal symptom, no-reflow or large distal embolization. The reason is that the patient did tolerate the acute transient occlusion and survive, so the transient occlusion of a balloon should cause hypotension of catastrophic level. It is the same rationale for PCI in ACS patients with elevated level of troponin (non-Q MI). This rationale does not apply to ACS patients who do not have cardiac enzyme elevation (unstable angina). The case report below illustrates the rationale and tactics during PCI of these extremely high-risk patients.

Case report

PCI of the acutely transient total occlusion due to non-Q AMI: A patient came to the emergency room with chest pain, acute ST-segment elevation in V1-V4 and a blood pressure of 80–90 mmHg. When the patient arrived at the cardiac interventional laboratories, the pain subsided and the ECG changes were less prominent. However, the blood pressure was still in the region of 80–90 mmHg. The coronary angiogram showed old total occlusion of the RCA and LAD. The

LCX was acutely occluded with minimal collaterals to the distal segment. The LVEDP was 30 mmHg. After surgery was declined due to extreme high risk, the patient underwent successfully PCI of the mid-LCX with IABP, and pacemaker on standby. The lesion was predilated with an undersized balloon, then a full-size stent was successfully deployed. The tactic was that the balloon should be undersized so there was less chance for dissection and distal embolization. The first inflation was short (10 seconds), of lower pressure, and the speed of inflation slow and gradual. The goal was to open a channel for stent position (Figure 8-3 A–C).

**Do *not* close atrial septal defect and PCI at the same session: In a case report from Tomai *et al.* a patient had PCI of lesions in the LAD and LCX, then had closure of an atrial septal defect with an Amplatzer. After the procedure, the patient was transferred to the ICU. One hour later, the patient developed severe shortness of breath, rales, and pulmonary edema requiring intubation and mechanical ventilation. Slowly, 12 hours later, the patient recovered with medical treatment. The problem is that closure of ASD can cause abrupt increase in LV preload and myocardial oxygen consumption, on an LV with possible dysfunction from slow flow or no-reflow. The lesson is not to perform PCI at the same time as closure of ASD.[31]

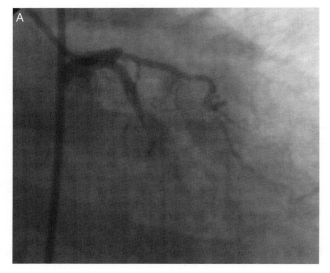

Figure 8-3: Strategy and tactics for PCI in patient with triple vessel disease and AMI. (A) The LAD was occluded at its ostium. It was seen as a stump. The LCX was acute occluded. Only a ramus intermedius was patent. *(Continued)*

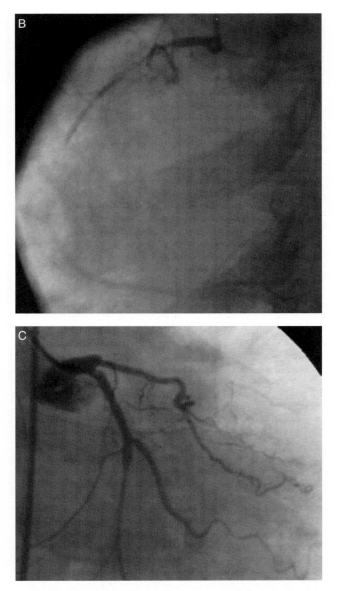

Figure 8-3 B,C: (B) The RCA was severely and diffusely diseased. (C) The LCX was predilated with balloon and successfully stented.

DIABETES MELLITUS

Diabetic patients are older, have more multiple vessel disease, and have other hematologic and metabolic factors with prothrombotic tendency, which frequently complicates the interventional procedure.[32] They have higher incidence of LV dysfunction, which can become more severe and result in hemodynamic collapse if the dilated artery is occluded. In addition to more acute complications, diabetics have significantly more late restenosis. When undergoing PCI, diabetic patients have more extensive atherosclerotic disease (more multiple vessel disease, prior MI, ACS, or peripheral vascular disease, etc.). Despite similar angiographic success, diabetic patients experience more in-hospital mortality and MI and poorer long-term survival.[33]

However, with the advent of DES, PCI for diabetic patients in the new era has a different meaning.

EVIDENCE-BASED MEDICINE APPLICATIONS

The Bypass and Angioplasty Revascularization Investigation (BARI) trial: In this trial, which randomized patients with multivessel disease between 1988 and 1991 (in the pre-stent era), the diabetic group had significantly worse 5-year mortality with angioplasty compared with surgery (35% vs 19%, respectively).[34] A recalculation of the BARI data showed the 5-year mortality of patients who had the left internal mammary artery (LIMA) graft was 13% compared with 45% in patients who received only saphenous vein grafts (SVGs).[35] At seven years, the benefits of CABG over PCI were more pronounced among patients with treated diabetes mellitus. There was no treatment difference among non-diabetic patients.[36]

One explanation for the difference of the BARI results is that surgery bypasses a series of lesions in one vessel and also bypasses the minor lesions which can become significant in the future. In contrast, PCI has to deal with every lesion individually. Many diabetics in this trial had poor glycemic control. However, with optimal diabetic control, as evidenced by an HbA1c of less than 7%, diabetic patients in the Scandinavian Simvastatin Survival study (4S) had the same mortality as the nondiabetic population.[37]

The effect of glycoprotein 2b3a inhibition in diabetic patients is proved from the pooled data of the PURSUIT, Gusto IV, and Paragon B trials. For diabetic patients with acute coronary syndrome, undergoing PCI, mortality was 1.2% compared with 4.2% in patients receiving placebo. For the first time, stenting strategy with adjunctive glycoprotein 2b3a therapy closes the gap between diabetic and nondiabetic patients with respect to 30-day mortality.[38–41]

Stenting results in better late outcomes than PTCA in diabetics, but a higher restenosis rate is still observed, compared with nondiabetic patients: 27% versus 22%, respectively.[42] The difference is in part due to unfavorable lesion characteristics of the diabetic patient population.[43] The most significant indicator for restenosis in diabetics is the small vessel size.[44] The diabetics had smaller coronary arteries by angiography. However, IVUS imaging showed similar absolute vessel size compared with nondiabetic patients. These observations confirmed the presence of a large plaque burden in the reference segments that cannot be detected by coronary angiography.[45]

EVIDENCE-BASED MEDICINE APPLICATIONS

Drug-Eluting Stent: The SIRollmUS-Eluting Stent in De Novo Native Coronary Lesions (SIRIUS) trial (diabetic subgroup): In this trial, 279 diabetic patients were randomized between bare and drug-coated stent (sirolimus, n = 131; control, n = 148), with an average lesion length of 14.5 mm and reference vessel size of 2.75 mm. For all clinical and angiographic indices, including late loss (in-stent and in-segment), restenosis (in-stent and in-segment), target lesion revascularization (TLR), and major adverse cardiac events (MACE), the difference between the two groups was highly significant in favor of the sirolimus group (P <0.001) compared with control. While the rate of restenosis and TLR are generally higher in diabetic patients, those treated with DES in the SIRIUS-Cypher stent had a 12-month MACE of 9.2%.[46]

EVIDENCE-BASED MEDICINE APPLICATIONS

Stenting or CABG in diabetic patients in the DES era: At the 52nd annual scientific meeting of the American College of Cardiology in April 2003, the results of the SIRIUS-Cypher stent were released and showed a 12-month MACE of 9.2% compared with 39.3% of the ARTS-Stent (bare stent) and 17.7% in the CABG branch of the ARTS trial. Practical applications with DES or surgery in patients with DM are suggested in Table 8-11.[47]

To confirm further the new gain of the DES in diabetic patients, the FREEDOM trial will enroll 2300 type II diabetic patients with multivessel disease, eligible for stent or surgery. These patients will be randomized between multivessel PCI with sirolimus-coated stent and abciximab and CABG with or without cardiopulmonary bypass (CPB). The end-points will be MACE/stroke at 12 months and 5-year mortality. The results will not be available until late 2004.[46]

Table 8-11
Practical applications for PCI and CABG in patients with DM

Factors favoring PCI

1. Lesions in large arteries (>3 mm)
2. Short, discrete lesion (<20 mm)
3. Double vessel disease rather than triple vessel disease
4. No albuminuria
5. Complete revascularization by PCI

Factors favoring CABG

1. Multivessel disease with LM disease
2. Long lesions (>20 mm) in small arteries (<3 mm)
3. Severe LV dysfunction
4. Single stenosis supplying >50% of viable myocardium
5. Diffuse disease

Aggressive and comprehensive medical management[48]

1. Tight glycemic control to achieve Hb A1c <7%
2. Blood pressure control to achieve BP <130/80
3. Control cholesterol to achieve LDL <100
4. ACE inhibition

REFERENCES

1. Davidson C, Ricciadi MJ. Complex Angioplasty. In: *Cardiac Catheterization and Interventional Cardiology Self Assessment Program*. American College of Cardiology, 2001: 53–8 .

2. Daniel WC, Lester SB, Jones P *et al*. Risk factors predicting in-hospital mortality following balloon angioplasty versus stenting. *J Am Coll Cardiol* 1999; **33** (Suppl A): 24A.

3. Califf RM, Philips HR *et al*. Prognostic value of a coronary artery jeopardy score. *J Am Coll Cardiol* 1988; **5**: 1055–63.

4. Ellis SG, Myler RK, King SB *et al*. Causes and correlates of death after unsupported coronary angioplasty: Implications for use of angioplasty and advanced support techniques in high risk settings. *Am J Cardiol* 1991; **68**: 1447–51.

5. Leon, M. *Complex Angioplasty*. Transcatheter Coronary Therapeutic Meeting, WDC, 2000.

6. Vogel RA, Shawl F, Tommaso C *et al*. Initial report of the national registry of the elective cardiopulmonary bypass supported coronary angioplasty. *J Am Coll Cardiol* 1990; **15**: 23–39.

7. Colombo A, Tobis J. The high risk patients. In: Colombo A, Tobis J, eds. *Techniques in Coronary Artery Stenting*. Martin Dunitz, 2000: 297–306.

8. Kollar A, Misra V, Pierson III R. Postoperative coronary revascularization on LVAD support for surgically inacces-

sible myocardial ischemia. *Cathet Cardiovasc Interv* 2002; **55**: 381–4.

9. Denk S, Syeda B, Beran G *et al*. Combined use of retrograde myocardial and distal coronary protection for last vessel intervention in an aorto-coronary vein graft. *Cathet Cardiovasc Interv* 2001; **54**: 342–5.

10. Shaw F. *When death is imminent*. Transcatheter Coronary Therapeutic Meeting, WDC, 2000.

11. Fragmin and Fast Revascularization during InStability in Coronary artery disease (FRISC II) Investigators. Long term low-molecular-mass heparin in unstable coronary artery disease: FRISC II prospective randomized multicentre study. *Lancet* 1999; **354**: 701–7.

12. Topol EJ, Ferguson JJ, Weisman HL *et al*. Long-term protection from myocardial ischemic events in a randomized trial of brief integrin beta3 blockade with PCI. *J Am Med Assoc* 1997; **278**: 479–84.

13. The EPILOG Investigators: Platelet glycoprotein IIb/IIIa receptors blockade and low dose heparin during percutaneous coronary revascularization. *N Engl J Med* 1997; **336**: 1689–1696.

14. The EPISTENT Investigators. Randomized placebo-controlled trial of platelet glycoprotein IIb-IIIa blockade with primary angioplasty in AMI. *Circulation* 1998; **98**: 734–741.

15. Ellis S. Elective coronary angioplasty: Techniques and complications. In: Topol, ed. *Textbook of Interventional Cardiology*, 3rd edition. WB Saunders, 1999.

16. Porter GA. Contrast medium-associated nephropathy: Recognition and management. *Invest Rad* 1993; **4**: 811–8.

17. Solomon R, Warner C, Mann D *et al*. Effects of saline, mannitol and furosemide on acute decreases in renal function induced by radiocontrast agents. *N Engl J Med* 1994; **331**: 1416–20.

18. Cigarroa RG, Lange RA, Williams RH *et al*. Dosing of contrast material to prevent contrast nephropathy in patients with renal disease. *Am J Med* 1989; **86**: 649–52.

19. McCullough PA, Wolyn R, Rocher LL *et al*. Acute renal failure after coronary intervention: Incidence, risk factors, and relationship to mortality. *Am J Med* 1997; **103**: 368–75.

20. Noto TJ, Johnson LE, Krone R *et al*. Cardiac catheterization 1990: a report of the registry of the Society for Cardiac Angiography and Interventions. *Cathet Cardiovasc Diagn* 1991; **24**: 75–83.

21. Briguori C, Manganelli F, Scarpato P *et al*. Acetylcysteine and contrast agent-associated nephropathy. *J Am Coll Cardiol* 2002; **40**: 298–303.

22. Mueller C, Buerkle G, Buettner HJ *et al*. Prevention of contrast media-associated nephropathy. *Arch Intern Med* 2002; **162**: 329–36.

23. Tepel M, van der Giet M, Scharzfeld C *et al*. Prevention of radiographic-contrast-agent-induced reductions in renal function by acetylcysteine. *N Engl J Med* 2000; **343**: 180–4.

24. Lepor N. A review of contemporary prevention strategies for radio-contrast nephropathy: A focus on Fenoldopam and N-acetylcysteine. *Rev Cardiovasc Med* 2003; **4** (Suppl 1): S15–S20.

25. Maydoon H. Clinical experience in the use of fenoldopam for prevention of radio-contrast nephropathy in highrisk patients. *Rev Cardiovasc Med* 2001; **2** (Suppl 1): S26–S30.

26. Rihal C, Textor S, Grill D *et al*. Incidence and prognostic importance of acute renal failure after percutaneous coronary intervention. *Circulation* 2002; **105**: 2259–64.

27. Gruberg L, Mehran R, Hong MK *et al*. Stents do not improve acute and long term clinical outcomes in patients with CRF and coronary diseases. *J Am Coll Cardiol* 1999; **33** (Suppl A): 28A.

28. Orford J, Fasseas P, Denkas A. *et al*. Anterior ischemia secondary to embolization of the posterior descending artery in a patient with CTO of the LAD. *J Invasive Cardiol* 2002; **14**: 527–30.

29. Meier B. Balloon angioplasty. In: Topol E, ed. *Textbook of Cardiovascular Medicine*. Lippincott-Raven Publishers, 1998: 1983.

30. Tanaka T, Oka Y, Tawara I *et al*. Effect of time interval between two balloon inflations on ischemic preconditioning during coronary angioplasty. *Cathet Cardiovasc Diagn* 1997; **42**: 263–67.

31. Tomai F, Gaspardone A, Pappa M. *et al*. Acute LV failure after transcatheter closure of a secundum ASD in a patient with CAD: A critical reappraisal. *Cathet Cardiovasc Interv* 2002; **55**: 97–9.

32. Stein B, Weintraub WS *et al*. Influence of diabetes mellitus on early and late outcome after percutaneous transluminal coronary angioplasty. *Circulation* 1995; **91**: 979–89.

33. Kip KE, Faxon DP, Deire KM *et al*. Coronary angioplasty in diabetic patients: The National Heart, Lung, and Blood Institute Percutaneous Transluminal Coronary Angioplasty Registry *Circulation* 1996; **94**: 1818.

34. The Bypass Angioplasty Revascularization Investigation (BARI) Investigators. Comparison of coronary bypass surgery with angioplasty in patients with multiple disease. *N Engl J Med* 1996; **335**: 217–25.

35. The Bypass Angioplasty Revascularization Investigation (BARI) Investigators. The influence of diabetes on 5-year mortality and morbidity in a randomized trial comparing angioplasty PTCA and bypass surgery (CABG) in patients with multivessel disease. *Circulation* 1997; **96**: 1761–9.

36. The BARI investigators seven-year outcome in the Bypass Angioplasty Revascularization Investigation (BARI) by

treatment and diabetic status. *J Am Coll Cardiol* 2000; **35**: 1122–9.

37. Haffner SM, Alexander CM, Cook TJ *et al*. Reduced coronary events in simvastatin treated patients with coronary artery disease and diabetes or impaired fasting glucose level. Subgroup analysis in the Scandinavian Simvastatin Survival study. *Ann Inter Med* 1999; **59**: 2661–7.

38. Roffi M, Chew DP, Mukherjee D *et al*. Platelet glycoprotein 2b3a inhibitors reduce mortality in diabetic patients with non-ST segment elevation acute coronary syndromes. *Circulation* 2001; **104**: 2767–71.

39. The PURSUIT Trial Investigators. Inhibition of platelet glycoprotein IIb/IIIa with eptifibatide in patients with acute coronary syndromes. *N Engl J Med* 1998; **338**: 436–43.

40. The Global Utilization of Streptokinase and t-PA for Occluded Coronary Arteries IV in Acute Coronary Syndrome (GUSTO-ACS) Investigators: Effects of glycoprotein 2B3A receptor blocker abciximab on outcome in patients with acute coronary syndromes without early coronary revascularization: the GUSTO-ACS randomized trial. *Lancet* 2001; **357**: 1905–14.

41. The PARAGON B Investigators. Randomized, placebo-controlled trial of tirated intravenous lamifiban for acute coronary syndromes. *Circulation* 2001; **105**: 316–21.

42. Navarro F, Iniguez A *et al*. Fate of conventional versus stenting angioplasty in diabetic patients (abstract). *Eur Heart J* 1998; **19**: 193.

43. Moussa I, DiMario C *et al*. Do patients with diabetes mellitus have an increased risk of restenosis after coronary stenting? A matched comparison to patients without diabetes (abstract). *Eur Heart J* 1998; **19**: 190.

44. Gregorio JD, Kobayashi N, Adamian M *et al*. A comparison of diabetics with restenosis to diabetics without restenosis. *J Am Coll Cardiol* 1999; **33** (Suppl 2): 82A.

45. Moussa I, Moses J, Wang X *et al*. Why do the coronary vessels in diabetics appear to be angiographically small? *J Am Coll Cardiol* 1999; **33** (Suppl 2): 78A.

46. Leon M. *The SIRIUS Trial*. Presented at the 52th Annual Scientific Meeting of the American College of Cardiology Meeting. Chicago, April 2003.

47. Loutfi M, Marco J. Particularities of percutaneous coronary revascularization in diabetic patients. In: Marco J, Serruys P, Biamino G *et al*. eds. *Syllabus for the Paris Course on Revascularization*, 2003: 173–91.

48. Chobanian A, Bakris G, Black H *et al*. The seventh report of the Joint National Committee on prevention, detection, evaluation and treatment of high blood pressure. *J Am Med Assoc* 2003; **289**: 2560–2571.

Chapter 9
Complex Lesions

Thach Nguyen, Cayi Lu, Shiwen Wang

---

*Basic; **Advanced; ***Rare, exotic, or investigational.

From: Nguyen T, Hu D, Saito S, Grines C, Palacios I (eds), *Practical Handbook of Advanced Interventional Cardiology*, 2nd edn. © 2003 Futura, an imprint of Blackwell Publishing.

**Selection of balloons
The RAVEL and SIRIUS trials

GENERAL OVERVIEW

In general, the decision to select a lesion for percutaneous coronary intervention (PCI) is predicated on the operator's assessment of his or her ability to safely treat the ischemia-producing lesion and achieve long-term patency and symptomatic relief.[1] With currently advanced technologies and appropriate selection of patients, the procedural success rate can be achieved in more than 95% of elective interventions. Compared with the early 1990s, PCI is more commonly attempted in lesions with prior stent, longer lesions, and smaller arteries. Abrupt closure was rare (1%), so was emergency coronary artery bypass graft surgery (CABG) (0.4%) and death (1.4%).[2] As many patients present with complex lesions with features predisposing to imperfect lumen reconstruction and complications, their intervention requires higher operational skills and level of experience, depends on non-balloon devices, and is time-consuming. Their long-term outcome may not parallel the acute success. In any case, the risk-benefit analysis should be cautiously assessed so the patient may be selected wisely for the best achievable short- and long-term results.[1] These lesion types and their problems are listed in Table 9-1.[3]

Table 9-1
Complex angiographic features

---

1. **Left main lesion:** large amount of myocardium in jeopardy
2. **Bifurcated lesions:** difficult to have perfect lumen reconstruction, high restenosis rate
3. **Ostial lesions:** late elastic recoil, difficult to find exact location of the ostium, retrograde embolization
4. **Saphenous vein graft lesions:** high risk of distal embolization and restenosis
5. **Angulated lesions:** difficult to have perfect lumen reconstruction and high risk of dissection or acute closure
6. **Long and diffuse lesions:** high risk of restenosis and no-reflow
7. **Heavily calcified lesions:** suboptimal lesion expansion and high risk of dissection
8. **Chronic total obstructions:** low success rate and high restenosis rate
9. **Small vessel:** high subacute occlusion and restenosis rate with stenting
10. **In-stent-restenosis:** recurrent restenosis after POBA, stenting, need brachytherapy (VBT)

Basic preprocedural analysis for success and complications

To facilitate the risk assessment of an interventional procedure, the coronary stenosis angiographic morphology was classified by the American Heart Association/American College of Cardiology Task Force.[4] In this classification schema, procedures of the type A lesions have high success rates and infrequent complications. In the type B lesions, if there is only one characteristic present, it is the type B1 lesion, which has a slight increase in the chance of complications. If two or more characteristics are present, this is the type B2 lesion and the predicted success rate drops to 75% with an approximately 10% chance of major complication.[4] The advent of stent and effective antiplatelet medications have lessened the predictive value of these characteristics.[5] Angiographic factors to be evaluated prior to intervention for procedural success are listed in Table 9-2.

New preprocedural model analysis

Extensive changes have occurred since the beginning of PCI, allowing treatment of more complex lesions with higher overall risk. A new classification schema was proposed and validated in a patient population reflecting current utilization practice (stenting in 64% and glycoprotein 2b-3a inhibitors in 41%).[5] The two major angiographic features that predict high mortality and complications are degenerated saphenous vein graft and nonchronic total occlusion (Table 9-3). The overall success rate was high at 95%, the mortality was low at 1%, and the rate for emergency CABG was 0.9%. These results were derived from outcomes at a major referral center of procedures performed by experienced operators who were assisted by another physician (even just a fellow-in-training) and had emergency help from senior partners if needed. These luxuries are not available in the real-world interventional laboratories where the practicing interventionalist performs the procedure alone, on a tight schedule. In performing interventions on patients with large ischemic burden, the strategy is not to cause prolonged ischemic time due to devices across the lesion, and to allow ample time for coronary perfusion between inflations. The new risk assessment schema is shown in Table 9-3.

LONG LESIONS

A long lesion is defined as a lesion of more than 20 mm in length. The rate of abrupt closure in long lesions may be as high as 6% and the rate of restenosis with bare stent increased up to 55%.[7] A number of factors may contribute to the increase of intimal hyperplasia, including: more metal causing an increase in foreign body reaction; and an unfavorable change in

Table 9-2
Evaluation of complexity prior to interventions[6]

Factors affecting the ability to access the lesion

Left main disease
Proximal tortuosity
Origin, size, and course of artery potentially influences guide selection, backup
Compliant vessel proximal to the target lesion (no calcification)
Non-critical lesions proximal to the target lesion
Presence of branches affecting wire passage

Factors affecting the ability to cross the lesion with a wire or a balloon

Degree of stenosis and length of lesion
Lesion morphology: eccentricity, thrombus, presence of calcium, complexity

Lesion characteristics that affect the outcome

Characteristics associated with increased incidence of dissection
Characteristics associated with increased incidence of thrombotic occlusion

Lesion characteristics that affect the reconstruction of a "perfect" lumen

Bifurcated lesions
Ostial lesion
Angulated lesions
Small vessel

Lesion or arterial characteristics associated with decreased ability to deliver a stent (in the case of emergency management of complication: dissection, perforation, acute closure, slow flow, etc.)

Diffuse disease
Severe calcification (stiff, non-accommodating channel)
Marked tortuosity or angulation

---

shear stress at the exit of the newly stented area following the straightening of the vessel.[7] Different options in the treatment of long lesion are listed in Table 9-4.

TECHNICAL TIP

Long or short balloons: Long balloons can dilate long lesions with one balloon placement rather than doing repeated inflations with a short balloon, thus avoiding plaque shifting and giving a better, smooth initial result. Dilating a

Table 9-3
New risk assessment schema

Risk factors

Strongest correlates	Non-chronic total occlusion Degenerated saphenous vein graft (SVG)
Moderately strong correlates	Length >10 mm Lumen irregularity Large filling defect Calcium + angle >45° Eccentric Severe calcification SVG age >10 years

Results

Highest risk	either of the strongest correlates
High risk	≥3 moderate correlates without strongest correlates
Moderate risk	1–2 moderate correlates without strongest correlates
Low risk	no risk factors

Table 9-4
Strategies of long lesion interventions

1. Pretreatment with antiplatelet agents
2. Ample use of intracoronary (IC) nitroglycerine to prevent distal vessel spasm
3. Avoid excessive particle embolization during rotablation
4. Avoid vessel-flow mismatch
5. Debulking prior to stenting
6. Drug-eluting stent
7. Brachytherapy (VBT)

long lesion with a short balloon can disrupt the plaque in multiple places and allow blood to enter the channel behind the plaque causing dissection. For long lesions located on bends, there is less occurrence of dissection with the use of a long balloon placed entirely around the bend.[8] The rate of restenosis, however, continues to be quite high in PCI of any long lesion.[7]

Rotational atherectomy was considered desirable for debulking long and superficially calcified lesion but it should be used with caution because of the large amount of atheromatous debris removed and released. It may cause excessive distal microembolization with subsequent no-reflow and ischemic events.[9]

The data from the New Approaches to Coronary Intervention (NACI) registry showed that each 1-mm increase in lesion length was associated with an increased relative risk of 1.014 (95% CI, 1.004–1.025) for target lesion revascularization (TLR) at 1 year.[10] With drug-eluting stent (DES), spot stenting is the technique of the past.

EVIDENCE-BASED MEDICINE APPLICATIONS

Drug Eluting Stent: The SIRollmUS-Eluting Stent in De Novo Native Coronary Lesions (SIRIUS) trial: In this trial, for the control group, the rate of restenosis was 29.7% for 8-mm bare stents and 52.4% for bare stents measuring 40 mm. By contrast, the rate of restenosis of the sirolimus-eluting stents of <8 mm length was only 1.7%. It was 6.5% in lesions treated with 40-mm stents. In general, for every 10 mm of bare metal stent implanted, the rate of restenosis increased by 13%. In the sirolimus group, this increase was 1.6% for every additional 10-mm stent used from a baseline of 1.7% (Table 9-5).[11]

CALCIFIED LESIONS

A calcified lesion is defined as any angiographically apparent calcium in the target vessel. Its level of calcification is classified as mild if cardiac motion is required to see the calcium, moderate when it is obvious without cardiac motion, and severe. Heavy calcification is a predictor of dissection that occurs at a hinge point where calcified and pliable vessel segments are subject to barotrauma. The reason is that the pressure is concentrated on the most resistant area (the calcified segment) and the tissue next to the calcified area. The mechanism of acute lumen gain after PTCA in calcified lesion is dissection while it is plaque compression and vessel expansion in fibrotic lesion. Higher pressure inflation also increases

Table 9-5
Restenosis versus stent length

Stent length	In-segment restenosis	
	Control (%)	Sirolimus (%)
10 mm	31.3	7.3
20 mm	37.5	8.5
30 mm	44.0	10.1
40 mm	51.5	11.8

the risk of balloon rupture (14%),[7] perforation, or balloon material entrapment.[12]

The selection of devices in calcified lesion depends on vessel size, tortuosity, presence of thrombus, bifurcation, lesion length, eccentricity, ostial location, vein graft and diabetes. Ideally, a patient with heavily calcified lesion should have IVUS to locate the calcium and its extent. If it is deep then there are no problems with PTCA. If it is superficial, the patient should have rotational atherectomy. However, because of excessive distal embolism, rotational atherectomy is not as commonly used as before.

TECHNICAL TIPS

**Device selection: First, predilate a lesion with POBA. If the lesion can be dilated then stenting would be feasible. Most lesions with mild calcifications respond to this; simply try. If a lesion cannot be fully dilated at 18 ATM then stent placement is contraindicated since incomplete stent expansion increases the risk of subacute thrombosis and restenosis. Then rotablation or cutting balloon angioplasty can be tried. However, if the lesion is distal and the proximal segment is severely calcified and tortuous (>60° angulation), then it is difficult to advance a cutting balloon to the lesion site. In these heavily calcified lesions, primary rotablation is suggested.[13]

**Advancing a stent in a tortuous artery: Even after rotablation and balloon dilation, stenting of severely calcified lesions is still difficult because hard and eccentric plaque in a proximal tortuous segment may still prevent the advancement of stent. In these circumstances, it is important not to force the stent into the lesion since this maneuver may result in stent deformation and inability to remove the stent later, if needed. In order to advance the stent, the guide backup should be optimal, the "buddy wire" technique may be used to straighten the proximal segment, to shift the stent over the edge of the plaque. Complete predilation of the lesion or further debulking of the lesion with rotablation may be needed.[13]

**Expanding a stent with CB after failure of high pressure inflation: Even after being advanced to the lesion area, not every stent can be fully deployed due to unexpected severe calcification of the lesion. In a case report by Colombo *et al.*, while a stent was being deployed in the proximal LAD, the distal part of a stent could not be opened even at 30 ATM. So the balloon was exchanged with a cutting balloon (CB) that was advanced into the distal segment and inflated at 12 ATM. The CB was withdrawn and exchanged for a non-compliant balloon that fully expanded the stent at 28 ATM.[14]

CAVEAT: Avoid stent embolization while exchanging a balloon in a tortuous and calcified segment: While exchanging a balloon on a half deployed stent, the stent is easier to be dislodged backward, especially if the stent has a funnel shape (the proximal end is larger than the distal undeployed end). Make an extra effort to keep the stent immobile while removing the old balloon and advancing the new balloon inch by inch. These situations happen in the following situations: (1) angulated segment; (2) sharply tapered vessel with distal segment much smaller than proximal segment; and (3) insertion site between saphenous vein graft or internal mammary artery graft to the native vessel.

In summary, in PCI for calcified lesions, the results are usually suboptimal because only 24% of cases achieved 90% cross-sectional area of the reference lumen.[15] Even with higher pressure inflation (>18 ATM), some stents are still underdilated. Without prior calcium removal, it may not be possible to fully expand a stent, because of severe calcification or large plaque burden. In order to advance the stent through calcified and rigid lumen, extensive manipulation would denude the endothelial layer and cause more intimal hyperplasia and restenosis. Cutting balloon angioplasty or plain balloon angioplasty with one or two buddy wires can help to break the plaque and allow full stent deployment. Rotational atherectomy is the method of choice for debulking the calcified lesion with adjunctive angioplasty or stenting, however, the restenosis rate after bare stent and rota-stent was still high. There are no new data with DES or brachytherapy on calcified lesions.

ANGULATED LESIONS

An angulated lesion is defined as a lesion on a bend of 45° or more. With simple POBA, the success rate was 70% with 13% ischemic complications.[16] The risk of acute closure was 2% if the bend was less than 45°, and 8% if the bend was between 45° and 90°; it was 13% if the bend was more than 90°.[7]

BEST METHOD

Advance a wire through angulated segments:

1. **First maneuver – select a balanced wire:** At first a floppy wire seems to navigate easily the tortuous segments. It does not cause pseudo-lesions or wire bias. However, after a few excessive turns, it is impossible to advance

a too floppy wire further. It behaves like a wet noodle. In contrast, it may be difficult to make a first extensive twist and turn with a very firm wire. Furthermore, a stiff wire may cause "bias" while passing through heavily calcified and angulated segment and shift interventional devices against the wall of the artery, making their passage difficult. In most cases a moderately firm wire is appropriate.[17]

2. **Add a second wire:** On many occasions, a floppy wire is able to be advanced though tortuous segments; however, it is not strong enough to tract a device. Then a second, soft or stiffer wire may need to be advanced parallel to the first one by wrapping around the first one (the "buddy wire").

3. **Add a second device:** Sometimes, a wire may be advanced at best to the proximal end of a distal segment of an artery. Then, advance a balloon as far as possible, then the wire, to the distal end.

TECHNICAL TIPS

**Advance a second, stiffer wire along the first wire through angulated segments: On many occasions, a floppy wire is not strong enough to tract a device. Then a second soft or stiffer wire may need to be advanced parallel to the first one. In this case, advance the second wire as usual, then, at the bend, twist it more, for example by wrapping it around the first wire three or four times. By that, the second wire will be advanced to the same branch or distal segment of the first wire as intended. If the second wire is not planned to be positioned at the same branch or distal end, just wrap the first wire around the second one once or twice so the first wire can turn around the bend and be directed separately to its own branch.

**Advance a stiff wire with the help of a balloon: Ideally, in many PCIs, it is best to have a wire advanced deeply to the distal end of any instrumented artery. However, in many real-life situations, a wire could easily cross the lesion at the mid-segment (e.g. of the RCA or LCX) and at best, might only be advanced just to the proximal end of the distal segment (e.g. before the PDA or after a large OM). Advance a balloon near the tip of the wire then advance the wire. If the balloon can be advanced across the lesion, then inflate the balloon at low pressure, thus avoiding dissection. While the balloon is inflated, advance the wire to the distal end. The shaft of the balloon catheter will straighten the proximal segment and a wire indwelled inside an inflated balloon can be advanced without much difficulty to the distal end, providing a better support for later device tracking (Figure 9-1 A–C).

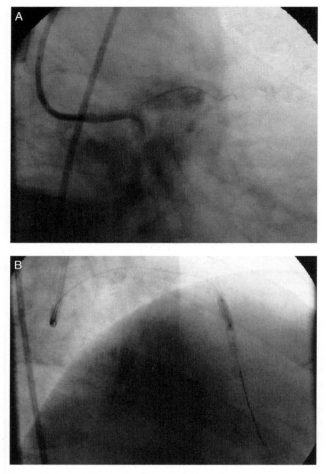

Figure 9-1: (A) There is difficulty in advancing the wire. (B) The wire can be advanced only to the mid-segment of the LAD. While the balloon is inflated, the wire can be advanced further. *(Continued)*

BEST METHOD

Avoiding perforation while advancing a balloon around a bend: should we add a new wire or change the balloon? Sometimes, if the wire is too soft and the currently available high-pressure balloons may have a very stiff tip that is not flexible enough to make a turn around the bend, its tip keeps pointing straight to the lateral wall. The reason is the tip of the balloon catheter is stiffer than the shaft of the wire. So the

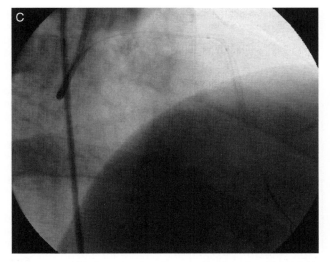

Figure 9-1: (C) The wire is advanced to the distal LAD, thus securing an excellent wire position and support for further movement of bulkier devices.

balloon-wire complex would have to follow the direction of its stiffer component (the tip of the balloon), pointing toward the wall, rather than curving around the bend. A further push may puncture the wall. In this case, either insert a second stiffer wire (buddy wire) to make the curve more rounded and so less bias for the balloon, or choose a lower profile and more flexible balloon.[17] In any circumstance, a second, stiffer wire is preferred because, as in this case, if a balloon cannot be advanced, how can a stent be advanced through the angulated segment? The stent may succeed to be advanced on the second, stiffer wire rather the first, softer wire.

BEST METHOD

Guess the chance for success of device advancement before and after wiring: With the advent of DES, there are more patients eligible for stenting even their anatomy is not favorable. Many elderly patients have very tortuous and calcified arteries.

1. **First maneuver – look at the angiogram – no calcium:** Before wiring, the first factor predictive of success for advancing any interventional device (wire, balloon, stent or thrombectomy, etc.) across a tortuous segment is the lack of calcification (e.g. in young patients). These arteries can let any stiff device slide through without problem.

2. **Second maneuver – look at the angiogram – large arteries:** The second factor is the size of the artery. If the artery is quite large, the wire can bypass the angles and connect all these segments on a straight line or a round curve that facilitates a lot the advancement of devices (Figure 9-2 A–C).

3. **Third maneuver – look at the angiogram – the angle after wiring:** After wiring, if the wire is able to stretch on a straight-line form or round curve, then the chance for the devices to move forward is much higher.

4. **Fourth maneuver: The usual requirements:** Finally, one cannot overemphasize the optimal backup of a guide, the trackability by a stiffer wire and the flexibility of the interventional device. All of these will help to advance the device to the area needed (Table 9-6).

**How long a balloon should be when wrapping around a bend: There is less occurrence of dissection with the use of a long balloon placed entirely around the bend because the longer the balloon, the greater the force required to

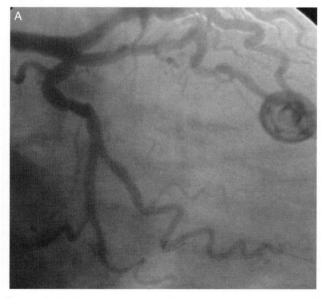

Figure 9-2: Advancing a wire through tortuous arteries. (A) The tortuous LCX with 90° angle from the LM. There was a severe lesion at the ostium of the large OM. There was a broken tip of a wire in the distal segment of the OM. This was the result of the jailed wire technique when a wire was jailed at the OM when a stent was deployed at the mid-LCX across the OM. *(Continued)*

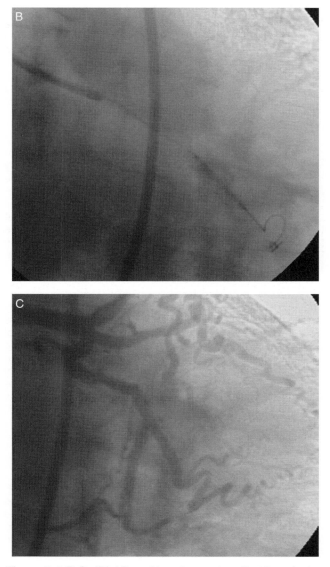

Figure 9-2 B,C: (B) After wiring, it was clear that the wire by-passed all the angles and formed a straight line from the tip of the guide to the OM. There was no sharp angle between the left main and LCX. This straight line facilitated the advance-ment of a balloon or stent. (C) The ostium of the OM after stenting was wide open.

Table 9-6
Factors that guarantee success of device advancement in angulated segments

---

1. Lack of calcification (accommodating vessel)
2. Large size of vessel so the wire can bypass the angles
3. Possibility of wiring on a straight-line form or round curve
4. Excellent guide support, wire trackability and device flexibility

---

straighten it.[18] A long balloon covers the lesion and adjacent areas so the stress pressure may be spread evenly over the lesion, rather than concentrated at the edge of the lesion. Short balloons may avoid the curve altogether in lesions not directly located on the angle. If the balloon does not cover the whole plaque, inflation of the balloon could result in plaque fracture and seepage of blood behind the plaque starting a dissection. Ideally, the balloon should be long enough such that there is a 10-mm margin of balloon extending beyond the bulk of the atheroma.[17]

Even so, it is difficult to have excellent results in sharply angulated lesions with simple POBA. Rotational atherectomy can be used if there is superficial calcification but the success rate is lower. In a more angulated bend, there is increased risk of perforation due to preferential ablation. Some stents can curve along the mildly angulated contour of an arterial segment. If the angle is too sharp, more than 90°, a stent cannot be sufficiently bent; rather, it straightens the angulated segment. The restenosis rate for these lesions straightened by a bare stent was not higher when compared with stented lesions not on a bend.[19] There are no new data with DES or VBT on angulated lesions.

LESIONS WITH THROMBUS

Thrombus is recognized angiographically as filling defects, irregular surfaces, or overhanging edges surrounded by contrast (Figure 9-3 A,B). With IVUS, a thrombus is seen as a mobile, pedunculated, hypoechoic mass; a brightly speckled mass, or by channels or flow within the plaque. However, the angiographically-labeled thrombotic lesions, when seen under IVUS, showed only 50% truly thrombotic. One-third of these so-called thrombotic lesions were purely calcified or they were just soft plaque without calcium or thrombus.[20] In patients undergoing PCI, the presence of pre-existing thrombus did not bear a poor prognosis for in-hospital (0.8% vs 0.6%, P=NS) or 6-month mortality (2.1% vs 1.8%, P=NS). However, the major ischemic events, including death/MI,

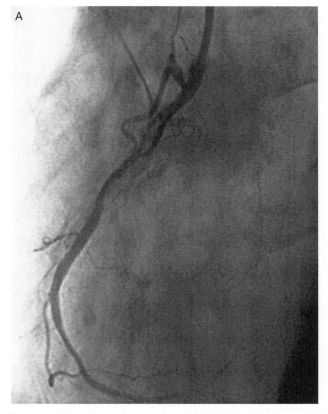

Figure 9-3: Lesion with thrombus. (A) Small round lucent object, surrounded by contrast in the mid RCA. *(Continued)*

and/or repeat revascularization, were higher in patients with thrombus (15.4% vs 11.2%, P<0.001).[20]

In patients with excellent coronary flow and stabilized symptoms, treatment with intravenous heparin for 24–48 hours prior to any definitive intervention has reduced complication rates. In many instances, significant thrombus can be squeezed by a balloon, embolized distally without long-term effect, or spread to the wall by a stent.

In a report by Douglas *et al.*, an attempt to remove the thrombus was made by first twisting a 0.014" wire and a balloon-on-a-wire to trap fibrin strands and subsequently withdrawing both wires into a deeply seated guide catheter. This maneuver yielded a large amount of thrombus, and subsequent angiography showed an excellent result with

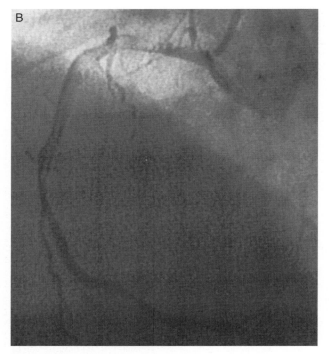

Figure 9-3: (B) Diffuse, large thrombi in the proximal RCA.

no evidence of residual thrombus.[21] Rarely, large proximal thrombi have been aspirated into a soft deep-seated guide.

The administration of thrombolytic agents can lead to deformity and/or fragmentation of large clots, with resultant abrupt closure or ischemia related to distal thromboembolization. On many occasions, it has been either ineffective or resulted in paradoxical vessel occlusion.[21] When urokinase was no longer available in the US, rPA was used instead, with similar results; however, it could cause stroke. In the presence of thrombus, the use of glycoprotein 2b3a inhibitor is strongly advocated. In instances of refractory or large thrombi, mechanical thrombectomy is indicated.[22]

TECHNICAL TIPS

**Maneuvering the AngioJet: The AngioJet catheter is a 5F device operated on 0.14" or 0.18" guidewire. The catheter is advanced over the guidewire until it reaches the thrombotic area. Then it is activated by pressing the foot switch on the drive unit. It is advanced at 2–3 mm/second, sweeping towards the distal end. Alternatively, the device can be advanced towards the distal end, crossing the thrombotic area without being activated. Once in the distal area, the catheter is activated and withdrawn slowly while still in action. This retrograde method may cause less debris embolization, although there was no firm evidence of its effectiveness. These passes can be repeated until the thrombus burden is cleared.[23]

Experiences with the X-SIZER device: The X-Sizer (Endicor Medical, Valkenswaard, The Netherlands) is a simple device combining vacuum technology with a patented helix cutter housed in the tip of a small catheter. When engaged, the slow-spinning blades serve to entrain the thrombus or soft material, which is then macerated and sucked out.

In the X-TRACT trial, at 30 days, the overall MACE rates were similar (17% in the X-Sizer group and 17.4% in the control group). However, large MIs, defined as a CPK-MB greater than 8 times normal limits, were reduced by 46%; 8.3% in the control group compared to 4.5% in the X-Sizer group. There was 1 perforation in the X-Sizer group and 4 in the control group.[24]

***Off-label maneuvering of the distal filtering device: Extraction of large thrombus in the Fogarty maneuver. In a case report by Eggebrecht *et al.*, a 6.0 mm filter Angioguard (Cordis Sunnyvale, CA) was deployed in the distal LAD with thrombus seen in the mid-segment. In an off-label maneuver, the expanded filter was withdrawn from the distal segment to the proximal segment in a Fogarty maneuver. In the first attempt, a 2×2 mm thrombus was found. The Fogarty maneuver was repeated three times. After that, PCI was carried on as usual.[25] In this case, the passage of an umbrella-type device could break the culprit plaque and trigger distal embolization and dissection. The authors were right when they chose the title of their article: "Abuse of a novel device".

SMALL VESSEL INTERVENTIONS

A small vessel is defined as a vessel with a minimum lumen diameter of less than 2.5 mm by quantitative coronary angiography. The procedural problems encountered during PCI of small vessels are listed in Table 9-7. There was no difference in restenosis rate between PTCA or stenting in the Benestent trial.[26] The reason is that in small vessels, although there is no difference in intimal hyperplasia, the loss index is still higher, relatively speaking, in the smaller lumen of a vessel with diameter <2.5 mm.

Table 9-7
Procedural problems with PCI of small vessels

1. Occlusion of the blood flow by still deflated balloon
2. Difficulty in advancing devices (wire, balloon, stent, etc.)
3. Inflation of compliant balloon can cause perforation
4. Dissection more likely occlusive
5. More significant residual stenosis
6. Higher rate of restenosis
7. More difficult to stent
8. Suboptimal results after stenting
9. Small area of myocardium in jeopardy

TECHNICAL TIP

**Wire selection and manipulation: In a small vessel, when manipulated, the wire's tip is straightened more by the confined diameter of the small vessel, so steering is more difficult. The tip curve should be short and is curved as dictated by the diameter of the vessel. The distal tip is soft rather than stiff because this is a poor area for manipulation and it is easier to exit the true lumen, causing perforation.[27]

TAKE-HOME MESSAGE

Stenting in a small vessel: [27]

1. Do not attempt stenting without excellent coaxial alignment and good backup support of the guide.
2. Do not attempt stenting if the lesion is not fully dilated after high pressure inflation (>15 ATM).
3. Use moderate push to advance the stent. Avoid forceful or prolonged manipulation of stent catheter to cross the lesion.
4. If the lesion cannot be easily crossed, try deeper intubation of the guide without aggressive manipulation.
5. Carefully assess the stent position in several projections before inflating the balloon.
6. Once deploying the stent, angiogram in multiple views to assess the result and to be sure that the distal part of the lesion is covered by the stent, without residual distal dissection.
7. In a small vessel, do not leave the stent with incomplete dilation, and/or residual distal narrowing or dissection.
8. In case of residual narrowing distal to the stent, repeated long inflation at low pressure with a balloon catheter matched to the vessel size is advised.

**Selection of balloons: Non-compliant balloons are suggested because small vessels usually have hard lesions, thus high pressure may be needed, making the proper size balloon critical. If the balloon is expanding its size with increasing pressure, then it is oversized and can change greatly the balloon:artery ratio. In lesions located in tapered vessels, balloon selection based upon proximal reference diameter may result in increased risk of dissection, whereas balloon sizing based on distal reference segment may yield suboptimal results but seems to be recommended as the first choice in small vessels. Additional inflation of only the proximal part with a short balloon will be the second step of the process.[27]

EVIDENCE-BASED MEDICINE APPLICATIONS

The RAVEL and SIRIUS trials: small vessels analysis: The randomized study with the sirolimus-eluting Bx Velocity-Expandable stent (RAVEL) trial compared DES with bare stent in all vessel sizes (<2.36 mm, 2.36–2.84 mm and >2.84 mm). At 6 months follow-up, there was 0% restenosis in all vessels with DES, while it was much higher in the bare stent group (Table 9-8). In the SIRollmUS-Eluting Stent in De Novo Native Coronary Lesions (SIRIUS) trial, there was a sizable rate of restenosis of 8% in small vessels with diameter <2.3 mm, while it was acceptable in larger size vessels (Table 9-9).[28]

The contradictory results among the DES trials (Table 9-10) can be explained by different lesion and patient characteristics as well as different procedural parameters. Stenting of short focal lesions in truly small vessels is su-

Table 9-8
Vessel size and restenosis rate in the RAVEL trial[28]

Mean radial diameter	DES	Bare stent
2.05 mm	0%	37.1%
2.56 mm	0%	20.6%
3.21 mm	0%	20%

All groups P<0.001

Table 9-9
The SIRIUS trial : vessel size sub-analysis

In-stent restenosis	TLR (up to 270 days)		
Vessel size	Sirolimus	Control	Sirolimus
Small (2.3 mm)	15%	23.1%	8.8%
Medium (2.8 mm)	7.5 %	13.4%	3.0%
Large (3.25 mm)	2.4%	14.5%	1.8%

Table 9-10
Differences between the RAVEL and SIRIUS trials

	SIRIUS	*RAVEL*
Study lesion length	15–30 mm	<18 mm
Allowed number of stents per lesion	(2 or 3)	1
Duration of anti-platelet therapy	3 months	2 months
Definition of non-q MI	FDA	WHO

perior to balloon angioplasty and cost-effective. Stenting of long lesions and small vessels in pseudo-small vessels with diffuse disease can have very good results with the DES.

REFERENCES

1. Douglas J. Percutaneous coronary interventions. In: Nguyen T, Hu DY, eds. *Advances and Challenges in Today's Cardiology.* Griffith Publishing, 1997.
2. Williams D, Vlachos H, Kelsey S *et al.* Procedural strategies and outcomes of PCI in 1999: Results of the dynamic registry. *J Am Coll Cardiol* 2000; **35** (Suppl A): 30A.
3. Nguyen T, Tresukosol D, Pham HM *et al.* Percutaneous coronary interventions for complex lesions and high-risk patients. In: Nguyen T, Hu DY, Saito S *et al.*, eds. *Management of Complex Cardiovascular Problems.* Futura Publishing Co, 2000.
4. Ryan TJ, Faxon DP, Gunnar RM *et al.* Guidelines for percutaneous transluminal coronary angioplasty: A report of the American College of Cardiology/American Heart Association task force on assessment of diagnostic and therapeutic cardiovascular procedures (subcommittee on PTCA). *J Am Coll Cardiol* 1988; **12**: 529–45.
5. Ellis S, Guetta V, Miller D *et al.* Relation between lesion characteristics and risk with percutaneous intervention in the stent and glycoprotein IIb/IIIa era: An analysis of results from 10,907 lesions and proposal for new classification scheme. *Circulation* 1999; **100**: 1971–6.
6. Holmes D, Berger P. Complex and multivessel treatment. In: Topol E, ed. *Textbook of Interventional Cardiology,* 3rd edition. WB Saunders, 1999.
7. Tan KH, Sulke N, Taub N *et al.* Lesion morphological determinants of coronary balloon angioplasty success and complications: Time for a reappraisal. *J Am Coll Cardiol* 1994; **23** (4): 222A.

8. King III SB. Complications of angioplasty. In: King III SB, Douglas JS, eds. *Atlas of Heart Disease*. Mosby, 1997.

9. Reisman M, Cohen B, Warth D *et al*. Outcome of long lesions with high speed rotational atherectomy. *J Am Coll Cardiol* 1993; **21**(4): 443A.

10. Saucedo JF, Kennard ED, Popma JJ *et al*. Importance of lesion length on new device angioplasty of native coronary arteries. NACI Investigators. New Approaches to Coronary Interventions. *Cathet Cardiovasc Interv* 2000; **50**: 19–25.

11. The SIRIUS Trial: Presented by M. Leon at the TransCatheter Therapeutics meeting, Washington DC, 2002.

12. Fitzgerald PJ, Sudhir K *et al*. Localized calcium is a major risk for arterial dissection during angioplasty: A catheter ultrasound study. *Circulation* 1991; **84** (Suppl II): II-722.

13. Reifart N. PTCA of calcified lesion. In: Fajadet J, ed. *Syllabus for EuroPCR*, 2001: 107–112.

14. Colombo A, Stankovic G. Cutting balloon angioplasty: Areas of application. In: Colombo A, Stankovic G, eds. *Colombo's Tips and Tricks in Interventional Cardiology*. Martin Dunitz, 2002: 29.

15. Vavuranakis M *et al*. Stent deployment in calcified lesions. Can we overcome calcific restraint with high pressure balloon inflation (abstract)? *Circulation* 1998; **17**: I-160.

16. Ellis S, Topol E. Results of percutaneous transluminal coronary angioplasty of high-risk angulated stenoses. *Am J Cardiol* 1990; **66**: 932–7.

17. Ellis S. Management of angulated lesions. In: Ellis S, Holmes Jr D, eds. *Strategic Approaches in Coronary Interventions*, 2nd edn. Lippincott Williams Wilkins, 2000: 207–10.

18. Douglas JS Jr. Percutaneous interventional approaches to specific coronary lesions. In: King III SB, Douglas JS, eds. *Atlas of Heart Disease*. Mosby, 1997: 11.10.

19. Hadjimiltiades S, Gourassas J *et al*. Effect of stent location, relative to a coronary bend, on restenosis (abstract). *Eur Heart J* 1998; **19**: 2845.

20. Kotani J, Mintz G, Pregowski J *et al*. Does a thrombotic lesion detected by coronary angiography always contain a thrombus? An IVUS study. *J Am Coll Cardiol* 2003; **41**(6): 9A.

21. Singh M, Reeder G, Ohman M *et al*. Does the presence of thrombus seen on a coronary angiogram affect the outcome after PCI? An angiographic trial pool data experience. *J Am Coll Cardiol* 2001; **38**: 624–30.

22. Douglas JS Jr. Management of coronary lesion with associated thrombus. In: Ellis S, Holmes Jr D, eds. *Strategic Approaches in Coronary Interventions*, 2nd edn. Lippincott Williams Wilkins, 2000: 266–74.

23. Dohad S, Parris T, Setum C. AngioJet® Rheolytic™ Thrombectomy: An important tool for percutaneous coronary interventions in high-risk patients; VEGAS II Trial. *Am J Cardiol* 2002; **89**: 326–30.

24. Ischinger T. Thrombectomy with the X-SIZER catheter system in the coronary circulation: Initial results from a multi-center study. *J Invasive Cardiol* 2001; **12**: 81–8.

25. Eggebrecht H, Baumgart D, Naber C *et al.* Extraction of Large Intracoronary Thrombus in AMI by percutaneous Fogarty Maneuver. Intentional abuse of a novel interventional device. *Cathet Cardiovasc Interv* 2002; **55**: 228–32.

26. Sawada Y, Nasaka H, Kimura T *et al.* Initial and six-month outcome PS stent implantation: STRESS/BENESTENT equivalent vs non-equivalent lesions. *J Am Coll Cardiol* 1996; **27**(Suppl I): 252A.

27. Marco J, Sousa JP, Boccallatte M *et al.* Coronary stenting in small vessels. In: Fajadet J, ed. *Syllabus for EuroPCR*, 2001: 159–74.

28. Regar E, Serruys P, Bode C *et al.* for the RAVEL Study Group. Angiographic findings for the multicenter randomized study with the sirolimus-eluting stent Bx Velocity Balloon expandable stent (RAVEL). *Circulation* 2002; **106**: 1949–56.

Chapter 10

Chronic Total Occlusion

*Kazuaki Mitsudo, Thach Nguyen,
Jui Sung Hung*

GENERAL OVERVIEW

    Chronic total occlusion (CTO) is defined as total occlusion (TIMI 0 or I) with either known duration of more than 3 months or

---

*Basic; **Advanced; ***Rare, exotic, or investigational.

From: Nguyen T, Hu D, Saito S, Grines C, Palacios I (eds), *Practical Handbook of Advanced Interventional Cardiology*, 2nd edn. © 2003 Futura, an imprint of Blackwell Publishing.

presence of bridging collaterals.[1] A chronically occluded artery with good collateral supply has the functional significance of 90% stenosis.[2] Percutaneous interventions (PCI) of the CTO lesion present great challenges including low success rate, prolonged procedure time, large amount of contrast use, high re-occlusion rate, and costs. In the past, the results of revascularization of CTO were disappointing.[3] However, with improved wire design, advanced imaging techniques, and increased operator skills, the primary success has been as high as 90%.[4]

The goal of intervention in CTO is to penetrate the total occlusion and place the wire in the true lumen of the distal vessel without causing intimal dissection. Crossing a CTO segment consists of penetrating a proximal fibrous cap, then a long segment of heterogenous (atheromatous or old thrombotic) material, and finally a distal fibrous cap. If the CTO evolves from acute occlusion, it contains large quantity of thrombotic material, with the old fracture plaque forming the distal cap. If it progresses from occlusion of a severe stenotic lesion, then a large amount of atheromatous plaque would be present. Shortly after PCI, silent reocclusion occurred in a small percentage of patients due to sufficient recruitment of collaterals. The use of glycoprotein 2b3a inhibitors did not improve the outcome. The factors predicting procedural success are shown in Table 10-1.[5]

TECHNICAL TIPS

*Selection of guides: The choice of the guide is very important because, without adequate support, it is impossible to push a wire or balloon through a CTO lesion. Usually, a left Judkins (short-tip, for easier deep intubation), left Amplatz, left extra-backup (left Voda, Boston Scientific, USA; EB, eXtra Back-up, Cordis USA; EBU, Extra Back-Up, Metronic, USA; or GL, Geometric Left, Guidant USA) guides are chosen for cannulation of the LCX or LAD, and a right Judkins, left Amplatz, Multipurpose or extra-backup guide for the RCA according to the size of the ostium and the orientation of the proximal segment of the vessel. In

---

Table 10-1
Factors influencing the success of CTO interventions

1. Duration of occlusion (75% if <3 months, 37% if >3 months), worst if the duration is unknown.
2. Presence of antegrade flow (76%), absence of antegrade flow (58%).
3. Angiographically tapered occlusion (77%) versus without a stump (50%).
4. Absence of bridging collaterals (71% versus 23%).
5. Lesion length <20 mm.

general, guides with side holes are not recommended because of poor vessel opacification and wastage of contrast. However, if persistent wedging of the vessel cannot be avoided, a guide with side holes can provide limited antegrade flow with ischemic relief.

**Optimal angiograms: Adequate visualization of the distal vessel beyond the CTO lesion is essential in mapping the direction where the wire should be pointed and also for confirming its position in the distal true lumen. If there is no visible distal flow from bridging collaterals or due to insufficient ipsilateral collaterals, a contralateral angiogram can be done to opacify the distal lumen through retrograde collaterals. These proximal and distal angiograms will help to direct a wire across the fibrous caps or a long occluded segment. The wire position should be always confirmed by two projection angles. When single-plane fluoroscopy is used, mistakes are often made regarding the wire route. Therefore, biplane cine-angiography is more accurate than bi-directional angiography in single-plane because the wire position and direction can be better recognized and confirmed at any time with use of less contrast.

**Optimal projection angles: The best projection angles differ according to the region of interest (ROI). The operator should explore the angles in which the stump can be seen most clearly, especially at the entry point. In general, it is desirable for the two projection angles to be perpendicular to the vessel axis of the ROI (Figure 10-1), and also perpendicular to each other (orthogonal projection). Because the summation of the blind area is smallest in the orthogonal projection (Figure 10-2), it will be easier to lead the wire tip to the distal true lumen.

**Entry point: If there is an angiographically tapered occlusion, the tapering stump is the starting place to probe the occlusion. It frequently contains small recanalized channels or neochannels (160–230 microns in diameter),[6] which are potential routes for wire crossing. However, if the stump is eccentrically oriented, the chance of crossing the CTO is lower, while the risk of subintimal wire passage is higher. When the stump cutoff is abrupt and flat, and the entry point is not identified by an angiogram, the center of the stump should be tried as entry point. In this situation, the invisible dimple of the probable entry point is explored by using the tip of a conventional wire, not a sleek hydrophilic-coated tip. If the artery is large enough and the entry point is at a side rather at the end of a stump, intravascular ultrasound (IVUS) can be used to identify the entry point (Figure 10-3). When there are extensive bridging collaterals (caput medusae), the chance of wire crossing is also lower. The

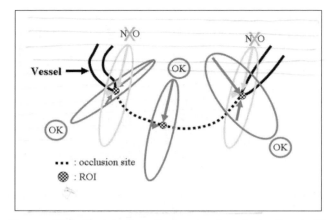

Figure 10-1: Required projection angles. Projections with perpendicular angles to the occlusion site of the vessel or guidewire tip site of the occluded part are recommended. Each ROI (region of interest) has its suitable projection angle (O). The angle optimal for the central ROI is not always suitable for the other ROI (X). For example, for viewing a proximal RCA site, the LAO/caudal or RAO/cranial is best. For the mid-RCA site, it is the straight LAO or RAO view. For the distal RCA site, the LAO/cranial or RAO/caudal projections are the most suitable.

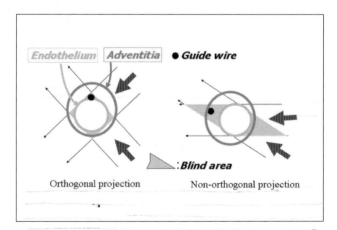

Figure 10-2: Orthogonal projections. Because the summation of the blind area, not projected by each view, is smallest in the orthogonal projections, it is very useful for leading the wire into the true lumen and to confirm successful wire entry in the true lumen.

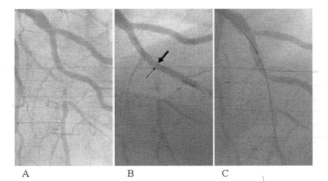

A   B   C

Figure 10-3: Identifying entry point using IVUS. (A) Obscured entry site of occluded LAD. (B) IVUS use in finding LAD occluded site. Upon identifying entry point, transducer (dot mark indicated by arrow) is left in place as a landmark. This technique can be applied when the artery is large enough for an IVUS catheter and the entry site is at a side (rather than at the end stump). (C) Use of Conquest guidewire to explore the small dimple at the transducer area results in successful crossing of CTO lesion.

reason is that these intracoronary collaterals consist of dilated vasa vasorum, which are very fragile and easily perforated. When there is a side branch near the stump, the natural tendency of any wire is to seek an easy escape that is a side branch and this would lower the chance of penetrating the long occluded lumen.[5] However, in experienced hands, when a super-stiff wire (e.g. Conquest Pro wire, Asahi Intec Co, Seto, Japan) is used, the presence of a side branch near the stump or of bridging collaterals may not be too relevant, and the success rate of crossing the CTO could reach 90%.[3]

CROSSING STRATEGIES

There are two strategies for crossing a CTO: the drilling and the penetrating strategy. The drilling strategy can be used first, then the penetrating one, or vice versa. In any situation, a conventional wire of intermediate level of stiffness is tried first. If it fails to progress across the lesion, then a standard wire is selected. If the second wire fails again, then a stiff wire or one with hydrophilic coating can be tried. Very experienced operators may simply bypass the intermediate wires and go straight to the stiff or hydrophilic-coated wires.

Drilling strategy: Initially, a 0.014" intermediate wire is used to cross the lesion. If it cannot cross the lesion, then a stiffer wire, i.e. a High Torque Standard wire (ACS Santa Clara CA, USA) or a Jowire, Miracle 3.0, 4.5, 6.0 or 12.0 g wire (Asahi Intec Co, Seto, Japan), with the small tip curved to form an abrading tool can be used (Figure 10-4, upper panel). A 180° back and forth rotation often causes the tip to grind through the lesion. If the wire buckles, it should be retracted, reoriented, and then rotated rather than forced through the lesion. Constant forward pressure on the wire is more successful than aggressive tapping against the occlusion ("jack-hammering"), which does not transmit additional force.[7] Once the wire enters the distal lumen, its tip should show easy free movement and smooth retraction or advancement. If there is

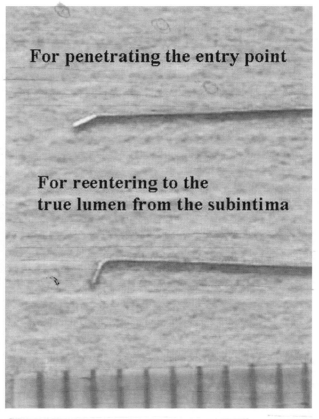

Figure 10-4: Typical tip shapes of the tapered-tip wire (Conquest Pro™ or Cross It™). For penetrating entry point, its 1.5–2.0 mm tip is bent at a curve of about 15–30° (upper panel). For re-entering the true lumen from the subintima, an almost 90° angle bend is required (lower panel).

no free rotation and no smooth advancement or retraction, the wire may lie subintimally or in a small branch along the main vessel. If the stiffer wires fail to cross the lesion, the next step is to try steeper and stiffer wire, i.e. a Conquest Pro wire (Asahi Intec Co, Seto, Japan) or a Cross It 400 wire (ACS Santa Clara CA, USA).

**Penetrating strategy: The first step is similar to the drilling strategy by using an intermediate wire. If it fails to cross the lesion, a stiffer wire such as the Conquest Pro wire (Asahi Intec, Seto Japan) or a Cross It 400 wire (ACS Santa Clara CA) with its 1.5–2.0 mm tip bent at a curve of about 15–30° is used to penetrate rather than drill the lesion (Figure 10-4, lower panel). The rotating motion should be minimized (<90° back and forth) to maintain directional control. At the outset, if the lesion is not hard, a gentle pushing force with a feather-light touch should be applied. If the lesion is hard, the pushing force should be gradually increased. If the direction is incorrect, the wire tends to go into the subintimal space or perforate the vessel because of the strong penetrating force. On the other hand, if the direction is correct, the chance of successful penetration of the fibrous cap is very high.[8]

WIRES

As a wire attempts to go through a CTO lesion, the first goal is to penetrate the hard proximal fibrous cap, so the wire has to be sharp and stiff. Once it enters the long atheromatous or thrombotic segment, then it should be sleek and flexible to be steered inside the occlusion with little friction resistance and without creating or seeking a subintimal pathway. Once it is near the distal lumen, the wire again needs to be sharp and stiff in order to cross the distal fibrous cap and re-enter the distal patent lumen.

Engineering evaluation of wires: When evaluating a wire for CTO lesion, there are two parts to look at: (1) a central shaft of stainless steel or Nitinol, and (2) a distal flexible tip shaped as a spring coil made of platinum or tungsten. Most wires have a strong shaft to push farther and a flexible tip to steer the wire to different directions upon subtle proximal torque movement by the operator. The wires made of Nitinol are more kink-resistant while those of stainless steel are more susceptible to kinking. The similarities and differences between wires are highlighted in Table 10-2.

TECHNICAL TIPS

Selection of wire: (1) **A blunt tip to grind: At the beginning of a PCI for CTO lesion, the most commonly used wire is the BMW (balanced middle weight) wire (Guidant, St Paul MN). It has a soft distal tip, a thin kink-resistant

Table 10-2
Characteristics of wires

Wires	Regular	Aggressive
Core extends to the tip	No	Yes
Increase pushability	No	Yes
Increase torqueability	No	Yes
Stiffer tip	No	Yes
Tapering tip	No	Yes
Sharper (short spring coil)	No	Yes
Long spring coil (increased steerability)	Yes	No

distal core and a strong stainless steel proximal shaft. This wire is good for the operator just to gain an initial feel of the CTO lesion. If the BMW wire fails to cross the lesion, some operators suggest the Intermediate or the Standard wire (Guidant, St Paul MN) to be tried next. All these three wires have almost the same long distal spring coil (i.e. good for steering), except the distal core becomes thicker (i.e. stronger) and not sharper (the core is untapered). In general, to be successful in drilling, these standard wires need to have a tip stiffer than 3 g. This 3 g or x g number means that 3 or x grams are necessary to bend the tip of the wire.

**Selection of wire: (2) A sharper tip to penetrate: Once the operator realizes that the three conventional wires are not able to cross the lesion, then he or she can choose a stiffer and sharper wire or a sleeker wire. A wire can be made stiffer by having a longer and bigger central core (i.e. stronger with shorter flexible tip), almost to the end of the tip. Then a wire with tapering distal segment (like an arrow, with a very short flexible tip) would become sharper. These two physical factors (i.e. increased stiffness and sharpness) would help the wire to penetrate any hard surface. A good example can be found in the design of the four wires of the Cross-IT XT family, (Guidant, Minneapolis, MN). The core of the shaft is extended to the distal tip, expanded longer, thicker, and becomes longest and thickest with the Cross-IT XT 400. Then the flexible tip has to become smaller (the shaft diameter is 0.014" while the tip is 0.010") and shorter as it cannot be the weak end of a sharp and stiff dagger-like wire. The shortest spring coil flexible segment is for steering. A wire with tapering tip is effective in the penetrating strategies as well as drilling strategies. The Conquest Pro (Asahi Intec, Seto, Japan) with a tip tapered from 0.014" to 0.009" has an effective hydrophilic coating in the shaft, sparing the tip ball. This design improves the wire movement without losing its efficacy in catching a small dimple at the entry point of the occlusion with no stumps.

**Selection of wire: (3) A strong shaft to increase pushability: In order to push a wire through a hard barrier, the central core of the body could be extended as far as possible next to the tip. The best example is the Miracle wire (Asahi Intec, Seto, Japan), which has a high torque transmission because the body shaft and the spring coil is a continuous core. This core can therefore transmit the pushing force generated at the proximal end to increase its pushability to 3, 4.5, 6, or 12 grams. This type of strong core is effective in penetrating any hard surface (i.e. increased pushability) and allows wire movement even it is operating in a very tight space (i.e. increased torqueability).

**Selection of wire: (4) Going through tight spaces by wearing a slippery coat: In order to navigate tight spaces, many wires are coated with slippery material such as the Crosswire (Terumo, Japan),[5] PT Graphics (Boston Scientific, USA), and Whisper (Guidant, USA). The main characteristic of these wires is that they have the lowest friction resistance against the vessel wall or lesions. Its main role is to help crossing the tiny 160–230 micron neo-channels. It does not help to drill or penetrate, because these wires have neither strong penetrating force nor drilling ability. The matter can become worse because these wires do not have a flexible spring coil, so they are not steerable, particularly in a tight long CTO segment. Without the ability to change direction, when facing a hard surface, the slippery tip of these wires just seeks an easy escape, creating subintimal false lumen. This is why these hydrophilic-coated wires should cross any lesion smoothly by themselves without being actively pushed against resistance. Once crossing the distal fibrous cap into the distal true lumen, these wires should be exchanged for a regular angioplasty wire, to prevent inadvertent distal exit and perforation.

TROUBLE-SHOOTING TIPS

**Shaping the tip: When trying to cross a hard surface or navigating the tight space inside the totally occluded segment, the tip of any wire should have a secondary bend just 1 or 2 mm from the tip (Figure 10-4, upper panel). The reason is that the typical 4–5 mm primary commercial J tip will be straightened when a balloon is advanced near the tip for added support. When the wire enters a long and totally occluded segment, its primary long tip will be straightened and entrapped in the tight confinement. Without a tiny secondary bend at the tip, the steerability of the wire will be lost.

**Delicate handling of the wire: When advancing a wire across a CTO lesion, buckling of the wire means that the wire tip is either in the wrong microchannel, or the tip is forced in a direction at an angle with the channel lumen. Applying additional force, or using a balloon for additional support to prevent the wire from buckling, would then only increase the risk of subintimal tracking. Handling of the wire is based on steering, rather than pushing the tip through the occlusion. This is a "trial and error" approach of carefully steering and redirecting the wire until a channel that connects the stump with the distal patent lumen is found. While the alignment of the wire with the target lumen is continuously monitored, the risk of subintimal tracking and dissection is significantly reduced. If the tip stiffness of the wire is not sufficient to pierce the distal fibrotic cap, the wire tip will be deflected and again forced into a subintimal layer. Continued maneuvering of the wire could then cause the wire to perforate the adventitia, resulting in a wire exit. The current wire has to be changed to a wire with a stiffer tip.

CAVEAT: How to navigate a wire: Without adequate visualization of the distal lumen, the operator will not be able to actively prevent the wire from choosing a subintimal pathway. The often very resistant nature of the distal part of an occlusion sometimes requires an exchange of the wire for, again, a wire with increased tip stiffness. However, it should be stressed that as long as the wire has not yet crossed into the distal lumen, an exchange of wire should never be facilitated by using a balloon or probing catheter. The reason is that a balloon catheter tip can damage the entry point (made with 160–230 micron diameter channels), thereby precluding additional attempts with different stiffer wires.[9] Also, if the wire has not yet crossed the occlusion because of subintimal position, an exchange catheter will sufficiently dissect the occluded segment as to preclude any additional guidewire attempts at recanalization. In case of an undetected wire perforation, the introduction of an exchange catheter could alter a benign wire exit into a potentially life-threatening perforation of the coronary arterial wall, requiring pericardiocentesis. Therefore, prior to advancing any device, either an antegrade or retrograde injection of contrast medium should angiographically confirm the distal, intraluminal position of the wire.[9]

**Parallel wire method (seesaw wiring): (Figure 10-5 A–H) When the wire tip goes into the subintimal space at the small branch or outside of the vessel, the second wire is advanced leaving the first wire in place (the parallel wire method). The first wire has two roles. One is to obstruct the incorrect pathway, and the other is to mark the route to the true lumen during wire manipulation. With the existence

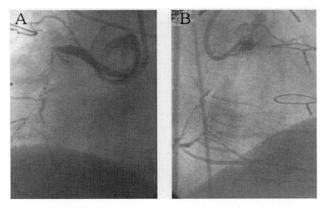

Figure 10-5: CTO lesion with bridging collateral in proximal RCA, shown in LAO (A) and LAO (B) views before intervention with seesaw wiring technique (Figure 10-6). *(Continued)*

of this landmark, the operator can lead the wire tip more easily to the direction of the true lumen. In the parallel wire technique, if the operator intends to use only one support catheter, the support catheter should be pulled back and re-inserted into the target vessel again with the second wire.

If the operator uses two support catheters at a time, the procedure becomes simpler. If it is difficult for the second wire to enter the true lumen, one can exchange the roles of two wires (Figure 10-6 A–D). Using the parallel wire method with two support catheters is called "Seesaw Wiring". The operator is able to move any of the two wires at any time. This method introduces fluid (blood) into the waterless occlusion site, triggering the hydrophilic mechanism (slippery when wet) and thus preventing the hydrophilic wires from sticking to each other.

**Support catheters: When there is a need to increase the stiffness of the tip of the wire, an over-the-wire balloon catheter (1.5-mm with surface coating) or a transport catheter (Excelsior, Boston Scientific, Boston or Transit, Cordis, USA) can be used. The catheter tip is advanced just near the entry point to enhance wire support and its torque control. This type of catheter facilitates wire exchange, which is frequently needed. While a softer and smaller diameter tipped catheter is preferred, kink resistance is mandatory to avoid difficulty in wire exchange. The balloon catheter can be advanced near the tip to increase the stiffness of the wire. Sometimes, the balloon and the wire can be advanced as a unit to increase the chance of crossing a hard surface.[10] Then, after removal of the wire, injection of contrast could be performed after blood has been aspirated through the

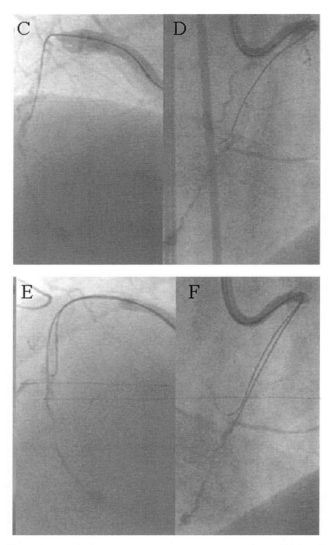

Figure 10-5: Parallel wire method or seesaw wiring. (C) (LAO view) and (D) (RAO view) show that the wire is deviated from the true lumen, a little rightwards in (C) and leftwards in (D). Leaving the first wire in place as a landmark, a second wire is advanced and directed into the true lumen. The second wire is viewed at the left and right of the first wire, respectively in (E) (LAO view) and (F) (RAO view).

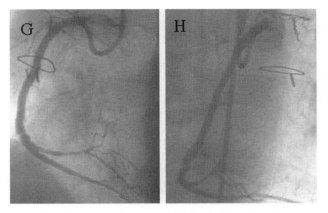

Figure 10-5: Parallel wire method or seesaw wiring (continued). (G) (LAO view) and (H) (RAO view) show post-stenting angiograms.

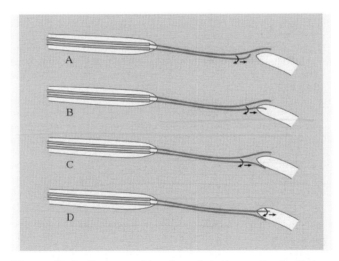

Figure 10-6: Seesaw wiring (parallel wire method with two support catheters). (A) When the first wire fails to cross into the distal true lumen, the first wire is left as a landmark, and the second wire is advanced into the occlusion site using the second support catheter. (B) The second wire is successfully manipulated into the true lumen. (C) Alternatively, the second wire fails to enter the true lumen. (D) Use of two support catheters facilitates role-exchange of the two wires. The first wire now is successfully engaged into the true lumen.

catheter to prevent bolus injection of air. Contrast should be diluted 50% with saline to decrease its viscosity. After the contrast injection, if there is non-opacification of the distal vessel, presence of a dissection, or visualization of a side branch, it is useful to continue the contrast injection while carefully pulling back the support catheter. This allows the operator to determine at which level of the occlusion the catheter entered a dissection or at which level the catheter deviated into a side branch.[10]

**Options for crossing the CTO lesion: Once there is difficulty in crossing a CTO (which happens frequently) there are different tactics to be used. They are listed in Table 10-3. One of the most aggressive (and dangerous) tactics is to inflate the balloon at the most distal position achievable, followed by powerful advancement of the wire while the balloon is inflated.[9] This maneuver does two things. As the balloon is inflated, the balloon catheter stays put so the guide can be held still by the operator without being pushed out by advancing the wire through the hard surface. The balloon also centers the wire so the wire can be advanced harder with lesser (and not without) chance of wire exit. Another variant of this aggressive maneuver is to advance a small balloon in a side branch proximal to the CTO lesion. Inflate the balloon to anchor (immobilize) the guide and advance the wire across the CTO lesion without backing out the guide.[11]

**Subintimal channel stenting: Passage of the wire before re-entry into the distal lumen is frequently observed during wiring of the CTO lesion and may result in procedural failure when antegrade flow cannot be established. Without the use of scaffolding stents, a subintimal passage has little chance of remaining patent, especially if the pathway is long. If re-entry of the wire into the distal true lumen can be achieved, it is possible to create a subintimal conduit using coronary

Table 10-3
Technical options when there is difficulty crossing a CTO

1. Deep-seating the guide
2. Advancing the balloon or transport catheter near the entry point
3. Using a stiffer wire
4. Using a steeper and stiffer wire
5. Using double wires and support catheters
6. Using larger guide for stronger backup
7. Inflating a balloon at the most distal location achieved or at a side branch proximal to the stump

stents that yield long-term vessel patency. To achieve success in a CTO lesion, the trick is to get the wire to recross
from this dissection plane back into the true distal lumen.[10]

COMPLICATIONS

Ischemic complications occur due to dissection, perforation at the occlusion site, or distal thrombotic embolizations.
Closure of a small side branch is often clinically insignificant.
However, distal thrombotic embolization can cause acute ST-
elevation MI by blocking the retrograde collateral flow from the
opposite coronary system. The attempt to cross a CTO lesion
or a re-entry from a subintimal space can require time and
patience. The procedure may have to be abandoned when the
fluoroscopic time has lapsed too long (>30 minutes) or when
too much contrast media has been used (>300 mL in a patient
with normal renal function). A further attempt a few days to a
few months later can be tried.

**Perforation: Perforation in an occluded segment may
not cause any clinical problem unless it is unrecognized
and enlarged by advancement or dilation of a balloon catheter. In order to prevent any bleeding, the support catheter
should not be advanced distal to the entry point prior to confirming wire entry into the distal true lumen. Bleeding can be
controlled by neutralizing heparin with protamine, with inflation of a balloon at low pressure in the proximal segment
to obstruct the antegrade flow. After pericardial drainage
and control of the vessel extravasation, the patient can be
given heparin again and the procedure may be continued.

Investigational devices
If the procedure is unsuccessful, investigational devices
could be used if available. They are listed in Table 10-4.
**The IntraLuminal Safe-Cross™ Guidewire with the
Optimal Coherent Reflectometry (OCR) and Radiofrequency ablation:** A new, novel wire system utilizes optical
coherent reflectometry (OCR) to guide the wire through the
occlusion. This new technology is based on the variable absorption and scattering of near-infrared light by substances
such as plaque, blood, tissue, and thrombus. Algorithms have

Table 10-4
Investigational devices for CTO

1. The IntraLuminal Safe-Cross™ Guidewire with optical coherent reflectometry (OCR) and radiofrequency ablation
2. The Frontrunner™ (LuMend)

been devised based on variable absorption rates and different scattering coefficients as a light beam of known intensity is introduced through the wire and illuminates the adjacent area of the tip. The direction of the tip of the IntraLuminal Safe-Cross™ Guidewire system is shown on a small monitor that is used to maintain the navigation of the wire system through the chronic occlusion, minimizing the possibility of perforating the arterial wall. The direction of the wire may be changed utilizing a 3.5F bidirectional catheter that also yields additional pushability for the wire. The wire advances by ablating the plaque by using the radiofrequency wave. In a small study, all stenoses were successfully crossed, without complications, using the wire system. This procedure also shows a reduction in the time required to cross these stenoses as well as an "early warning system" for detecting the arterial wall, therefore minimizing the risk of perforation.[12]

The LuMend Frontrunner™ CTO Catheter: The tip shape of the Frontrunner CTO Catheter resembles the tip of biopsy forceps without the blade. The mechanism of this catheter is a controlled micro-dissection by opening the forceps separating atherosclerotic plaque in various tissue planes to create a passage through the CTO. It uses elastic properties of adventitia versus inelastic properties of fibrocalcific plaque to create fracture planes.

REFERENCES

1. Ellis SE, Guetta V, Miller D. Relation between lesion characteristics and risk with percutaneous intervention in the stent and glycoprotein IIbIIIa era. *Circulation* 1999; **100**: 1971–6.

2. Flameng W, Schwartz F, Hehrlein FW. Intraoperative evaluation of the functional significance of coronary collateral vessels in patients with CAD. *Am J Cardiol* 1978; **42**: 187–92.

3. Nobuyoshi M, Shizuta S. Update on percutaneous management of chronic total occlusion. *J Interven Cardiol* 1998; **11**: II S42-S45.

4. Mitsudo K. Data on file.

5. Puma JA, Sketch MH, Tcheng JE *et al*. Percutaneous revascularization of chronic total occlusions: An overview. *J Am Coll Cardiol* 1995; **26**: 1–11.

6. Katsuragawa M, Fujiwara H, Miyamae M *et al*. Histologic studies in PTCA for CTO: Comparing tapering and abrupt types of occlusion and short and long occluded segments. *J Am Coll Cardiol* 1995; **7**: 259–64.

7. Freed M. Chronic total occlusion. In: Freed M, Grines C, Safian R, eds. *The New Manual of Interventional Cardiology*. Physician's Press, 1996.

8. Wong CM, Kwong Mak GY, Chung DT. Distal coronary artery perforation resulting from the use of hydrophilic guide-

wire in tortuous vessels. *Cathet Cardiovasc Diagn* 1998; **44**: 93–6.

9. Hamburger J, Holmes D. Treatment of chronic total coronary occlusions. In: Ellis S, Holmes D, eds. *Strategic Approaches in Coronary Intervention*, 2nd edn. Lippincott Wiliams Wilkins, 2000: 333–40.

10. Meier B. The chronic occlusion. In: Ellis S, Holmes D, eds. *Strategic Approaches in Coronary Intervention*, 2nd edn. Lippincott Wiliams Wilkins, Philadelphia, 2000: 325–33.

11. Saito S. Tips and tricks in angioplasty of CTO. *Russian J Interv Cardiol* (in press).

12. Koolen J, Bonnier H, Grube E. A novel guidance system for facilitating the crossing of plaque and chronic total occlusions. *J Am Coll Cardiol* 2000; **2** (Suppl A): 40A.

Chapter 11
Ostial Lesions

Thach Nguyen, Ho Thuong Dzung, Devan Pillay, Buxin Chen, Quan Fang

General overview
    **Selection and position of guides for ostial lesions
    **Disengagement of guides during aorto-ostial lesion interventions
    **Re-engagement of guides after stenting
    ***Two-guide techniques for aorto-ostial lesions
    ***Double wire to position ostial stent
    CAVEAT: Strategic concerns for interventions in ostial left anterior descending artery, left circumflex
    **Optimal balloon predilation
    **Selection of stent for aorto-ostial lesions
    **Positioning a stent for aorto-ostial lesions
    **Can we have perfect position of a stent for coronary ostial lesions?
    **Deployment of stent in aorto-ostial lesions
    **Post-dilation in stenting of an aorto-ostial lesion
    **Watermelon seeding effect of aorto-ostial lesions
    **Avoiding occlusion of side branch during main branch angioplasty
    ***Cutting balloon angioplasty of a jailed sidebranch ostial lesion
    ***Extraction of stent by cutting balloon at ostial lesion

GENERAL OVERVIEW

Ostial lesion is defined as a lesion of a native coronary artery or a bypass graft within 3 mm of the aortic wall or of a major vessel (branch vessel ostial disease). These lesions are commonly composed of a large amount of fibrocellular material and less often contain the compliant lipid-rich material that typifies

---

*Basic; **Advanced; ***Rare, exotic, or investigational.

From: Nguyen T, Hu D, Saito S, Grines C, Palacios I (eds), *Practical Handbook of Advanced Interventional Cardiology*, 2nd edn. © 2003 Futura, an imprint of Blackwell Publishing.

intracoronary lesions.[1] So during PCI of these lesions, complete predilation with balloon angioplasty followed by stenting is indicated. There were no new data of DES on ostial lesions.

TECHNICAL TIPS

**Selection and position of guides for ostial lesions: Because of the proximity of the lesion to the ostium, no guide should be fully engaged nor deep-seated. The usual Judkins guide may provide sufficient backup with coaxial alignment without aggressive intubation. A guide with side holes would help. However, waste of contrast media through side holes would mask the exact location and the severity of the ostial lesion. As long as coaxial alignment is maintained, the interventional device can be advanced, positioned, and checked with the tip of the guide positioned just outside the ostium.

**Disengagement of guides during aorto-ostial lesion interventions: Once the device catheter carrying the undeployed stent, balloon, or atherectomy blade is properly positioned, the guide is then gently withdrawn 1 or 2 cm into the aorta, so the balloon or the stent is not inflated or deployed inside the guide. Gentle forward pressure on the device catheter or low-pressure balloon inflation (1–2 ATM) may help to maintain proper balloon position while the guide is retracted. Frequent test injections should be done to verify that the tip of the guide does not inadvertently engage beyond the ostium and that the devices do not move outside the intended area (Figure 11-1).

**Re-engagement of guides after stenting: After deployment of a stent, a coronary angiogram is done in order to check the results. One particular helpful technique to readvance the guide into position is to inflate the balloon to 1 ATM inside the stent with 1–2 mm protruding into the aorta. With the balloon inflated and protecting the stent struts, the guide is manipulated to be coaxial with the tip pointing straight at the ostium (in the LAO view), then the guide is pulled over the balloon into position for final angiography. Once the coronary angiogram is done, the guide can be backed out by advancing the wire in further. This maneuver should be done under fluoroscopy so the wire is not advanced too far, perforating the coronary artery. If the balloon is pulled back, the guide should be pulled a little first, so pulling the balloon out will not move the guide forward into the ostium.

***Two-guide techniques for aorto-ostial lesions: Correct positioning of a stent at an ostial lesion can be difficult due to poor visualization once the guide is backed out of the artery to allow deployment. The simultaneous use of a diagnostic catheter allows optimal visualization of stent position, while maintaining a stable guide position well away from the stent.[2] In a case report by Lambros *et al.* which illustrates the technique of using a second diagnostic catheter to enhance visualization of the lesion during stent positioning, a patient successfully underwent interventions for an aorto-ostial lesion in the SVG to LAD. An 8F JR guide was stable and provided good support. However, with the guide in a position that would allow adequate visualization of the lesion, the tip of the guide sat on the lesion, precluding perfect stent deployment. When the guide was withdrawn slightly, visualization was poor and the proximal balloon remained within the guide, risking movement during deployment. Then a 6F diagnostic catheter was introduced from the opposite site and engaged, providing excellent vision for stent positioning.[2]

***Double wire to position ostial stent:** Difficulty in positioning the guide during stenting of an ostial RCA lesion is sometimes made easier by use of a second steerable wire placed in the aorta just above the coronary sinus. This second wire stabilizes the guide outside the coronary artery and prevents it from moving deeply into the guide. It also defines the junction of the coronary artery and aorta, an important landmark for stent placement (Figure 11-2).

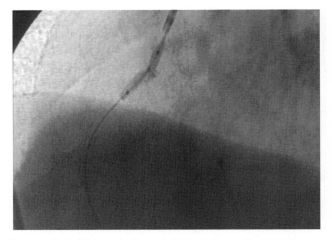

Figure 11-1: Before balloon inflation, the guide is retracted 1–2 cm into the aorta.

CAVEAT: Strategic concerns for interventions in ostial left anterior descending artery, left circumflex: Interventions of ostial LAD or LCX lesions pose many concerns, which are listed in Table 11-1.

**Optimal balloon predilation: Because of the extra rigidity and tissue elasticity in the ostial lesion, complete expansion of non-compliant and high pressure balloon is needed prior to stenting. If the balloon cannot be fully expanded with a pressure higher than 18 ATM, then cutting balloon angioplasty or rotablation may be needed.[3]

**Selection of stent for aorto-ostial lesions: A stent in the aorto-ostial lesion needs to have strong struts in order to prevent recoil. It should have markers at two ends so it can be positioned accurately. Overdilating a stent can shorten it, so a stent should be long enough that it does not leave the ostium uncovered. In large lesions such as the aorto-ostial saphenous vein graft, a biliary stent can cover the lesion. However, it has a large articulation gap. This is why this stent is not ideal for this location.

**Positioning a stent for aorto-ostial lesions: It is frequently difficult to identify the proximal end of an ostial lesion with certainty. The first reason is that the guide cannot be engaged deeply into the ostium or the lesion itself. The guide has to be seated outside the aorta, so during injection, part of the contrast enters the ostium and part swirls under and along the curve of the coronary sinus, thus masking the exact location and severity of the ostial lesion. The second reason is that there is a device across the lesion during positioning a balloon, stent or interventional device, so the minimal flow at the ostium may not be able to delineate the lesion and the location of the ostium. During

Table 11-1
Technical concerns with PCI of ostial LAD and LCX lesions

1. The balloon or stent can impinge on the origin of the non-dilated artery and obstruct flow.
2. If there is acute occlusion, there could be significant jeopardy to cardiac function or survival.
3. Possible difference of vessel size from the left main to the LAD or LCX.
4. Dissection at the proximal LAD and LCX could extend in a retrograde fashion into the LM segment.
5. Stent restenosis at the proximal end could result in restenosis of the LM.
6. Antegrade and retrograde embolization.

balloon inflation, if the waist is in the middle of the balloon then the position of the balloon is perfect. This is why the two markers at the ends of a stent help tremendously in positioning the stent. Different landmarks such as a fleck of calcium in the aortic wall may also help to identify the entry point of the ostium. The presence of a second wire curving along the coronary sinus may help to prevent deep engagement of the guide. However, the wire cannot locate the starting point of the ostial segment because the aortic wall is not a straight wall. The coronary sinus can curve deeper under the sinotubular ridge where the ostium is seen above, cannulated by the tip of the guide with the contrast flow swirling below (Figure 11-2). Once a stent is deployed, it is more difficult to evaluate the severity of the short ring size ostial segment that is left uncovered by a too short stent. A small guide can pass through it without causing any ventricularization of pressure and a coronary angiogram would not detect any abnormality because the ostial segment is covered with contrast from back flow. The situation can become worse if the ostial segment is not filmed on the best orthogonal projection. If viewed from an angled projection, the lesion may not be seen because the adjacent contrast-filled vessel segments are projected over the short napkin-ring size uncovered segment and mask it.

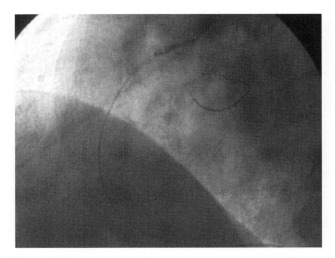

Figure 11-2: A second wire protrudes from the guide and curves along the coronary sinus. It will prevent the tip of the guide from engaging deeply in the ostium and marks the proximal boundary of the ostium.

**Can we have perfect position of a stent for coronary ostial lesions? In patients with ostial lesions of a side branch, such as the diagonal or obtuse marginal (OM), a stent can be positioned and deployed perfectly if the angle between the side branch and the main branch is 90°. If the angle is more or less than 90° (not perpendicular) then the proximal end of the stent can protrude into the main branch lumen or stay too far inside the side branch, leaving the ostium uncovered.

**Deployment of stent in aorto-ostial lesions: A stent premounted on a non-compliant balloon is preferred so there is no need to change the balloon for post-dilation. A second wire can be inserted and positioned in the coronary sinus. This wire will prevent the tip of the guide engaging deeply in the ostium and the location of the wire curving along the coronary sinus will mark the proximal boundary of the ostium. When deploying the stent, hold the guide and the balloon firmly to avoid any movement; the patient may be asked to hold their breath. After inflation and deflation of the balloon, remove the balloon while pulling the guide under fluoroscopy, to prevent it from advancing forward into the ostium and damaging the stent. Then perform adjunctive angioplasty with a high-pressure balloon to ensure full stent expansion and apposition.

**Post-dilation in stenting of an aorto-ostial lesion: When a stent is deployed in an ostial segment, it is ideal to have 1 mm of stent struts protruding from the ostium. This 1-mm strut will fence the atheromatous plaque of the aortic wall. This is why, after preliminary stenting, any stent should be postdilated with a larger balloon in order to flare its proximal struts against the aortic wall, thus preventing any difficulty with later re-engagement of guide or damage to the struts by the guide or by other interventional devices.

**Watermelon seeding effect of aorto-ostial lesions: In patients with ostial lesion, while inflating the balloon, it sometimes migrates proximally or distally. As a result, the balloon should be inflated more slowly, one ATM at a time, and the balloon catheter gently retracted to keep the balloon from migrating distally. Even so, there are cases of persistent watermelon seeding. Cutting the balloon will help to solve the problem, especially in in-stent restenosis.

**Avoiding occlusion of side branch during main branch angioplasty: It is not feasible to dilate every ostial lesion because of tortuosity of the proximal segment or because of the small size of the side branch. In such a situation, angioplasty of the main branch with a cutting balloon may prevent plaque shifting and occlusion of the side branch. This limited PCI is frequently applied to symptomatic relief of elderly and high-risk patients.

***Cutting balloon angioplasty of a jailed sidebranch ostial lesion:** When there is failure in dilating an ostial lesion with POBA, then CB could be used with extreme caution. In a case reported by Hongo *et al.*, repeated failures with POBA occurred when dilating an ostial lesion through the side struts. Then a CB was inserted, with the proximal segment well inside the main vessel lumen, and the balloon was inflated with excellent results.[4]

***Extraction of stent by cutting balloon at ostial lesion:** The CB is designed with blades mounted along its length. During inflation, the blades are protruded outwards and exposed. Then, during deflation, there is a mechanism of gradual rewrapping the balloon with multiple wings over the blades. During this process of rewrapping, there is a possibility of creating a recess in the form of an acute angle formed by the balloon and the blades.[1] This recess can get stuck into the stent struts and prevent withdrawal of the CB. If the CB is pulled strongly enough it could pull with it the stent or part of the stent. When the CB is withdrawn, the pulling force applied on the balloon catheter will not be parallel to the vessel axis. An anchoring point will then be formed at the stiff proximal edge of the blade and the soft proximal balloon catheter. This anchoring point can be easily caught on the proximal stent struts, especially at the RCA orifice, as an almost 90° curve is formed by the proximal RCA and the aortic wall.[2] In order to prevent this problem, after deflation the CB should be advanced first, then withdrawn gently. Other possibilities[3] include: stent struts fracture by the microblades, or – another possible catching point – an under-expanded stent with inadequate struts apposition.[5]

REFERENCES

1. Steward JT, Ward DE, Davies MJ *et al.* Isolated coronary artery stenosis: Observations of the pathology. *Eur Heart J* 1987; **8**: 917–20.
2. Lambros J, Fairshid A, Pitney MR. Simultaneous use of a diagnostic catheter to facilitate stent deployment in aorto-ostial stenosis: A case report. *Cathet Cardiovasc Diagn* 1997; **40**: 210–11.
3. Colombo A, Stankovic G. Ostial lesion. In: Colombo A, Stankovic G, eds. *Colombo's Tips and Tricks in Interventional Cardiology.* Martin Dunitz, 2002: 45.

4. Hongo R, Brent B. Cutting balloon angioplasty through the stents struts of a "jailed" sidebranch ostial lesion. *J Invasive Cardiol* 2002; **14**: 558–60.

5. Wang H, Kao H, Liau C *et al.* Coronary stent strut avulsion in aorto-ostial ISR: Potential complication after CB angioplasty. *Cathet Cardiovasc Interv* 2002; **56**: 215–19.

Chapter 12

Acute ST-elevation Myocardial Infarction

Thach Nguyen, Mintu Turakhia,
Pham Hoan Tien, Wang Lefeng,
C Michael Gibson

INTRODUCTION

ST-segment elevation acute myocardial infarction (STEMI) is caused by occlusion of a major coronary vessel. Prompt restoration of patency in the infarct-related artery (IRA) reduces the infarct size, minimizes the myocardial damage, preserves left ventricular function and reduces mortality. Different modalities of treatment and their combinations have been tested in small or large randomized clinical trials.

---

*Basic; **Advanced; ***Rare, exotic, or investigational.

From: Nguyen T, Hu D, Saito S, Grines C, Palacios I (eds), *Practical Handbook of Advanced Interventional Cardiology*, 2nd edn. © 2003 Futura, an imprint of Blackwell Publishing.

INTERVENTION AT THE EPICARDIAL LEVEL

Fibrinolytic therapy: Prior to the advent of percutaneous intervention (PCI), fibrinolysis was the mainstay of therapy for STEMI, and it continues to be the dominant strategy worldwide. All agents in this category activate plasminogen by cleaving it to form plasmin, which enzymatically cleaves fibrin strands that have caused platelet and red cell aggregation within the active thrombus. Fibrin degradation leads to clot dissolution and rapid restoration of flow within the IRA.

The Food and Drug Administration (FDA) has classified thrombolytic agents into two categories: fibrin-selective and fibrin non-selective. Fibrin selectivity refers to increased enzymatic activity of a plasminogen activator in the presence of fibrin.

Fibrin-selective agents are referred to as tissue plasminogen activators and include alteplase (tPA) and tenecteplase (TNK). These agents focus their activity preferentially at the clot surface, cleaving plasminogen to plasmin. As fibrin is degraded, the lysine-binding sites on fragmin molecules are continually exposed, which then facilitates continuing lysis of the clot. By this mechanism, the fibrin-selective agents induce thrombolysis without inducing a systemic lytic state or depleting circulating fibrinogen.

Agents with reduced fibrin specificity (fibrin non-selective) include streptokinase (SK), reteplase (rPA), and anistreplase. These agents activate free and bound forms of plasminogen and induce a systemic increase in fibrin degradation products (FDPs) and decrease circulating levels of fibrinogen and α-antiplasmin. The low level of fibrinogen and high level of FDPs with anticoagulant properties help to sustain thrombotic dissolution.

Efficacy of fibrinolytic therapy decreases as the time between initiation of treatment and onset of symptoms increases. Because of continued fibrin cross-linking, older clots are resistant to disruption and require greater plasmin activity to achieve clot dissolution. It is thought that fibrin-selective agents may have a greater ability to access and dissolve this complex mesh of cross-linked fibrin in the acute thrombus. Of the currently-available fibrin-selective agents, TNK-tPA has a 14-fold higher specificity for fibrin and an 80-fold higher resistance to plasminogen activator-inhibitor (PAI-1) compared with tPA.[1] Practically, in the subgroup analysis of the Assessment of the Safety and Efficacy of a New Thrombolytic (ASSENT) 2 trial,[2] significantly lower 30-day mortality was found among patients who presented more than 4 hours after onset of symptom (7% in TNK-tPA group and 9.2% in tPA group; P=0.018). This 2% absolute difference in mortality was maintained at 1-year follow-up, although the difference was no longer statistically significant.[3]

The TIMI flow: In order to evaluate the reperfusion achieved by fibrinolytic therapy, a grading system for coronary artery perfusion was developed.[4] If there is no antegrade flow, it is termed Thrombolysis In acute Myocardial Infarction (TIMI)-0 flow. If there is some penetration of the contrast across the lesion, it is TIMI-1 flow. If the artery is completely visualized but the flow is slower than the flow in the normal branch, then it is TIMI-2 flow. If there is a strong and brisk flow, this is TIMI-3 flow (Figure 12-1).[4] In this early TIMI-1 trial, a strong relation between TIMI flow and mortality was demonstrated. The higher percentage of TIMI-3 flow at 90 minutes angiography, the lower is the mortality. Successful reperfusion is then considered only when there is a TIMI-3 flow which conferred a 42-day mortality rate of 4.7%, compared with 7% for TIMI-2 flow patients and 10.6% for TIMI-0-1 flow patients.[5] From the 7% average 30-day mortality, in order to further decrease mortality by 1%, there is a need of an additional increase of 20% of TIMI-3 flow opening in the 90-minute angiogram.

More accurate flow evaluation: the corrected TIMI frame count: Further analysis among patients with TIMI-3 flow after reperfusion still revealed a divergence of mortality within the subgroup. An objective counting technique based on angiography was developed in an effort to provide a more quantitative, reproducible measure of reperfusion. The cor-

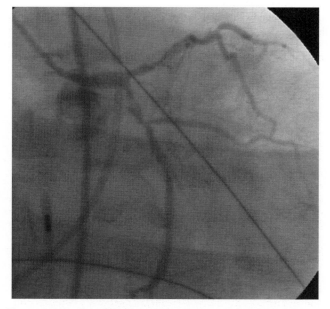

Figure 12-1: The TIMI flow. TIMI-0 flow: no antegrade flow (see Figure 3-15). TIMI-2 flow: the artery is completely visualized but the flow is slower than the flow in the normal branch. In the TIMI-3 flow, there is a strong and brisk flow.

rected TIMI frame count (CTFC) is defined as the number of angiographic frames needed for dye to traverse a coronary artery.[5] By convention, the frame count system uses a film speed of 30 frames per second (FPS), which is the standard in most cardiac catheterization laboratories. Frame 0 (the starting reference frame) is defined as the first frame in which injected contrast touches two borders (but does not fully opacify) of the proximal segment of the major coronary vessel. The end frame is defined as the first frame in which injected contrast appears in the distal bed of the reference vessel. The number of frames between the end frame and start frame is the CTFC (Figure 12-2 A, B-3).

CTFC is particularly useful because it can account for rate of coronary filling and difference in epicardial vessel size and length. Inter-observer variability is reduced because CTFC relies on objective definitions. The CTFC is an independent predictor of in-hospital mortality from AMI and can further stratify patients with TIMI-3 flow into low- and high-risk groups.[7]

Assessment of tissue perfusion: the myocardial perfusion grading system: The divergence in mortality among patients with TIMI-3 flow is also associated with degree of tissue perfusion. Specifically, restoration of flow in the IRA may not be a reliable predictor of restoration of tissue perfusion supplied by the IRA. Therefore a new technique to assess myocardial tissue perfusion independent of epicardial flow was developed. The TIMI myocardial perfusion grading (TMPG) system was designed and validated to further risk stratify patients in whom successful epicardial reperfusion

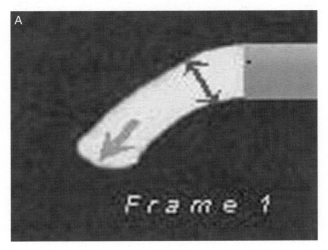

Figure 12-2: The corrected TIMI frame count. (A) The first frame is defined as the frame in which injected contrast touches the two borders, but does not fully opacify it. *(Continued)*

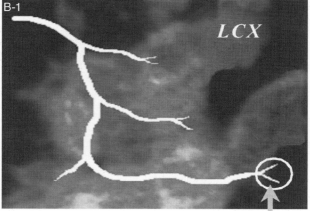

Landmark:
Last Branch off
Most Distal OM

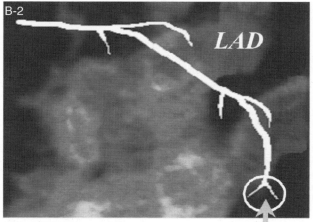

Landmark:
Bifurcation of
LAD at Apex

Figure 12-2 B: The end frame is defined as the first frame in which contrast appears in the distal bed of the reference vessel. (1) For the LCX, it is the last branch off the most distal OM; (2) for the LAD, it is the bifurcation of the LAD at the apex. (*Continued*)

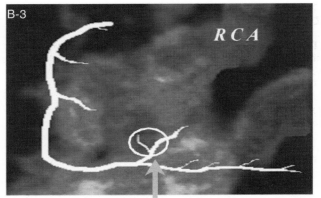

Landmark:
First Branch off
Posterolateral

Figure 12-2 B: (3) for the RCA, it is the first branch off the postero-lateral branch. (Adapted from Gibson CM, TIMI.TV website.)

(TIMI-3 flow) was achieved. The definitions of TMP grades are shown in Table 12-1 (see also Figure 12-3).[8]

TMPG is a multivariate predictor of 30-day mortality, independent of age, gender, admission pulse, anterior MI location, CTFC, or TIMI flow grade.[8] Patients with TIMI-3 flow in the IRA after PCI and poor myocardial perfusion (TMPG 0 or 1) have a mortality of 5.4%, which is significantly higher than patients with TIMI-3 flow and TMPG 2 (4.4%) or TMPG 3 (2.0%; P <0.01).[8] Thus, even among patients with TIMI-3 flow or normal CTFC, there is a 7-fold gradient in mortality depending on the extent of the microvascular perfusion. TMPG remains a strong predictor of mortality, independent of flow in the epicardial artery even two years after fibrinolytic therapy.[9] CTFC and TMPG are important predictors and continue to serve as primary endpoints in many ACS clinical trials.

TECHNICAL TIPS

**Angiographic technique to calculate the CTFC and TMPG: It is important to remember that CTFC is a marker of coronary flow and not simply epicardial stenosis. After the lesion is successfully treated, CTFC can remain abnormal and may reflect poor downstream perfusion. Cinefilming should continue long enough to determine if the dye reaches the distal vessel (i.e. to distinguish TIMI 1 versus TIMI 2 flow). In addition, pre-injection "puffs" under fluoroscopy for a "quick look" should be minimized. Alternatively,

Table 12-1
Definitions of TMP grades

TMP Grade 0: There is no dye entering the myocardium and there is minimal or no blush apparent in the distribution of the culprit artery, indicating lack of tissue-level perfusion.

TMP Grade 1: Dye slowly enters but fails to leave the microvasculature. There is a ground glass appearance ("blush") or opacification of the myocardium in the distribution of the culprit artery, that fails to clear from the microvasculature, and dye staining is present on the next injection (~30 seconds between injection).

TMP Grade 2: Delay entry and exit of dye from the microvasculature. There is a ground glass appearance ("blush") or opacification of the myocardium in the distribution of the culprit artery, that is strongly persistent after three cardiac cycles of the washout phase and either does not or only minimally diminishes in intensity during washout.

TMP Grade 3: Normal entry and exit of dye from the microvasculature. There is a ground glass appearance ("blush") or opacification of the myocardium in the distribution of the culprit artery, that clears normally and is either gone or only mildly/moderately persistent at the end of the washout phase (i.e. dye is gone or mildly/moderately persistent after three cardiac cycles of the washout phase and noticeably diminishes in intensity in the washout phase), similar to an uninvolved artery. Blush that is of only mild intensity throughout the washout phase but fades minimally is also classified as grade 3.

the operator may wait for 30 seconds prior to performing angiography to ensure that the dye has been washed from the artery. During angiography, the operator should continue the cinefilm until the dye has been completely washed out of the artery (at least five cardiac cycles after the dye begins to wash out of the artery). This will allow accurate assessment of the epicardial flow (CTFC) and myocardial perfusion (TMPG). The technical goals of the angiography are summarized in Table 12-2.[10]

**Cinefilm technique for the calculation of CTFC and TMPG: For evaluation of the left system, the first injection should be in the right anterior oblique (RAO) caudal position. The RAO cranial position should then be used to view the bifurcation. The usual views of the IRA and non-IRA can be performed after the first critical injection. Size 5F or 6F catheters are adequate, while 4F catheters are too small for quantitative angiography. The angiographic protocol of the first injection and the suggested projected angles are described in Tables 12-3 and 12-4.

TIMI Myocardial Perfusion (TMP) Grades

 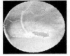

TMP Grade 3	TMP Grade 2	TMP Grade 1	TMP Grade 0
Normal ground glass appearance of blush Dye mildly persistent at end of washout	Dye strongly persistent at end of washout Gone by next injection	Stain present Blush persists on next injection	No or minimal blush

Figure 12-3: The Myocardial Perfusion Grading System. In TMP Grade 0, there is no dye entering the myocardium and there is minimal or no blush apparent in the distribution of the culprit artery. In TMP Grade 2, there is a ground glass appearance ("blush") or opacification of the myocardium in the distribution of the culprit artery, which is strongly persistent after 3 cardiac cycles of the washout phase and either does not or only minimally diminishes in intensity during washout. In TMP Grade 3, there is a ground glass appearance ("blush") or opacification of the myocardium in the distribution of the culprit artery, which clears normally and is either gone or only mildly/moderately persistent at the end of the washout phase (i.e. dye is gone or mildly/moderately persistent after 3 cardiac cycles of the washout phase and noticeably diminishes in intensity in the washout phase), similar to an uninvolved artery.

Table 12-2
Exploratory endpoints using digital subtraction angiography

- Size of the myocardial blush (cm^2)
- Brightness of the myocardial blush (gray scale)
- Rate of growth of the myocardial blush (cm^2/sec)
- Rate of growth of the brightness of the myocardial blush (gray/sec)
- Rate at which blush fades from peak (both gray/sec and cm^2/sec)

TECHNICAL IMPLICATIONS

Any patient with chest pain coming to the hospital within 12 hours from onset and with an electrocardiogram (ECG) suggestive of ST-elevation AMI can be offered to undergo emergency PCI. A catheterization laboratory team should be available to proceed with primary PCI within 45 minutes of activation (Tables 12-5 and 12-6).[11] It is reasonable to withhold thrombolytic therapy and transfer the patient for primary intervention if PCI can be completed within 2 hours.

Table 12-3
The critical first injection

1. The first injection should be in **a 9 inch mode**
2. In the 9 inch mode, do not pan
3. It is critical that **the camera should not move** so digital subtraction of the images can be done at a later date.
4. Have the patient **taking a deep breath and hold the breath** during injection so the ribs and the diaphragm will not move again allowing digital subtraction
5. Minimize pre-injection "puff" or small injection prior to the first critical injection as this may impact the assessment of the blush grades

Table 12-4
Recommended projected angles

Left coronary artery system			
RAO	0–30	CAU	20–25 (preferred view)
RAO	0–15	CRA	35–45
LAO	45–60	CAU	30–40
LAO	60	CRA	10–20
Right coronary system			
LAO	10–15	CRA	30–45 (preferred view)
LAO	45–60	Straight	0
RAO	30–45	Straight	

Table 12-5
Indications for primary PCI (11)

1. Symptomatic AMI in less than 12 hours
2. AMI 12–24 hours with continued chest pain
3. Cardiogenic shock <24 hours
4. Thrombolytic failure within 12 hours of chest pain, especially if anterior MI
5. Suspected re-occlusion after lytic therapy
6. Non-diagnostic ECG(LBBB, Paced rhythm, ischemic ST-T changes), with positive enzymes, refractory angina, or hemodynamic instability/CHF)

First, different views of the presumed non-infarct related arteries (non-IRA) are taken with a diagnostic catheter in order to estimate their patency and collateral flow to the diseased artery. Next, angiography and identification of the presumed IRA is performed with a guide so PCI can be started promptly if needed. If the IRA has a significant stenosis or thrombus with inadequate flow (TIMI flow <3) and there is no significant left

Table 12-6
Angiographic exclusions precluding performance of primary PCI

1. Unprotected LM >60% stenosis
2. IRA less than 70% stenosis with TIMI-3 flow
3. IRA supplies small amount of myocardium: risk> benefits
4. Inability to clearly identify the IRA
5. IRA with TIMI-3 flow and lesion morphology high risk for abrupt closure or no reflow
6. Asymptomatic patient with multivessel disease with TIMI-3 flow, and CABG is indicated

main coronary artery lesion, then the patient is prepared for emergency PCI. A left ventriculogram can be performed after PCI if the patient is hemodynamically stable. This will help to assess systolic function, extent of injury (wall motion abnormality), and evaluate valvular or mechanical abnormalities. The left ventriculogram should not be performed if the left ventricular end diastolic pressure (LVEDP) exceeds 30 mmHg.

In cases of hemodynamically unstable patients, consultation with anesthesia and surgery is advised because it may allow the interventional cardiologist to focus on the procedure itself while medical and supportive care are effectively performed by other skilled providers. A low threshold should be present for placement of an intra-aortic balloon pump in hemodynamically unstable patients.

TECHNICAL TIPS

**Crossing the lesion: Usually the IRA is occluded with a soft and fresh thrombus that can be crossed easily with a steerable floppy wire. Once this new total occlusion is crossed, some operators wait up to one minute to determine if the patient develops a reperfusion arrhythmia. The lesion can then be "dottered" by moving the uninflated balloon back and forth. This will allow flow of stagnant blood proximal to the occlusion to seep slowly into the distal vasculature. This maneuver prevents the abrupt opening of the occluded artery, which theoretically may minimize the chance of flooding of the distal vasculature with stagnant blood. This may decrease the probability of developing reperfusion arrhythmias, especially with interventions to the RCA. After completion of this maneuver, the operator may inject a small amount of contrast media to verify the position of the wire in the true lumen (and not in a side branch). If the wire position is still ambiguous, then the wire can be removed and dye can be injected through the central lumen of the balloon. This maneuver also aids in the assessment of the artery size for selection of balloon size.

**Avoiding vaso-vagal symptoms: Rapid restoration of flow, particularly to inferior-territory IRA, may lead to hypotension from reperfusion bradyarrhythmias. It is recommended to aggressively hydrate patients with an inferior MI prior to reperfusion. Administration of nitrates is contraindicated. Venous sheath access prior to intervention may be useful for rapid insertion of a temporary pacemaker if necessary. For unstable patients, or in cases where clinical suspicion is high for development of a bradyarrhythmia, the operator may place a temporary wire in the right atrium, ready to advance into the right ventricle for pacing if necessary.

**Balloon angioplasty: If the size of the distal artery is not known, a small (2.0 mm) balloon may be used to initially cross the lesion. Because artery occlusions often occur at epicardial vessel branchpoints, the size of the proximal artery may not reflect the true size of the distal vessel due to abrupt tapering of the vessel diameter at these branchpoints.

After restoration of flow with a 2.0-mm balloon, a balloon with a diameter equal to the reference size of the arterial segment proximal to the occlusion is positioned across the lesion. It is inflated until the indentation on its waist disappears. The balloon is then deflated and retracted into the guide. Oversizing the balloon may be associated with dissection and alpha-adrenergic "storm" (vasospasm) in the distal microvasculature.

LIMITATION OF PTCA

Although the mortality after plain PTCA was lower than after stenting, PTCA alone cannot seal off the ruptured plaque and turn off the thrombotic tendency by providing a smooth lumen with strong flow without shear stress. The adverse interactions between fibrinolytic agent and plain balloon angioplasty (not stenting) are listed in Table 12-7. The adverse outcomes were repeated again in the GUSTO-V and ASSENT-2 trials when elective PCI was discouraged by protocol.[12–13]

Table 12-7
Adverse interactions between fibrinolysis and POBA

1. Clot lysis triggers the coagulation cascade
2. Plaque rupture, injury to the arterial wall leads to mural thrombus
3. Unenven lumen with imperfect flow and heightened shear stress activates the platelet and the coagulation cascade

**Lesions with heavy thrombotic burden: In situations of small or moderate thrombotic burden, conventional angioplasty and/or stenting was tried first. Some operators advocate the use of an export catheter to aspirate thrombus prior to PCI in lesions with a large thrombotic burden. After the export catheter is positioned near the thrombus, continuous negative pressure is applied while advancing the export catheter across the lesion. This maneuver is repeated several times until no further thrombotic material can be aspirated.[12] In the PAMI trial, stenting resulted in angiographic resolution of thrombus in more than 80% of patients.[11] When an angiographic filling defect consistent with the presence of a thrombus after stenting is observed, repeat balloon dilatation with higher pressure should be attempted. Extrusion of the ruptured plaque may angiographically mimic the presence of thrombotic material. If angioplasty or stenting fail to dissipate all visible thrombi, other mechanical thrombectomy devices may be utilized. In a study of 66 patients with ACS (49 of whom had ST elevation MI), lesions with thrombus were randomized to thrombectomy with the X-Sizer catheter or to conventional PCI. Post-procedural TIMI-3 flow was similar in both groups, but the corrected TIMI frame count was lower in patients treated with the X-Sizer catheter (18.3% versus 24.7% among conventionally-treated patients ($P<0.05$)).[13]

**Avoiding antegrade embolization: Thrombotic burden is often large in patients with prolonged AMI symptom duration or if the IRA is a large-diameter vessel such as an RCA or a saphenous vein graft. There is a significant possibility of antegrade embolization due to strong contrast injection or during removal of catheter wires. Distal embolization in the IRA can occur after the dissolution of occlusive thrombus by balloon inflation or stenting and disruption of retrograde collateral flow, resulting in persistent, symptomatic ST-elevation. This is why manipulation of hardware in the IRA has to be gentle and minimal to avoid dislodgement of thrombus with detrimental retrograde or distal embolization resulting in new infarctions. In a pilot trial with distal filtering device (Angioguard) by LF Wang *et al.*, 40 patients undergoing primary PCI were randomized for conventional treatment or protection with the Angioguard device. There were no clinical differences at baseline or at follow-up. However, there was less distal embolization in patients receiving the Angioguard (5.2% vs 36.8%, P=0.042), better CTFC (19.9 vs 34.1, P=0.045) and higher blush grade 3 (73.3% vs 31.6%, P=0.022) (manuscript submitted for publication).

CAVEAT: Avoiding retrograde embolization: During PCI of the proximal segment of the LAD and LCX, fragments of large thrombi may be squeezed back and occlude the ostium of the adjacent vessel (Figure 12-4). Fragments

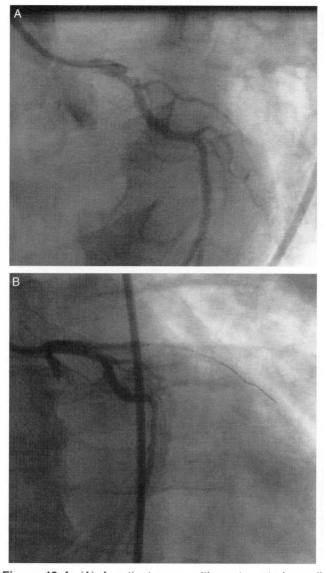

Figure 12-4: (A) A patient came with acute anterior wall MI. The LAD was closed at its origin. (B) During PCI of the proximal segment of the LAD, balloon angioplasty showed no problem with the flow to the LCX. This figure showed good flow to the LCX during inflation of the balloon. In reality, retrospectively, there was some haziness at the ostium of the LCX during inflation of the balloon. This haziness disappeared with balloon deflation. *(Continued)*

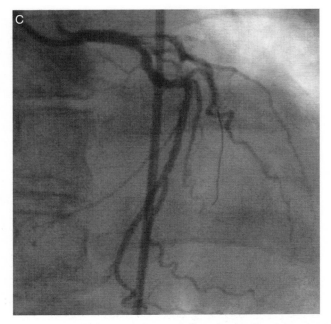

Figure 12-4: (C) The balloon was inflated at the distal segment of the total occlusion (thrombus) so there was no retrograde embolization to the LCX. Here an angiogram showed patency of the distal end of the lesion while there was still significant residual stenosis at the origin of the lesion. *(Continued)*

can even adhere to catheter balloons after deflation, which, when withdrawn or retracted into the guide, may lead to embolization and occlusion of proximal branches. Embolization may be dramatically minimized by first opening the Y-connector prior to injection of contrast agent and allow back flow to remove any free thrombotic material. Since then, stent placement in ostial LAD and LCX lesions has generally been avoided to minimize risk of left main complications or retrograde extrusion of clots. However, interventions may be necessary and even desirable in such lesions that demonstrate significant elastic recoil after conventional PTCA, which is not uncommon.[12] Moreover, with successful removal of thrombus at the ostial lesion by use of a thrombectomy device, use of drug-eluting stents may be an optimal strategy in the future.

**Primary stenting: After balloon predilation, the reference diameter following intracoronary nitroglycerin may be used to estimate the size of the stent, and the goal should be

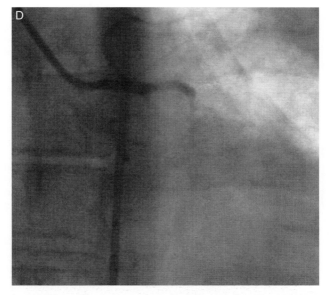

Figure 12-4: (D) After stenting, the thrombus was squeezed back and occluded the left circumflex causing cardiac arrest.

a stent:artery ratio of 1:1. Oversizing of the stent is associated with an increase in distal microvasculature embolization and precipitation of alpha-adrenergic storm. To minimize oversizing, semi-compliant balloons of the same diameter as the reference vessel (or non-compliant balloons slightly larger) may be used. Careful attention must be applied to ensure complete coverage of the fractured plaque and any residual intimal dissection. It is important to remember that not every lesion can be or should be stented. The reasons for performing conventional PTCA without stenting are listed in Table 12-8.

Table 12-8
PTCA rather than stenting due to technical problems

1. Excessive proximal tortuosity
2. Large thrombus
3. Proximity of major side branch
4. Very small vessel
5. Inability to take antiplatelet medication

CAVEAT: Did you miss the IRA? During the diagnostic angiogram all the major vessels and their large branches should be accounted for. In a PCI case performed by one of the authors, the LAD showed one moderate lesion in its mid-segment with typical angina and ST segment elevation in 2,3,AVF. The RCA was nowhere to be seen, even with the aortogram. It was explained to the patient by the junior staff that congenitally she had no RCA. Because the symptoms were so typical because of the ECG change, an extraordinary effort was made to locate the RCA. It was found to be in its usual location when the RCA is originated from the left sinus: anterior and superior to the LM ostium (Figure 12-5). The patient underwent successfully PCI of the artery. In another case, a patient with AMI was found to have patent LAD, LCX and RCA. So where was the IRA? Because there was only minor ST elevation in leads I and AVL, it was

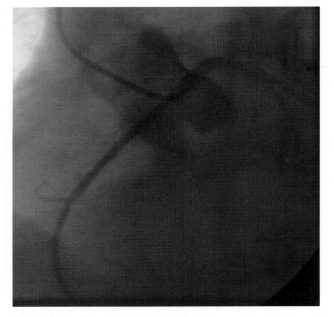

Figure 12-5: The missing RCA: A patient arrived with typical angina and ST segment elevation in 2,3,AVF. The LAD showed one moderate lesion in its mid-segment. The RCA was nowhere seen even with the aortogram. The RCA was found to be in its usual location when it is originated from the left sinus: anterior and superior to the LM ostium. (see Figure 3-15). The patient underwent successfully PCI of the artery: the left Judkins injection showed both the LM and the anomalous RCA.

suspected that the diagonal should be the IRA. A wire was advanced and probed the area suspected of being the possible origin of a large diagonal. The wire successfully entered and PCI of a large diagonal branch was performed successfully (Figure 12-6 A–C).

**Ensuring the IRA patency after stenting: In order to maintain patency and successful reperfusion of the IRA, it is important to achieve the best result possible: TIMI-3 flow, TMPG 3, low CTFC, large minimal lumen diameter (MLD), complete coverage of the plaque, and appropriate apposition of stent struts to the vessel wall. Pharmacologic management includes intravenous and oral antiplatelet and anticoagulant therapy. Intravenous heparin administration is continued after percutaneous intervention if there are many thrombi observed during intervention. However, with increasing use of glycoprotein 2b3a inhibitors, heparin administration is not continued after stent placement because clinical trials have shown no little benefit of continuing heparin following the procedure when a glycoprotein 2b3a inhibitor is used.

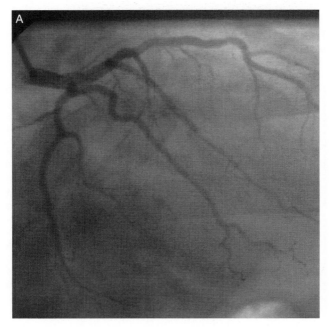

Figure 12-6: The missing diagonal. (A) A patient came with typical chest pain. There was mild ST segment elevation in I, AVL. In this RAO caudal view, the LAD, LCX arteries were patent. *(Continued)*

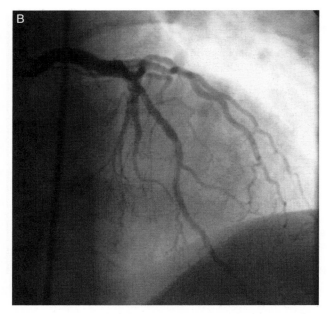

Figure 12-6: (B) In the AP cranial view, the LAD was seen patent. *(Continued)*

**Risk following stenting: IRA epicardial flow prior to percutaneous intervention is an important predictor of early and late mortality.[14] Even when TIMI-3 flow in the IRA was achieved after reperfusion, TIMI-0 or TIMI-1 flow before PCI is associated with a higher 30-day mortality (5.2%) compared to TIMI-2 or better flow (1.4%). In contrast to balloon angioplasty alone, angioplasty with stenting is associated with increased mortality among patients with baseline TIMI 0–1 flow. This difference in mortality is largest in the first month after PCI and is believed to be related to subacute thrombosis after stent placement, distal embolization or alpha-adrenergic storm downstream.[15] Despite excellent luminal scaffolding after angioplasty or stenting, aggressive and prolonged antiplatelet therapy with glycoprotein 2b3a inhibitors may be warranted for this high-risk subgroup. It is unclear if intravascular ultrasound (IVUS) may better guide stent placement and lead to improved outcomes.

**Identification of high-risk patients: In the emergency room, if patients present with a heart rate of less than 100 bpm and a blood pressure more than 100 mmHg, their in-hospital mortality is very low. In these patients, catheter-based intervention can be performed without surgical

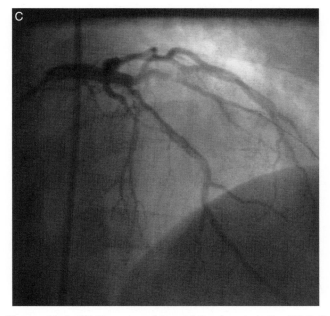

Figure 12-6: (C) Because of the subtle change in the ECG, it was suspected that a missing diagonal should be the IRA. A wire was advanced and probing the area suspecting the origin of a high diagonal. In this AP cranial view with deep inspiration and steep cranial in order to elevate the LCX above the LAD, a wire successfully entered a large diagonal branch and PCI was performed successfully.

stand-by if no further iatrogenic complications are made (perforation, dissection) (Figure 12-7).[16] The other high-risk patients are listed in Table 12-9. The mortality in high-risk patients undergoing stenting was higher at 9% while for PTCA it was only 4.9% (P=0.05). In the low-risk group, the mortality was only 0.6%.[17] The reason for the high mortality may be the lower rate of TIMI-3 after stenting or stenting itself causing subacute thrombosis.[18] In the PAMI-2 trial, only patients with persistent ischemia after PTCA benefit from IABP (Table 12-10).[19]

The rationale for adequate level of 2b3a inhibition and early mechanical revascularization: The results of GUSTO-5 and ASSENT-3 support the use of early percutaneous revascularization in patients with AMI receiving glycoprotein 2b3a inhibitors, regardless of symptomatology.[19] Early mechanical revascularization may reduce shear stress and decrease platelet activation. Additionally, early mechanical

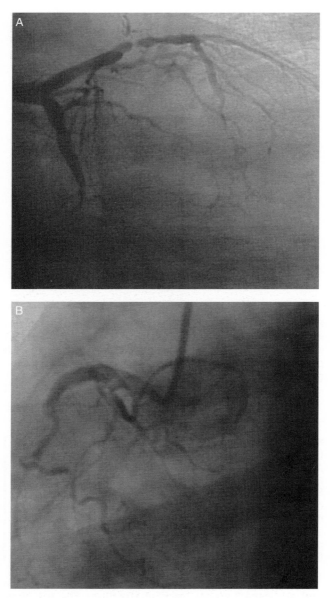

Figure 12-7: PCI of the only remaining IRA. A patient came with ST elevation in V leads. Blood pressure was 90/60 mmHg. (A) Occlusion of LCX. (B) Occlusion of the RCA. *(Continued)*

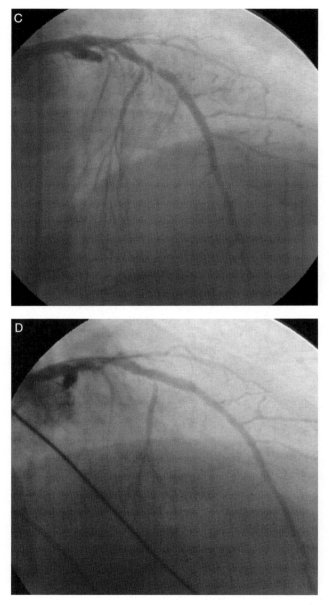

Figure 12-7: (C) Severe lesion in the LAD which is the IRA. (D) Successful stenting of the mid-LAD under support of an IABP and temporary pacemaker.

Table 12-9
The high-risk patient

1. >70 years of age
2. Ejection fraction <45%
3. Multivessel disease
4. Suboptimal PCI
5. Persistent arrhythmia

Table 12-10
Requisite conditions for primary PCI with no surgery on site

1. Experienced operators who perform regularly elective and primary PCI at tertiary centers.
2. Nursing and technical staff are experienced in handling acutely ill patients.
3. Catheterization laboratories must be well equipped with resuscitative equipment, IABP, etc.
4. Staff available 24/7/365.
5. Must have protocols for emergent transfer to surgical centers (high grade LM, unstable 3-vessel disease)
6. Protocols should address in whom to delay PTCA (TIMI-3 flow with >70% residual, etc.)[20]

revascularization may promote fibrosis or a "plaque sealing" effect and lower the rates of reocclusion.[20]

For maximal efficacy, glycoprotein 2b3a inhibition must inhibit more than 80% of platelets. Subtherapeutic platelet inhibition may lead to a paradoxical increase in prothrombotic effects, including death and MI.[21–26] Low levels of glycoprotein 2b3a inhibition may also promote inflammation via induction of platelet P-selectin expression, leading to increased serum levels of CD40 ligand. Conversely, a higher level of glycoprotein 2b3a inhibition reduces this inflammatory effect.[19]

Adverse effects of glycoprotein 2b3a inhibitors generally require long-term exposure to low levels of platelet inhibition (such as with oral glycoprotein 2b3a inhibitor agents) or short-term (>12 hours) exposure to glycoprotein 2b3a inhibitors in the absence of mechanical revascularization (GUSTO IV).[24,26]

Management of tissue malperfusion: After the IRA is opened, its coronary blood flow (CBF) should increase. One small study by Escobar et al. demonstrated that, after the first balloon angioplasty, the CBF increased. Then, after stenting, one-third of patients had substantially diminished CBF, while the other two-thirds had increased flow or no change.[27–28] The flow was then restored after infusion of vasodilators. The same phenomenon was also observed in fibrinolytic-treated patients.[29] In the TIMI trials, even though the residual stenosis was only 16% following stenting, normal flow was not restored in up to one-third of patients.[4] By the CTFC, in the absence of AMI, it normally requires 21 frames for the dye to traverse a coronary artery. In the setting of AMI, the average frame count of an IRA is 36 frames. After mechanical interventions, the flow of the IRA reversed to the level of the non-IRA, over 30 frames. It does not reverse to the normal level of a patient without AMI (21 frames).[30] This paradoxical flow fluctuation was observed also in the non-IRA, where the patient can have stable lesions with similar severity.[30] The new understanding is that AMI is not a focal disease; rather it is a systemic thrombophilic phase[31,32] precipitating simultaneous plaque rupture, causing simultaneous acute occlusion or slow flow in multiple major coronary or peripheral territories (stroke or acute limb ischemia due to thrombus).

With pharmacologic or mechanical opening of the IRA, distal micro-embolization occurs, with subsequent platelet activation and release of potent vasoconstrictors including serotonin, which induces microvascular spasm. In a study by Leosco et al., at baseline, the patients had low serotonin in the coronary sinus. Following intervention with balloon angioplasty, the level of serotonin increased 30-fold.[33] Following intracoronary stenting, the serotonin level increased more than 120-fold, causing vasoconstriction downstream. It was reversed by intracoronary infusion of any vasodilating agents such as alpha-adrenergic blockers, adenosine, nicorandil, calcium channel blockers, or nitroprusside. However, a blanket use of adenosine in the AMISTAD I and II trials did not result in better outcomes.[34-35]

Unfractionated heparin: In patients undergoing primary interventions, with the concomittant use of glycoprotein 2b3a inhibitors, it is now common to give 70 units/kg of UFH to achieve an activated clotting time (ACT) of 200–250 seconds.[36] If the glycoprotein 2b3a inhibitors are not used, high dose UFH to achieve ACT >350 seconds has been associated with reduced subacute thrombosis. UFH is not continued after the procedure because it has not been proven to decrease the rate of reocclusion or ischemia, unless there are a lot of residual thrombi. In patients with UFH-induced thrombocytopenia, either recombinant hirudin, bivalirudin, or argatroban should be used during PCI.[37]

Low molecular weight heparin (LMWH): The ASSENT-3 trial examined the combination of a fibrinolytic and a platelet glycoprotein 2b3a inhibitor (specifically half-dose TNK-tPA and full-dose abciximab), with a second experimental arm, which examined enoxaparin and full-dose TNK-tPA.[38] Although there was no difference in mortality between treatment arms, there was a trend toward lower mortality in the LMWH group in the subgroup of patients that received primary PCI.

Rescue angioplasty for failed thrombolysis: Since clinical signs and electrocardiographic data of reperfusion are not precise, the guidelines of the ACC/AHA task force suggest that catheterization be performed in any thrombolytic patients with ongoing chest pain or hemodynamic instability, or in asymptomatic patients who are less than 12 hours of symptom onset with persistent ST elevation, after 90 minutes of thrombolytic therapy.[37] However, the patients who require rescue angioplasty due to failed thrombolysis remained at increased risk for reocclusion, because they possibly had higher resistance to pharmacologic reperfusion, large thrombus burden or platelet-rich thrombi, factors unfavorable to the performance of mechanical intervention.

Rescue PCI should be performed on high-risk lesion (>75%) with TIMI of 2 or less. The mortality of patients who failed rescue PTCA was high, in the 30% range, while it was only 7–11% in patients with persistent occluded IRA treated conservatively. There was no indication for PCI of the IRA if the TIMI flow is 3 following lytic treatment. However, there are exceptions, which include the patients with high-risk of reocclusion or severe complications if there is occlusion of the IRA, and patients with >90% residual stenosis, prior MI, decreased LV ejection fraction, or multivessel disease.

Non-IRA lesion: Stenosis of non-IRA vessels should not be treated by emergent PCI unless there is evidence of persistent ischemia or cardiogenic shock after adequate reperfusion of the IRA.

PCI for saphenous vein graft: Patients with prior coronary artery bypass grafting who present with AMI are equally likely to occlude native vessels and bypass grafts, although LIMA grafts have a lower rate of stenosis. AMI after CABG usually affects smaller territories and presents with milder symptoms.[36] In comparison to native vessels, SVG thrombosis typically has a suboptimal response to fibrinolytic therapy. Vein grafts lack side branch vessels that would normally deliver the fibrinolytic agent to the site of occlusion.[37] In the case of mechanical intervention, because of the large size of the SVGs and high thrombotic burden, there is a significant risk of distal embolization. In the PAMI-2 trial the overall in-hospital and 6-month mortality of patients with prior CABG was higher compared with patients without prior CABG. Patients with CABG had lower rates of TIMI-3 flow after PCI, and mechanical intervention was less frequently attempted.[38] Recently, catheter-based filter devices were found to be effective in preventing distal embolization in primary PCI of SVG lesions.

Left main PCI in AMI: In a small study by Marso et al., in which 40 patients with AMI due to LM occlusion were treated with emergent PCI, the angiographic success rate was 88%. In-hospital mortality was 55%, and CABG was performed in 10% of patients. The 12-month mortality after left main PTCA with stenting was high (58%) but substantially lower than PTCA without stenting (78%; P <0.05).[39] All hospital deaths were a result of cardiogenic shock. Therefore, although PCI strategy for AMI from left main disease is feasible, short- and long-term mortality is high.[40] If LM occlusion is a result of aortic dissection, then PCI of the LM may be performed as a bridge toward hemodynamic stability before proceeding with definitive surgery.[41]

CONCLUSION

Despite numerous advances in management of STEMI, the treatment goal remains unchanged: prompt restoration of patency in the infarct-related artery (IRA) can reduce myocardial infarct size, minimize myocardial damage, preserve ventricular function, and significantly reduce mortality. The dominant and benchmark reperfusion strategy worldwide remains fibrinolytic therapy. However, rapid restoration of patency by catheter-based percutaneous intervention can result in excellent outcomes,[42] and the use of an early interventional strategy continues to increase.

If experienced operators are available at an institution with a large procedure volume, and if the interval between door and balloon (reperfusion) is less than 120 minutes, primary PCI has been shown to be superior to pharmacologic reperfusion, mostly by virtue of reducing recurrent MI and ICH. This benefit is mitigated by a number of factors and adjunct therapies, including glycoprotein 2b3a receptor antagonists, antithrombotics and antiplatelet agents, and low-dose fibrinolytics. These agents help to increase the opening rate of the IRA, increase tissue perfusion, and sustain patency after the acute event.[43] Female sex, age >65, presence of left bundle branch block, and advanced time of presentation (>12 hours) represent high-risk factors, and early mechanical intervention should be considered in these patients even in the absence of chest pain. In subgroups where PCI is comparable to thrombolysis in reducing mortality, mechanical reperfusion may still have an important role in prevention of ventricular remodeling, dilatation, and dysfunction that could impact the long-term prognosis of patients with AMI.

REFERENCES

1. Keyt BA, Paoni NF, Refino CJ et al. A faster-acting and more potent form of tissue plasminogen activator. Proc Natl Acad Sci USA 1994; **91**: 3670–4.
2. Single-bolus tenecteplase compared with front-loaded alteplase in acute myocardial infarction: the ASSENT-2 double-blind randomised trial. Assessment of the Safety and

254 Practical Handbook of Advanced Interventional Cardiology

Efficacy of a New Thrombolytic Investigators. *Lancet* 1999; **354**: 716–22.
3. Sinnaeve P, Granger C, Barbarsh G. Single bolus tenecteplase and front-loaded alteplase remain equivalent after one year: follow-up results of the ASSENT-2 trial. *Eur Heart J* 2000; **21**: 481.
4. The TIMI Study Group. The Thrombolysis in Myocardial Infarction (TIMI) trial. Phase I findings. *N Engl J Med* 1985; **312**.
5. Gibson CM, Cannon CP, Daley WL *et al*. TIMI frame count: a quantitative method of assessing coronary artery flow. *Circulation* 1996; **93**: 879–88.
6. Cannon CP, Braunwald E. GUSTO, TIMI and the case for rapid reperfusion. *Acta Cardiol* 1994; **49**: 1–8.
7. Gibson CM, Murphy SA, Rizzo MJ *et al*. Relationship between TIMI frame count and clinical outcomes after thrombolytic administration. Thrombolysis In Myocardial Infarction (TIMI) Study Group. *Circulation* 1999; **99**: 1945–50.
8. Gibson CM, Cannon CP, Murphy SA *et al*. Relationship of TIMI myocardial perfusion grade to mortality after administration of thrombolytic drugs. *Circulation* 2000; **101**: 125–30.
9. Gibson CM, Murphy SA, Barron HV. Relation of epicardial blood flow and myocardial perfusion to long term outcomes 2 years following thrombolysis in AMI: A TIMI 10B substudy. *Circulation* 2000; **102**: 435.
10. Gibson CM. How to do the Corrected TIMI Frame Count. Instruction to the investigators of the TIMI trials. **www.timi.tv** accessed May 28 2003.
11. Stone G, Grines C. Beyond primary PTCA: New approaches to mechanical reperfusion therapy in AMI. In: Stack RS, Roubin GS, O'Neill W, eds. *Interventional Cardiology Medicine, Principles and Practice*. Churchill Livingstone, 2002: 301–62.
12. Wang HJ, Kao HL, Liau CS, Lee YT. Export aspiration catheter thrombosuction before actual angioplasty in primary coronary intervention for acute myocardial infarction. *Cathet Cardiovasc Interv* 2002; **57**: 332–9.
13. Beran G, Lang I, Schreiber W *et al*. Intracoronary thrombectomy with the X-Sizer catheter system improves epicardial flow and accelerates ST-segment resolution in patients with acute coronary syndrome: a prospective, randomized, controlled study. *Circulation* 2002; **105**: 2355–60.
14. Ross AM, Coyne K, Reiner J. Very early PTCA of IRA with TIMI flow is associated with improved clinical outcomes. *J Am Coll Cardiol* 2000; **35**: 403.
15. Lansky A, Stone G, Mehran R. Impact on baseline TIMI flow on outcome after primary stenting versus primary PTCA in AMI: Results of the PAMI trials. *J Am Coll Cardiol* 2000; **35**: 368A.
16. Wharton TP, Jr, McNamara NS, Fedele FA, Jacobs MI, Gladstone AR, Funk EJ. Primary angioplasty for the treatment of acute myocardial infarction: experience at two community

hospitals without cardiac surgery. *J Am Coll Cardiol* 1999; **33**: 1257–65.

17. Grines CL, Cox DA, Stone GW *et al*. Coronary angioplasty with or without stent implantation for acute myocardial infarction. Stent Primary Angioplasty in Myocardial Infarction Study Group. *N Engl J Med* 1999; **341**: 1949–56.

18. Stone GW, Marsalese D, Brodie BR *et al*. A prospective, randomized evaluation of prophylactic intraaortic balloon counterpulsation in high risk patients with acute myocardial infarction treated with primary angioplasty. Second Primary Angioplasty in Myocardial Infarction (PAMI-II) Trial Investigators. *J Am Coll Cardiol* 1997; **29**: 1459–67.

19. Quinn MJ, Plow EF, Topol EJ. Platelet glycoprotein IIb/IIIa inhibitors: recognition of a two-edged sword? *Circulation* 2002; **106**: 379–85.

20. Kern MJ, Meier B. Evaluation of the culprit plaque and the physiological significance of coronary atherosclerotic narrowings. *Circulation* 2001; **103**: 3142–9.

21. The PRISM Investigators. A comparison of aspirin plus tirofiban with aspirin plus heparin for unstable angina. Platelet Receptor Inhibition in Ischemic Syndrome Management (PRISM). *N Engl J Med* 1998; **338**: 1498–505.

22. The PRISM-PLUS Investigators. Inhibition of the platelet glycoprotein IIb/IIIa receptor with tirofiban in unstable angina and non-Q-wave myocardial infarction. Platelet Receptor Inhibition in Ischemic Syndrome Management in Patients Limited by Unstable Signs and Symptoms (PRISM-PLUS) Study Investigators. *N Engl J Med* 1998; **338**: 1488–97.

23. The PURSUIT Trial Investigators. Inhibition of platelet glycoprotein IIb/IIIa with eptifibatide in patients with acute coronary syndromes. The PURSUIT Trial Investigators. Platelet Glycoprotein IIb/IIIa in Unstable Angina: Receptor Suppression Using Integrilin Therapy. *N Engl J Med* 1998; **339**: 436–43.

24. Simoons ML. Effect of glycoprotein IIb/IIIa receptor blocker abciximab on outcome in patients with acute coronary syndromes without early coronary revascularisation: the GUSTO IV-ACS randomised trial. *Lancet* 2001; **357**: 1915–24.

25. The PARAGON Investigators: Platelet IIb/IIIa Antagonism for the Reduction of Acute coronary syndrome events in a Global Organization Network. International, randomized, controlled trial of lamifiban (a platelet glycoprotein IIb/IIIa inhibitor), heparin, or both in unstable angina. *Circulation* 1998; **97**: 2386–95.

26. Topol EJ. Reperfusion therapy for acute myocardial infarction with fibrinolytic therapy or combination reduced fibrinolytic therapy and platelet glycoprotein IIb/IIIa inhibition: the GUSTO V randomised trial. *Lancet* 2001; **357**: 1905–14.

27. Escobar J, Marchant E, Fajuri A. Stenting could decrease coronary blood flow during primary angioplasty in acute myocardial infarction. *J Am Coll Cardiol* 1999; **33**: 361A.

28. Lincoff AM, Topol EJ. Illusion of reperfusion. Does anyone achieve optimal reperfusion during acute myocardial infarction? *Circulation* 1993; **88**: 1361–74.

29. Gibson CM, Ryan KA, Murphy SA *et al*. Impaired coronary blood flow in nonculprit arteries in the setting of acute myocardial infarction. The TIMI Study Group. Thrombolysis in myocardial infarction. *J Am Coll Cardiol* 1999; **34**: 974–82.

30. Garbo R, Steffenino G, Dellavalle A, Russo P, Meinardi F. Myocardial infarction with acute thrombosis of multiple major coronary arteries: a clinical and angiographic observation in four patients. *Ital Heart J* 2000; **1**: 824–31.

31. Leosco D, Fineschi M, Pierli C *et al*. Intracoronary serotonin release after high-pressure coronary stenting. *Am J Cardiol* 1999; **84**: 1317–22.

32. Mahaffey KW, Puma JA, Barbagelata NA *et al*. Adenosine as an adjunct to thrombolytic therapy for acute myocardial infarction: results of a multicenter, randomized, placebo-controlled trial: the Acute Myocardial Infarction STudy of ADenosine (AMISTAD) trial. *J Am Coll Cardiol* 1999; **34**: 1711–20.

33. Late breaking trials: AMISTAD-2. In: Scientific Session of the American College of Cardiology. Atlanta, GA; 2002.

34. Platelet glycoprotein IIb/IIIa receptor blockade and low-dose heparin during percutaneous coronary revascularization. The EPILOG Investigators. *N Engl J Med* 1997; **336**: 1689–96.

35. The ASSENT 3 Investigators. Efficacy and safety of tenecteplase in combination with enoxaparin, abciximab, or unfractionated heparin: the ASSENT-3 randomised trial in acute myocardial infarction. *Lancet* 2001; **358**: 605–13.

36. Grines CL, Booth DC, Nissen SE *et al*. Mechanism of acute myocardial infarction in patients with prior coronary artery bypass grafting and therapeutic implications. *Am J Cardiol* 1990; **65**: 1292–6.

37. Reiner JS, Lundgren CF, Kopecky SL. Ineffectiveness of thrombolysis for AMI following vein graft occlusion (abst). *Circulation* 1996; **94**: I-570.

38. Stone GW, Brodie BR, Griffin JJ *et al*. Clinical and angiographic outcomes in patients with previous coronary artery bypass graft surgery treated with primary balloon angioplasty for acute myocardial infarction. Second Primary Angioplasty in Myocardial Infarction Trial (PAMI-2) Investigators. *J Am Coll Cardiol* 2000; **35**: 605–11.

39. Marso SP, Steg G, Plokker T *et al*. Catheter-based reperfusion of unprotected left main stenosis during an acute myocardial infarction (the ULTIMA experience). Unprotected Left Main Trunk Intervention Multi-center Assessment. *Am J Cardiol* 1999; **83**: 1513–17.

40. Neri R, Migliorini A, Moschi G, Valenti R, Dovellini EV, Antoniucci D. Percutaneous reperfusion of left main coronary disease complicated by acute myocardial infarction. *Cathet Cardiovasc Interv* 2002; **56**: 31–4.

41. Barabas M, Gosselin G, Crepeau J, Petitclerc R, Cartier R, Theroux P. Left main stenting – as a bridge to surgery – for acute type A aortic dissection and anterior myocardial infarction. *Cathet Cardiovasc Interv* 2000; **51**: 74–7.

42. Timmis G, Timmis S. The restoration of coronary blood flow in acute myocardial infarction. *J Interv Cardiol* 1998; **11**: S9-S17.

43. Smith SC Jr, Dove JT, Jacobs AK *et al*. ACC/AHA guidelines for percutaneous coronary intervention: a report of the American College of Cardiology/American Heart Association Task Force on Practice Guidelines (Committee to Revise the 1993 Guidelines for Percutaneous Transluminal Coronary Angioplasty). *J Am Coll Cardiol* 2001; **38**: 2239i.

Chapter 13
Bifurcation Lesions

Samuel J Shubrooks, Jr

*Basic; **Advanced; ***Rare, exotic, or investigational.

From: Nguyen T, Hu D, Saito S, Grines C, Palacios I (eds), *Practical Handbook of Advanced Interventional Cardiology*, 2nd edn. © 2003 Futura, an imprint of Blackwell Publishing.

GENERAL OVERVIEW

Bifurcation lesions present some of the most difficult challenges in percutaneous coronary interventions. Treatment of such lesions is associated with reduced procedural success and increased complications as well as increased restenosis risk. Several factors are likely to contribute to these poorer outcomes. Plaque and endothelial characteristics of ostial lesions appear to lead to increased recoil and increased risk of dissection with compromise of side branches and/or main vessel. Intervention in either branch of a bifurcation lesion frequently leads to "snow plowing" with shifting of plaque, compromising the opposing branch. Because of these concerns, such lesions are often treated less aggressively, leading to greater residual stenosis and therefore greater restenosis.

TECHNICAL CONSIDERATIONS

True bifurcation lesions are generally considered to be those in which a single lesion involves both main vessel and branch vessel with greater than 50–70% stenosis in both. Lesions in which a side branch originates from within a significant lesion in the main vessel, but without apparent significant disease in the branch itself, may also be considered as bifurcation lesions since the branch vessel may require treatment as well. Situations in which a branch without apparent disease originates near, but not within, a lesion in a main vessel rarely require treatment of the branch vessel. However, treatment of branch vessels with severe ostial lesions may, at times, result in compromise of the main vessel, requiring bifurcation intervention.

Because treatment of bifurcation lesions with balloon angioplasty alone frequently gives suboptimal results, experience has developed in the use of other technologies, including directional coronary atherectomy (DCA), rotational atherectomy, and stenting. These newer devices generally provide improved procedural results, though with the potential of increased complications, with continuing uncertainty as to the long-term outcomes. In our laboratory, we studied 70 consecutive patients with true bifurcation lesions, 30 treated with conventional PTCA alone and 40 with either DCA or rotational atherectomy with adjunctive PTCA.[1] Use of atherectomy resulted in lower immediate residual stenosis in both the main and the branch vessels and a decreased 1-year target vessel revascularization (TVR) (28% vs 53%). Independent predictors of need for TVR were side branch diameter >2.3 mm, lesion length, and treatment with PTCA alone. This experience suggests that more aggressive debulking techniques should be considered for larger side branches, although they may be of no benefit for smaller ones.

BALLOON ANGIOPLASTY (PTCA)

Dilatation of main vessel only: A strategy of dilatation of the main vessel only may be suitable if the side branch has no apparent ostial disease, or if there is no more than moderate disease that does not require treatment, with the side branch originating adjacent to, but not within, the main vessel lesion. Under these circumstances, risk of side branch compromise is minimal, and if it occurs, it can be easily treated.[2] This strategy may also be suitable if an involved side branch is of small caliber and diffusely diseased such that loss would have little, if any, clinical significance. Loss of septal branches, except those of very large caliber, rarely results in adverse clinical outcomes, probably because of collateral septal supply. Unless the artery is very large with excellent final MLD after POBA, it is difficult to justify POBA alone because of lower restenosis rates with atherectomy and bare stenting.

Treatment of main vessel and side branch using a double wire technique: If a branch arises from within the lesion in the main vessel, there is an increased risk of branch occlusion with dilatation of the main vessel alone, with a reported incidence of 38–41% if there is greater than 50–70% stenosis of the branch origin.[2-4] This may occur as a result of plaque shifting, dissection involving the branch origin, or embolization. Therefore, side branches considered to be clinically important, and particularly those with ostial disease, should be treated as well as the main vessel. Follow-up of patients treated with PTCA of both branches have been reported as having an angiographic restenosis rate at 6 months of 37%[5] and a clinical restenosis rate of 42%.[4]

TECHNICAL TIPS

**Double balloon angioplasty: When treatment of the side branch is anticipated, a double wire technique should be used with a guidewire advanced into each branch, being careful that the wires do not twist during manipulation. Although some operators use a triport hemostasis valve, both wires and balloons can be easily advanced through the same opening of a single hemostasis Y adaptor. The main vessel and side branch can be sequentially dilated using either rapid exchange or over-the-wire dilating catheters. Sequential dilatations will permit the use of a smaller guiding catheter, but this strategy frequently results in shifting of plaque toward the undilated vessel with failure to achieve optimal results in both vessels. A more optimal result can usually be obtained using a "kissing balloon" strategy with simultaneous dilatations in both branches (Figure 13-1). Since both balloons will inflate together in the main vessel proximal to the bifurcation, it is important that these balloons not be oversized for the vessel diameter or inflated

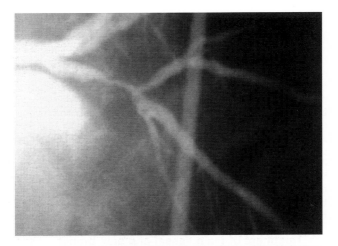

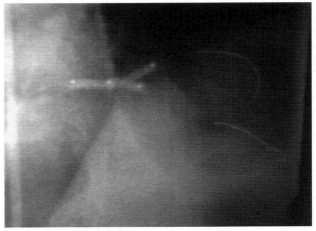

Figure 13-1: Severe lesion in proximal LAD involving first diagonal branch. PTCA of LAD alone would likely have compromised the diagonal. A 3.5-mm balloon in the LAD and a 3.0-mm balloon in the diagonal were inflated simultaneously, giving a good final result in both branches. *(Continued)*

to high pressures. The dilating diameter of the two balloons together will be less than the nominal diameters of the balloons individually, depending on balloon and vessel compliance and inflation pressure, and this must be considered subjectively. This technique may, therefore, not be suitable if the proximal vessel diameter is not larger than that of the branches involved. In this case, both branches may be di-

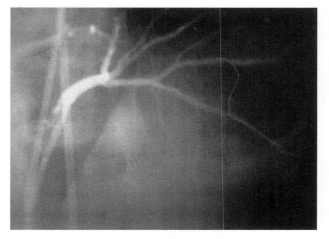

Figure 13-1 *(Continued)*

lated more aggressively sequentially with a final low-pressure kissing dilatation to limit plaque shifting. Unfortunately, many ostial side branch lesions, because of their plaque characteristics, are poorly dilatable, resulting in a significant residual stenosis. Cutting balloon (CB) angioplasty can give better acute results without plaque shifting.

 **Selection of guides in double balloon technique: It is important that the guide has a sufficiently large lumen to permit passage of both balloons simultaneously with adequate vessel visualization. Required minimal guide lumen diameter may be calculated by adding 0.006" to the combined diameters of the largest portion of the shafts of the two dilating catheters. With presently available low-profile balloon catheters, this can be accomplished with a large lumen 8F guide with most over-the-wire catheters and with a large lumen 7F guide with some rapid exchange catheters. The guide must also be carefully selected to provide the best possible support for device delivery.

 **Which branch to wire first? To avoid wire crossing, the most difficult branch should be wired first. Usually, it is the SB which needs more manipulation. Then the second wire can be inserted to cross the lesion with gentle torquing. An easy way to identify the wire is by having a steering device of a different color on each wire.

DIRECTIONAL CORONARY ATHERECTOMY (DCA)

 The removal of plaque with DCA has potential advantages in treatment of bifurcation lesions in decreasing the amount of plaque shifted toward side branches, possibly decreasing the incidence of dissection, and providing a larger, smoother lumen that could decrease restenosis without the necessity of stenting with its technical challenges.[6]

EVIDENCE-BASED MEDICINE APPLICATIONS

The CAVEAT trial: Analysis of data from the CAVEAT I trial indicated a larger post-procedure lumen in main vessels in bifurcation lesions treated with DCA as opposed to PTCA, but with an increased risk of side branch occlusion associated with an increase in small non-Q myocardial infarction with no difference in restenosis at 6 months.[7]

TECHNICAL TIPS

**Indications and contraindications: DCA may be particularly beneficial in larger vessels, with side branches >2.5 mm diameter, and with bulky and eccentric lesions. Its use may provide a lumen as large as that obtained with stenting without the technical difficulties of bifurcation stenting. In addition, when stenting becomes necessary because of an unsatisfactory result with DCA alone, the initial treatment with DCA may decrease the amount of plaque shifted into a side branch. DCA should be avoided with heavily calcified lesions and in situations where use of a 10F guide is not feasible. DCA of side branches is unlikely to be successful with side branches of >2.5 mm diameter, in those severely diseased, or with an acute takeoff angle from the main vessel.

**Selection of cutter and guide for DCA: It is important that there is good guide support prior to beginning bifurcation treatment. The older DCA cutters require a 10F guide. The newer Flexicut cutters can be used with 8F guides with an inner diameter of at least 0.087". A 6F DCA cutter or a small flexicut cutter should be used for treatment of vessels 2.5–2.9 mm diameter, a 7F device or a medium Flexicut cutter for vessels 3.0–3.4 mm diameter, with consideration of a 7F graft cutter or a large Flexicut cutter for vessels larger than 3.5 mm.

**Wiring technique: A wire is first passed beyond the lesion in the main vessel. Use of an extra support wire will frequently help in delivery of the device.

The double wire technique, which uses Nitinol wires placed in both branches with both wires left in place while DCA is performed first in the main and then in the branch vessel, has been described.[8] This technique has the potential risk of the guidewire becoming trapped in the cutter during operation and is rarely required since side branch access with a guidewire is rarely difficult.

**Cutting technique: Cuts should be made as in routine DCA in the direction of plaque. At least some cuts in the direction of the bifurcation may be helpful in maintaining branch patency and providing access with a wire into the branch. Side branch occlusion with DCA has been associated with branches originating within the main vessel lesion and having greater than 50% branch ostial disease, as well as branches located on bends, within long lesions, or involved in dissection.[7,9] In our laboratory, there is an increased incidence of side branch occlusion with DCA as compared to PTCA,[1] but with aggressive management by experienced operators it is rare not to obtain a final good result in both branches of the bifurcation.

**DCA in side branch: When a satisfactory result has been obtained, the DCA device is removed from the coronary artery and the wire removed from the main vessel and repositioned in the branch vessel. This is generally not difficult even if a side branch occlusion has occurred. DCA is then performed in the branch vessel using an appropriate sized cutter. If the side branch is small, it may be appropriate to treat this with PTCA rather than DCA, although as previously noted, ostial lesions may not dilate satisfactorily. If an excellent result is obtained in both branches with DCA alone, adjunctive final balloon dilatation may not be necessary, but generally a smoother, larger lumen is obtained if the procedure is completed with a low-pressure "kissing" balloon dilatation.

ROTATIONAL ATHERECTOMY

Lesion debulking with rotational atherectomy rather than DCA may be of particular benefit in smaller vessels, vessels that are heavily calcified, and those with significant ostial side branch lesions. Use of rotational atherectomy may decrease the incidence of dissection and side branch loss. As with DCA, rotational atherectomy followed by adjunctive PTCA may provide a satisfactory smooth lumen and thus avoid the need for bifurcation stenting or decrease the incidence of side branch occlusion if main vessel stenting alone is performed (Figure 13-2).

TECHNICAL TIP

**Strategies for rotational atherectomy: A guiding catheter of sufficient size to permit passage of the largest anticipated burr should be used. A Rotablator wire is

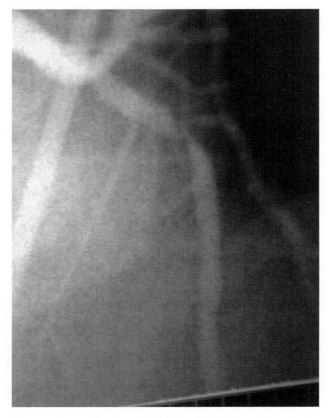

Figure 13-2: Severe LAD/diagonal bifurcation lesion. Because of severe ostial involvement of the diagonal, rotational atherectomy was first performed with a 1.75-mm burr, followed by "kissing" balloon inflations with a 2.5-mm balloon in the diagonal and a 3.5-mm balloon in the LAD, followed by placement of a 3.5-mm stent in the LAD. Because of the initial atherectomy treatment of the branch, there was no compromise of this following stenting in the LAD.

generally passed first across the lesion in the main vessel into the distal vessel and rotational atherectomy with the smallest burr to be used performed in the main vessel lesion. If the branch lesion is much more severe than that in the main vessel and it is anticipated that wire access in the main vessel will not be difficult, initial treatment of the branch lesion may be done. As each branch is treated, the wire must be removed from the opposing branch. With

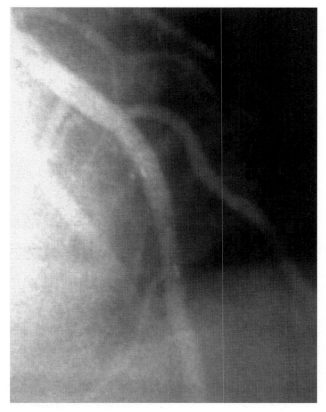

Figure 13-2 *(Continued)*

progressive increases in burr size, it is generally preferable
to treat first one branch and then the other with the same
burr, redirecting the guidewire from one branch to the other.
In some situations in which it is felt that access to the side
branch with the guidewire will not be difficult, the main
vessel may be treated first with progressively increasing
burr sizes with subsequent treatment of the side branch.
Wire bias resulting in dissection and/or perforation are of
particular concern in side branches with an acute angle of
takeoff. This may be reduced by use of a small burr and
careful attention to wire bias. Since rotational atherectomy
alone usually results in a suboptimal lumen, the procedure
is generally completed with a "kissing" balloon inflation that
can usually be accomplished with low-inflation pressures
(Figure 13-3).

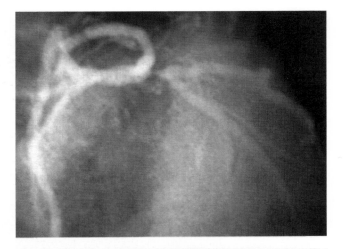

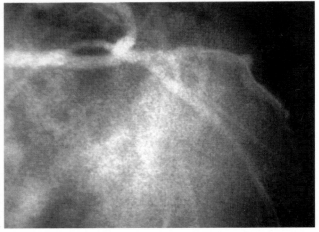

Figure 13-3: Severe ostial stenosis of the circumflex artery with ostial involvement of a large marginal branch (not well seen). PTCA alone or stenting into either branch would likely have compromised the opposing branch. Because of the ostial location of the lesion, PTCA would have given a sub-optimal result and the angle of origin was into both circumflex branches, followed by a low-pressure balloon inflation, giving a good final result.

STENTING

There is now increasing experience with stenting of bifurcation lesions. Stenting may be performed as an initial strategy or used as a "bail-out" if the previously described techniques fail to provide a satisfactory result. When stenting is planned, adjunctive initial use of debulking techniques may permit a better stenting outcome (Figure 13-2). Numerous techniques have been devised, all with technical challenges and often less than optimal results and uncertain long-term outcomes.[10,11] In a recently reported series of 70 patients having bifurcation stenting, the simplest strategy of stenting a main vessel across the side branch with rescue of the branch as needed was compared with several complex stenting strategies. Procedural outcomes were similar but a greater frequency of long-term adverse coronary events was seen in patients undergoing complex stenting.[12] Available stents and operator experience with new techniques may improve stenting outcomes in the future.

TECHNICAL TIPS

**Stenting of main vessel alone: The simplest stenting strategy involves deployment of a stent in the main vessel lesion, resulting in "jailing" of the side branch. Predictors of side branch occlusion are similar to those found with PTCA and atherectomy and include side branches arising within the main vessel lesion and having ostial lesions >50%. Side branch occlusion most commonly occurs during high-pressure inflation with stent deployment. Late occlusion or progression of disease at the side branch origin appears to be rare and some occluded side branches may actually reopen with time.[13,14]

**Interventions of side branch: Compromise of small side branches of <2 mm diameter is frequently of no clinical significance and may require no particular treatment. With loss of a larger side branch, a second guidewire can usually be passed through the stent into the compromised branch. This can usually be accomplished with any wire, although in difficult situations, success is sometimes greater with a wire having a stiffer tip or a hydrophilic coating (Choice PT, Scimed, Minneapolis, MN and Shinobi, Cordis Miami, FL). Some operators leave a guidewire in the side branch at the time of stent deployment as a marker for the site of origin of the branch. The wire may occasionally, however, become entrapped with stent deployment and this technique is usually not necessary in locating the origin of the branch occlusion. Care must be taken to avoid passing the wire behind the stent rather than through a cell into the side branch. Proper positioning of the wire within the stent lumen is confirmed by easy, unobstructed passage beyond the stent. Positioning of the wire under the stent may be indicated by inability to advance a balloon catheter. A balloon catheter can usually be easily advanced over the wire across the ostial lesion and dilatation performed. Occasionally, use of a fixed wire balloon may be successful when an over-the-wire balloon fails to cross. It is important to maintain the proximal shoulder of the balloon within the stent since passage of the entire balloon into the side branch may result in entrapment. If no balloon will cross into the side branch and treatment is felt necessary, or in the case of some severe side branch lesions seeming unlikely to respond to balloon dilatation, rotational atherectomy through the stent struts into the branch can be performed. When this is done, a small burr should be used initially with slow advancing to assure ablation of any stent struts and with gradual increase in burr size to prevent burr entrapment in the branch. Frequency and severity of side branch compromise may be decreased by PTCA, rotational atherectomy, or DCA of the side branch prior to stent placement, although redilatation is frequently required following stent deployment. With a poor result in the branch despite these procedures, bail-out T stenting as described below can be performed.

**Crossing a stent at its side strut: With rescue of side branches "jailed" within a stent, it is important to recognize differences in stent design and the result of dilatation of stent cells. In slotted tube and repeating cell stents, the stent struts are stretched and displaced with side lumen dilatation, resulting in a progressively larger lumen as balloon size increases, although not all stents respond equally. With the NIR stent (Boston Scientific), the side lumen increases little more than 2 mm until balloon size reaches approximately 4 mm, at which point strut rupture occurs. This stent should, therefore, not be used with anticipated need to dilate a side branch >2 mm diameter. It has also been demonstrated that side branch dilatation through a stent consistently results in narrowing of the main stent lumen immediately downstream from the side branch; this narrowing increases in severity with the increasing size of the balloon used for side branch dilatation. Redilatation of the main stent lumen then results in some reduction of size of the side lumen. This problem can best be avoided by ending the procedure with "kissing" balloon dilatation of both the main lumen and side branch, although with caution to keep the proximal balloon margin within the stent and to avoid overdilatation of the proximal stent.[15]

**T stenting: In T stenting of bifurcation lesions, a guide-wire is placed in both the main lumen and the side branch and a stent is deployed first in the side branch with the proximal stent edge at the origin of the side branch, being careful this does not protrude into the main lumen. The wire is then removed from the side branch and a stent placed over the wire in the main lumen across the origin of the side branch.[10–12,16] It is probably then optimal to recross from the main lumen stent into the side branch and to dilate the ostium to provide a larger cell opening into the branch.

An alternative approach to T stenting is to deploy the first stent in the main lumen after prior treating with PTCA, DCA, or rotational atherectomy. If, after placement of the main lumen stent, results in the side branch are poor and appear to require stenting, a wire is passed through the main lumen stent into the side branch, the origin dilated, and a stent is then passed into the side branch and deployed with its proximal margin just at the origin of the branch.

T stenting can provide excellent results when the side branch originates at a right angle from the main lumen (Figure 13-4 A). With other than a right angle takeoff, there will be either an unstented gap at the origin of the branch, or protrusion of a portion of the side branch stent into the main lumen (Figures 13-4 B,C). When the latter occurs, it may be possible to advance a guidewire through the protruding stent struts and dilate these to the diameter of the main vessel lumen.

**"Kissing" stents: "Kissing" stents may be placed in both branches of a bifurcation with overlapping of the proximal stent portions.[10,11,17] Guidewires are placed in both branches and, with or without predilation, stents are deployed in both branches with proximal overlap. This may be done with either simultaneous stent deployment with equal pressure in both balloons or with sequential stent deployment followed by final simultaneous inflations of both stent balloons (Figure 13-4 D). This provides good access to both branches of the bifurcation but should be used only in larger arteries and where the size of the proximal vessel will permit simultaneous high-pressure balloon inflations. With this technique, a double-barreled lumen is created in the proximal vessel with a metallic carina not opposed to any vessel wall. Although this procedure has been reported and used in our laboratory with procedural success, the long-term outcome is uncertain.

**V stenting: Guidewires are placed in both branches of the bifurcation with predilation performed as necessary. Stents are then sequentially deployed in each of the branches with the proximal stent margins carefully positioned so as not to enter the bifurcation itself. This should then be finished with a simultaneous "kissing" balloon inflation (Figure 13-4 E). This technique provides good access into both of the branches but leaves uncovered any disease in the bifurcation itself or proximal to the bifurcation.[10–12]

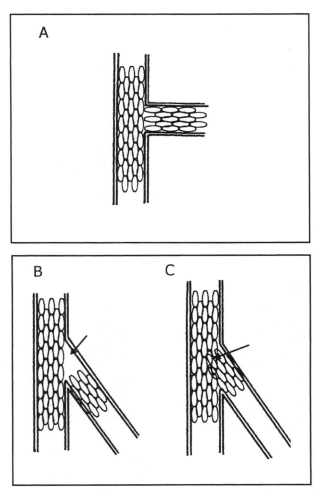

Figure 13-4: Types of bifurcation stenting. (A) T stenting with the right angle takeoff of side branch providing good coverage of lesion. (B) T stenting with acute angle takeoff of side branch leaving an unstented gap at origin of branch (arrow). (C) T stenting with a similar acute angle takeoff of the side branch with coverage of origin but protrusion of the stent into the main lumen (arrow). *(Continued)*

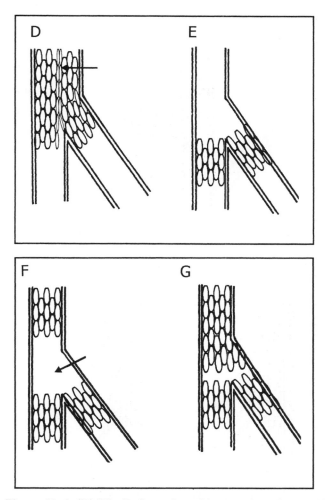

Figure 13-4: (D) "Kissing" stenting with stents in main vessel and side branch and creation of double-barrel lumen in proximal vessel (arrow). (E) V stenting, providing good coverage of main lumen and side branch just beyond the bifurcation but leaving the bifurcation itself uncovered. (F) Y stenting similar to (E), but with placement of a third stent in the proximal vessel, the bifurcation itself remaining unstented (arrow). (G) "Trousers stenting" with the third stent advanced over 2 balloons into both distal branches overlapping the distal stents. *(Continued)*

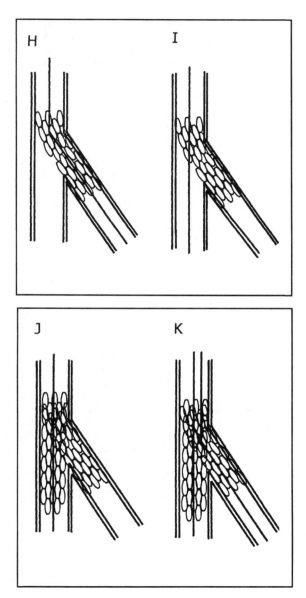

Figure 13-4: (H) "Culotte stenting" with placement of first stent in the most angulated branch, followed by (I) advancing a guidewire through this stent into the opposing vessel, (J) stenting this vessel through the first stent after predilation, and finishing by (K) recrossing the initial stent with a guidewire and doing simultaneous "kissing" balloon dilatations in both branches.

**Y or "trousers" stenting: V stenting, as described above, is performed. The wire is then removed from the branch vessel and a third stent advanced over the guidewire in the main lumen and deployed with the distal stent margin just at the proximal border of the side branch origin so as not to "jail" it. This should again be finished with "kissing" balloon inflations.[10–12,18] This technique has the advantage of stenting disease proximal to the bifurcation but, of necessity, leaves a small unstented gap at the origin of the branch vessel (Figure 13-4 F).

A further variation of this technique is "trousers" stenting in which a third stent is free mounted on the proximal portions of two balloons with the distal portions of the balloons uncovered with stent.[10–12] Guidewires are left in both branches following V stenting and over these wires the two balloons on which the third stent are mounted are advanced until the distal portions of the balloons enter each of the side branches and the distal stent margin reaches the proximal margins of the previously placed V stents. The third stent is then deployed with simultaneous "kissing" balloon inflations (Figure 13-4 G). Although this technique permits coverage of the entire bifurcation, it is extremely technically difficult and requires a sufficiently large proximal vessel to permit the simultaneous inflations.

**"Culotte" stenting: In "culotte" stenting, a stent is placed in one branch with a second stent placed through a cell of the first stent into the branch vessel with overlapping of the proximal portions of both stents (Figures 13-4 H–K)). Guidewires are initially placed in both branches and predilation is performed, either sequentially or simultaneously. A stent is then placed in one vessel covering a segment proximal and distal to the bifurcation across the opposing branch. Generally the larger, more important branch is stented first, although consideration must also be given to angulation at the bifurcation. If there is marked angulation, it is preferable to stent the more angulated branch first to permit easier access into the opposing branch. Another guidewire is then advanced across the deployed stent into the unstented vessel as previously described. Some operators prefer leaving the initial guidewire in the branch vessel during stenting of the first vessel as a guide to recrossing, although this has the disadvantage of possibly entrapping this wire. Once the unstented branch has been crossed with a wire, this is dilated with a balloon to open the stent cell in preparation for stenting of the branch. The balloon is then removed and the second stent advanced over the branch wire and positioned so as to cover the branch lesion and widely overlap the proximal portion of the previously placed stent. The guidewire in the first branch, having been pulled back prior to deployment of the second stent, is then readvanced across the struts of both stents into the first vessel and balloons advanced over both wires to finish with a "kissing" balloon inflation. During this final inflation, it is important to be certain that both balloons are within the proximal stent and that they are inflated at relatively low pressure, being careful not to oversize the overlapped balloons.

This technique has the advantage of completely covering the bifurcation and permitting access into both branches. A series of 50 patients treated in this manner resulted in 94% procedural success and 12.5% target lesion revascularization at 6 months if a final "kissing" balloon inflation could be performed, vs 44% if this was not possible.[19]

**True bifurcated stents: True bifurcated stents are currently being developed but none are thus far available for general clinical use. A single case using the Bard XT Carina stent (Bard, Galway, Ireland) has recently been reported.[20] This consists of a bifurcated stent mounted on a dual balloon delivery system. Further developments of such a stent may lead to better coverage of true bifurcation lesions than any other technique presently available.

PRACTICAL CONSIDERATIONS

Many bifurcation lesions may be treated with PTCA alone with satisfactory results, particularly if the branch vessel is small or not more than mildly diseased, with best results obtained by use of "kissing" balloon inflation. For branch vessels >2.5 mm in diameter with ostial involvement, and for longer lesions, debulking with DA or rotational atherectomy provides a better acute lumen gain and lower need for TVR. Ostial lesions are particularly resistant to PTCA alone, and DA or rotational atherectomy will provide more optimal results. In many cases, stenting will result in a larger lumen in the main vessel, although with the risk of branch compromise. This may be treated with side branch "rescue" with PTCA or by various complex stenting techniques. Regardless of approach to bifurcation lesions, it is critical to: (1) obtain optimal angiographic views to adequately define the bifurcation anatomy, (2) choose a guiding catheter with an adequate lumen size and optimal backup support, (3) carefully plan an initial strategy most appropriate for vessel size and lesion morphology, and (4) consider the best subsequent options if the initial approach fails to provide satisfactory results.

REFERENCES

1. Dauerman HL, Higgins PJ, Sparano AM *et al*. Mechanical debulking versus balloon angioplasty for the treatment of true bifurcation lesions. *J Am Coll Cardiol* 1998; **32**: 1845–52.

2. Meier D, Gruentzig AR, King SB *et al*. Risk of side branch occlusion during coronary angioplasty. *Am J Cardiol* 1984; **53**: 10–14.

3. Boxt LM, Meyerovitz MF, Taus RH *et al*. Side branch occlusion complicating percutaneous transluminal coronary angioplasty. *Radiology* 1986; **161**: 681–3.

4. Weinstein JS, Baim DS, McCabe CH, Lorell BH. Salvage of branch vessels during bifurcation lesion angioplasty: Acute and long-term follow up. *Cathet Cardiovasc Diagn* 1991; **22**: 1–6.

5. Renkin J, Wijns W, Hanet C *et al*. Angioplasty of coronary bifurcation stenoses: Immediate and long-term results of the protecting branch technique. *Cathet Cardiovasc Diagn* 1991; **22**: 167–73.

6. Safian RD, Schreiber TL, Baim DS. Specific indications for directional coronary atherectomy: Origin left anterior descending coronary artery and bifurcation lesions. *Am J Cardiol* 1993; **72**: 35E–41E.

7. Brener SJ, Leya FS, Apterson-Hinsen C *et al*. A comparison of debulking versus dilatation of bifurcation coronary arterial narrowings (from the CAVEAT I trial). *Am J Cardiol* 1996; **78**: 1039–41.

8. Lewis BE, Leya FS, Johnson SA *et al*. Acute procedural results in the treatment of 30 coronary artery bifurcation lesions with a double-wire atherectomy technique for side-branch protection. *Am Heart J* 1994; **127**: 1600–7.

9. Vaska KJ, Franco I, Whitlow PL. Risk of side-branch occlusion following directional coronary atherectomy (abstract). *Circulation* 1991; **84** (Suppl II): II-81.

10. Baim DS. Is bifurcation stenting the answer? *Cathet Cardiovasc Diagn* 1996; **37**: 314–16.

11. Di Mario C, Columbo A. Trousers-stents: How to choose the right size and shape. *Cathet Cardiovasc Diagn* 1997; **41**: 197–9.

12. Pan M, de Lezo JS, Medina A *et al*. Simple and complex stent strategies for bifurcated coronary arterial stenosis involving the side branch origin. *Am J Cardiol* 1999; **83**: 1320–5.

13. Aliabadi D, Tilli FV, Powers TR *et al*. Incidence and angiographic predictors of side branch occlusion following high-pressure intracoronary stenting. *Am J Cardiol* 1997; **80**: 994–7.

14. Fischman DL, Savage MT, Leon MB *et al*. Fate of lesion-related side branches after coronary artery stenting. *J Am Coll Cardiol* 1993; **22**: 1641–6.

15. Ormiston JA, Webster MWI, Ruygrok PN *et al*. Stent deformation following simulated side-branch dilatation: A comparison of five stent designs. *Cathet Cardiovasc Interv* 1999; **47**: 258–64.

16. Carrie D, Karouny E, Chouairi S, Puel J. "T"-shaped stent placement: A technique for the treatment of dissected bifurcation lesions. *Cathet Cardiovasc Diagn* 1996; **37**: 311–13.

17. Colombo A, Gaglione A, Nakamura S, Finci L. "Kissing" stents for bifurcational coronary lesion. *Cathet Cardiovasc Diagn* 1993; **30**: 327–30.

18. Teirstein PS. "Kissing" Palmaz-Schatz stents for coronary bifurcation stenoses. *Cathet Cardiovasc Diagn* 1996; **37**: 307–10.

19. Chevalier B, Glatt B, Royer T, Guyon P. Placement of coronary stents in bifurcation lesions by the "culotte" technique. *Am J Cardiol* 1998; **82**: 943–9.

20. Carlier SG, van der Giessen WJ, Foley DP *et al*. Stenting with a true bifurcated stent: Acute and mid-term follow-up results. *Cathet Cardiovasc Interv* 1999; **47**: 361–9.

Chapter 14

Approach to the Patient with Prior Bypass Surgery

John S Douglas, Thach Nguyen, Tan Huay Cheem

---

*Basic; **Advanced; ***Rare, exotic, or investigational.

From: Nguyen T, Hu D, Saito S, Grines C, Palacios I (eds), *Practical Handbook of Advanced Interventional Cardiology*, 2nd edn. © 2003 Futura, an imprint of Blackwell Publishing.

**Cause of failure of PCI in LIMA graft
**PCI in the subclavian artery
Conclusions

GENERAL OVERVIEW

Patients who experience recurrence of ischemia after coronary artery bypass graft surgery (CABG) have lesions in diverse anatomic distributions (saphenous vein graft (SVG), native arteries, internal mammary, radial, gastroepiploic graft, or proximal subclavian artery). The results of percutaneous coronary interventions (PCI) depend on the types of conduits (native artery, arterial or saphenous vein grafts) or the locations on the conduits (proximal, mid-, distal or at the anastomotic sites) and the age of the grafts.[1] Despite the use of new interventional devices, SVG intervention was still associated with significant in-hospital mortality (8%) and Q-wave myocardial infarction (MI) (2%).[2] The clinical and technical problems encountered during PCI of SVG are listed in Table 14-1.

Early postoperative ischemia (<1 month): The most common cause of ischemia within hours or days of surgery is acute vein graft thrombosis (60%). Other causes are incomplete surgical revascularization (10%), kinked grafts, and focal stenoses distal to the insertion site and at the proximal or distal anastomotic sites, spasm or injury, insertion of graft to a vein causing AV fistula, or bypass of the wrong vessel (Figure

---

Table 14-1
Clinical and technical problems during PCI of SVG

Problem	Corrective measure	Adverse outcome
Diffuse disease	Long stent	High rate of restenosis
Thrombus	Thrombectomy	Distal embolization
Degenerated SVG	Distal protection	Distal embolization
Restenosis	Drug-eluting stent (DES)	?% restenosis
	Brachytherapy (VBT)	?% restenosis after VBT

Problems without solution yet:

- Progression of disease in other areas of the graft
- Retrograde embolization during PCI of aorto-ostial lesions
- Distal protection in bifurcation lesions: one or two devices? Which branch?

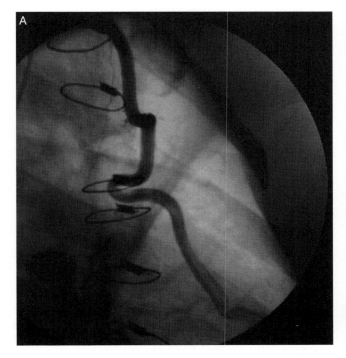

Figure 14-1: LIMA to large cardiac vein: (A) The LIMA at its origin. *(Continued)*

14-1).[3] The patients at increased risk for early postoperative ischemia include those undergoing technically demanding minimally invasive and "off-bypass" techniques.[4]

Early postoperative ischemia (1 month–1 year): Recurrent angina between 1 month and 1 year after the surgery is most often due to peri-anastomotic stenosis, graft occlusion, or mid-SVG stenosis from fibrous intimal hyperplasia. Recurrence of angina at about three months postoperatively is highly suggestive of a distal graft anastomotic lesion and should, in most cases, lead to evaluation for PCI.

Late postoperative ischemia (>3 years after surgery): At this stage, the most common cause of ischemia is the formation, in vein grafts, of new atherosclerotic plaques which contain foam cells, cholesterol crystals, blood elements, and necrotic debris as in native vessels. However, these plaques have less fibrocollagenous tissue and calcification, so they are softer, more friable, of larger size, and frequently associated with thrombus.

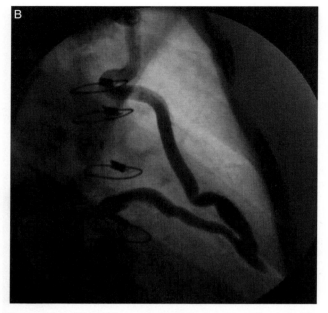

Figure 14-1: (B) LIMA inserted into the large cardiac vein. The proximal vein was closed. The distal vein (which is larger) was seen flowing back to the left atrium.

INDICATIONS FOR REVASCULARIZATIONS[1]

Indications for percutaneous interventions: PCI offers a less invasive alternative for revascularization in symptomatic post-bypass patients, including many who were not candidates for repeat surgery because of contraindications (pulmonary and renal failure, old age, malignancy). Other patients who can undergo PCI with acceptable risks are patients with patent arterial grafts that would be jeopardized by reoperation, patients with relatively small amount of ischemic, symptom-producing myocardium, and patients with no arterial or venous conduit available for graft.

The status of the left anterior descending artery (LAD) and its graft significantly influences the selection process because of its impact on long-term outcome and lack of survival benefit of repeat surgery to treat non-LAD ischemia.[5] A patent left IMA (LIMA) to LAD improves the safety and so favors the selection of PCI in the right coronary artery (RCA) or left circumflex artery (LCX) distributions. Thus selection of lesions for PCI must be based on careful analysis of the probabilities of initial success, complications, and for long-term safety and

Table 14-2
Anatomic factors influencing revascularization decisions in post-bypass patients

Often lead to PCI	*Often lead to CABG*
Patent arterial graft (especially LAD)	Diseased SVG to LAD
≥ 2 patent grafts	Ejection fraction: 25–35%
1–3 culprit lesions	>3 culprit lesions
Inadequate conduit	Multiple SVG lesions
Near-normal left ventricle	Available arterial conduits

Difficult surgical access

- Posterior lateral target vessel
- Mediastinal scarring secondary to radiation, infection, or pericarditis
- Prior muscle transfer closure of unhealed sternotomy

Future cardiac surgery anticipated

- In-situ prosthetic valve
- Mild to moderate aortic or mitral valve disease

efficacy compared with competitive surgical strategies and medical therapies.

Indications for surgical revascularization: Reoperation is frequently recommended for severe disease of vein graft to the LAD. Multiple vessel involvement, small number of patent grafts, severe vein graft disease, and a damaged ventricle are factors more likely to lead to repeat surgery (Table 14-2).[1] In the past, PCI was not preferred for bulky atheromatous lesions or thrombus-laden grafts. With the advent of distal protection devices, the acute results are more promising. However, the long-term data on a large scale are still lacking.

CLINICAL APPLICATIONS

Interventions within hours of coronary bypass surgery: In the very early hours after surgery, because of symptomatic ischemia, urgent coronary angiography may reveal a compromised graft. During intervention, extreme care is warranted and balloon sizing should be conservative because of the possibility of suture line disruption and severe hemorrhagic complications.[1] Once a graft is thrombosed, opening of the native vessel is preferable. However, if the native vessel is not a reasonable target, balloon interventions on the graft are also effective if thrombus formation is not extensive. Intracoronary thrombolytic therapy, although technically feasible, is reported only in rare cases, with one-third requiring mediastinal drainage due to bleeding.[6] Therefore, removal of thrombus by a thrombectomy device is preferred. In general, no PCI could ever be done without the patient being anticoagulated.[7] However, after removal of any obstruction, a good TIMI-3 flow may prevent any further thrombotic formation with an oral antiplatelet drug alone, without long-term anticoagulant.

Native coronary interventions:[1] One year after bypass surgery, patients begin to develop new atherosclerotic plaques in the graft conduits or to show atherosclerotic progression in the native coronary arteries. Whenever possible, native artery lesions are targeted first because of their lower rate of restenosis. Their procedural success is high (approximately 90%). Their outcome is quite favorable, with in-hospital mortality of 1%, Q-wave myocardial infarction (MI) 1%, non-Q-wave infarction 4%, and emergency surgery 2.8%.[1] Approaches to native vessel sites in post-bypass patients include the treatment of protected left main disease, recanalization of old total occlusion, or native artery via venous or arterial grafts.

Saphenous vein graft interventions: One to three years after surgery, patients begin to develop atherosclerotic plaques in the SVG and, after 3 years, these plaques appear with increased frequency. At the early stage, dilation of the distal anastomosis can be accomplished with little morbidity and good long-term patency (80–90%). Dilation of the proximal and mid-segment of the vein graft was highly successful at 90%, with a low rate of mortality (1%), Q-wave MI, and CABG (2%). The rate of non-Q-wave MI was 13%. The length of time since surgery was an important factor for restenosis, as was the location of the lesion. The lowest target lesion revascularization (TLR) rate by bare stent [25% with plain angioplasty (POBA) and 14% with stenting] was noted for lesions that occurred at the distal anastomosis within one year of surgery.[8] There are no data on DES yet available.

When evaluating the SVG lesions for intervention, the interventional cardiologist must consider possible consequences of atheromatous embolism, considering that the entire lesion and accompanying thrombus may be fragmented, dislodged, and embolized. If the risk of major atheroembolization, which could be decreased by distal protection devices, is acceptable, compared with other therapeutic options, PCI may be appropriate.[1] Also, the relatively high subsequent coronary event rate and restenosis potential must also be factored into this decision. If the lesion is relatively bulky, pretreatment with diltiazem or verapamil in 200–300 µg increments intracoronary up to 1 mg (or nitroprusside 40 µg bolus) seems to minimize slow and no-flow states, but these strategies are of limited effectiveness in preventing enzymatic leak compared with the distal protection devices.[1]

Intervention of the aorto-ostial lesion: There is not much difference in the technique of PCI for aorto-ostial lesion of the SVG. However, because there is increased fibrotic change and more spasm, there is a question about need of prior debulking followed by stenting or stenting alone of the aorto-ostial lesion. In a study by Ahmed *et al.* for both groups of patients with or without prior debulking, the TLR rate after one year was similar at 19%. The technical concern during PCI of large and bulky aorto-ostial lesion is the antegrade and retrograde embolization. There is distal protective device for antegrade embolization but there is none for retrograde embolization.[9]

Intervention in degenerated saphenous vein grafts: The lesions that are bulky or associated with thrombus are considered to be high-risk. The complications include distal embolization, no-reflow, abrupt closure, and perforation. So different approaches were devised because there is much to lose from the standpoint of distal embolization causing non-Q MI and increasing long-term mortality. In the case of perforation of SVG, usually there is contained perforation rather than cardiac tamponade due to the extrapericardial course of the grafts and extensive post-pericardiotomy fibrosis.

EVIDENCE-BASED MEDICINE APPLICATIONS

The Vein Graft AngioJet Study (VEGAS) Phase II Trial: In this trial, the patients were randomized to have either local infusion of urokinase or underwent thrombectomy with the AngioJet device (Possis Medical Inc, Minneapolis, MN) in SVG lesions with demonstrable thrombus or in native arteries.[10] The results showed that the AngioJet was found to be superior for patients undergoing high-risk PCI with large thrombus burdens. However, despite efficient removal of thrombus as evidenced by lower angiographic thrombus score, the rate of significant elevated CK-MB was still high at 11%.[10]

EVIDENCE-BASED MEDICINE APPLICATIONS

The X-TRACT trial: This trial enrolled 800 patients who had a target lesion in a native coronary artery with definite angiographic thrombus or a strong suspicion of thrombus, or a lesion in any SVG with or without obvious thrombus. At 30 days, there were no differences in cardiac death, MI, or TVR. The overall, 30-day MACE rates were similar (17% of the X-Sizer group and in 17.4% of the control group). However, large MIs, defined as CK-MB leak greater than 8 times normal limits, were reduced by 46% (8.3% in the control group compared to 4.5% in the X-Sizer group). There was one perforation in the X-Sizer group and four in the control group.[11]

In general, the X-Sizer system (EndiCOR Medical, Inc, San Clemente, CA) is more effective in removing thrombus and atheromatous debris while the AngioJet system was effective only in the removal of fresh thrombus, and not the friable, grumous vein graft material or older organized thrombi.[12]

EVIDENCE-BASED MEDICINE APPLICATIONS

The Saphenous Vein Graft Angioplasty Free of Emboli Randomized (SAFER) Trial: In this trial, the patients with SVG interventions were randomized to have usual PCI without or with the PercuSurge GuardWire system (Percu-Surge, Medtronic AVE, Sunnyvale, CA).[13] This distal protection device uses standard 8F guide and as the primary wire, a 0.014" GuardWire, which is ended with flexible coils. An elastomeric balloon (on-the-wire) is mounted proximal to the coils. This balloon is passed beyond the area to be treated and inflated at low pressure to block blood flow and entrap embolic debris. In the meantime, PCI is carried on accordingly. When PCI is finished, an export catheter for aspiration of debris is delivered near the distal balloon and debris is aspirated by suction. Following 10–15 seconds of aspiration, the distal occlusion balloon is deflated and debris-free blood flow is returned to the distal vessel. Before using this device, procedural considerations include (1) selection of appropriate landing zone for the distal occlusive balloon so there is no local dissection due to balloon inflation, (2) complete obstruction of distal flow, (3) the size of conduit, and (4) patient's tolerance of prolonged occlusion. The results of the SAFER trial showed there was a 50% decrease of in-hospital and 30-day MACE (17.4% for the GuardWire group and 10.4% for the control). The major angiographic predictors at baseline for MACE in PCI of SVG are thrombus, long lesion, diffuse disease and impaired baseline flow. Embolization can happen to any PCI on SVG, even in lesion <10 mm. With the distal protection device, the MACE was reduced but still at 10% with 6% angiographic flow-related complications (ARFC) (final TIMI flow <3, distal embolization or no-reflow).[13]

EVIDENCE-BASED MEDICINE APPLICATIONS

Distal protection with the FilterWire: The FIRE trial: In a study with 650 patients comparing the BSC/EPI FilterWire EX (a polyurethane filter bag) (Boston-Scientific-Embolic Protection, Santa Clara, CA) versus the PercuSurge GuardWire to trap embolic debris in SVG, although reduced flow was common (36.1%) when the FilterWire was in place, there were no sustained episodes of abrupt closure and only one case of no-reflow after removal of the Filter-Wire. Even so, distal branch vessel occlusion was found in 11%.[14] The advantages and disadvantages of the two kinds of distal protection device are listed in Table 14-3.

Table 14-3
Advantages and disadvantages of distal protection devices

Advantages	Disadvantages
Balloon occlusive devices	
Easy to use	No antegrade flow
Aspirate large and small particles	Balloon-induced injury
Reliably trap debris	Not as steerable as PTCA wire
More tolerable with intermittent occlusion	Difficult to image during procedure
	Balloon can move during PCI
Distal embolic filter devices	
Preserve antegrade flow	May not capture all debris
Contrast imaging possible throughout the procedure	Difficult to evaluate the retrieval of debris during procedure
	Filters may clog
	Delivery catheters may cause embolization before filter deployment
	Cannot remove emboli intermittently in order to relieve overload

TECHNICAL TIPS

**How to ensure there is total distal protection: After position and inflation of the distal balloon of the protection device [e.g. PercuSurge (Medtronic AVE, Sunnyvale, CA) or an ACE balloon as above], before performing PCI, inject a column of contrast into the lumen to mark the location of the balloon. The proximal end of the column should be around the lesion to be dilated. While performing PCI, if the distal column of contrast does not move, and there is no contrast seeping distally, then it is assured that the balloon is being kept immobile and the distal protection is intact.

**Long PCI with intermittent distal balloon occlusion: Before PCI, advance, inflate the distal protection balloon and do some extensive aspirations to decrease the thrombotic burden. Deflate the occlusion balloon to permit some distal flow. Then the balloon is reinflated, the transport catheter removed and PCI could be started. During the procedure, intermittent aspiration can be done as above until the PCI is completed. In this way the patient can have intermittent perfusion to the distal territory, temporary relief of ischemia, and triggering of ischemic preconditioning. The key factor for success is to have good aspiration before deflating the occlusion balloon. Once the balloon is deflated to have some distal perfusion, there is no movement of hardware across the lesion so the chance for spontaneous distal embolization is lower (Figure 14-2 A–C).

**No flow with distal filter devices: During PCI of SVG, the filter can be overloaded with thrombi and atheromatous material and the distal flow can be cut off. In a case report by Tan HC *et al.* (unpublished), after predilating angioplasty of an SVG lesion, repeat angiography showed no flow, with the contrast holding up at the filtering device (Figure 14-3 A). The differential diagnoses were distal embolization despite use of distal protection device, or that the Filterwire was "choked" with embolized atheromatous materials. An aspiration catheter was loaded and delivered to the EPI filter site (Figure 14-3 B). An export catheter syringe was first filled with saline to "agitate" the filtered materials. This was followed by vacuum aspiration. Repeat angiography showed restoration of TIMI-2 flow with filling defect visualized within the EPI Filterwire indicative of large embolized atheromatous material (Figure

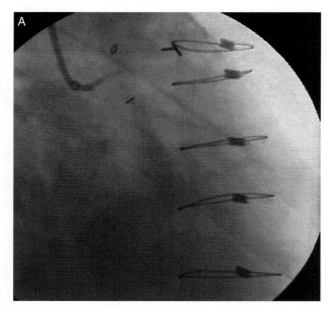

Figure 14-2: PCI of SVG with intermittent balloon occlusion by PercuSurge. (A) Complete obstruction of the SVG. *(Continued)*

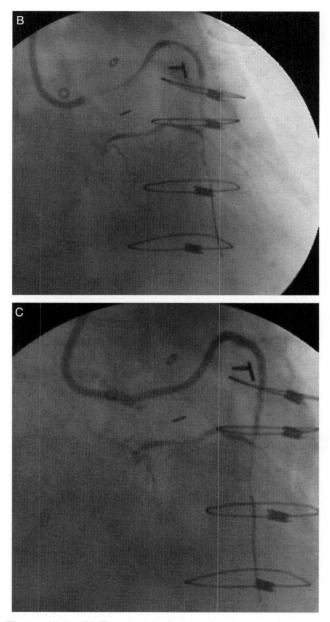

Figure 14-2: (B) Transient deflation of balloon for ischemic relief. The balloon is seen as a dot distally. (C) Successful removal of debris, angioplasty and stenting of the SVG at its mid-segment.

14-3 C). The EPI Filterwire was then confidently captured by the retrieval device with a final angiography showing excellent results and TIMI-3 flow.

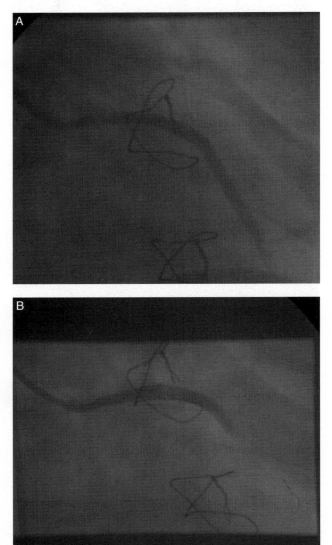

Figure 14-3: (A) The baseline angiogram showed severe ostial lesion of an SVG. (B) After predilating angioplasty of the SVG lesion, repeat angiography showed no flow with the contrast holding up at the distal filtering device. *(Continued)*

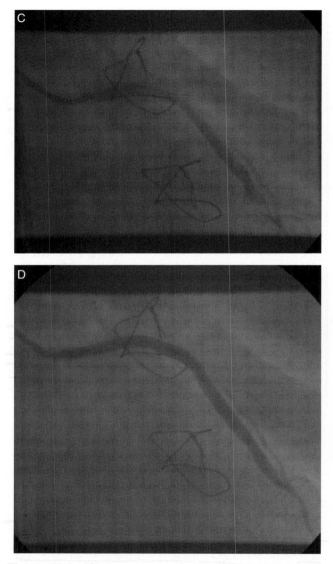

Figure 14-3: (C) An export catheter was advanced to the filter device and the filtered materials were aspirated. Repeat angiography showed restoration of TIMI-2 flow with filling defect visualized within the EPI Filterwire indicative of large embolized atheromatous material. (D) The filter device was removed and final angiogram showed a good result. (Courtesy of the Cardiac Catheterization Laboratories of National University Hospital, Singapore.)

In the case of a filter device full of embolized material, only the proximal part of the filter should be withdrawn into the capture sheath, since a forceful pull of the filtering device may squeeze out emboli. Then, during withdrawal, the Y adapter should be opened for full back bleeding so that any emboli particle released during transit can be flushed out.

**Avoid distal occlusive device in SVG ostial lesion: Because of lack of antegrade flow when the distal occlusive balloon is inflated, debris from PCI of the ostial SVG could embolize to the brain and cause stroke. So the use of distal occlusive balloon should be avoided.[15]

**Double wire technique with distal occlusive device: The SVG is cannulated with one PTCA wire and one Guardwire for distal balloon occlusion. When the balloon is inflated, PCI can be done over the PTCA wire. When the balloon has to be inflated or deflated, then the Guardwire is used. In this way, less time to exchange balloon or transport catheter is needed.[15]

***Improvised distal protection devices: In any laboratories without the dedicated distal protection device, Stein *et al.* suggested the use of available material to protect from embolization in patients with degenerated SVG undergoing PCI. Advance distally beyond the index lesion a deflated over-the-wire balloon (e.g. the ACE balloon, Boston Scientific/Scimed, Quincy, MA). Inflate it to block the flow. Perform PCI. Be sure the patient can tolerate the ischemia due to inflation of balloon. After PCI, advance a large transport catheter with many side holes and aspirate the debris from the distal blood column.[16]

TECHNICAL IMPLICATIONS

PCI in the SVG grafts
In general, in search for the location of the insertion site, the more posterior the destination of the left-sided grafts, the higher they are located on the aorta. The top graft generally goes to the distal LCX, and the lowest graft goes to the LAD. Most left-sided grafts arise in a cranial direction from the aorta. Right coronary grafts are usually placed on the anterior aspect of the aorta and travel in a caudal direction.[1]

TECHNICAL TIPS

**Guides for left bypass grafts: The right Judkins coronary or left venous bypass or hockey stick catheters are effective guides for grafts arising anteriorly (the LAD and diagonals). However, the left Amplatz and the hockey stick guides often provide the best backup for grafts arising in the inner curvature of the aorta (to the LCX). Engagement is best achieved by advancing the guide into the ascending aorta at the level of the aortic cusps then gently withdrawing with clockwise rotation of the guide to orient the tip to the ostium in the LAO view. When the tip of the guide catches the ostium, the guide is then advanced to obtain optimal backup.[17]

**Guides for right bypass grafts: For grafts arising from the outer curve of the aorta (usually to the RCA), the Multipurpose guide is the best to provide excellent coaxial alignment. Engagement into the ostium is achieved by advancing the guide into the aorta while doing a clockwise rotation in order to point its tip towards the right, in the LAO projection.[17] In the case of a right Judkins or small Amplatz right (AR-1), the guide is turned clockwise so it will point toward the outer curvature, then is slowly turned counterclockwise to engage the graft with its tip pointing down. If the aorta is relatively large, a posteriorly located RCA graft may be difficult to reach with a Multipurpose or right Judkins guide but an Amplatz left (AL-2) will usually be successful in this situation.

**Balloon angioplasty for vein grafts: Balloons are generally sized 1:1 to venous grafts and slightly oversized for suboptimal initial results, or when dealing with restenotic lesions. Long (30–40 mm) balloons are frequently used when the lesions are long and bulky or when thrombus is present. The extra fibrosis of mature vein graft lesions often requires dilation to higher pressures >12 ATM.

**Stenting for vein grafts: The saphenous vein grafts have a high degree of elastic recoil that can be overcome by stenting. Aorto-ostial vein graft lesions are most often treated with placement of stents or with DCA. Nondilatable aorto-ostial or distal anastomotic lesions have been successfully treated with rotational or directional atherectomy. However, their long-term restenotic results are still disappointing. There are no hard data for DES on PCI of the SVG.

**Size and length of stent: If a small stent is deployed in a friable and fragile atheromatous segment of an SVG, any further attempt to recross it with a large balloon would have increased risk of stent embolization. Deployment of too large a stent would cause distal embolization due to excessive plaque extrusion. This is the same reason why overdilating a balloon should be avoided. The length of the stent should be longer than the measured length of the lesion by QCA. The reason is the soft atheromatous content of a plaque will be squeezed farther and rearranged along its length as a result of pressure from a stent. When multiple stenting is planned, the distal stent is deployed first, then the proximal one. This strategy is to avoid recrossing a newly deployed stent. However, if there is very tight proximal lesion, then crossing it can cause distal debris embolization. A proximal tight lesion can decrease distal contrast flow and so hammers the optimal visualization of stent position and deployment. The risk and benefit of each strategy (to stent a distal or a proximal lesion first) should be assessed well before embarking on a selected path.

CAVEAT: Mismatch and risk of dislodgment during PCI at the insertion site: Problems with interventions at the anastomotic site include: tortuosity of the arterial segments proximal and distal to the insertion site; difference in diameter of the segment proximal and distal to the target lesion; the degree of size mismatch between the distal vein graft and native vessel; and the angle of insertion of the vein graft into the native vessel. In case of stenting at the anastomotic site, the proximal part of the stent can be bigger, so the stent can have a funnel shape and can more easily be dislodged backwards. The size of the balloon is the size of the native segment distal to the insertion site.[1]

PCI of chronic total occlusion: With better distal protection devices, another provocative thought is to recross the chronic total occlusion of an SVG, insert the distal protection device beyond the lesion, perform PCI with debulking and stenting, then bring the patient back more than a month later for brachytherapy.

PCI in the arterial grafts

Balloon angioplasty and stenting are feasible in arterial in-situ (left or right IMA) or arterial grafts removed from the radial site. In PCI of IMA grafts, hydrophilic steerable wire is helpful in the presence of tortuosity. Care must be taken to ensure that there is sufficient catheter length to reach distal sites with extra-long (145 cm) balloon catheters or short guides (80 cm), or the guide can be shortened and capped with a flared, short sheath 1 size smaller.[17]

TECHNICAL TIPS

**Guides for right and left internal mammary artery graft: On many occasions, the Judkins Right guide can more easily engage the subclavian artery because its primary curve is less acute. Then it is exchanged for the LIMA guide over a 0.038" wire. The usual view for cannulation of the LIMA is the AP view, with the patient's arms down by the side. Selection of the subclavian artery is achieved by placing the guide, with or without the wire protruding, around the arch beyond the origin of the desired artery. The guide is then gently withdrawn and rotated counterclockwise to direct the tip superiorly until the wire or guide tip enters the subclavian origin. An angled hydrophilic wire may facilitate passage through a tortuous subclavian. The guide can then be advanced over the wire beyond the origin of the internal mammary artery, which is usually situated inferior to the thyrocervical trunk and distal to the vertebral artery. Small flush injections of contrast media and gentle withdrawal of the guide can identify the location of the ostium. Gentle counterclockwise rotation of the catheter tip directs it anteriorly and enables it to enter the vessel selectively. If it is difficult to see the ostium, a 60° LAO or 45° RAO projection would elongate the aortic arch, allowing excellent visualization of the origin of the IMA, so the guide tip can be engaged with precision (see Figure 3-9 B–C).

***Engaging a LIMA guide with a wire:** If the IMA is difficult to be engaged, a slippery hydrophilic or a very steerable soft wire can be used to superselect the IMA. It then functions as a guide rail for cannulation of the angioplasty guide. This has been necessary more commonly in the right IMA with the tip of the guide nearby. Be very gentle when cannulating the IMA because it is prone to spasm and dissection. Intracoronary nitroglycerin or verapamil can be given generously. If the subclavian artery is very tortuous, guide cannulation can be achieved through the ipsilateral radial or brachial approach.

***Engaging the RIMA with a pigtail catheter:** After failing to engage the very tortuous right subclavian artery from the femoral approach and from the brachial approach with standard IMA catheter, a new approach with a pigtail was tried by Lapp *et al.* A 5F pigtail catheter (Expo, Boston Scientific Scimed, Boston, MA) was placed distally to the RIMA ostium and a long 0.014" coronary wire (Choice PT Extra Support, Boston Scientific Scimed) was advanced through the catheter. The more the catheter was moved distally, the more the loop of the pigtail catheter straightened. With this maneuver, the curvature of the pigtail could be adjusted to intubate selectively the RIMA ostium. Then the wire was advanced into the distal part of the vessel, across the lesion. Then the pigtail catheter was exchanged for an IMA guide for PCI. This technique using a coronary wire in a 5F pigtail catheter allows the tip of the catheter to be shaped according to the specific anatomy.[18]

TAKE-HOME MESSAGE

Management of patients with IMA graft:[19]

1. Check the subclavian or the IMA in patients who are anticipating to go for CABG if there is a 20 mmHg difference of blood pressure between the two arms.[20]

2. Always check the subclavian artery in post-CABG patients with angina.

3. In evaluating the LIMA check the 90° lateral view. It may be the only view that shows the distal insertion site adequately.

4. Watch out for spasm and pseudostenosis of the LIMA when instrumenting that vessel.

5. Watch for guide catheter deep intubation of the LIMA. Watch the pressure tracing. Do not inject into the LIMA if you are not sure of the position of the guide. Too deep intubation may cause dissection.

***Femoral or radial approach:** The LIMA or RIMA can be approached by the radial approach if the takeoff and proximal course of the two IMAs is descending vertically or internally. Use the femoral approach if the IMA takeoff is descending externally.[21]

**Cause of failure of PCI in LIMA graft: The most common cause of failure of IMA graft angioplasty is mild, moderate, and severe tortuosity of the IMA graft.[23] Mild tortuosity is defined as an isolated curve or series of curves in the graft <90°, moderate tortuosity when the bends make an angle between 90° and 150°, and severe tortuosity is when the graft produced a series of angles in the graft of more than 150° or an isolated turn of 360°. In the majority of IMA graft angioplasty the tortuosity is mild to moderate and does not affect the outcome. Severe tortuosity is associated with technical failure.[22]

**PCI in the subclavian artery: On many occasions, in symptomatic patients after CABG, non-invasive studies point towards ischemia in the distribution of a left or right IMA graft. The usual sites of obstruction include the IMA graft itself, the lesion at the insertion site, or the subclavian artery. Obstructive lesion of the subclavian artery proximal to the origin of the LIMA graft can happen, though it is rare (Figure 14-4). The lesion can be corrected by stenting the subclavian artery.[23] A suspicion of the subclavian lesion is suggested when there a difference of more than 20 mmHg between the pressure of the two arms.[20]

Iatrogenic occlusion of the IMA side branch in order to treat coronary steal syndrome? In a few patients with

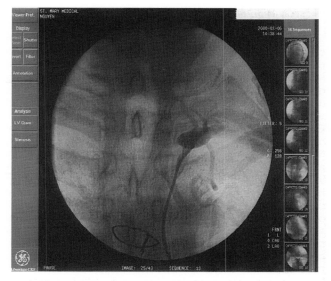

Figure 14-4: Occlusion of the subclavian artery.

unstable angina after bypass surgery, a diagnostic coronary angiogram could show a patent LIMA graft with large thoracic side branch. Because of suggestion of flow diversion from the LIMA into the thoracic artery causing ischemia in the LIMA graft territory, should coil embolization of this thoracic branch be performed?[24]

The LIMA side branches to the chest wall are found in 9–25% of patients.[25] After surgery, reversed blood flow through a LIMA, from a coronary artery, a true steal phenomenon, occurs only if pressure is lower than or proximal to the IMA origin.[26] If there is diversion of blood flow, it will be in systole since systemic arterial flow is predominantly systolic while the coronary circulation is mainly diastolic.[27] Even systolic flow diversion would have a trivial effect, since coronary systolic flow is minimal. This noncompetitive physiology was demonstrated by measuring flow through a large pectoralis artery branch and the patent IMA at rest and during hyperemia.[28] Balloon occlusion of a large LIMA side branch did not alter the measured LIMA flow to the LAD.[29] Using Doppler wires, a trial of balloon occlusion of the LIMA side branch prior to permanent occlusion can easily demonstrate whether flow through the LIMA would increase from the intervention.[28] Therefore, therapeutic LIMA side branch occlusion is unwarranted unless it can be demonstrated to increase LIMA flow or objectively reduce myocardial ischemia, as described above.

CONCLUSIONS

Following successful SVG intervention, there is a high cardiac event rate for most patient subgroups. Lasting success and long-term patency of PCI in the distal anastomotic lesions is an exception. The restenotic process in vein grafts does not plateau as it does in native coronary arteries, and mild-to-moderate non-target vein graft lesions are associated with recurrent ischemic events in about one-third of patients. Even with careful selection of patients, emphasizing focal disease and absence of thrombus, as with the SAVED trial, 6-month cardiac event rates were 38% for balloon angioplasty and 26% after stent implantation.[30] The 5-year event-free survival rate was 31% and survival was less favorable than with native interventions. If one moves from these relatively ideal candidates to the treatment of diffuse disease, recent total occlusions, the prospects for long-term patency and clinical stability diminish, while the acute risk of thromboembolic myocardial infarction, bleeding, and costs escalate. At present, continued study is needed to develop methods (membrane covered stent, distal protection device, thrombectomy, brachytherapy, etc.) to prolong the functional life of degenerating venous grafts, and after thoughtful cost-conscious consideration of risks and benefits and of resource consumption, day-to-day application of percutaneous strategies to these difficult problems must be done with caution. The data from the DES studies are eagerly awaited.

REFERENCES

1. Douglas J. Approaches to the patient with prior bypass surgery. In: Topol EJ, ed. *Textbook of Cardiovascular Medicine.* Lippincott-Raven Publishers, 1998: 2101–18.
2. Keeley E, Velez C, O'Neill W *et al.* Long term clinical outcome and predictors of major adverse cardiac events after PCI for SVG. *J Am Coll Cardiol* 2001; **38**: 659–65.
3. Broderick TM, Wolf RK. Coronary angioplasty to relieve a kinked venous bypass conduit. *Cathet Cardiovasc Diagn* 1995; **35**: 161–4.
4. Hartz RS. Minimally invasive surgery. *Circulation* 1992; **94**: 2669–70.
5. Brener SJ, Ellis SG, Dykstra DM *et al.* Determinants of the key decision for prior CABG patients facing need for repeat revascularization: PTCA or CABG? *J Am Coll Cardiol* 1996; **27**(Suppl A): 45A.
6. Holmes DR, Chesebro JH, Vlietstra RE *et al.* Streptokinase for vein graft thrombosis: A caveat. *Circulation* 1981; **63**: 729.
7. Colombo A, Stankovic G. Massive air embolism. In: Colombo A, Stankovic G, eds. *Colombo's Tips and Tricks in Interventional Cardiology.* Martin Dunitz, 2002: 15.

8. Gruberg L, Hong MK, Mehran R *et al*. In-hospital and long term results of stent deployment compared with ballon angioplasty for treatment of narrowing at the saphenous vein graft distal anastomosis site. *Am J Cardiol* 1999; **84**: 1381–4.

9. Ahmed JM, Hong MK, Mehran R *et al*. Comparison of debulking followed by stenting alone for saphenous vein graft aorto-ostial lesions: Immediate and one-year clinical outcomes. *J Am Coll Cardiol* 2000; **35**: 1560–8.

10. Dohad S, Parris T, Setum C. AngioJet® Rheolytic™ Thrombectomy: An important tool for percutaneous coronary interventions in high-risk patients; VEGAS II Trial. *Am J Cardiol* 2002; **89**: 326–30.

11. Stone G, Cox D, Babb G. *et al*. Safety and efficacy of a novel device for treatment of thrombotic and atherosclerotic lesions in native coronary arteries and saphenous vein graft: Results from the Multicenter X-Sizer for treatment of thrombus and atherosclerosis in coronary applications trial (X-TRACT) study. *Cathet Cardiovasc Interv* 2003; **58**: 419–27 and *J Am Coll Cardiol* 2003; **41** (Suppl A): 43A.

12. Stone G, Grines C. Beyond primary PTCA: New approaches to mechanical reperfusion therapy in AMI. In: Stack RS, Roubin GS, O'Neill W, eds. *Interventional Cardiology Medicine, Principles and Practice*. Churchill Livingstone, 2002: 301–62.

13. The SAFER trial: Presented at the TransCatheter Therapeutics meeting in Washington DC, 2002, by Ross Prpic MB BS.

14. Stone G, Rogers C, Hermiller J *et al*. A prospective randomized multicenter trial comparing distal protection during SVG intervention with a filter-based device compared to balloon occlusion and aspiration: The FIRE trial. *J Am Coll Cardiol* 2003; **41** (Suppl A) 43A.

15. **www.summitmd.com**, accessed June 29, 2003.

16. Stein B, Moses J, Terstein P. Balloon occlusion and transluminal aspiration of SVG to prevent distal embolization. *Cathet Cardiovasc Interv* 2002; **51**: 69–73.

17. King III SB. Approaches to specific sites. In: King II SB, Douglas Jr JS, eds. *Atlas of Heart Diseases: Interventional Cardiology*. Mosby, 1997: 10-1–10-17.

18. Lapp H, Haltern G, Kranz T *et al*. Use of a pigtail catheter to engage a difficult internal mammary artery. *Card Cathet Interv* 2002; **56**: 489–91.

19. Paul Terstein Fix. The stent session at the TransCatheter Therapeutic meeting in Washington DC, 2002.

20. Osborn L, Vernon S, Reynolds B *et al*. Screening for subclavian artery stenosis in patients who are candidates for coronary bypass surgery. *Cathet Cardiovasc Interv* 2002; **66**: 162–5.

21. Shimshack TM, Giorgi LV, Johnson WL *et al*. Applications of PTCA to the internal mammary artery graft. *J Am Coll Cardiol* 1988; **12**: 1205–14.

22. Singh M. Internal mammary artery stenosis. In: Ellis S, Holmes Jr D, eds. *Strategic Approaches in Coronary Interventions*, 2nd edn. Lippincott Williams Wilkins, 2000: 476–80.

23. Kugelmass AD, Kim DS, Kuntz R *et al*. Endoluminal stenting of a subclavian artery stenosis to treat ischemia in the distribution of a patent left IMA graft. *Cathet Cardiovasc Diagn* 1994; **33**: 175–7.

24. Eisenhauer MD, Mego DM, Cambier PA. Coronary steal by IMA bypass graft side-branches: A novel therapeutic use of a new detachable embolization coil. *Cathet Cardiovasc Diagn* 1998; **45**: 301–6.

25. Singh RN, Sosa JA. Internal mammary artery-coronary artery anastomosis: Influence of the side-branches on surgical result. *J Thorac Cardiovasc Surg* 1981; **82**: 909–14.

26. Ayres RW, Lu C, Benzuly KH *et al*. Transcatheter embolization of an IMA bypass graft side-branch causing coronary steal syndrome. *Cathet Cardiovasc Diagn* 1994; **31**: 301–3.

27. Kern M. Does a LIMA side branch ever need occlusion? (Why I don't think so.) *Cathet Cardiovasc Diagn* 1998; **45**: 307–9.

28. Kern MJ, Bach RG, Donohue TJ *et al*. Role of large pectoralis branch artery in flow through a patent left internal artery conduit. *Cathet Cardiovasc Diagn* 1995; **34**: 240–4.

29. Abhyankar AD, Mitchell AS, Berstein L. Lack of evidence for improvement in internal mammary graft flow by occlusion of side branch. *Cathet Cardiovasc Diagn* 1997; **42**: 291–3.

30. Savage MP, Douglas JS Jr, Fischman DL *et al*. Stent placement compared with balloon angioplasty for obstructed coronary bypass grafts. The Saphenous Vein Graft De Novo trial investigators. *N Engl J Med* 1997; **337**: 740–7.

Chapter 15
Left Main Lesions

Seung Jung Park, Thach Nguyen

---

*Basic; **Advanced; ***Rare, exotic, or investigational.

From: Nguyen T, Hu D, Saito S, Grines C, Palacios I (eds), *Practical Handbook of Advanced Interventional Cardiology*, 2nd edn. © 2003 Futura, an imprint of Blackwell Publishing.

GENERAL OVERVIEW

In the past, patients with severe stenosis in the left main (LM) coronary artery were referred for coronary artery bypass graft surgery (CABG) because of improved survival compared to medical therapy alone.[1] With increased operator's experience, better equipment, and more effective antiplatelet drugs, elective stenting for unprotected LM stenosis, with or without debulking, has been performed with success.[2] However, the outcomes reported for PCI of the LM differ from center to center.

In the US, the typical patients who underwent PCI for LM were old, with a mean age of 82, and had an average ejection fraction of 31%. However, their lesions were less complex (ostium: 25%, body/distal: 60%, and bifurcation: 15%).[3] In Europe, the typical patients were slightly younger (mean age of 74), with a good EF of 57%. However, their lesions were much more complex (ostium: 26%, mid-shaft: 21%, and distal bifurcation: 53%).[4] The acute and long-term outcomes reflected these approaches. All the US patients (except one) were discharged alive after 5 days, while in Toulouse, the in-hospital mortality included 7 deaths and 8 MIs in a group of 214 patients. After one year or five years, the mortality was high, in the 10–15% range, reflecting the old age of these patients. There was no difference in outcome of patients with LM disease treated by PCI or CABG.[5] The cardiac mortality was highest in the complex distal bifurcation lesions (19% versus 11%). The majority of the events occurred in the first 6 months, suggesting the important role of in-stent restenosis.[4]

In general, the procedural success rate was good in experienced centers. Subacute stent thrombosis occurred in less than 1%. The angiographic restenosis rate (>50% diameter stenosis) was 15.8% (11.1% in the debulking group vs 18.0% in the non-debulking group, P=NS). The target lesion revascularization (TLR) rate was 11%. The event-free survival rate was 81.57% after 2 years of follow-up.[2]

The patients with LM disease can be stratified according to the risk of the procedure (Table 15-1). The patients with LM lesion in whom PCI should be avoided are listed in Table 15-2.[6]

STANDARD TECHNIQUES

The lesion at the mid-shaft can be predilated and then stented as any discrete lesion. The ostial LM lesion is dilated and stented with the guide tip positioned in the aortic sinus. The proximal end of the stent is left protruding outside the ostium and expanded against the aortic wall as in stenting for any aorto-ostial lesions. The most technical difficulty is to debulk, dilate, and stent the distal lesion, which is technically a bifur-

Table 15-1
Risk classification of patients with LM

High-risk patients

Not eligible for CABG
Age >75
Renal failure
Poor distal run-off
Severe respiratory problem
LVEF <30%

Low-risk patients

Large reference diameter
Without heavy calcification
Lesion location:
• Ostial lesion
• Body lesion
• Distal bifurcation where compromise of LCX is acceptable
No contraindication for CABG

Table 15-2
Contraindications for PCI and indications for CABG

Reduced LV function
Distal bifurcation, reduced LV function and good candidate for CABG
Distal bifurcation, good candidate for surgery and occluded RCA
MVD with reduced LV function and good candidate for surgery
Heavily calcified LM disease
Short (<8 mm) LM

cated or trifurcated lesion. In the highly litigious climate of the US medical environment, this technique should be restricted to highly skilled interventionalists working with patients who understand and accept the risk/benefit ratio of this percutaneous approach.[7] The technically favorable factors for PCI in LM lesion are listed in Table 15-3.[6]

TECHNICAL TIPS

*Selection of guides: As in PCI of any aorto-ostial lesion, a small 6F guide can be seated atraumatically outside the left main ostium. This position helps to reduce the risk of dissection, especially in LM stem with heavy calcification and diffuse disease. However, a large guide of 7F size is needed to accommodate the two 3.0 and 3.5-mm balloons

---

Table 15-3
Technically favorable factors in PCI of LM

EF >50%
No calcification
Anatomically suitable for stenting:
  Ostial LM with   >8 mm in length
                       >3.6 mm in diameter
  Mid-shaft LM   >3.6 mm in diameter

---

for the final kissing maneuver. For patients who require debulking with DCA or rotablation, larger guides of 8 to 9F size are needed.

**Indications for intra-aortic balloon pump (IABP): Patients with normal LV function can tolerate global ischemia well during balloon occlusion. IABP is not routinely used during LM intervention. However, it should be ready for emergency use although it is not inserted prophylactically. If the LV function is poor, prophylactic IABP and PCI with a perfusion balloon should be performed to prevent life-threatening hemodynamic collapse.

DEBULKING

Directional coronary atherectomy (DCA) helps to remove plaque. However, it does not completely eliminate acute recoil and late negative vessel remodeling. Its restenosis rate was found to be similar to those of balloon angioplasty alone, despite better initial angiographic results.[8] On the contrary, optimally deployed coronary stents can reduce the rate of restenosis compared with balloon angioplasty alone by preventing acute elastic recoil and negative chronic vessel remodeling.[9] DCA combined with stenting, when compared to stenting alone, was reported to result in larger post-procedural lumen gain and significantly lower angiographic restenosis. Therefore, this combined approach may be reasonable to overcome the limitations of DCA, with improved angiographic results of stenting for the management of unprotected LM stenosis. It was found to be especially useful for the treatment of unprotected LM with eccentric lesions and large plaque burden at the distal bifurcation (Figure 15-1). At the present time, DCA is routinely performed prior to stenting if the lesion is suitable for debulking. Rotational atherectomy prior to stenting is also performed if the plaque has diffuse superficial calcification.

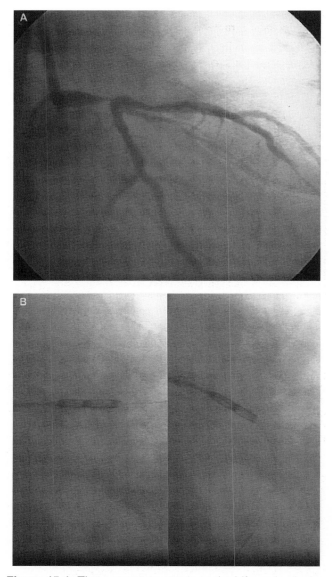

Figure 15-1: Three separate stents on the bifurcation lesion (kissing stent technique). (A) Coronary angiogram (RAO view) demonstrated tight stenosis at the LM bifurcation site. The lesion involved the distal LM and proximal left anterior descending artery (LAD). (B) Directional coronary atherectomy (DCA) was performed on the distal LM and proximal LAD and left circumflex (LCX) ostium. *(Continued)*

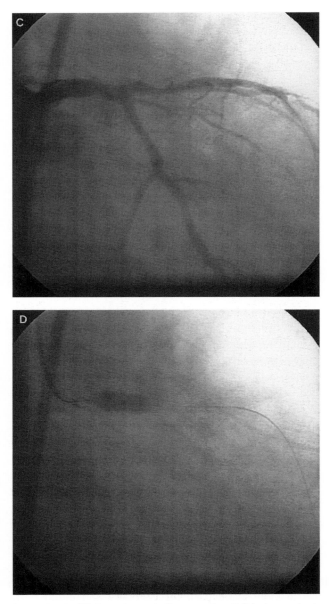

Figure 15-1: (C) Coronary angiogram after DCA showed relatively good angiographic results; however, more than 30% of residual stenosis remained. (D) A 1.0-mm Nir stent was deployed first in the LM area, which was dilated up to 4.6 mm in diameter. *(Continued)*

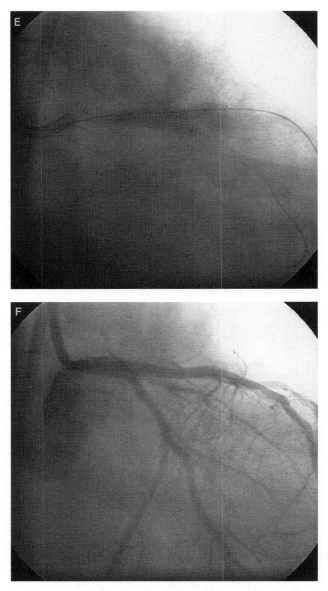

Figure 15-1: (E) After stenting in the LM area, a kissing stenting with 2 Nir stents on the LAD and LCX ostium was performed through the stented LM segment, which could make a new carina of the distal LM area. (F) Final angiogram after stenting on the LM bifurcation lesion, showing good results without residual stenosis. *(Continued)*

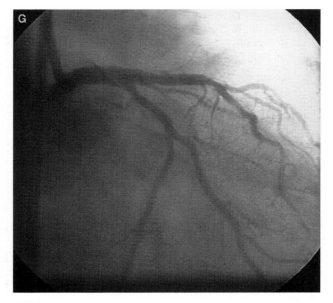

Figure 15-1: (G) Follow-up angiogram at 6 months after the procedure showed no evidence of restenosis and quite good patency on the stenting site.

**Directional atherectomy: With the conventional 7F Atherocath GTO system (Guidant, Temecula, CA) this is a complex procedure. The insertion of these large inflexible catheters requires extra-stiff 9 to 10F guiding catheters, rigid wires, and achieves insufficient tissue removal in calcified lesions and vessels with large reference diameters. However, the newly designed Flexicut (Guidant, Temecula, CA) is characterized by a shaft diameter slightly smaller than 6F (0.076", 1.94 mm). The shaft does not increase in size to adapt to large vessels (cf. the GTO device: 5F, 6F, 7F). This is accomplished by increasing the size of the urging balloon (2.5, 3.0, and 3.5 mm). The Flexicut is compatible with large lumen (>0.87") 8F guiding catheters. The rigid part of the cutting chamber is shorter than in the GTO catheter (13 vs 16 mm), improving tip flexibility while maintaining the length of the cutting window (9 mm). The cutting chamber is more efficient with an increased opening angle of 149° (119° in the GTO model) and the cutter is coated with titanium nitride, which in vitro can effectively cut blocks of calcium hydroxyapatite. To accommodate the material retrieved, a longer (29 mm) tapered distal collection chamber (nose cone) has replaced the shorter nose cone of the GTO.[10]

**Who can do DCA? The choice between stenting and DCA in PCI of LM lesion should be made based upon the operator's experience and the anatomy to be treated. Because the long-term effect of the strategy of debulking by DCA prior to stenting has not been reported, this strategy should be reserved for centers where the operators are well experienced with DCA. Further clarification of the role of DCA and stenting in a randomized trial are needed.[6]

**Rotational atherectomy: During the procedure, keep a systolic blood pressure above 120 mmHg. Have a vasodilator cocktail with nitrate (3 mg), verapamil (125–250 μg) and adenosine to prevent and limit the no-flow/slow-flow phenomenon. Keep a high rotational speed of 180,000 rpm. If the speed drops, the burr should be withdrawn slightly until the speed returns to baseline. Each run should be less than 30 seconds. After rotational atherectomy, perform low-pressure (8 ATM) balloon angioplasty. After the balloon is deflated, withdraw the winged balloon and reinsert it to test the possible access for the stent. If there is difficulty with reinserting the winged balloon, then redilate the LM with higher pressure. Once the access is fine, stent the LM.[10]

**When not to debulk: Usually routine DCA is performed prior to stenting, which facilitates optimal stent expansion and hopefully reduces the rate of in-stent restenosis. However, in some patients, negative remodeling is the cause of LM stenosis. In this situation, only stenting is performed because further debulking with DCA may cause perforation. Current tubular stents designed with much higher radial strength can easily overcome vessel recoil and shift away large plaque burden on the radial axis. They are able to provide a large lumen compatible for optimal flow. Under the guidance of IVUS, adjunctive high-pressure non-compliant balloon dilation is performed so the stent can be fully expanded. This strategy is applied in the majority of the patients without the need for prior debulking. The long-term results of this strategy need close follow-up and validation by prospective and randomized trials.

**Need for intravascular ultrasound (IVUS): IVUS is an important adjunctive imaging modality for optimal intervention of LM stenosis. Routine use of IVUS helps the operator to assess the size and length of the lesions, and decide what type of stent should be selected and what additional adjunctive procedures should be performed. After IVUS, about 25% of lesions require additional inflation due to incomplete strut apposition and/or suboptimal stent expansion.[6]

**LM interventions without debulking and IVUS: In a recent report of LM intervention, 99% of the lesions were dilated and stented without prior debulking (except one case with rotablation) and without routine IVUS (except 4 out of 55 patients).[11] The stent was dilated empirically to a size of half a millimeter larger than the largest diameter of either the LCX or LAD. The length of the LM was measured by the radiopaque spring tip of the wire or the double marker balloon. The restenosis rate in this non-debulking group was similar to the same group of our above study (20% vs 18%), which was higher than the debulking group (11.1%), even though it was not statistically significant. Further studies are needed.[11]

STENTING

The selection of stenting strategies was determined by the location and characteristics of the lesion. Stenting of the ostial and mid-shaft lesions is discussed in detail in Chapters 11 and 7 respectively. Stenting of the distal LM depends on the complexity of the lesion, with or without involvement with the LAD, LCX, or both. Stenting of the LM alone is simple, however, the most feared complication is side branch occlusion due to plaque shifting causing acute closure of the LAD or LCX. The best method of PCI for distal lesions including bifurcation lesions is highlighted below.[12]

BEST METHOD

Which technique is the best for LMCA bifurcation stenting?

Best strategy: Main branch stenting with provisional side branch angioplasty: Stenting of the LM and a large SB across a diminutive non-dominant SB or an SB without ostial lesion, is the simplest and preferred method. If there is plaque shifting to the SB then subsequent balloon angioplasty of the SB through the stent strut can be done with a final kissing balloon technique. This scenario is usually seen in patients with LM and severe ostial LAD while a diminutive non-dominant LCX has no lesion. This technique is still valid in the DES era as illustrated in the SIRIUS bifurcation study (see below).

Second best strategy: Main branch stenting with preventive sidebranch balloon inflation: Stenting of the LM and a large LAD across a diminutive non-dominant LCX or an LCX without ostial lesion is the best and simplest method. In order to prevent plaque shifting from the LM or LAD toward the ostial LCX, a kissing balloon inflation is performed: an SB balloon is inflated first at low pressure (e.g. 2 ATM), then the MB balloon is fully inflated. The role of the SB balloon is to prevent plaque shifting from the MB lesion.

Third best strategy: Main branch stenting with provisional sidebranch stenting: The simplest technique of stenting a bifurcation lesion is to deploy a stent in the main lumen after prior treatment with PTCA, DCA, or rotational atherectomy. If, after placement of the main lumen stent, results in the SB are poor even after rescue balloon angioplasty, then stenting of the SB is needed. Final kissing balloon inflation is performed to correct the deformation of the LM stent due to SB dilation.

EVIDENCE-BASED MEDICINE APPLICATIONS

The SIRIUS Bifurcation Study: In this study, 50 consecutive patients with bifurcation lesions were treated with rapamycin eluting stent. The lesions were located as follows: 26 on the LAD-diagonal, 1 on LAD-septal, 14 on the LCX-obtuse marginal, 7 on the RCA, and 2 on the LM. Ten lesions were treated with only one stent on the MB with PTCA on the SB, while in the remaining 40 cases both branches were stented with the modified T stenting technique. In all cases, a final kissing balloon inflation was performed. The 6-month follow-up showed 16–18% of total MACE for both strategies. The rate of restenosis is seen in Table 15-4. The treatment of bifurcation lesions with T stenting or with MB stenting using the Cypher stent is feasible, with low rate of restenosis in the MB. The rate of restenosis in the side branch still occurs at high rate (20%) with both strategies and is located at the ostium, most likely due to incomplete ostial coverage.[12]

TECHNICAL TIPS

**Preventive side branch balloon inflation in order to avoid plaque shifting: The best way to intervene in a bifurcation lesion is to stent the MB without compromising any SB. Since dilation of the MB can cause plaque shifting even when there is no lesion at or near the ostium of the

Table 15.4
The 6-month restenosis rates

	Main branch		Side branch	
	Stent+Stent	Stent+PTCA	Stent+Stent	Stent+PTCA
Restenosis	0%	5.3%	19%	21%

SB, prevention of plaque shifting with low-pressure balloon inflation in the SB may help to improve the result of PCI at the bifurcation lesion. Usually both branches are wired and both balloons are advanced into the MB and the SB. If there is no lesion in the SB, in anticipation of plaque shifting from the MB, the SB balloon is inflated first at low pressure (e.g. 2 ATM). Full inflation of the MB balloon is then performed. The role of the SB balloon is to prevent plaque shifting from the MB lesion. This is the preventive kissing balloon technique. After successful inflation, both balloons are deflated, and removed proximally so a good angiogram can be performed in order to evaluate the result. The key point is that the inflation of the MB balloon should be optimal so there is complete rearrangement of plaque material when the SB balloon is still inflated. This technique should prevent further plaque shifting during final stent deployment.

**How to manipulate a wire to cross a side strut of a stent: The tip of the wire is shaped to approximately 90° and advanced past the opening of the SB. Then the wire is pulled back with a curved tip positioned at the opening of the SB. A slight pull to straighten the tip with a small twist will advance the wire deeper across the opening of the SB. The tip should be shaped according to the severity of the angulation of the SB and the length of the curved tip is equal to the diameter of the MB. In an "extreme angulated" lesion, the shape of the tip with a wider, >90° curve is very important for success in accessing the SB. Hydrophilic-coated wire might find less friction in crossing the struts, but the risk of dissecting the SB increases. If unsuccessful, a 1.5-mm, over-the-wire balloon or an open-end catheter can be advanced near the origin of the SB to increase the torquing ability of the wire and support of the wire to cross the struts. This technique is especially useful for a reverse (>90°) angle of origin of an SB.[13]

**Risk and benefits of a "jailed wire": In some cases, a hydrophilic-coated wire can be voluntarily "jailed" – left in the SB while the MB is stented. In case of occlusion, this wire can be a valuable landmark to re-cross with another wire into the SB. According to some experienced operators, this technique is very useful because it helps to maintain the SB open and to favorably modify the angulation between both branches. Access to the SB after MB stenting is, therefore, facilitated. After stenting the MB, the wire in the MB is pulled back and, ideally, the most distal cell of the stent at the opening of the SB is crossed and the wire is advanced distally in the side branch. Then the "jailed" wire is withdrawn from the SB with risk of deep intubation of the guide and pushed into the MB. Intervention at the SB can now be continued.[13]

**Selection of stents: Tubular stents are routinely used for treatment of LM ostial or mid-shaft lesions. At the distal bifurcation, the strategy of stenting depends on the size of the secondary branch. In intervention of the distal LM and the LAD, if the LCX is small (<2.5 mm) with a dominant RCA, then a tubular stent will be positioned from the distal LM to the LAD, across the LCX. If the LCX is large, then Y or T stenting with a combination of tube and coil stents is performed (Figure 15-2). The angiographic restenosis rate is similar among all locations and types of LM stenting.[14] The stent should be at least 4 mm in diameter.

**Advance a stent with wire ready across its side strut: The Brazilian technique. After pushing a wire in each branch of the bifurcation, predilation with balloon is performed. The balloon is removed with two wires well positioned across the lesion and in the two branches. Then a premounted stent is prepared as follows. Hold the distal half of the stent while inflating the balloon to expand the proximal half of the stent. Once the proximal half of the stent is inflated, the proximal end of the SB wire is introduced

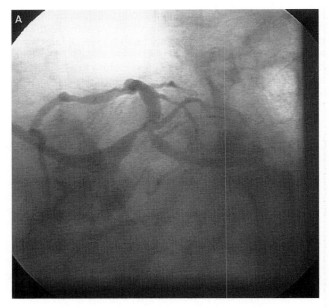

Figure 15-2: Combination of coil and tube stents (Y stents technique). (A) Left coronary angiogram (LAO caudal view), showing severe eccentric narrowing at the bifurcation of the LM coronary artery. DCA was performed first from the distal LM area to the proximal LAD. *(Continued)*

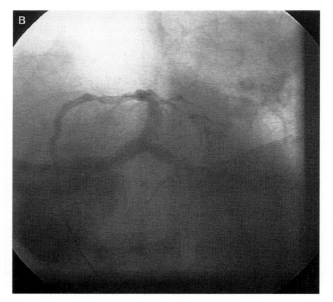

Figure 15-2: (B) After the debulking procedure, a Crossflex coil stent (4.0 × 9 mm) was deployed first, from the distal LM to the left circumflex artery, and another tube stent (4.0 × 9 mm) was deployed on the proximal LAD lesion site. From a technical viewpoint, the coil stent was used for the negotiation of an acute angle from the distal LM to the left circumflex, and then another short tube stent was deployed on the proximal LAD through the space of the coil stent strut. *(Continued)*

backward through a stent strut. The stent is then manually recrimped on the balloon. Now the stent is ready, with the MB wire in the main lumen and the SB wire going through its side strut. The stent is advanced on two wires up to the bifurcation lesion. The stent is deployed as usual with a wire ready at its side for intervention of the SB lesion. The main advantage of this technique is that both wires are in the right position during the whole procedure. Optimal pre-dilation with kissing balloon inflation should be performed in order to secure stent access and to check that wires are not crossed. This technique is also applied for the newly designed AST SLK-View bifurcation stent (Advanced Stent Technologies, San Francisco, CA) that has a side opening for the bifurcation lesion.[13]

**Which branch to be stented first? Generally the larger, more important branch is stented first, although consideration must also be given to angulation at the bifurcation.

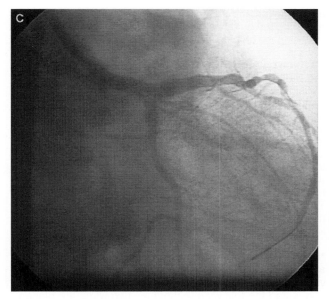

Figure 15-2: (C) Follow-up coronary angiogram at 6 months after the procedure showed no evidence of angiographic re-stenosis.

(1) If there is marked angulation, it is preferable to stent the more angulated branch first to permit easier access into the opposing branch. (2) If an important dissection or occlusion is present in one branch, this branch should be stented first, since wire removal might be risky. (3) When the lesion remains T-shaped after wiring, access to the SB is difficult, or the SB lesion is long and severe or dissected, the SB should be stented first. (4) Visualization of the origin of the SB ostium is sometimes difficult and before stent deployment it is important to check stent positioning using multiple orthogonal views.[13]

**Balloon angioplasty of a side branch: The balloon should not be advanced completely through the stent into the SB for inflation because this increases the risk of balloon entrapment. The inflation pressure should also be kept well under the rated burst pressure because balloon rupture within a stent strut can also cause balloon entrapment. If it is impossible to advance an over-the-wire or rapid exchange balloon across a side strut, then a fixed wired balloon may cross because there is minimal transition between wire and balloon. Furthermore, only one device needs to be inserted. If the balloon fails to advance, repeated, quick forward and backward movement ("Dottering") of the balloon, while adjusting the guide catheter position by deeper intubation, may help the balloon to cross.[13]

**Which balloon to be inflated *first* and *last* during kissing balloon technique? After deploying a stent through the side strut of an MB stent, a kissing balloon inflation is needed. The SB balloon should be inflated first in order to facilitate rotation of the stent towards the right direction. Then the MB balloon is inflated. If the diameter of the MB is not too big, full inflation of both balloons can excessively overstretch the MB. Then inflate alternatively the two balloons with high and low pressure in order to accommodate their size in the MB. At the end, after a full inflation of the SB balloon, deflate it to 2 ATM, then inflate fully the MB balloon. The lower pressure inflation of the SB balloon prevents further final deformation of the SB stent while expanding the MB stent at maximum. This is the final kissing inflation.

***Prevention of ostial restenosis of SB after DES stenting: the crushing stent technique: In order to prevent ostial restenosis of the SB after DES, Colombo *et al.* suggested the following technique. Two wires are placed in the two branches of the bifurcation lesion. The SB is stented first, with the proximal end completely covering the SB ostium. A distal half of the proximal end of the stent is protruding into the MB lumen. The SB wire is removed. An MB stent is advanced across the lesion while fully covering the ostium of the SB. The MB stent is deployed, crushing the proximal end of the SB stent into the arterial wall around the SB ostium. Hopefully, this technique delivers enough drug to the ostium of the SB that it prevents its restenosis.[12]

EXTREMELY HIGH-RISK INTERVENTIONS

As PCI becomes more successful, with improved interventional equipment, more effective antiplatelet drugs, and increased operator's experience, older and sicker patients are requesting PCI for LM lesions. In these situations, indications should be reviewed and risks and benefits discussed in detail with patients and families. Usually in these very elderly patients, for whom surgery is not an option due to LM and diffuse disease, the strategy is to stent the LM only. If the patient has LM and LAD or LCX lesion, then the LM has to be stented first before performing PCI distally in other lesions. In the case of patients with LM and an EF <40% plus an occluded RCA, Fajadet J *et al.* suggested the following important technical points (without any guarantee of a perfect outcome).[6] The mortality was 75% for patients in this group of LM and three-vessel disease.[6]

1. The systolic BP must be maintained at above 120 mmHg.
2. IABP should be available in the laboratory at any time.
3. Place the wire in the distal LAD.
4. Predilate the lesion with an undersized balloon to ensure the stent passes through and avoids distal dissection. Use a short inflation time (10–15 seconds) at high pressure (16–18 ATM).
5. Wait for 30–45 seconds or more for recovery of blood pressure and triggering of ischemic preconditioning.
6. Stent the lesion with shorter inflation time (<20 seconds) and higher pressure (16–18 ATM).
7. Carefully evaluate the result with multiple cine projections to confirm perfect deployment.

REFERENCES

1. Taylor HA, Deumite NJ, Chaitman BR *et al.* Asymptomatic LM coronary artery disease in the Coronary Artery Surgery Study (CASS) registry. *Circulation* 1989; **79**: 1171.

2. Park SJ, Park SW, Lee CW *et al.* Stenting of unprotected left main coronary stenosis: Acute and long-term results of the first 100 cases: Elective intervention of left main coronary artery stenosis. *J Am Coll Cardiol* 2000; **35** (Suppl A): 61.

3. Sharma S, Kini A, Mitre C *et al.* Unprotected LM coronary stenting: Predictors of restenosis and long term follow-up results. *J Am Coll Cardiol* 2003; **41**: 6–27A.

4. Boccalatte M, Mulvihill N, Gottilla R *et al.* Does lesion location have an impact on long term clinical outcome after unprotected LMCA stenting? *J Am Coll Cardiol* 2003; **41**: 6–27A.

5. Boccalatte M, Mulvihill N, Loufti M *et al.* CABG and stent to treat LMCA: Direct comparison of revascularization strategies. *J Am Coll Cardiol* 2003; **41**: 6–27A.

6. Fajadet J, Black A, Hayeruzadeh B *et al.* Unprotected left main stenting. In: Fajadet J, ed. *Syllabus for EuroPCR*, 2001.

7. Zoltan T. LM angioplasty goes "main stream." *Cathet Cardiovasc Interv* 1999; **46**: 160–1.

8. Topol E, Leya E, Pinkerton C *et al.* A comparison of directional atherectomy with coronary angioplasty in patients with coronary artery disease. *N Engl J Med* 1993; **329**: 221–7.

9. Serruys PW, de Jaegere P, Kiemeneij F *et al.* A comparison of balloon-expandable stent implantation with balloon angioplasty in patients with coronary artery disease. *N Engl J Med* 1994; **331**: 489–95.

10. Park SJ. DCA for the LM. **www.summitmd.com**, accessed 4 December 2003.

11. Wong P, Wong V, Tse KK *et al.* A prospective study of elective stenting of unprotected LM coronary disease. *Cathet Cardiovasc Interv* 1999; **46**: 153–9.

12. The SIRIUS Bifurcation Study. Presented by A. Colombo at the AHA Scientific meeting, Chicago, October 2002.

13. Lefevre T, Louvard Y, Morice MC. Current approaches for stenting bifurcation lesion. In: Fajadet J, ed. *Syllabus for EuroPCR*, 2001.
14. Park SJ, Lee CW, Kim YH *et al*. Technical feasibility, safety and clinical outcome of stenting of unprotected left main coronary artery bifurcation narrowing. *Am J Cardiol* 2002; **104**: 1609–14.

Chapter 16

Removal of Embolized Material

Kirk Garratt, Thach Nguyen

INTRODUCTION

Percutaneous techniques for treatment of coronary artery disease (PCI) have evolved and diversified dramatically, but they all have at least one common feature: all involve technical manipulation of complex equipment in the confines

---

*Basic; **Advanced; ***Rare, exotic, or investigational.

From: Nguyen T, Hu D, Saito S, Grines C, Palacios I (eds), *Practical Handbook of Advanced Interventional Cardiology*, 2nd edn. © 2003 Futura, an imprint of Blackwell Publishing.

of coronary arteries, and are operated from a significant distance. When traversing severely diseased coronary arteries and manipulating equipment, particularly devices with detachable components, the opportunity for loss or embolization of material in the coronary circulation presents itself. In this chapter we will review and discuss the management strategies for embolized material.

GENERAL PRINCIPLE

When a problem with defective equipment (unexpandable stent, uncoiling wire, asymmetrically bulging balloon due to metal fatigue, twisted guide, etc.) arises inside the coronary artery or the ascending aorta, the ideal is to remove the entire system below the level of the renal arteries so the problem can be corrected without risk of cerebral embolization or to any vital organ.

In the case of a stent that slips off the delivery balloon inside the coronary artery, it cannot be brought to the iliac artery simply by withdrawing the whole system, even as a unit. Pulling the indwelling angioplasty wire will leave a loose, free stent behind. So all efforts are concentrated on keeping the wire inside the stent and across the lesion for prompt access of rescue devices. As a stent slips off the delivery balloon, there are two options: either to retrieve it or to deploy it in a safe, non-target location. Retrieval should be attempted if threatening malposition occurs, or if the stent is loose in the aorta or in another location in which deployment cannot be undertaken safely. In the retrieval strategy, the stent should be brought safely below the renal arteries so there is no chance for systemic embolization. Once below the renal arteries level, the next important step is to remove the embolized stent from the femoral sheath without injuries to the femoral artery or need of arterial cut-down. Everything should be done within an acceptable time frame, with a wire still across the lesion. In the meantime, the patient has to be watched closely and the clinical condition remain stable, so the scheduled PCI can be continued and finished.

Sometimes peripheral embolization of stents can be the best option. Systemic embolization does not cause any severe clinical sequelae, except to the cerebral circulation. Short wire fragments retained in a totally occluded artery do not pose any long-term side effects.[1] There are many reports of embolized stents into the lower extremities and periphery, without evidence of untoward long-term event effects. Use of long-term anticoagulation with coumadin used to be recommended in such cases, but there are insufficient data to be certain of the need for this; 6–9 months of therapy with aspirin and a thienopyridine drug should be sufficient. Any foreign materials that are retained more than 1 week should not be

Table 16-1

Procedural options in the management of embolized material

1. No treatment for peripherally embolized small stents.
2. Deploy the embolized stent in inconsequential location.
3. Remove a tubular stent with a snare.
4. Remove a broken wire segment with a snare.
5. Remove embolized material with a snare made with a loop of angioplasty wire emerged from a transport catheter.
6. Remove a tubular stent with two twisted wires.
7. Secure a stent by inflating a small balloon distal to it and removing the whole system.
8. Remount the stent with a balloon through a transport catheter.
9. Grasp a stent with a biopsy forceps at the ostium of a coronary artery.

removed percutaneously because they may be covered and incorporated by fibrous tissue. Aggressive extraction of the embolized material may injure and perforate the vessel.

All of the techniques discussed in this chapter are used only as references. They range from the standard methods with the commercial snares to the improvised techniques, which become lifesaving if the procedure is successful. The selection of a particular method or equipment depends on the patient's clinical condition, familiarity of the operators with the retrieval equipment, and availability of the equipment in the cardiac catheterization laboratories. The discussion focuses more on coronary stent, but the retrieval technique may be applied to any embolized device or fragments. Different options in the management of embolized materials are listed in Table 16-1.

RETRIEVAL OF EMBOLIZED CORONARY STENT

The significant majority of stents used in contemporary North America, Europe, and Asia are of the slotted tube design. These stents are generally constructed of surgical stainless steel hypodermic tubing which is fashioned (usually through a laser-cutting method) into a specific configuration. They differ from self-expanding stents, which are generally constructed out of multiple interlacing strands of wire, or flexible coil stents, which are usually formed from a single compliant filament. The Wallstent and Radius stents (Boston Scientific, Quincy, MA) are examples of self-expanding stents, while the Gianturco-Roubin stent (Cook Inc, Bloomington, IN) and the Wiktor stent (Medtronics, Minneapolis,

MN) are examples of flexible coil stents. Flexible coil stents are essentially not used in contemporary PCI practices, and self-expanding stents have very limited application. Since coronary stents represent a detachable component of a PCI system, stents are, by their nature, prone to accidental release from the overall apparatus. Significant coronary calcification, tortuosity, and suboptimal guide position can contribute to stent embolization.

Stent embolization: This typically occurs in one of three scenarios. First, the stent may be successfully introduced into the coronary circulation, but it cannot be advanced into the target area. This is usually due to proximal tortuosity, rigid and calcified segment, or insufficient predilation of the target lesion. Second, in an attempt to direct stenting without predilation, unexpected difficulty in advancing a stent may be encountered. In these cases, the stent should be gently retracted back into the guide, removed and the lesion predilated. If the distal tip of the stent has engaged the lesion, it is possible that manipulation to advance the stent may strip the stent off the balloon, such that it remains imbedded in the lesion when the balloon is retracted. In this case, the coronary wire is generally still in place, indwelling through the stent lumen and the lesion.

Most frequently, stents also become dislodged from the deployment balloon when they are retracted from the coronary artery back into the guide. At that time, the tip of the guide may catch the proximal edge of the stent, and strip it off the deployment balloon. The stent will be left dangling on the coronary wire at or near the ostium of the vessel under treatment.

TECHNICAL TIP

**How to withdraw a stent without embolizing it:[2] When a stent is unable to arrive at the target area because of tortuous proximal segment or because it is unable to cross a tight lesion, it has to be withdrawn into the guide. Then the tip of the guide should be lined up well coaxially with the indwelling wire and its straddling stent. If the guide cannot provide an excellent coaxial relationship with the stent, then the guide should be retracted until a favorable alignment between the guide and stent can be achieved. Sometimes, removal may require retracting the guide to the tip of the femoral sheath in order to straighten the tip of the guide.

REMOVAL OF A STENT WITH A SNARE

Standard equipment: The GooseNeck Amplatz Microsnare catheter (Microvena Co, White Bear Lake, MN) is a Nitinol retrieval device that includes a transport end-hole catheter and loop snares. The wire, which moves freely in the catheter, extends from the proximal end of the catheter, out the distal end, and then it is folded and re-enters the distal lumen and extends back to the proximal end. Retraction of one or both ends of the wire causes it to retract into the distal tip. The 4F catheter tapers to a 2.3F tip. The snares are available in 2, 4, and 7 mm diameter. Once emerged from the catheter, the loop is at a right angle to the tip, thus facilitating the grasping of target object. The 4F transport catheter can easily fit inside a 6F guide.[3]

Retrieval of a tubular stent from the coronary artery: Once a stent slips off the delivery balloon, the indwelling wire is advanced as far as possible into the distal vasculature and the balloon removed. A 4F transport catheter with a GooseNeck snare is assembled. The loop of the snare, emerging from the transport catheter, is passed over the angioplasty wire, encircles it, and is advanced up to the coronary ostium. The snare is manipulated into the artery to loop around the unexpanded stent under fluoroscopic guidance. An effort should be made to grab the proximal part of the stent. Once the loop is in the right position, the transport catheter is advanced to tighten the loop around the stent. Then the guide, with the stent secured by the snare, is withdrawn to the iliac artery as a unit. If extraction of a stent through the usual 6F or 7F femoral sheath is difficult or impossible, then the sheath is changed to a larger (9F) one through which the embolized stent can be removed. An embolized broken wire segment or any embolized device can be snatched by the snare with the same technique.

Improvised equipment: Assembling a snare from angioplasty wire: The snare is formed by folding a 300-cm long 0.014" wire and introducing it through a 4F transport catheter. Once it arrives near the tip of the catheter, one end of the wire is pulled while the other end is advanced slightly to position the sharp point of the tight fold within the catheter so that it will not injure the vessels or cardiac wall during movement of the snare. By advancing one end of the wire while holding the other end until a desired diameter is achieved, a workable loop snare emerges from the tip of the catheter (Figure 16-1). The embolized material is trapped by the snare using the usual technique. After the loop is tightened successfully at the distal end, a hemostat is used to fix the wire in position at the proximal end and the entire system is pulled as a unit to the iliac artery.

The art of loop snaring:[4] The important difference between the commercial and the improvised snare is the angle of the snare at the tip of the transport catheter. The GooseNeck loop is at a right angle with the catheter while the improvised snare loop is parallel to it. This difference is absolutely vital in positioning the loop and assessing its position in the technique of snaring.

Once a stent slips off the delivery balloon, the wire should be kept indwelling inside the stent so the free movement of the stent is limited to the longitudinal axis of the wire. That

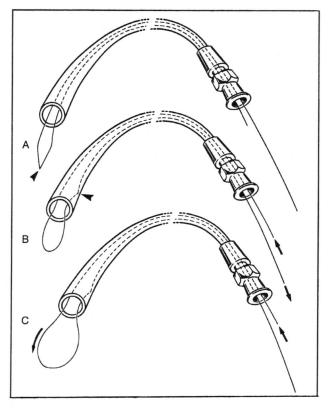

Figure 16-1: Making a snare from angioplasty wire. By advancing one end of the wire while holding the other end until a desired diameter is achieved, a workable loop snare emerges from the tip of the catheter. (Adapted from Gerlock AJ, Mirfakhraee M. Foreign body retrieval. In: Gerlock AJ, Mirfakhraee M, eds. *Essentials of Diagnostic and Interventional Angiographic Techniques.* WB Saunders, 1985: 27–38. With permission from the publisher.)

position of the wire will tremendously help the rescue effort by giving prompt access to the defective stent. The GooseNeck Microsnare is inserted into the guide with its loop encircling the angioplasty wire. Once it arrives at the right position, its loop is encircling the proximal end of the stent. Then the loop is tightened by advancing the transport catheter, and the whole stent-snare-wire complex is ready to be pulled out. The improvised snare can achieve the same result but requires more skillful manipulation because the loop is not at a right angle to the catheter. In the case of a broken wire segment or a free stent not on an angioplasty wire, their capture depends on correct alignment of the loop to the free end of these free fragments.

TECHNICAL TIPS

**Which end to loop?[4] The loop snare technique is effective if the embolized fragment (wire or stent) has a free end for ensnarement. The patient is positioned under the fluoroscope for locating both ends of the fragment and to identify its free end, which usually pulsates.

**Identify the position of the snare:[4] The snare is held at a right angle to the calculated plane of the embolized fragment. To do this, the patient must be positioned under the fluoroscope in such a way that the wire is seen in its full length. This implies that the wire or stent is vertical to the X-ray beam. Then the snare is held in such a way that it is shown under fluoroscopy as a straight line or a closed loop, confirming its vertical plane in relation to the wire or stent fragment. Then the free end of the wire can be captured. If the snare loop plane is parallel to the plane of the broken wire or stent, ensnarement is impossible (Figure 16-2).

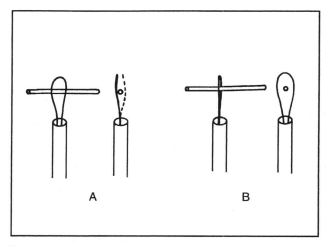

A   B

Figure 16-2: The significance of the plane of the snare loop in relation to the broken wire or embolized stent. The snare is held in such a way that it is shown under fluoroscopy as a straight line or a closed loop, confirming its vertical plane in relation to the wire or stent fragment. (Adapted from Gerlock AJ, Mirfakhraee M. Foreign body retrieval. In: Gerlock AJ, Mirfakhraee M, eds. *Essentials of Diagnostic and Interventional Angiographic Techniques.* WB Saunders, 1985: 27–38. With permission from the publisher.)

**Securing the embolized wire fragment:[4] The next important step is to make sure that the snare has encircled the embolized wire or stent. The transport catheter is advanced, causing the broken wire fragment or stent to bend when the snare is engaged. Withdrawing the ends of the wire to capture the embolized wire or stent is not suggested because it can cause disengagement (the stent or the wire fragment can get out of the encircling loop) (Figure 16-3).

***How to manipulate a pointed loop:[4] If the stiff folded end of the loop cannot be withdrawn in the catheter to make a round loop outside the tip of the catheter, then the pointed loop is kept inside the transport catheter during transit. When the tip of the catheter arrives near the embolized object, it is positioned with its tip cephalad to the object, and the wire loop, still well inside the catheter, is at the upper level of the object. While the wire loop remains in place, the catheter is withdrawn to expose the loop. This technique is helpful in preventing vascular injury from the stiff, folded end of the pointed loop (Figure 16-4).[4]

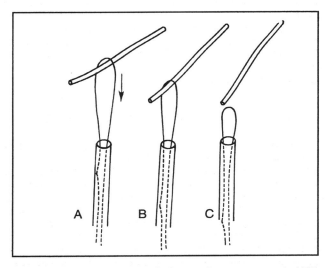

Figure 16-3: Improper technique of ensnarement. Withdrawing the ends of the wire to capture the embolized wire or stent can cause disengagement. (Adapted from Gerlock AJ, Mirfakhraee M. Foreign body retrieval. In: Gerlock AJ, Mirfakhraee M, eds. *Essentials of Diagnostic and Interventional Angiographic Techniques*. WB Saunders, 1985: 27–38. With permission from the publisher.)

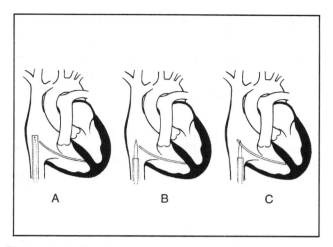

Figure 16-4: Technique of ensnarement with a pointed loop. When the tip of the catheter arrives near the embolized object, it is positioned with its tip cephalad to the object and the wire loop, still well inside the catheter, at the upper level of the object. While the wire loop remains in place, the catheter is withdrawn to expose the loop. (Adapted from Gerlock AJ, Mirfakhraee M. Foreign body retrieval. In Gerlock AJ, Mirfakhraee M, eds. *Essentials of Diagnostic and Interventional Angiographic Techniques.* WB Saunders, 1985: 27–38. With permission from the publisher.)

REMOVAL OF A STENT WITH A BALLOON

The technique is to advance a small 1.5 or 2.0-mm balloon over the wire and through the stent, and inflate the balloon distal to the stent. Retracting it back then will bring the stent back into the guide. If the balloon cannot be advanced all the way through the stent, low-pressure inflation of the balloon when it is at least partially within the stent will suffice. In many cases, the system may be removed without loss of the coronary wire position or removal of the guide. This will be easiest if a 7F or 8F guide has been used. In some cases, the stent may be contained within the distal tip of the guide, but the inflated balloon cannot be retracted into the guide. In this case, the guide and balloon should be removed as one unit over the wire. An extension wire will allow preservation of coronary access. The removal of an inflated balloon from a coronary artery is not without danger. The balloon should be of very low profile and the artery should be large enough to easily accommodate the movement of an inflated balloon.

REMOVAL OF A STENT WITH TWO WIRES

When a snare is not available to remove the embolized stent, there is a possibility of withdrawing the free stent with a second wire twisting around the stent to immobilize it to the first wire.[5,6]

TECHNICAL TIP

***Manipulation of wires to remove an embolized stent:
Once a stent slips off the delivery balloon, the wire should be kept indwelling inside the stent so the free movement of the stent is limited to the longitudinal axis of the wire. In order to remove this free-standing stent with wires, a second wire should be advanced and pass through the struts of that unexpanded stent and not through the central lumen. The 0.014" coronary wire is unable to pass through the cells of a Palmaz-Schatz stent, which are only 0.012" wide, so it has to go through the 1-mm gap at the articulation site. If the stent is half-expanded, then the size of the cell is bigger, to accommodate the tip of a second wire. Once the second wire is advanced as far as possible, then the two wires are twisted proximally with the stent straddling their stiff segment. The stent is then trapped between the two entangled wires and removed.

In order to be successful in entrapping the stent, both wires should be advanced deeply so the stent is straddling their stiff part. A soft floppy distal tip is not strong enough to entrap a stent when twisted. As the wires are removed slowly, the guide engages deeper into the ostium. This is the sign that the stent has been properly snared. In theory, if the second wire goes through the central lumen of the stent, both wires can be easily pulled out, leaving the free stent behind. So the second wire should strategically go through the side-struts and not the central lumen. With gentle and persistent pulling, the whole system (guide, stent entwisted between two wires) will be successfully withdrawn.[6]

DEPLOYMENT OF AN EMBOLIZED STENT

**Deployment of an embolized stent: Proper management of this situation is generally straightforward. The deployment balloon should be advanced back over the wire and fully into the stent. Even if the stent is not advanced completely through the lesion, it should be expanded where it is to its fullest possible dimension using the deployment balloon. If the deployment balloon is unable to be advanced through the stent, a lower profile, flexible-tipped balloon catheter should be inserted instead. Use of a very small diameter (1.5–2.0 mm) balloon will facilitate subsequent larger balloon entry, if a nominally sized balloon will not pass through. It is virtually always possible to advance a balloon at least part way through the stent, and open it partly. The remainder of the stent can be expanded sequentially. Occasionally, a new, smaller balloon will be needed to pass through the unopened portion of the lost stent. Predilation of the target lesion (usually possible with the balloon used to expand the initial stent) will assure success with additional stent implantation efforts.

CAVEAT: To deploy or to remove an embolized stent? It is important to make a decision whether to deploy or to remove an embolized stent right at the beginning, because once a stent is partially deployed, the stent will have to be perfectly deployed with its struts well apposed to the arterial wall (as in any standard stenting procedure). A half-deployed stent that obstructs the flow will cause early or late acute vessel occlusion. So either the stent is perfectly deployed or it should be removed. It is easier to remove an intact (not-yet-deployed) stent than to remove one later with its struts sticking out or after being crushed or disfigured. It is also easier to deploy a stent at the present time when the patient is still stable, rather than recross later an acutely occluded artery due to thrombus obstructing a partially deployed stent. If the operator attempts to open the proximal half of a stent, try to open it as wide as possible because another balloon will have to be re-inserted at the imperfect opening that is just being opened. If the opening of the stent is small or crooked, then the attempt to re-insert a second larger balloon will be difficult. Once the stent is deployed, it will be recrossed by other interventional devices (including a new stent) to dilate and to stent the distal index lesion. If the first (embolized) stent is not well deployed and the lumen is not large enough, PCI of the distal index lesion would be very hard and almost impossible. Contemplating all these challenges beforehand will help the operator to make a wise decision, whether to remove an embolized stent with a snare or to perfectly deploy it.

REMOVAL OF FRACTURED WIRES

Virtually every coronary angioplasty device is advanced into the coronary system over a wire. The soft, atraumatic tips of coronary wires have been known to fracture off if being manipulated excessively and embolize in the coronary circulation. This most frequently occurs when the shapable wire tip becomes lodged in an atherosclerotic plaque and separates from the body of the wire when the wire is retracted. This occurred rather more frequently in the past, when nearly all wires were manufactured by bonding a flat forming ribbon to the round end of a wire. Current coronary wires are constructed of a gradually tapering filament that is an extension of the shaft of the wire, so solder points and other relatively weak junctions are minimized in contemporary wire design. Nonetheless, fracture of wire tips may still occur.

TECHNICAL TIP

**Removal of wire fragment: Recovery of wire fragments is generally accomplished relatively simply through insertion of two or more additional angioplasty wires into the coronary artery under treatment. By twisting these wires together, the retained fragment can become entrapped in these angioplasty wires, and the entire system can be removed as one block. When this technique fails, a retrieval device is needed for removal of these wire fragments.

REMOVAL OF EMBOLIZED MATERIAL FROM THE ILIAC ARTERY

Once the embolized object is brought to the iliac artery, the main problem is to remove it through the vascular sheath without the need for arterial cut-down. If the 6F or 7F sheath is too small, the sheath should be changed for a 9F sheath (Figure 16-5). Biliary forceps, alligator forceps, or cardiac bioptome are suitable for retrieving the stent in the common iliac artery or at the tip of the arterial sheath. Coil stents such as the Wiktor stent have been successfully retrieved by using the alligator forceps,[7] and tubular stents such as Palmaz-Schatz stents have been successfully retrieved by using the bioptome.[8] The disadvantages of these instruments are (1) the need to directly grasp the relatively small stent, (2) the likelihood of damaging the stent itself, (3) the possibility of endovascular trauma, and (4) the loss of guidewire position during stent retrieval.[14] Hence innovative techniques are developed for stent retrieval using easily available instruments. Most of the stents available today are radiopaque and not difficult to locate under fluoroscopy. They are mainly used when the device is brought to below the renal artery level. Familiarity with each can be extremely useful in the rare event of stent misplacement (Figure 16-6).

Basket retrieval device: The basket retrieval device is designed for capturing biliary stones and other irregularly shaped elements from within tubular biologic structures. This device consists of helically arranged loops which can be collapsed or expanded by retracting or advancing a lever on the proximal end of the system. When a stent is dangling from a coronary wire, advancement of a basket retrieval device over the wire will bring it into close proximity to the stent. Retraction

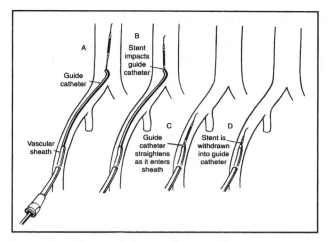

Figure 16-5: Removal of a stent from the iliac artery. Attempts to withdraw a stent into a guide require excellent coaxial relations between the stent and the tip of the guide. Sometimes the guide needs to be retracted into the arterial sheath so the tip can be straightened out.

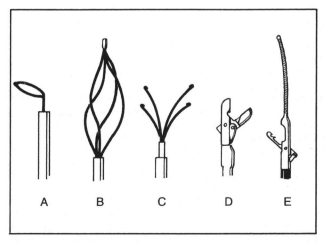

Figure 16-6: Different equipment for removal of embolized material.

of the basket traps the stent and the system can be retrieved safely.

TECHNICAL TIP

***Best use for basket retrieval device:** It can be used to catch a stent from one side and pull it free from a deployment balloon. It works best if the stent has been damaged and misshaped such that a portion of the stent projects laterally away from the deployment balloon (Figure 16-6 B).[2]

Biliary stone forceps device: The biliary stone forceps device is a very effective but potentially hazardous tool. Consisting of a set of curved finger-like projections that extend from the distal tip of a plastic catheter, the system can be used to hook irregularly shaped objects in biologic tube structures (Figure 16-6 C). These systems were originally designed to assist in the removal of obstructive stones in the biliary tree. It is difficult to advance this catheter in perfect alignment with a coronary wire. Occasionally it is useful to remove the finger-like components of the system inside the transport catheter and advance the catheter over a separate wire to bring it into proximity with the coronary stent. Then readvance the finger-like component to grasp the embolized material. However, because of its sharp finger-like projections, it is generally not advised to use this within the coronary system or within vein grafts. These catheters are available in lengths of 130 to 150 cm, with catheter bodies of 4F and 5F diameter. The retracted device has reasonably good fluoroscopic visibility, but the finger-like projections are quite thin and have poor radiopacity. It is best used to catch a partially deployed stent or in situations where a portion of a stent has become separated from the balloon.[2]

Biopsy or alligator forceps: Alligator forceps are familiar to most cardiologists. The design of standard myocardial bioptomes follows the design principles of alligator forceps. This type of forceps device is used widely throughout medicine and surgery. The "biting jaws" action of these devices makes them attractive for capturing embolized material. A variety of these devices are available in most hospital settings, but most are not suitable for use within the vascular tree because the catheter bodies have insufficient length, the shaft diameter is too large, or the devices are too rigid to be advanced safely into the coronary arterial system. Thinner, softer disposable bioptomes are generally immediately available in catheterization laboratories and can be used, but they are still generally too rigid for use beyond the ostium of a vessel. Bioptome jaws are quite sharp, so gripping any device

must be attempted with great care to avoid severing thin metallic structures (Figure 16-6 D).[2]

Cook Retained Fragment Retrieval Tool: (Cook Inc,
Bloomington, IN) This is a device that resembles a fixed-wire
angioplasty balloon catheter with an articulating arm. The arm
is operable from the proximal hub. Activating this arm opens
the device in a "trapdoor" fashion. Advancing this system
alongside a retained fragment can be very useful for recovery
of the lost material, but this device is too bulky and too rigid for
safe use within the coronary tree. It is available in lengths of 80
and 145 cm (Figure 16-6 E).[2]

TECHNICAL TIPS

**Retraction of a stent into a guide: Once the stent is
brought to the iliac artery, it is manipulated to be withdrawn
into a guide, if there is a favorable alignment between the
stent and the guide. In these situations, the guide may
be retracted into the arterial sheath to straighten its tip. If
there is no excellent coaxial relationship, the stent can be
stripped off the balloon (Figure 16-5).

*****Stent removal from the iliac artery with a commercial
snare:** Position the snare above the stent and tighten it at the
distal end of the stent under fluoroscopic control. The stent can
now be pulled into the guide and retrieved. The stent should
be snared at the distal end, which is close to the operator. By
pulling this end, the operator can manipulate this end to enter
the tip of the femoral sheath and be removed from the body. If
the stent is snared at the proximal end, it is more difficult to manipulate the stent to enter the guide. If the stent is crushed from
the proximal end, the whole stent will collapse and its large
mass is difficult to pass through the femoral sheath. If the stent
is crushed at the distal end, there is only a small area of damage, and it can still be manipulated into the sheath. Changing
to a larger size (9F) sheath will help to get the stent to enter the
sheath (Figure 16-5).

CONCLUSION

Embolization of equipment into the coronary tree is domi-
nated by loss of stents in today's interventional practice. Loss
of stents typically occurs because of inadequate predilation
of the target lesion, and/or improper guide alignment with the
coronary ostium. Extreme tortuosity and extensive plaque
calcification also contribute to the odds of coronary stent loss.
The most important consideration in avoiding complications
associated with stent embolization is to select appropriate

tools and strategies for managing the planned intervention. Use of routine predilation of a target lesion, careful guide alignment with the ostium of the target vessel, and appropriately supportive wires will minimize opportunities for stent loss. Specific retrieval techniques to recover lost stents are described. The most consistent device, easiest to use and readily available, are the coronary loop snares, but all of the devices described above may have an important role to play in the event of embolized coronary equipment. Familiarity with, and immediate access to, these devices is important in contemporary practice.

REFERENCES

1. Hartzler G, Rutherford B, McConahay D. Retained percutaneous transluminal coronary angioplasty components and their management. *Am J Cardiol* 1987; **60**: 1260–4.

2. Garratt K, Bachrach M. Stent retrieval: Devices and technique. In: Heuser R, ed. *Peripheral Vascular Stenting for Cardiologists*. Martin Dunitz, 1999: 27–37.

3. Eisenhauer AC, Piemonte TC, Gossman DE *et al*. Extraction of fully deployed stents. *Cathet Cardiovasc Diagn* 1996; **38**: 393–401.

4. Gerlock AJ, Mirfakhraee M. Foreign body retrieval. In: Gerlock AJ, Mirfakhraee M, eds. *Essentials of Diagnostic and Interventional Angiographic Techniques*. WB Saunders, 1985: 27–38.

5. Veldhuijzen FLMJ, Bonnier HJRM, Michels HR *et al*. Retrieval of undeployed stents from the right coronary artery: Report of two cases. *Cathet Cardiovasc Diagn* 1993; **30**: 245–8.

6. Wong PHC. Retrieval of undeployed intracoronary Palmaz-Schatz stents. *Cathet Cardiovasc Diagn* 1995; **35**: 218–23.

7. Eckhout E, Stauffer JC, Goy JJ. Retrieval of a migrated coronary stent by means of an alligator forceps. *Cathet Cardiovasc Diagn* 1993; **30**: 166–8.

8. Berder V, Bedossa M, Gras D *et al*. Retrieval of a lost coronary stent from descending aorta using a PTCA balloon and biopsy forceps. *Cathet Cardiovasc Diagn* 1993; **28**: 351–3.

Chapter 17

Complications

*Thach Nguyen, Damras
Tresukosol, Vo Thanh Nhan,
Mingzhong Zhao, Hong Zhao*

---

*Basic; **Advanced; ***Rare, exotic, or investigational.

From: Nguyen T, Hu D, Saito S, Grines C, Palacios I (eds), *Practical
Handbook of Advanced Interventional Cardiology*, 2nd edn. © 2003
Futura, an imprint of Blackwell Publishing.

Table 17-2
Differential diagnoses of dissection

Causes	Corrective techniques
1. Streaming of contrast	More forceful and steady injection
2. Deep guide intubation	Withdrawal of guide
3. Stiff wire straightening the vessel	Withdraw the wire with the flexible tip proximal to the new lesion
4. Overlapping of radiopaque wire	Withdraw the tip proximal to the new lesion

residual stenosis, and impair flow are considered severe, and should be stented promptly, especially if the vessel diameter is >2.5 mm. The important take-home message regarding precautionary measures and tactics for prompt reversal of acute closure can be found below. Securing and maintaining wire access across the occluded artery is the single most important consideration in managing acute abrupt vessel closure.[2] In the case of spiral dissection, stent the distal end to stop further propagation of the dissection and the entry site to stop the source of dissection. However, some dissections cannot be stented (2–3%) because of severe proximal tortuosity, small size of the vessel, etc. The majority of dissections not resulting in acute ischemic complications heal with time, leaving no negative impact on restenosis rate.[6]

TAKE-HOME MESSAGE

Precautionary measures and tactics for prompt reversal of acute closure:

1. Ready access to contralateral artery and vein with 5F sheaths, in case hemodynamic support is needed.
2. Prior to PCI, perform lower abdominal aortogram to identify patients who may not tolerate intra-aortic balloon pump (IABP) placement.
3. IABP may be inserted prophylactically in selected patients or on standby for immediate insertion in case of hypotension or ischemic complication.
4. Maintaining wire across lesion.
5. Prompt balloon reinflation.
6. Primary perfusion balloon should be considered early.
7. Prompt placement of stent to stop the dissection.

CAVEAT: Does the origin of the dissection make a difference in management and prognosis? During PCI, a dissection can happen locally due to excessive plaque fracture from balloon angioplasty or it is originated proximally

at the LM or RCA ostium by a guide and propagated distally
to the angioplasty site. The management of the locally dissected lesion is prompt local stenting. The management of
the ostial dissection that propagates distally is by stenting
of the ostial LM or RCA first, then the distal dissected segment. In these two situations, the wire has to be maintained
across the lesion. The third scenario happens when a
wire is manipulated to cross a stented area and in fact is
advanced outside a stent, behind its stent struts. When the
balloon is advanced behind the stent and inflated distally, a
dissection can occur and can be propagated in a retrograde
or antegrade fashion. In this situation, a new wire has to enter the true lumen in order to secure a persistent true lumen
access. In any situation, do not remove the wire across the
lesion unless there is strong evidence that it is in the false
lumen. Careful review of the angiographic film will show the
origin of the dissection (local or ostial) and whether or not
the wire is in the true lumen. Summary of these three scenarios is shown in Table 17-3.

**CAVEAT: Does the site of the dissection make a dif-
ference in management and prognosis?** During PCI,
dissection can happen anywhere. The dissections that can
propagate distally in a retrograde and antegrade fashion are
from the LM, the RCA, the LIMA and the SVG graft. When
there is dissection in these locations, hand injection of contrast in the coronary sinus will help to confirm the absence
of retrograde aortic involvement. The dissections from the
ostium can be due to angioplasty of an ostial lesion or due
to a guide tip. It can be propagated very far distally, to the
mid- or distal segment of the dissecting artery. The management includes prompt stenting at the site of origin. Then a
propagating dissection could possibly stop at a previously
stented area due to compression of the three layers of the
arterial wall by the stent. If a dissection happens in the proxi-

Table 17-3
Management of dissection according to site of origin

Site of origin	Wire	Management
Ostium	Keep in place	Stent ostium first
Local (non-ostial)	Keep in place	Stent local dissecting area
Local, in false lumen	Keep in place	• Insert second wire in true lumen • Remove first wire only after firm evidence that it is in a false lumen • Stent the narrowing area of true lumen

mal and mid-segment of the LCX that is encased inside the AV groove, the dissection may not commonly be propagated very far distally. However, because dissection is confined in a tight space (narrow corridor), so the luminal encroachment by the dissection is more severe (Figure 17-1 A–E). It is different from the LAD or RCA that lie and so dissect freely to the distal segment, without causing flow disturbances on the epicardial surface. These situations are summarized in Table 17-4.

TECHNICAL TIPS

*Stent edge dissection: If there is only minor dissection, there is no need for treatment. In the case of edge dissection following stent deployment, it is not imperative to cover all the edge dissections that are considered minor, with a residual lumen by IVUS larger than 50%, or not in a strategic location (not in the left main or at the ostium of a major branch).[7]

*Preventing dissection: In order to prevent dissection, usually the patient would have low-pressure (6–8 ATM) predilation.[8] However, in cases of lesion with unexpected heavy calcification, due to inadequate balloon predilation, some stents cannot be deployed completely. Other strategy includes minimal manipulation of interventional

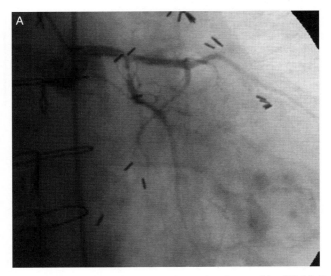

Figure 17-1: Anatomy of an LM dissection by a guide. (A) A left coronary injection showed severe in-stent restenosis of the proximal LCX and ostial lesion of the LAD. *(Continued)*

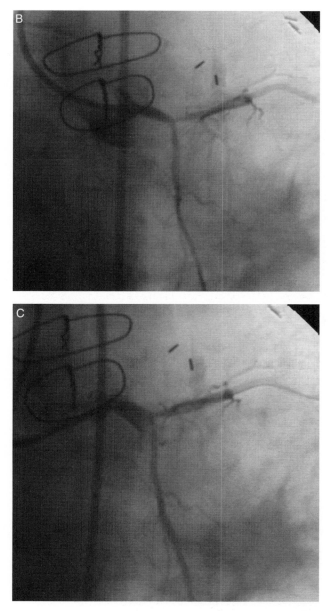

Figure 17-1: (B) After a small balloon inflation at the proximal LCX, a coronary angiogram was done to check the result. This is frame #3 of the injection. (C) At frame #5, there was a lift of the entry site at the LM, that propagated distally. *(Continued)*

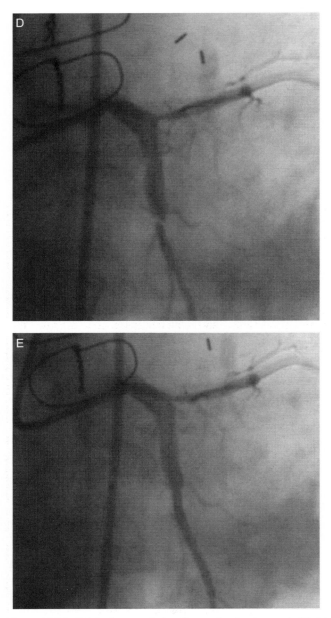

Figure 17-1: (D) At frame #7, the dissection is stopped. (E) At frame #8, the dissection is completed.

Table 17-4
Possible extent of a dissection according to site of origin

Site of origin	Extent of propagation
Ostial LAD, LCX, RCA, LIMA, SVG	Distally in an antegrade and retrograde fashion, flow possibly diminishes
LCX	Proximal and mid-segment encased in the AV groove with OM branch in horizontal position so the dissection can be stopped at the mid-segment; however, the lumen encroachment can be higher

devices prior to stent placement in order to limit the occurrence of dissection at the ostium or at the segment proximal to the lesion.[8] Then prompt stenting would prevent further propagation of dissection.

**Recrossing the dissected segment: Once the wire position is lost, try to recross the lesion with a very soft wire rather than a stiff wire. The post-angioplasty angiogram should be reviewed carefully. Look for the plane of dissection and the most likely location of entrance to the true lumen by many different orthogonal views. Then the tip of the wire is positioned at that location and manipulated to enter the true lumen. If there is a problem with recrossing the segment, or entry in the false lumen, an IVUS study should be done and the artery recrossed by a second wire parallel to the IVUS so it can be advanced under IVUS guidance. The dissection is identified as the two lumens separated by a large tissue flap. The true lumen is confirmed by the presence of contrast agent during injection while the false lumen has no flow during injection of contrast. A stent is to be deployed and seal the entry of the dissecting plane.

CAVEAT: Causes of acute occlusion after stenting: If stenting is the best strategy for prevention or treatment of occlusion, how can occlusion happen after stenting?[9] The usual causes of occlusion after balloon angioplasty and stenting were distal dissection (13%) and thrombus (13%). However, after stenting, 8% of patients had protrusion of tissue compromising the lumen and causing occlusion.

The common denominator in these occlusions was a compromised distal blood flow promoting thrombotic formation. In such cases a perfect outflow after stenting is the best way to prevent any complications.[9]

LEFT MAIN DISSECTION

Left main (LM) dissection is the forerunner to catastrophic vessel closure. It can be precipitated by manipulation of interventional hardware in the LM ostium or during intervention of the ostial lesion of the left anterior descending (LAD) artery. Sharp angulation at the LM-LAD junction appears to be a risk factor for LM dissection when the inflated balloon partially covers the LM.[10] The usual management of LM injury is coronary artery bypass surgery (CABG). However, it is necessary to keep the patient stable while waiting for emergency surgery. Unprotected LM revascularization is not a common procedure for the majority of US operators. Even so, to save the life of the patient, the acutely occluded LM has to be opened as a bailout emergency procedure, similar to pericardiocentesis in cardiac tamponade. The strategy is to open the LM even before inserting the temporary pacemaker and the intra-aortic balloon pump. The whole emergency procedure should be finished in a matter of minutes in order to reverse the process of hemodynamic collapse, shock, or impending death. Once the patient is stabilized, the decision about CABG can then be entertained (Figure 17-1).

CAVEAT: Can the LM main dissection be missed by a small guide? On many occasions, there is a clear discrepancy between the dramatic clinical presentation (severe chest pain, hypotension, ST-T change) and the paucity of the coronary artery findings. In these situations, additional orthogonal views need to be taken to confirm the noninvolvement of the coronary system or the presence of aortic dissection or LM dissection masquerading as AMI. In a report by Sakurai *et al.*, a small guide can cross the ostial lesion of the LM without causing ventricularization of pressure, so the ostial lesion or dissection of the LM is missed. In situations with strong suspicion of LM dissection by ST elevation in the anterior leads and hemodynamic collapse, repeat angiogram is to be performed with a larger guide in order to detect the ostial lesion caused by dissection.[11]

INTRAMURAL HEMATOMA

Not infrequently, after inflation of a balloon, there is fracture of the atherosclerotic plaque, including rupture of the vasa vasorum causing formation of intraplaque, periplaque, and extraluminal and intramyocardial hematoma. The compression of these hematoma on the blood flow depends on their size. The obstruction was evident, as the flow was obviously impeded although there was no sign of endoluminal dissection or thrombotic formation. Its cause is to be evidenced by IVUS. The incidence of intramural hematoma per artery was averaged at 6.7%. The entry site was identified in 86% and had the appearance of a dissection into the media, while the site of re-entry into the true lumen was identifiable only in 8%. In 60%, the angiogram had the appearance of a dissection, in 11% it appeared to be a new stenosis, and in 29% there was no abnormality detected.[12] The management is to stent the hemodynamically significant obstructed segment.

ACUTE THROMBOTIC CLOSURE

Even when the technical aspect of a PCI is almost flawless, the possibility of acute closure by uncontrolled platelet aggregation and new occlusive thrombotic formation still exists, not infrequently with superimposed vascular spasm. A thrombus is recognized as a progressively enlarging or mobile intraluminal lucency, surrounded by contrast. Its incidence is low in stable angina patients. However, in patients with acute coronary syndrome, lesions with thrombus, long and diffuse lesions, or in degenerated vein grafts, the probability of having an acute occlusion due to thrombotic formation or distal embolization is high.[13] After stenting, acute closure due to subacute thrombosis happens if there is not complete apposition of stent struts into the vessel wall and unrecognized mechanical obstruction proximal or distal to the stent.

To prevent thrombotic formation, in the case of a short procedure with minimal injury to the endothelium, prior treatment with oral antiplatelet drugs such as aspirin plus clopidogrel is effective. A maintenance dose of oral antiplatelet agents should be given for at least 48 hours or a loading dose of 300 mg of clopidogrel prior to the procedure. In the case of extensive injury to the endothelium by interventional hardware, the prospect of recurrent thrombosis could also be preempted by prior infusion of glycoprotein 2b3a inhibitors.[14] This is why minimal manipulation of the artery lumen prior to stent placement limits the depth and extent of vessel wall injury at the segment proximal to or around the lesion.[2]

BEST METHOD

Dissolution or removal of occlusive intracoronary thrombus:

During an interventional procedure, if there is mild haziness at the lesion site or at the proximal segments, this is the early sign of thrombotic formation. At that moment the main goal is to have TIMI-3 flow, because a perfect flow is the best prevention against thrombotic formation and against shear stress which activates platelet aggregation.

1. **First maneuver:** When there is new thrombus occluding the proximal or mid-segment of an artery, some operators would make forceful injection of contrast to dislodge the thrombus.
2. **Second maneuver:** Use the balloon to squeeze it, spread it to the wall.
3. **Third maneuver – rule out dissection:** Then occult dissection at the lesion site or in its proximal segment has to be ruled out. If there is mechanical obstruction that impedes the flow, stenting could secure a perfect flow and reverse the process of thrombotic formation.
4. **Fourth maneuver:** Removal of thrombus with thrombectomy devices.
5. **Fifth maneuver – treatment of underlying causes:** During PCI, any instrumentation of an arterial segment could break the integrity of the endothelial barrier and cause formation of thrombus. The appearance of thrombus is not the cause of the problem, it is the effect of any mechanical injury. So definitive treatment of thrombus needs to address these mechanical problems such as therapeutic plaque rupture, recognized or unrecognized dissection, intimal denudation due to forceful jamming of stent, distal thrombotic embolization, distal traumatic push by a tip of a wire which rolls into a ball, or intramural hemorrhage with opening into the lumen.
6. **Nitroglycerin:** Intracoronary (IC) nitroglycerin can be given to reverse any superimposed spasm that might rarely (5%) occur.

While the thrombus is being taken care of, usual emergency measures have to be taken to keep a decent blood pressure with IABP, temporary pacemaker, IV fluid, etc. ACT has to be checked to be sure it is above 200 seconds. Other exotic options are listed in Table 17-5.

Table 17-5
Other options in the treatment of newly formed intracoronary thrombus

1. Crossing the lesion with a wire and "jack-hammering" the clot
2. Aspirate the thrombus with a transport catheter
3. Aspirate the thrombus with a deeply inserted guide (as a last resort)
4. Aspirate small debris through the guide during deflation of balloon

*****Aspiration of thrombus through a guide:** Several operators describe the technique of aspirating thrombus through a guide, most often at the proximal segment of an RCA because of its large size so its thrombotic burden is larger and it is easier to deep-seat a guide. Usually, an 8F Judkins Right (JR) or a Multipurpose guide is manipulated to be engaged deeply in a favorable anatomy, or downgoing proximal segment. It is advanced over a guidewire or a balloon catheter to minimize injury to the vessel wall. This technique is not advocated as a routine procedure but as a last resort attempt to stop the acute infarction with ongoing shock in a limited number of patients. The benefits of the technique have to outweigh the risks of dissection and acute closure in the proximal segment.[15] If there is large thrombus and available equipment, removal of thrombus with mechanical atherectomy is strongly suggested.

NO-REFLOW

No-reflow is defined as stagnant contrast agent in the distal vasculature without apparent proximal obstruction. The incidence is 2% with PTCA, 7% in patients undergoing rotational atherectomy, and 12% for primary angioplasty and much higher at 42% for PCI of degenerated SVG. The cause is mainly embolization of atheromatous material (gruel) and aggravated by microembolization of platelet-rich thrombi that release vasoactive agents (e.g. serotonin), causing intense arteriolar vasospasm in the distal vasculature. The mortality of patients who developed no-reflow was 8%.[16]

TECHNICAL TIP

****Differential diagnoses of no-reflow:** The differential diagnosis of an apparent no-reflow phenomenon is dissection or acute thrombotic formation in the proximal segment, which is not well appreciated by conventional angiography. If in doubt, a transport or infusion catheter can be inserted through the wire and advanced to the distal segment of the no-flow area. Then the wire is removed. Pressure gradient is measured, and contrast injection through the end-hole will help to make the distinction between no-reflow or proximal obstructive lesions. Then injection of 3–5 cc of contrast agent with slow withdrawal of the catheter into the guide is useful to reveal any proximal disease, however hemodynamically insignificant. The results are classified into three categories and the managements are summarized in Table 17-6.[17]

Table 17-6
Differential diagnoses of no-reflow

Diagnosis	Proximal lesion	No-reflow	Distal lesion
Pressure gradient	(+)	(−)	(−)
Distal flow	Patent	No flow	Slow flow due to distal lesion

Results:

1. If there is a pressure gradient, the cause could be proximal vessel obstruction or extensive intragraft pathology. The injection of contrast in the distal vasculature will show a patent distal artery. The treatment is correction of the proximal obstructive lesion.

2. If there is no pressure gradient and no single large embolus to explain the reduction of the flow, and the contrast washout remains poor in the distal bed, then the patient has no-reflow. This diagnosis of distal microvascular spasm and obstruction is a diagnosis of exclusion.

3. If there is no gradient, however, the pullback angiography could show a distal severe lesion that was not seen by conventional antegrade angiography through the guide. The absence of the pressure gradient suggests that the disease is not flow-limiting. Correction of the lesion should resolve the no-reflow phenomenon and the symptoms of the patient.

MANAGEMENT OF NO-REFLOW

The treatment includes forceful injection of blood through the guide catheter in order to raise driving pressure across the capillary bed. Another approach is to inject small boluses of nitroglycerin (100–200 μg) (very quick try) and/or calcium channel blockers (100–200 μg of verapamil) or adenosine (12–18 μg). Verapamil is effective in 67% of cases in alleviating arteriolar spasm and restoring antegrade flow. Nitroprusside 40 μg bolus up to 100–200 μg can also be given with action to be seen in 2 minutes.[18] Epinephrine can be given especially in patients with hypotension. The dosage ranges between 50 and 200 μg and multiple doses can be given and adjusted according to the presence and severity of hypotension.[19] It is important to deliver these agents into the distal artery through a balloon catheter or drug delivery catheter. Glycoprotein 2b3a inhibitors can be given as a bolus and a maintenance dose. For patients undergoing rotational atherectomy, this problem can be prevented by having shorter runs, slower speeds, smaller initial burr size with small stepwise increases in burr size, and with infusion of nitroglycerin and calcium channel blocking agents.

**Preparation of nitroprusside: One ampule of 100 mg nitroprusside (Nipride) is diluted with 250 mL of 5%DW. With a 20 cc syringe, withdraw 1 cc of the above solution and fill it with 19 cc of 5%DW (400 μg of nitroprusside). Then give patient bolus of 3–4 cc (with 1 cc=40 μg).[18]

AIR EMBOLISM

The incidence of air embolism should be virtually none if meticulous safety measures are practiced. Once it happens, the patient will experience pain and hypotension similar to occlusion of a coronary artery in AMI. A small air embolus will be dissipated quickly.

TECHNICAL TIPS

**Management of air embolism: Strong hand injection of contrast may help to dissipate the air bubble into the distal microvasculature. Chest pain will disappear in less than 1 minute. However, if it is a large air bubble, with an over-the-wire balloon catheter ready in the guide, the operator can advance the catheter to the air bubble and aspirate the air embolus through its central lumen.[20]

**Management of massive air embolism: In a case report of Colombo *et al.*, 35 cc of air was injected into the LV during LV angiogram. The patient received CPR for 45 minutes then recovered with percutaneous cardiopulmonary support (CPS).[21] In case of air embolism in the right atrium or ventricle due to air entry during the subclavian or jugular vein cannulation, the patient should be put in the left lateral position so the air can be moved to the top of the RV or RA. A catheter then is inserted in the area and the air sucked out. In case of air embolism in the LV, then the patient should be put in the right lateral position, a pigtail catheter advanced into the LV and the air withdrawn while CPR is given.

CORONARY PERFORATION

Perforation of a coronary artery with a wire can be innocuous as long as the perforation is not inadvertently enlarged by a balloon. With new devices and attempts to cross chronic total occlusion (CTO), stiffer wires and laser wires harbor the risk that the wire will be forced through unrecognized subadventitial pathways into the true distal lumen. The subsequent dilation may then lacerate the adventitia and cause coronary perforation. In the most devastating scenario, there are actual rents or lacerations of the epicardial arteries with free communication of blood into the pericardial sac. This vessel rupture almost universally results in immediate hemodynamic collapse. Without control of bleeding and drainage of the pericardial sac, fatality may result.[22]

The incidence of perforation was only 0.4% (20% due to guidewire, 74% due to devices).[23] The manifestation of perforation was delayed (5–24 hours) in 20% of patients, as seen in PCI with cutting balloon.[24] Angiographic features associated with higher risk of perforations are listed in Table 17-7.[24]

In spite of the use of glycoprotein 2b3a inhibitors, the risk of perforation and tamponade did not increase. A classification scheme is shown in Table 17-8.[25]

The treatment includes immediate inflation of the balloon at low pressure for 10 minutes (artery/balloon ratio 0.9 to 1:1) at the site of the type III perforation. For the type II perforation, without tamponade, some operators would inflate a perfusion balloon for 10–15 minutes to seal the perforation. Because of the catastrophic effect of perforation, it is critical

---

Table 17-7
Risk factors of perforations

1. Oversizing balloon (balloon:artery ratio >1.2)
2. High-pressure balloon inflation outside the stent
3. Stenting of tapering vessel
4. Stenting of contained perforations from other devices
5. Stenting of lesions that are recrossed after severe dissection or abrupt closure
6. Stenting of total occlusion when there has been unrecognized subintimal passage of the wire
7. Stenting of small vessels (<2.6 mm)

Table 17-8
Classification of perforation

Class	Definition	Risk of tamponade
I	Extraluminal crater without contrast extravasation	8%
II	Pericardial or myocardial "blush" without contrast agent "jetting"	13%
III	Contrast agent "jetting" through a frank (>1 mm) perforation A: Directed toward the pericardium B: Directed toward the myocardium	63%

for interventional cardiologists to be experienced in the peri-cardiocentesis technique. If bleeding continues, inflate a perfusion balloon for 15–30 minutes. Prolonged balloon inflation is successful in 60–70% of perforations.[26] If sealing is not successful, start giving protamine in incremental doses of 25–50 mg over 10–30 minutes until ACT <150 seconds; this should also be done in cases of jet extravasion and cav-ity spilling, because reversal of anticoagulation could lead to acute arterial occlusion or stent thrombosis. So the risk and benefit of anticoagulant reversal should be considered care-fully. Pericardiocentesis is to be performed if there is hemody-namic compromise. A covered stent to seal the perforation, now available in the US (JoStent Graft-JoMed International, Helsingborg, Sweden), is the best treatment.[27] Once there is no further dye extravasation, the patient is admitted for obser-vation, and echocardiography should be repeated to check for further effusion. Detailed management of perforation is listed in Table 17-9.

TECHNICAL TIPS

**Preventive measures – perforation by a wire: To avoid perforation, the tip of a wire is advanced gently, without forcing against resistance. It should move freely. Once in the distal segment, avoid placing the tip in small branches, for it can be inadvertently moved forward and perforate the artery. Its position should be checked frequently.

**Preventive measures – perforation due to balloon inflation: After inflation of a balloon, keep the deflated bal-loon in place, watch the ECG to see whether it reverses to baseline and ask the patient to check the relief of chest pain

---

Table 17-9
Strategies in the management of coronary perforation: A step-by-step approach

1. First: prolonged balloon inflation at low pressure, 2–6 ATM for 10 minutes. If bleeding continues, inflate perfusion bal-loon for 20–30 minutes.
2. Pericardiocentesis with a side hole catheter inside the pericardial space if tamponade.
3. If bleeding continues: reversal of anticoagulation:
   (a) 1 mg of protamine for every 25 units of heparin given in the previous 4 hours: maximum 25–50 mg IV over 10–30 min until ACT <150 sec.
4. Covered stent for proximal or mid-segment of the perfo-rated artery.
5. Coil (material) embolization for perforation of distal end.

caused by balloon inflation. Then make a small injection to check for severe dissection and perforation. If there is good flow distally and no obvious extravasation of blood, then the balloon is removed proximal into the guide. If there is any problem, dissection or perforation, then the balloon is ready to be re-inflated. Do not remove the balloon unless everything is clear. Wait for more than two minutes before the next inflation for ischemic precondition to kick in: the patient should have less chest pain with the second and subsequent balloon inflation compared with the first one. If there is perforation, then inflate the balloon at low pressure. Once the patient is stabilized or has ischemia, then change to a perfusion balloon if there is an old one on the shelf (perfusion balloons are no longer produced because of little daily use).

**Management of perforation at the proximal and mid-segment: The treatment with prolonged balloon inflation, in some fortunate cases, may permanently cover the defect with a tissue flap and solve the problem. Reversal of anticoagulation can be done with protamine. Nevertheless, in patients with substantial tears or lacerations, a covered stent offers a viable option. Tamponade can still happen even rarely after PCI in patients with previous CABG. The reason is that there is scar formation in the pericardial area so there is more contained perforation, with intramuscular or mediastinal hemorrhage rather than frank bleeding or effusion. If there is covered stent available, a large perforation can be successfully stopped by delivering a covered stent at the perforated site. Because the PTFE covered stent is bulkier, the proximal segment should be predilated, the guide position should be optimal and extra buddy wire may be needed. The stent should not be pushed hard because it can be embolized.

**The disadvantage of perfusion balloon catheter: In case of perforation, in order to stop the extravasation, the perfusion catheter can seal the lesion and permit distal perfusion. However, the perfusion catheter has important disadvantages:

1. Since they rely on intrinsic blood pressure to maintain perfusion, they are of limited use in patients with systemic hypotension. In order to have effective perfusion through the balloon, the systemic blood pressure should be at least above 80 mmHg.
2. They have high profile so they are not easy to be advanced through tortuous or calcified segments.
3. If the balloon covers a large side branch, inflation time will be limited by ischemia.[28]

***How to make a covered stent with a venous segment:**
In case of perforation and if there is no PTFE-covered stent
available, then a segment of a vein can be harvested. A tour-
niquet should be placed around the patient's left arm, so the
vein can be seen clearly and determined for its size. Then
the left antecubital fossa is prepared and the area around
the vein infiltrated with 1% xylocaine. An incision is created
sagittally over the vein that is carefully dissected from the
surrounding tissue. Side branches are ligated with 4-0 silk
sutures. Once a sufficient segment of the vein is isolated,
it is ligated proximally, then distally, and divided. The harvested vein is then placed over a stent so that the endothelium faces toward the stent. The distal struts of the stent are
gently released from the balloon as the tip of the balloon is
reflected downward. This allows the distal edge of the vein
to be secured using two interrupted 7-0 Prolene sutures
(Ethicon, Somerville, NJ) while avoiding damage to the
underlying balloon. The proximal edge is secured in similar
fashion. The time taken to harvest the vein and to secure it
on the stent is approximately 20 minutes. After that, the vein-
covered stent is delivered to the site and deployed.[29]

***How to make a covered stent with balloon material:**
In case of perforation and if there is no PTFE-covered stent,
then Pienvichit *et al.* suggested cutting both ends of a lightly
inflated balloon in order to have a cylinder of balloon material. Then crimp a stent over another premounted stent with
the balloon cylinder in between. This results in a makeshift
covered stent.[30]

**Reversal of glycoprotein 2b3a inhibition: The degree of platelet inhibition by the small molecule inhibitors
(Eptifibatide, tirofiban) is maintained through high plasma
concentration which is proportional to platelet inhibition.
So its effect disappears with discontinuation of the drug.
In contrast, abciximab is mostly platelet-bound with low
plasma level. In order to reverse the effect of abciximab,
platelet infusion is needed.

BEST METHOD

**Management of perforation at the distal end of an ar-
tery:** If the perforation is at the distal end of a large vessel or
a branch, the treatment is by reversing the anticoagulation
state, balloon tamponade of the more proximal segment
if the patient can tolerate the ischemic injury, injection of
thrombin to the distal branch, and closure of the perforated
branch with embolized material (including platelet infusate,
clotted blood, or coil material).

1. **First maneuver – balloon tamponade:** Prolonged balloon tamponade at proximal segment, if tolerated, then perfusion balloon tamponade if needed.
2. **Second maneuver:** If sealing is unsuccessful, then reverse anticoagulation with protamine.
3. **Add new drug: platelet product:** If the distal end needs to be sealed off, then injection of 3–4 cc of platelet infusate at the distal perforated end through the transfer catheter or through the lumen of an over-the-wire balloon. Do not inject platelet infusate at the ostium of the main artery. The whole artery can clot. There is risk of delayed bleeding (investigational).
4. **Add new device:** Covered stent can be used to block the opening of the side branch with perforation at its distal end.
5. **Add new drugs:** Injection of thrombin, gelatin sponge (Gelfoam) or polyvinyl alcohol form (PVA) to distal segment to thrombose the distal vessel (investigational).
6. **Add new device:** Closure of the distal branch with coil material.

**In case of perforation, which one is better: covered stent or prolonged balloon inflation? After perforation, there are choices either to inflate a regular balloon with reversal of anticoagulation by heparin or to deploy a PTFE-covered stent. If the patient still needs anticoagulation to keep the just dilated or stented lesion open, then covered stent is best. If anticoagulation may not be needed after PCI, then reversal of heparin and prolonged inflation of a balloon to seal off the perforation is an acceptable choice. In a case report by Colombo *et al.*,[31] full reversal of heparin and prolonged ischemia due to continuous balloon inflation caused slow flow in the distal bed. Later they contributed to the early thrombosis of the covered stent. So it is better to deploy a covered stent without full reversal of heparin and glycoprotein 2b3a inhibition. However, the covered stent is of higher profile, bulkier, and so cannot be always advanced in distal or through tortuous segment.

CAVEAT: The decision whether to send the patient for CABG after perforation: After perforation, if there is no covered stent and no embolizer, and if the bleeding does not stop after long local tamponade, the patient may need surgery. However, it is not an easy and simple procedure. Many times, the area around the perforation has intramural hematoma so the whole myocardial area is edematous and swollen. In that situation, it is almost impossible to locate the perforated branch, so the surgeon just ligates the more proximal segment and bypasses any other diseased arteries. Surgery does not reperfuse the perforated branch we try to save. Surgery may not be needed if the patient can

Table 17-10
Important procedural considerations for prevention of perforation

1. Constantly monitor distal wire.
2. Treat suspected perforation seriously, especially in patients on glycoprotein 2b3a inhibitors.
3. Perform pericardiocentesis in the cardiac catheterization laboratory. Insert a 6F pigtail catheter for drainage.
4. Local measures to seal perforation before leaving the cardiac interventional laboratories.
5. Admit to ICU, frequent echocardiography follow-up.

tolerate clinically the closure of a small branch or the distal end of a large vessel (Table 17-10).

RETROGRADE AORTIC DISSECTION

Retrograde aortic dissection secondary to coronary dissection is a nightmare for the interventionalist. Usually it happens after inflation of the proximal RCA (more common) or the LAD (Figure 17-2). Even though it is rare, it must be positively ruled out when there is unexplained chest pain or hypotension after angioplasty or stenting of any ostial or proximal lesion. If it is detected early, prompt corrective measures including prompt stenting of the ostial lesion which is the entry site to seal off the dissection. Surgical consultation is needed, when there is significant aortic regurgitation, involvement of the supra-aortic vessels, and progression of the index dissection. If none of these problems is present, a watchful waiting is the best attitude.[32] Follow-up CT scan of the chest may identify the medically stabilized patient who needs no further treatment or the complicated patient who may need surgery.[33]

CEREBROVASCULAR ACCIDENT

During the interventional procedure, embolized material to the central nervous system can cause transient ischemic attack (TIA) or disabling stroke. The less-known problems are transient or permanent blindness or seizure.

Embolic stroke: The incidence of embolic stroke secondary to coronary interventions is 0.38%.[34] This low frequency is due to meticulous adherence to safety measures and appropriate anticoagulation. The patients with stroke were older (72 versus 64 years of age, P<0.001), had lower ejection fraction, diabetes, and experienced a higher rate of intraprocedural complications necessitating emergency use of intra-aortic balloon pump (23% versus 3%, P<0.001). The

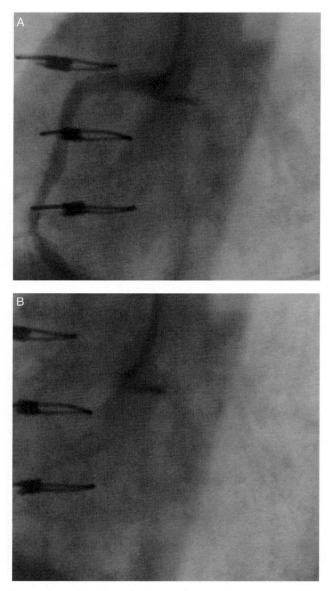

Figure 17-2: (A) After a balloon inflation of the proximal RCA, an angiogram showed dissection of the proximal segment at the first curve and persistent contrast staining at the ostium on the aortic wall area. (B) Persistent staining at the base of the ostium.

in-hospital and 1-year mortality was dramatically high (26 versus 1.5% and 56 versus 6.5%, P<0.001, respectively).[38] Compared with hemorrhagic stroke, ischemic stroke patients had higher rate of in-hospital MACE (57% versus 25%, P<0.03).[34] The strongest independent predictors were use of thrombolytic prior to PCI, heparin before and after PCI, low creatinine clearance, past history of CVA, and diabetes.[35]

With the advent of intravenous thrombolytic therapy, direct injection of a fibrinolytic agent (investigational), or intracranial vessel angioplasty (investigational), the management of embolic stroke is changing drastically. Once embolic stroke is confirmed, fibrinolytic drugs can be given intravenously: tPA 0.9 mg/kg for a maximum of 90 mg, 10% as a bolus and the rest to be infused in one hour.[36]

Transient and permanent blindness: Occipital blindness occurs rarely and usually disappears within a few hours. However, with emboli, the patient can develop permanent blindness. The MRI findings show contrast agent extravasation, without cerebral ischemia or hemorrhage. These findings are also seen in posterior leukoencephalopathy syndrome. The mechanism is a transient vasculopathy with disruption of blood-brain barrier as a cause of transient cortical blindness after contrast angiography. The main treatment is aggressive hypertension control and symptomatic treatment of headache.[37]

VENTRICULAR TACHYCARDIA OR FIBRILLATION

Cardiac arrest can be caused by VT, VF, or asystole. While the patient is being resuscitated with intubation, external cardiac massage, or IABP, pacemaker being inserted, usually the blood pressure is sustained at an unacceptable level of 50–60 mmHg.

BEST METHOD

The one and only maneuver: Coronary perfusion during CPR. During CPR, the blood pressure is low, as evidenced by aortic pressure. If there is good LV function prior to cardiac arrest the chance for good recovery is high. A coronary angiogram during CPR in a patient with asystole shows almost no flow to the coronary system. The interventional cardiologist can help coronary perfusion by keeping the guide inside the LM, gently pull it out, withdraw oxygenated blood to a large syringe connected to the guide and inject this blood into the coronary system. Mix this blood with some contrast and inject to check the flow to the distal coronary vasculature and feeble movement of the LV. With good oxygenation from the ventilator (the patient is intubated), correction of electrolyte, acid-base imbalance, and opening of the acute occluded artery (which causes the cardiac arrest), coupled with forced coronary perfusion by injection of oxygenated blood, the chance for the patient to recover is higher. Try not to cause dissection of the LM with movement of the guide.

***How to differentiate between ventricular tachycardia and supraventricular tachycardia by intracardiac electrocardiogram (ECG):

To record an intracardiac ECG, a 0.014" Choice Floppy angioplasty wire (Boston Scientific/Scimed Maple Grove, MN), is placed in the lumen of a 6F Multipurpose catheter with the wire tip minimally protruding. The proximal end of the wire is attached to a surface V1 ECG lead with a sterile alligator clamp. During continuous ECG and pressure monitoring, the catheter is manually withdrawn from the right ventricle and right atrium.[38] The RV ECG complex is wider and the RA ECG complex is smaller. VT is seen as RV wide complex with AV dissociation. RA ECG complex is seen in accordance with RV complex in SVT.

REFERENCES

1. Ellis S. Elective coronary angioplasty: Techniques and complications. In: Topol EJ, ed. *Textbook of Interventional Cardiology*, 3rd edn. Lippincott-Raven Publishers, 1998: 147–62.
2. Raizner A, Kaluza G. Acute closure. In: Nissen S. *et al. Cardiac Catheterization and Interventional Cardiology Self-Assessment Program*. The American College of Cardiology, 2001: 147–9.
3. Meier B. Balloon angioplasty. In: Topol EJ, ed. *Textbook of Cardiovascular Medicine*. Lippincott-Raven Publishers, 1998: 1977–2010.
4. Huber MS, Mooney JF, Madison J *et al*. Use of a morphologic classification to predict clinical outcome after dissection from coronary angioplasty. *Am J Cardiol* 1991; **68**: 467–71.
5. Ziada KM, Tuzeu M, Nissen SE. The role of intravascular ultrasound imaging in contemporary stenting. *Intravascular Imaging* 1997; **1**: 73–9.
6. Savage M, Dischman D, Bailey S *et al*. Vascular remodeling of balloon-induced dissection: Long-term angiographic assessment. *J Am Coll Cardiol* 1995; **25**: 135A.
7. Reimers B, Spedicato L, Sacca S *et al*. Residual dissection after coronary stent implantation not covered by additional stent. *J Am Coll Cardiol* 1999; **33** (Suppl 2): 12A.
8. Briguori C, Sheiban I, De Gregorio J *et al*. Direct coronary stenting without predilation. *J Am Coll Cardiol* 1999; **34**: 1910–15.

9. Cheneau E, Mintz G, Leborgne L *et al*. Mechanism of abrupt vessel closure after coronary angioplasty: Results of a systematic IVUS study. *J Am Coll Cardiol* 2003; **41**: 6–8A.

10. Sathe S, Sebastian M, Vohra J *et al*. Bailout stenting for LM occlusion following diagnostic coronary angiography. *Cathet Cardiovasc Diagn* 1994; **31**: 70–2.

11. Sakurai H, Saburi Y, Matsubara K *et al*. A pitfall in the diagnosis of left main coronary obstruction due to aortic dissection. *J Invasive Cardiol* 1998; **10**: 545–6.

12. Akiko M, Mintz G, Bui A *et al*. Incidence, morphology, angiographic findings and outcomes of intramural hematomas after PCI. *Circulation* 2002; **105**: 2073–42.

13. Bergelson BA, Fishman RF, Tommaso CL. Abrupt vessel closure: Changing importance, management, and consequence. *Am Heart J* 1997; **134**: 362–81.

14. Haase KK, Mahrholdt H, Schroder S *et al*. Frequency and efficacy of glycoprotein 2b3a therapy for treatment of threatened or acute vessel closure in 1332 patients undergoing PTCA. *Am Heart J* 1999; **137**: 234–40.

15. Lablanche JM, Fourrier JL, Gommeaux A *et al*. Percutaneous aspiration of a thrombus. *Cathet Cardiovasc Diagn* 1989; **17**: 97–8.

16. Kaplan BM, Benzuly KH, Kinn JW *et al*. Treatment of no-reflow in degenerated SVG interventions: Comparison of intracoronary verapamil and nitroglycerin. *Cathet Cardiovasc Diagn* 1996; **39**: 113–18.

17. Sherman JR, Anwar A, Bret JR *et al*. Distal vessel pull-back angiography and pressure gradient measurement: An innovative diagnostic approach to evaluate the no-reflow phenomenon. *Cathet Cardiovasc Diagn* 1996; **39**: 1–6.

18. Hillegass W, Dean N, Laio L *et al*. Treatment of no-reflow and impaired flow with the nitric oxide donor nitroprusside following PCI: Initial human clinical experience. *J Am Coll Cardiol* 2001; **37**: 1335–43.

19. Skelding K, Goldstein J, Mehta L *et al*. Resolution of refractory no-reflow with intracoronary epinephrine. *Cathet Cardiovasc Interv* 2002; **57**: 305–9.

20. Haraphongse M, Rossall RE. Large air embolus complicating angioplasty. *Cathet Cardiovasc Diagn* 1989; **17**: 244–8.

21. Colombo A, Stankovic G. Massive air embolism. In: Colombo A, Stankovic G, eds. *Colombo's Tips and Tricks in Interventional Cardiology*. Martin Dunitz, 2002: 15.

22. George B. Coronary artery rupture: An interventional complication on the rise. *Cathet Cardiovasc Diagn* 1995; **36**: 155.

23. Ellis S, Ajluni S, Arnold AZ *et al*. Increased coronary perforation in the new device era: Incidence, classification, management and outcome. *Circulation* 1994; **90**: 2725–30.

24. Maruo T, Yasuda S, Miyazaki S. Delayed appearance of coronary artery perforation following cutting balloon angioplasty. *Cathet Cardiovasc Interv* 2002; **57**: 529–31.

25. Liu F, Erbel R, Haude M *et al*. Coronary arterial perforation: Prediction, diagnosis, management and prevention. In: Ellis S, Holmes Jr D, eds. *Strategic Approaches in Coronary Interventions*, 2nd edn. Lippincott Williams Wilkins, 2000: 500–14.

26. Grines C, Savu M, Tejada LA. Appendix 1. In: *Interventional Cardiology: The Essentials for the Boards*. Futura Publishing Co., 1999: 283.

27. Wedge D, Hauge M, von Birgelen C. *et al*. Treatment of coronary artery perforation with a new membrane covered stent. *Z Kardiol* 1998; **87**: 948–53.

28. van der Linden LP, Bakx ALM, Sedney MI *et al*. Prolonged dilation with an autoperfusion balloon catheter for refractory acute occlusion related to PTCA. *J Am Coll Cardiol* 1993; **22**: 1016–23.

29. Bates M, Shamsham F, Faulknier B *et al*. Successful treatment of iatrogenic renal artery perforation with an autologous vein-covered stent. *Cathet Cardiovasc Interv* 2002; **57**: 39–43.

30. Pienvichit P, Waters J. Successful closure of a coronary artery perforation using makeshift stent sandwich. *Cathet Cardiovasc Interv* 2001; **54**: 209–13.

31. Colombo A, Stankovic G. Coronary rupture. In: Colombo A, Stankovic G, eds. *Colombo's Tips and Tricks in Interventional Cardiology*. Martin Dunitz, 2002: 13–27.

32. Colombo A, Stankovic G. In: Colombo A, Stankovic G, eds. *Colombo's Tips and Tricks in Interventional Cardiology*. Martin Dunitz, 2002: 13.

33. Jessurun GA, Van Boven AJ, Brouwer RM *et al*. Unexpected progressive opacification of the ascending aorta during coronary angioplasty: Diagnostic and therapeutic sequelae. *J Invasive Cardiol* 1997; **9**: 540–3.

34. Fuchs S, Stabile E, Kinnaird T *et al*. Stroke complicating PCI: Incidence, predictors and prognostic implications. *Circulation* 2002; **106**: 86–9.

35. Dukkipati S, Deo D, Sadeghi M *et al*. CVA after PCI: Incidence, predictors, outcomes. *J Am Coll Cardiol* 2003; **41**: 6–2A.

36. The National Institute of Neurological Disorders and Stroke rt-PA Stroke Study Group. Tissue Plasminogen Activator for acute ischemic stroke. *N Engl J Med* 1995; **333**: 1581–7.

37. Zwicker JC, Sila C. MRI findings of a case of transient cortical blindness after cardiac catheterization. *Cathet Cardiovasc Interv* 2002; **57**: 47–9.

38. Holmes D, Kern M. Simplified intracardiac electrocardiography for Ebstein's anomaly. *Cathet Cardiovasc Interv* 2002; **57**: 367–8.

Chapter 18

Vascular Brachytherapy

Moo-Huyn Kim,
Phong Nguyen-Ho,
Thach Nguyen, Greg L Kaluza

GENERAL OVERVIEW

Restenosis after balloon angioplasty (POBA) is mainly due to late constriction of the arterial wall (negative remodeling) while restenosis after stenting (ISR) is due to intimal hyperplasia (IH).[1] The rate of ISR averaged 20% for focal lesion and up to 50% in patients with diabetes and/or complex lesions.[2] There were many interventional modalities and more than 20 drugs tested to treat restenosis and ISR. Although they were promising *in vitro* and in animal studies, almost all were failures or of too little efficacy when tried in humans.[3] At this present time, the preventive strategy for restenosis after percutaneous coronary interventions (PCI) is by drug-eluting stent (DES), while the main treatment for ISR is brachytherapy (VBT).

---

*Basic; **Advanced; ***Rare, exotic, or investigational.

From: Nguyen T, Hu D, Saito S, Grines C, Palacios I (eds), *Practical Handbook of Advanced Interventional Cardiology*, 2nd edn. © 2003 Futura, an imprint of Blackwell Publishing.

BASIC RADIATION PHYSICS

Radioactivity is the spontaneous process in which an unstable nucleus, with either too many or too few neutrons, turns to a stable state (ground state) whereby superfluous energy is released. The release of energy is called radiation, in which β particles are lightweight high-energy electrons, while gamma rays are protons originating from the center of the nucleus.[4] This process is often called the disintegration of an atom.[4] The amount of energy absorbed by tissue is the radiation dose and expressed in Gray (Gy). For therapeutic purposes, the radiation (prescription) dose is calculated according to the activity of the radiation source, the exposure (dwell) time, the type of radiation, and inversely to the distance from the source.

Mechanism of action: Radiation kills cells directly through ionizing deoxyribonucleic acid (DNA) and causing double-stranded breaks, or indirectly through ionizing water and generating injurious free radicals.[5] If repair mechanisms do not correct the chromosomal mutations, the cell cannot function normally or undergo reproduction. In general, the mitosis or M phase of the cell cycle is the most radiosensitive when the radiation dose necessary to prevent cell division is lower than that required to destroy a differentiated cell.

During VBT, β-emitting isotopes produce much less energy per nuclear disintegration, so they penetrate only the tissue closest to them, within a radius of less than 1 centimeter. γ-photons penetrate several meters farther with high and homogenous level of energy. Therefore, β-radiation can be blocked by a few millimeters of plastic while γ-radiation requires several centimeters of lead shielding. In order to produce enough β-energy to achieve adequate tissue penetration, very high-activity beta sources are required; on the other hand, only low-activity gamma sources are needed.[4] The advantages of β VBT are shorter dwell time (2–4 minutes) because of high activity, and less shielding, less adjacent tissue radiation because of low energy; laboratory staff can remain in the vicinity of the patient. However, with a rapid dose fall-off within millimeters from the source with β-radiation, positioning the source in the middle of the vessel lumen (centering) is important in reducing dose heterogeneity. Also, radiation of large diameter (>4 mm) vessels might be inadequate.[6,7] In contrast, γ VBT requires longer dwell times (15–20 minutes) because of low activity and more shielding because of high energy; furthermore, adjacent tissues receive significant radiation and laboratory staff must leave the room during treatment. Large vessel diameter and centering of the source are less important issues with γ VBT.

Delivery: Several types of devices have been developed for VBT, of which the FDA-approved ones are the removable, catheter-based linear sources. Radioactive isotopes are manufactured into small metallic canisters, or seeds, and incorporated into the distal end of a 0.014–0.040" wire. Radio-opaque markers at both ends of the radioactive segment facilitate positioning of the source. The distal end of the catheter lumen is closed (blind) to maintain isolation of the radioactive source from the bloodstream. After a PCI procedure, the delivery catheter is positioned across the target lesion; the source-wire is then introduced, or afterloaded, from the proximal end of the catheter and advanced distally until the radioactive source spans the injured segment totally. The afterloading process can be manual (performed by the physician) or automated (performed by a motorized unit), depending on the commercial system. Besides the catheter-based linear sources, other methods of delivery include the liquid isotope-filled balloon, the gas-filled balloon system (^{133}Xe), the radioactive coil (^{186}Re), the ^{32}P-coated balloon, and the ^{32}P-radioactive stents.[8,9]

Clinical trials: Because of its complexity and safety concerns, VBT has been subjected to a scrutiny that has by far exceeded those required for earlier interventional device-based therapies. Three major US-based randomized clinical trials provided the safety and efficacy data for the FDA approval of the three current clinically available VBT systems.

- **The GAMMA-1 trial:** This trial for in-stent restenosis included 252 patients and has been the largest randomized study with gamma radiation so far. Patients were assigned to receive VBT from a ribbon containing a sealed source of ^{192}Ir or a placebo non-radioactive ribbon. As in the SCRIPPS trial, radiation dose was prescribed with IVUS guidance to deliver a dose between 8 and 30 Gy to the adventitia. At six-month follow-up, the restenosis rate was significantly lower after VBT compared to the placebo (32.4% vs 55.3% respectively, P=0.01). After nine months, the composite primary end-point (death, myocardial infarction, TLR) was significantly lower in the ^{192}Ir group (28.2% vs 43.8% in the placebo group, P=0.02). The rate of TLR was significantly lower in the ^{192}Ir group (24.4% vs 42.1% in the placebo, P<0.01), as was the rate of TVR (31.3% vs 46.3 % in the placebo, P=0.01).[10]
- **The Stent And Restenosis Trial (START) trial:** This trial examined the effectiveness of the Novoste BetaCath system (^{90}Sr/Y) in 476 patients (50 sites) with ISR and lesion length <20 mm. As such, it is the largest intracoronary radiation trial completed to date. It has confirmed the usefulness of beta radiation in stented vessels, yielding a 42% reduction in target lesion revascularization (TLR) and 34% reduction in target vessel revascularization (TVR). Restenosis in the entire analysis segment including edges was reduced by 36%. Most importantly, due to a relatively low amount of newly placed stents (22%) and more prolonged use of the antiplatelet treatment during the course of the

trial, no late thrombosis was observed. However, a relatively high incidence of edge stenosis was still noted, due to
the frequent occurrence of "geographic miss" (34%).[11]

- **The INHIBIT trial:** The Intimal Hyperplasia Inhibition with
Beta In-stent Trial (INHIBIT) enrolled 332 patients with ISR
randomized to receiving 0 (control) or 20 Gy of radiation
with the Guidant system of a centered ^{32}P source. The restenosis rate was reduced from 52% in the placebo group to
26% in the radiation group, a 50% reduction. Overall MAC-
Es including TVR were reduced by 36%. Late thrombosis in
patients subjected to VBT was low at 1.8% and similar to the
control group (0.6%, P=NS).[12]

- **The Beta-Cath Trial:** In contrast to the positive experience of VBT in ISR, results in de novo lesions have been
somewhat discouraging. The Beta-Cath trial, with 1455 patients, was the largest, multicenter study of brachytherapy
in de novo lesions and assessed the safety and efficacy
of ^{90}Sr/^{90}Y in conjunction with angioplasty or provisional
stenting. Initially, this trial had a high rate of stent thrombosis in patients receiving 30 days of antiplatelet therapy;
subsequently, prolongation of antiplatelet therapy for >60
days corrected this problem. However, no significant differences in MACE defined as death, MI, and TVR were found
between the VBT and control groups, mainly due to a significant incidence of new stenoses at the edges of radiation
zones, suggesting that brachytherapy for de novo lesions
may not be as successful as it is in ISR.[13]

COMPLICATIONS

Late thrombosis: Early clinical trials of VBT suffered
unexpectedly high rates of late thrombotic occlusion, particularly when a new stent was placed in conjunction with
VBT[14,15] or when the patient had discontinued thienopyridine
therapy.[10,16] Thus, to prevent late thrombosis, the implantation
of new stents is discouraged, and patients need to take aspirin
and clopidogrel for an extended period of 12 months.[17,18] As
many as 20% of INHIBIT trial patients received a new stent
and the late thrombosis was nevertheless minimal.[12]

Edge restenosis: Successful inhibition of neointima in
the center of the radiation treatment zone is frequently offset
by new stenoses at the proximal or distal edges. The angiographic appearance of this paradoxical narrowing is called the
edge effect, or "candy wrapper". This observation was a major
shortcoming of radioactive stents and is also seen in catheter-
based VBT.[8] The reason is that the vessel segment dilated
by the balloon is longer than the segment subjected to VBT.
Failure of the radioactive source to encompass this segment
is termed "geographic miss" and results in inadequate or ab-

sent delivery of the prescribed radiation to the distal ends of the injured zone.[19,20]

TECHNICAL TIPS

Baseline angiography: Baseline angiography is to identify the lesion, the target segment, and different strategies for PCI and VBT. The segment for VBT should be filmed without being foreshortened and side-branch overlapping. Then a few best views are selected and the whole PCI procedure should be filmed in these identical projections, with an optimal position of the image intensifier between the lead shields. The baseline angiogram will help to determine the level of radiation energy needed (dose prescription) according to the length and the size of the vessel. The angiograms with the PCI devices and the radiation source in place are performed with contrast agent, to document the exact location of the injured segments.[4]

PCI strategies: As in any PCI, the baseline angiogram determines the complexity of the PCI and the anticipated movement of the radiation source. Then PCI has to be performed with satisfactory results: minimal residual stenosis and optimal distal flow. After that, VBT can be started, because instrumentation after VBT inevitably carries the risk of geographic miss.[4] The guide should have a stable position, so that the radiation source does not move after being positioned. If it is too deeply engaged, it can obstruct the flow and cause ischemia. It can advance further when the source is withdrawn during positioning and repositioning. If it is too far outside the ostium, it may slip during the procedure and move the source ribbon.[4] Then the radiation delivery catheter should be advanced gently, because it is very fragile without the inserted ribbon, so it may be kinked during transit or caught by a stent strut. After VBT, the source is removed. Blood should then be withdrawn back into the injection syringe, and the guide flushed prior to contrast injection for an angiogram because of possible thrombus formation during a long dwell time (15–20 minutes).[4] A final angiogram should confirm the persistent patency of the instrumented segment, without dissection or thrombus.

Procedural complications: The most common peri-procedural complications are myocardial ischemia due to high profile of the device and dissection or inability to advance the delivery catheter due to its stiffness. Furthermore, radiation increases local thrombogenicity, so heparin is given according to standard protocol and glycoprotein 2b3a inhibitor should be given more liberally. If because of angina refractory to usual treatment, the entire catheter should be withdrawn and placed in a bail-out box. If that is not successful, then move the source to a larger diameter artery while arranging for further PCI or bypass surgery. In any case, the source is removed and placed in the bail-out box prior to further manipulation of the index vessel. VBT can be resumed later when the clinical condition allows.[4]

TAKE-HOME MESSAGE

How to avoid geographic miss:[4]

1. Geographic miss is associated with the device injury prior to VBT, not with the original lesion length. Therefore always select a source length that is 10 mm beyond the ends of the *injured* area (*not* original lesion length) or one to two times the length of the lesion. Avoid instrumentation (e.g. additional stents) after VBT (Figure 18-1).
2. To get an accurate estimate of the injured segment, film the position of all devices (balloon, stent, atherectomy, etc.) with contrast in the same projection and respiratory position, without foreshortened projection or overlapping side branches. Use a proximal or distal branch as an index anatomical landmark to assess the distance from it to the markers on the angioplasty balloon or on the source.
3. Film the dummy and active source in the same projection and respiratory position.
4. Do not perform VBT before a satisfactory PCI result. Check the proximal segment of the lesion. Be sure the radiation source can be advanced to the intended area. Avoid post-VBT endovascular manipulation and instrumentation.
5. "Watermelon seed" effect, i.e. slippage of the angioplasty balloon, may add to the injury length and should be taken into account when positioning the source. Cutting balloon angioplasty may help to avoid slipping and limit the injury length.

DELIVERY SYSTEMS

The Food and Drug Administration (FDA) has approved three catheter-based intracoronary brachytherapy systems that differ in type of isotopes, delivery catheters, and methods and are not interchangeable.

The CheckMate™ system: The CheckMate™ system (Cordis, Miami Lakes, FL) uses a γ-radiation source. The source-wire is a nylon ribbon containing variable numbers (6, 10 or 14 corresponding to 23 mm, 39 mm and 55 mm total source length) of ^{192}Ir seeds. The system label allows treating vessels of 2.7 to 4.0 mm in diameter and a length up to 45 mm. When placed across the treatment zone, the source-delivery

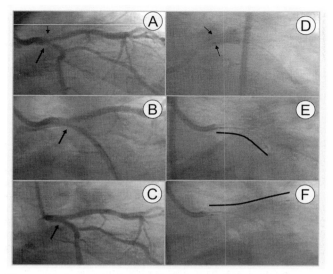

Figure 18-1: Brachytherapy for left main bifurcation in-stent restenosis. A 58-year-old male patient, who had a stent deployed in the ostial LAD (S670 3.0 × 12 mm) in August 2001. Six months later, in April 2002, main bifurcation restenosis remained, so two stents were deployed in the ostia of the LAD (S670 3.5 × 15 mm) and LCX (Bx velocity 3.0 × 8 mm). (A) Three month later, in July 2002, there was again ISR of the LM bifurcation and the ostia of the LAD and LCX. (B) The patient underwent cutting balloon angioplasty in both ostial sides of LAD and LCX. (D) This was followed by kissing balloon technique. (E,F) The patient underwent VBT with holmium-DTPA liquid balloon at the target dose of 18 Gy at 1 cm from the intima (3.0 × 30 mm balloon, solid line) for 220 seconds with 4 fractionations each. (C) April 2003: Nine-month follow-up angiogram showed both arteries patent with no evidence of intimal hyperplasia by IVUS.

catheter is not centered in the vessel lumen but conforms to the curvature of the vessel. The source-wire is afterloaded manually using a hand-cranked device. Dosimetry can be either fixed (14 Gy to 2 mm from the source center) or guided by IVUS, and the dwell time is generally 15–25 minutes.

TECHNICAL TIPS

1. The gamma-VBT with ^{192}Ir is the only one with a documented effect on saphenous vein grafts.
2. The fixed dose prescription makes the oncologist's work easier.

3. The simplicity of the Cordis system makes it safe and reliable. Of 12 system failures reported to the Nuclear Regulatory Commission since market approval through December 2002, the majority were human errors (e.g. wrong dose calculations, source mishandling) and not technical failure.
4. The source is exchanged once a month.
5. Treatment can be interrupted in an event of ischemia resulting from a catheter occluding the vessel. It should be resumed in order to deliver the prescribed dose (underdosing may exacerbate restenosis).

The BetaCath system: The BetaCath system (Novoste, Norcross, GA) uses a β-emitting radioisotope, $^{90}Sr/^{90}Y$. The 5F delivery catheter contains 3 lumens: one to accommodate the guidewire, one for the radioactive source-wire and one to provide a means of hydraulic fluid return. The catheter is not centered in the coronary lumen but its relatively large shaft size (1.67 mm) affords some degree of passive centering. With this hand-held system, the physician hydraulically propels the radioactive beads down the delivery catheter using a fluid-filled syringe. Three $^{90}Sr/^{90}Y$ seed train lengths, 30 (12 seeds), 40 (16 seeds) and 60 (24 seeds) mm, are available to treat lesion lengths up to 40 mm in vessels 2.75–4.0 mm in diameter. A 3.5F catheter is available in 30-mm length to treat discrete lesions (treatable with 20-mm balloon). The dose prescription is fixed at 18.4 or 23 Gy (below or above 3.25 mm vessel diameter, depending on the vessel caliber) at radial distance of 2 mm from the source with dwell time of 3–4 minutes.

TECHNICAL TIPS

1. The fixed dose prescription makes the oncologist's work easier.
2. There are three technical details to observe to ensure the smooth movement of the delivery catheter:
   a. Avoid overtightening of the hemostatic valve (Touhy-Borst valve) as it compromises source movement, particularly source return.
   b. Saline must not be used as a hydraulic fluid because it causes corrosion.
   c. Use of the internal mammary artery (IMA) guide is discouraged with the 3.5 F system as it may impede source's movement.
3. The 5 F system is available in extended length (267 vs 155 cm) which allows the radiation personnel to work outside the sterile field and obviates the need to bag the device in a sterile fashion.
4. Manual tandem positioning of the source is off-label but has been performed successfully to treat extremely long lesions.

5. Treatment can be interrupted in the event of ischemia resulting from catheter occluding the vessel. It should be resumed in order to deliver the prescribed dose (under-dosing may exacerbate restenosis).

The Galileo III™ system: The Galileo III™ system (Guidant, St Paul, MN) is characterized by solid ^{32}P imbedded into the distal 20 mm of the source-wire delivered through a centering balloon catheter. The wire is automatically stepped within the centering balloon to provide 40 (2 steps) or 60 (3 steps) mm of total source length. The centering balloon is available in two lengths (32 and 53 mm between markers) to accommodate the stepping source. When inflated, the balloon centers the catheter in the vessel lumen, and its specially designed shape (three longitudinal chambers separated by three parallel channels for blood flow) allows blood to perfuse the distal vessel and side branches, thereby minimizing ischemia. The source-wire is advanced and withdrawn by a fully automated, remote afterloading system, without the need for physician handling of the isotope. A touch-screen technology guides the operator through the whole procedure. A dose of 20 Gy is prescribed to a depth of 1 mm beyond the lumen surface (requiring the vessel diameter estimation) and applied for 2–4 minutes. Lesions up to 47 mm in length and vessels 2.4–3.7 mm in diameter can be treated. Because ^{32}P has a half-life of 14 days, the source needs to be exchanged every month.

TECHNICAL TIPS

1. The system is fully automated and as such is potentially ideal for a cardiologist operator to use alone, should the presence of an oncologist be no longer mandated.
2. In contrast to the other two systems described above, the dose is tailored to the vessel diameter (20 Gy to 1 mm beyond lumen surface, NOT from the source center). Yet the only parameter that needs to be keyed in is the vessel diameter – the unit calculates the dwell time based on a given day's source activity and the index vessel diameter.
3. Although not officially recommended, it is prudent to select the centering balloon diameter smaller than the vessel caliber in the distal portion of the vessel segment planned for treatment. The centering may be less ideal, but undesired over-dilatation of the vessel with the centering balloon can be prevented and, consequently, unnecessary injury at the (distal) end of the radiation zone, minimizing the potential for an "edge effect".
4. The ideal tool to determine vessel size for the centering catheter selection and for dose prescription is IVUS. However, online QCA or visual estimate is also acceptable.

5. Treatment can be interrupted in the event of ischemia resulting from the centering catheter obstructing the blood flow. It should be attempted to resume in order to deliver the prescribed dose (underdosing may exacerbate restenosis).

The Liquid Balloon System: With the success of the catheter-based VBT mentioned above, there are efforts to improve, simplify the delivery system and make it more affordable. One of the promising devices in its phase 2 trial is the radioactive liquid balloon system.[21]

CLINICAL TRIAL

The Brite II Trial: A multicenter randomized study of a novel ^{32}P deployable balloon system for the treatment of in-stent restenosis. The Brite II trial looked at brachytherapy for instent restenosis with either ^{32}P balloon-based radiation or PTCA. The new balloon is called RDX (produced by Radiance Medical Systems Inc, Irvine, CA) and has the ^{32}P incorporated into the material of the balloon. The 33-mm balloon system is designed to deliver 20 Gy of beta radiation at 1 mm beyond the lumen of the balloon into the vessel wall for single or stepped irradiation. All the patients had stable or unstable angina, positive functional test, and a single restenotic lesion (50–100% restenosis). The average age in both groups was 62 years, with 37% diabetic and 20% prior CABG. The TVR rate was 25% in radiation vs 43% in the placebo. Nine-month MACEs were 24% in radiated segments vs 55% in placebo. Therefore, the ^{32}P brachytherapy system was associated with a 40% reduction in MACE.

During VBT, there is no need for change in shielding when using the liquid balloon systems for VBT with rhenium-188(186) and holmium-166. It is necessary to have a lead shielding box (pig) with remote control device of a three-way stopcock (Figure 18-2). The preparation is simple and the most important part in the delivery of VBT is complete evacuation of air inside the balloon. In contrast to conventional gamma or beta sources, residual air bubble inside the balloon of the liquid balloon system can cause edge restenosis or focal under-radiation areas. The residual air bubble can not be identified if radioactive source is not mixed with contrast agent. However, dilution of radioactive liquid with contrast requires increase in dwell time and may cause instability of the radioactive source with deviated target dose.[22–24]

TECHNICAL TIPS

1. The delivery balloon should be tested outside the body with nominal pressure inflation to check for leakage. An-

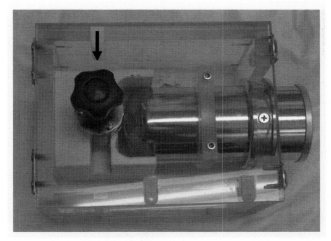

Figure 18-2: Box with lead shielding and remote controlling three-way stopcock (arrow).

other reason for this testing is possible better removal of air bubble from the balloon.

2. The balloon length is between 20 and 40 mm. A perfusion balloon catheter can be used to provide continuous minimal distal flow.

3. Complete removal of air bubble is absolutely required because residual air trapping in the balloon results in focal under-irradiation and restenosis.

4. Careful manipulation of the three-way stopcock is necessary to prevent minor isotope leakage. Additional protection with a vinyl towel is required in the manipulation field.[25]

5. In order to avoid geographic miss, VBT should cover a safety zone ranging from 5 to 7 mm at the both ends because there is 86% radiation dose reduction at the ends of balloon and there is only 16% radiation at 2.5 mm from these ends.[26]

6. The contrast media can be mixed with radioactive rhenium and holmium.

7. Balloon inflation pressure should be at nominal level because the dose calculation is based on balloon nominal size. Lower pressure may result in under-radiation (Figure 18-3).

8. Long ischemic time: fractionation is allowed in intolerable cases because the average dwell time of the liquid balloon system, which blocks blood flow, is between 3 and 5 minutes.

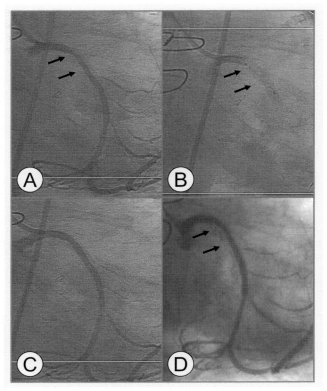

Figure 18-3: (A) Before VBT, there was in-stent restenosis at the proximal segment of the LCX. (B) The ISR received VBT with Ho-DTPA filled balloon. The length of the balloon is longer than the lesion. (C) After VBT. (D) Angiogram one year later without restenosis. The balloon inflation pressure should be at nominal level because the dose calculation is based on balloon nominal size. Lower pressure may result in under-radiation.

Safety issues in catheterization laboratories: The Nuclear Regulatory Commission (NRC) and the Food and Drug Administration (FDA) regulate the medical use of radioisotopes. The NRC ensures adequate protection of public health and safety in all aspects of nuclear material use, handling, storage, and disposal through issuance of regulations and licensing. To be licensed for VBT, each facility must maintain a quality management program that guarantees compliance with the NRC regulations. During a VBT procedure, the interventional cardiologist is responsible for selecting patients, carrying out the PCI, and monitoring the patient's clinical condition. The radiation oncologist determines the dose prescription and dwell time. After the delivery catheter is positioned by the cardiologist, the radiation oncologist performs the delivery and removal of the radioactive source from the patient. A medical physicist works closely with the radiation oncologist to prepare and calibrate the source, help with calculating the dose, and ensure that NRC regulations for radioisotope handling and environmental monitoring are followed. A radiation safety officer is also in charge of determining environmental and personnel exposure to radiation and providing safety training and education for all personnel.[27,28]

Physical restructuring with additional shielding, especially with gamma VBT, is required to provide a safe environment for VBT. A storage room for radioactive sources should be near the catheterization laboratories to minimize transport time and distance; this room should have all the equipment necessary for the physicist to prepare, calibrate, and store the radioactive material. In all cases of emergency, the physicist's responsibility is to remain focused on safely retrieving the sources and minimizing unnecessary exposure to patient and staff. To allow for rapid and well directed action, contingency plans must be made in advance, discussed, and rehearsed for a variety of likely and unlikely occurrences.[4]

TECHNICAL TIPS

**Safety measures: The radiation source is brought to the cardiac catheterization laboratories in a shielding device (pig). To decrease the level of radiation exposure, the operators and staff should avoid touching the shielding device and the treatment catheter, and keep their distance from the source.[4]

**Equipment set-up: Before the procedure, the VBT equipment is checked by the radiation oncologist (mechanical integrity, flushing the system, dummy source, etc.) A bail-out box must be in the procedure room, consisting of long-handled instruments for grasping a source and of a shielded container (lead for gamma radiation, plastic for beta radiation). Radiation detectors are needed to survey the environment during the procedure and contamination monitors for source leakage after. During a gamma radiation treatment, additional sterile gowns and gloves should be open on a table ready for cases of emergency when staff need to rapidly approach the patient.[4]

PRACTICAL APPLICATIONS

As VBT becomes the treatment of choice for ISR, multiple secondary analyses of the VBT trials have shown its effect in patients with high-risk factors such as diabetes,[29] small vessel caliber and long lesions,[30] chronic total occlusions,[31] or ostial lesions.[32] The average restenosis rate after VBT was 20% or higher. With these results, VBT may find a niche for ISR and not for de novo lesions because it cannot compete with the 3–7% restenosis rate after DES.[33] There are two areas of potential possible benefit with VBT: the patient with ISR; and failure after prior VBT or with DES (especially in bifurcation lesions), while VBT may be detrimental to patients who have received a second stent.

Gamma therapy in ISR after failed VBT: Because there are no documented data in patients with repeat restenosis after prior VBT for ISR, a prospective registry was designed to follow and compare the outcomes of these patients. In this second round of VBT, 350 patients with a failure of VBT after ISR were offered either angioplasty alone (299 patients) or repeat VBT (51 patients). All patients in the VBT arm also received long-term (at least 6 months) clopidogrel therapy. None developed late thrombosis. These patients were able to tolerate 20 Gy of radiation up to 1 mm beyond the source while on average they had received only 15 or 16 Gy in their first VBT treatment. This insufficient dosing may account for the recurrence of ISR in these 350 patients.

At follow-up, the repeat VBT group had less TLR compared to the angioplasty-only group (19.6 vs 55%, respectively). The TVR rate was reduced from 57.7% to 21% in favor of the VBT patients.[34]

**Re-stenting and VBT: In the treatment of patients with ISR receiving VBT, additional stent deployment ("stent sandwich") provides a better acute angiographic result. However, the acute gain (larger lumen dimensions) is offset by late exaggerated intimal proliferation. IVUS studies showed that 79% of patients in the VBT group with newly placed stents had struts with neointima at follow-up while only 27% in the placebo group had the same observation (P<0.001). There was no change in the luminal diameter (MLD) in the non re-stented segments, while it was significantly decreased in the re-stented segments due to exaggerated neointimal hyperplasia. These observations suggested that the maximum effectiveness of ^{192}Ir radiation in treating ISR lesions was limited to non-restented segments. Regardless of supplementary iVBT, re-stenting strategies provide little advantage to improve long-term outcomes.[35]

DES for ISR: In the treatment of patients with ISR, the results of DES were compared with VBT, cutting balloons, and bare metal stents, in the Rapamycin-Eluting Stent Evaluated at Rotterdam Cardiology Hospital (RESEARCH) registry. The TLR rate was 12.3%, which is not negligible. The rate was higher at 21.4% if the index vessels received prior VBT. These real-world results showed that DES is not a promising modality of treatment for ISR.[36]

REFERENCES

1. Rankin JM, Spinelli JJ, Carere RG *et al.* Improved clinical outcome after widespread use of coronary-artery stenting in Canada. *N Engl J Med* 1999; **341**(26): 1957–15.

2. Mehran R, Dangas G, Abizaid AS *et al.* Angiographic patterns of in-stent restenosis: classification and implications for long-term outcome. *Circulation* 1999; **100**(18): 1872–8.

3. Kim MH, Cha KS, Han JY *et al.* Effect of antioxidant probucol for preventing stent restenosis. *Cathet Cardiovasc Interv* 2002; **57**: 424–8.

4. Sianos G, van der Giessen W, de Feyter P *et al.* Intracoronary radiation therapy. In: Marco J, Serruys P, Biamino G *et al.* eds. *Syllabus of The Paris Course on Revascularization*, 2003: 243–64.

5. Weinberger J. Radiation. In: Topol EJ, ed. *Textbook of Interventional Cardiology.* W.B. Saunders Co., 1999: 650–63.

6. Popowski Y, Verin V. Debate: centering is important. *J Interven Cardiol* 1999; **12**: 243–5.

7. Raizner AE. The centering debate: the importance of centering in endovascular brachytherapy. *Vascular Radiotherapy Monitor* 1999; **2**: 3–10.

8. Albiero R, Nishida T, Adamian M *et al.* Edge restenosis after implantation of high activity (32)P radioactive beta-emitting stents. *Circulation* 2000; **101**(21): 2454–7.

9. Albiero R, Colombo A. European high-activity ^{32}P radioactive stent experience. *J Invasive Cardiol* 2000; **12**(8): 416–21.

10. Leon MB, Teirstein PS, Moses JW *et al.* Localized intracoronary gamma-radiation therapy to inhibit the recurrence of restenosis after stenting. *N Engl J Med* 2001; **344**(4): 250–6.

11. Popma JJ, Suntharalingam M, Lansky AJ *et al.* Randomized trial of ^{90}Sr/^{90}Y beta-radiation versus placebo control for treatment of in-stent restenosis. *Circulation* 2002; **106**(9): 1090–6.

12. Waksman R, Raizner AE, Yeung AC *et al.* Use of localised intracoronary beta radiation in treatment of in-stent restenosis: the INHIBIT randomised controlled trial. *Lancet* 2002; **359**(9306): 551–7.

13. Kuntz RE, Speiser B, Joyal M *et al.* Clinical and angiographic outcomes after use of Sr-50 Beta radiation for the treatment of de novo and restenotic coronary lesions. Presented at the 50th annual scientific session of the American College of Cardiology, Orlando, March 2001.

14. Costa MA, Sabate M, van der Giessen WJ *et al.* Late coronary occlusion after intracoronary brachytherapy . *Circulation* 1999; **100**(8): 789–92.

15. Waksman R, Bhargava B, Mintz GS *et al.* Late total occlusion after intracoronary brachytherapy for patients with in-stent restenosis. *J Am Coll Cardiol* 2000; **36**(1): 65–8.

16. Raizner AE, Oesterle SN, Waksman R *et al*. Inhibition of restenosis with beta-emitting radiotherapy: report of the Proliferation REduction with Vascular ENergy Trial (PREVENT). *Circulation* 2000; **102** (9): 951–8.

17. Teirstein PS, Moses JW, Casterella PJ *et al*. Late thrombosis after coronary radiation may be eliminated by longer antiplatelet therapy and reduced stenting: the SCRIPPS III results. *J Am Coll Cardiol* 2001; **37** (Suppl A): 60A. Abstract.

18. Waksman R, Ajani AE, White RL *et al*. Prolonged antiplatelet therapy to prevent late thrombosis after intracoronary gamma-radiation in patients with in-stent restenosis: Washington Radiation for In-Stent Restenosis Trial Plus 6 Months of Clopidogrel (WRIST PLUS). *Circulation* 2001; **103** (19): 2332–5.

19. Sabate M, Costa MA, Kozuma K *et al*. Geographic miss: a cause of treatment failure in radio-oncology applied to intracoronary radiation therapy. *Circulation* 2000; **101**(21): 2467–71.

20. Kim HS, Waksman R, Cottin Y *et al*. Edge stenosis and geographical miss following intracoronary gamma radiation therapy for in-stent restenosis. *J Am Coll Cardiol* 2001; **37**(4): 1026–30.

21. The Brite II Trial: A Multi Center Randomized Study of a Novel P-32 Deployable Balloon System for the Treatment of In-Stent Restenosis. Presented at the 52nd annual scientific meeting of the American College of Cardiology, Chicago, April 2003.

22. Coussement PK *et al*. Intracoronary beta-radiation of de novo coronary lesions using a (186)Re liquid-filled balloon system: six-month results from a clinical feasibility study. *Cathet Cardiovasc Interv* 2002; **55**(1): 28–36.

23. Hoher M *et al*. Intracoronary beta-irradiation with a liquid (188)Re-filled balloon: six-month results from a clinical safety and feasibility study. *Circulation* 2000; **101**(20): 2355–60.

24. Park SW *et al*. Treatment of diffuse in-stent restenosis with rotational atherectomy followed by radiation therapy with a rhenium-188-mercaptoacetyltriglycine-filled balloon. *J Am Coll Cardiol* 2001; **38**(3): 631–7.

25. Hausleiter J L, Makkar R, Berman D *et al*. Leakage of a liquid [188]Re-filled balloon system during intracoronary brachytherapy: A case report. *Cardiovasc Radiat Med* 2000 **2**: 7–10.

26. Hong MK *et al*. Impact of geographic miss on adjacent coronary artery segments in diffuse in-stent restenosis with beta-radiation therapy: angiographic and intravascular ultrasound analysis. *Am Heart J* 2002 **143**(2): 327–33.

27. Kaluza G, Masur W, Raizner A. Radiotherapy for prevention of restenosis. *Cathet Cardiovasc Interv* 2001; **52**: 518–21.

28. Nguyen-Ho P, Kaluza G, Zymek P *et al*. Intracoronary brachytherapy. *Cathet Cardiovasc Interv* 2002; **56**: 281–8.

29. Gruberg L, Waksman R, Ajani AE *et al*. The effect of in-tracoronary radiation for the treatment of recurrent in-stent restenosis in patients with diabetes mellitus. *J Am Coll Cardiol* 2002; **39** (12): 1930–6.
30. Ajani AE, Waksman R, Cha DH *et al*. The impact of lesion length and reference vessel diameter on angiographic restenosis and target vessel revascularization in treating in-stent restenosis with radiation. *J Am Coll Cardiol* 2002; **39** (8): 1290–6.
31. Sharma AK, Ajani AE, Garg N *et al*. Usefulness of gamma intracoronary radiation for totally occluded in-stent restenotic coronary narrowing. *Am J Cardiol* 2003; **91** (5): 595–7.
32. Ajani AE, Waksman R, Cheneau E *et al*. Impact of intra-coronary radiation on in-stent restenosis involving ostial lesions. *Cathet Cardiovasc Interv* 2003; **58** (2): 175–80.
33. The SIRolImUS-Eluting Stent in De Novo Native Coronary Lesions (SIRIUS) trial presented by Martin Leon at the Late-Breaking Trial session at the TransCatheter Therapeutics meeting in Washington DC, 2002.
34. Gamma therapy in ISR after failed radiation therapy: Presented by Walkman R, at the 52nd annual scientific meeting of the American College of Cardiology, Chicago, April 2003.
35. Morino Y, Limpijankit T, Honda Y *et al*. Late vascular response to repeat stenting for ISR with or without radiation: An IVUS volumetric analysis. *Circulation* 2002; **105**: 2465–8.
36. The results of the Rapamycin-Eluting Stent Evaluated at Rotterdam Cardiology Hospital (RESEARCH) presented by Saia F. at the 52nd annual scientific meeting of the American College of Cardiology, Chicago, April 2003.

Chapter 19

Rotational Atherectomy

Thach Nguyen, Mark Reisman, Ted Feldman

GENERAL OVERVIEW

The Rotablator atherectomy catheter is, in essence, a sanding device. A nickel-plated brass burr is coated with about 2500 20-micron diamond chips, with an exposure of 5 microns over the burr surface. The burr is welded to a spring coil shaft that is coupled to a gas-driven turbine. The turbine

*Basic; **Advanced; ***Rare, exotic, or investigational.

From: Nguyen T, Hu D, Saito S, Grines C, Palacios I (eds), *Practical Handbook of Advanced Interventional Cardiology*, 2nd edn. © 2003 Futura, an imprint of Blackwell Publishing.

drives the shaft and burr at rotational speeds of between 50,000 and 200,000 rpm. Contact of the diamond grit with atheroma results in sanding of the plaque and creating microparticulate debris. Eighty percent of particles are less than 4 microns and are thus carried away in the circulation. The remaining particles of larger size are partially responsible for many of the side effects and complications of this mechanism of atherectomy. Since atheroma removal is the primary mechanism of lumen enlargement (vs vessel stretching), there is no recoil on 24-hour angiography following PTCRA.[1]

CURRENT INDICATIONS

Calcification and very hard lesions remain the main indications for rotational atherectomy. Randomized trials in relatively simple lesion anatomy have not shown any differences in the long-term outcome of balloon angioplasty compared to rotational atherectomy. Many lesions, however, could not be considered for randomized trials and are treatable only with rotational atherectomy. Among the groups of patients most frequently in this category are those with prior bypass surgery in whom native lesions are very old, and calcification or extreme fibrosis is common. Similarly, dialysis patients typically have calcified, fibrotic, and long lesions with well-established diffuse atherosclerosis. At the extremes of the elderly population, such lesions are the rule and frequently vessels are too small for stenting or cannot reasonably have stents delivered unless the calcium is debulked to some degree.

Branch ostial stenosis and aorto-ostial stenosis are two particular indications for rotational atherectomy. Lesions on these sides tend to recoil when treated with balloon angioplasty alone, and particularly branch ostial stenosis often involves vessels that are too small to stent easily, and stent placement may impinge on the parent vessel. Debulking with a Rotablator in these lesions shows very stable results in contrast to the rubber band-like effects seen with PTCA alone. Aorto-ostial lesions are often calcified and often stent results are suboptimal unless debulking is performed at this location first. This is particularly true in protected left main disease.[3,4]

Chronic total occlusions represent another group for which debulking is particularly advantageous either prior to or in combination with stent implantation. Chronic occlusions have been shown to have a high recurrence rate after PTCA. Stent delivery is often difficult due to the extreme bulk of atheroma in these lesions. Special care must be taken to demonstrate that the wire is intraluminal distal to the occlusion segment before rotational atherectomy is undertaken.

TECHNICAL TIPS

**Selection of guides: The Rotablator is unique in that it is a front-cutting device and enters the lesion only during therapeutic intervention. The speed of rotation and coaxial tracking over the wire obviates the need to push or dotter the device, and thus excellent guide support is not as necessary and not as important as its coaxial position.[5] Guides with rounded curves for the left system are easier to get the burr through than the Judkins shapes. The large lumen guide will limit the contact between the burr and the inner lumen of the guide, so less local friction is generated. It can provide a good line-up with smooth transition between the guide and the aorto-ostial lumen. A small guide can intubate the ostium, so there is less debulking in the ostial segment. A firm tip may be beneficial since occasionally a soft tip guide can "fish mouth" and hinder advancement of the large burrs. The guides with side holes are recommended because they will provide increased perfusion that can promote particulate clearance.[2]

**Coaxial tip alignment: This will reduce the tension or pull required on the wire for advancing the burr. Significant support or deep intubation is not needed with this device since activation of the burr provides orthogonal displacement of friction, which will reduce drag to ease passage of the burr through the vessel. An example is the use of an Amplatz guide in the treatment of an ostial LCX lesion. An Amplatz guide can often be manipulated to "telescope" into the LCX, resulting in a centrally positioned wire. Judkins curves that are generally not directed toward the LCX will cause the burr to cut primarily on the inner curve of the ostial LCX lesion (i.e. the wall contiguous with the left main artery).[2]

**Selection of wires: In tortuous or rigid vessels, the stiff type C and Extra Support wire conform poorly to angles and bends so it is difficult to advance them while staying optimally center positioned. Use of a PTCA wire in exchange for the type C wire may be necessary. In a straight vessel with eccentric lesion (i.e. the LAD) they are preferred because they provide greater vessel contact with eccentric lesions in straight vessels.

In patients with proximal lesions and distal tortuosity, a RotaWire Floppy will be able to negotiate the distal segment while providing a platform for proximal ablation. In proximal tortuous vessels, the same RotaWire Floppy can successfully cross the tortuous vessels without causing too much wire bias or pseudolesions, but it provides inadequate support for the burr and makes traversing the lesion more difficult.[2] In patients with distal lesions, when support is required to advance the burr, the stiff type C or RotaWire

Extra Support wires may be better in delivering the burr than the soft and flexible RotaWire Floppy.

When a wire of the Rotablator system cannot cross a lesion, the best approach is to place a conventional angioplasty wire and then exchange it for a Rotablator wire through the transfer catheter.

**Wire manipulations: Once removed from the packaging loop, the wire should be maintained straight on the table. This position is to avoid inadvertent kinking and to retain its torquing capability. Rotate the wire while advancing by using the wire clip as a torque device. This maneuver can reduce the side contact and friction and improve its tracking ability.[2]

The distal tip must be placed distal to the lesion since the burr cannot track over the larger spring-coil segment of the wire. The tip should be positioned in a large branch that can absorb and carry away the debris. It should not be trapped in the vessel, especially in small branches, because any of its rotation once the burr is activated can result in wire fracture.[2]

**Wire bias: Since a stiff wire has the tendency to follow outside curves and bends,[6,7] and preferentially forces a burr into one side of the vessel wall, this problem is further complicated as greater tension on the wire is required to advance the burr. This tension can cause the wire to become taut, resulting in pseudolesions or wire bias. Wire bias may be favorable, displacing the burr into the greater part of the plaque mass in some eccentric lesions, or may be unfavorable, moving the burr toward an angle or a bifurcation point with greater risk of perforation, or away from the greater part of plaque mass in a particular lesion. In cases with unfavorable wire bias, manipulation of the wire position or guide catheter may correct the problem. In cases of favorable wire bias, a lumen larger than the size of the burr can be achieved and subsequent burr sizes should be predicated on these results, i.e. a larger burr may not be required.[2]

**Pseudolesions: Rotablator wires have a greater tendency to cause pseudolesions than conventional PTCA wires.[8] This is especially true in tortuous right coronary arteries or serpentine LAD vessels. If pseudolesions are prominent distally, the wire should be retracted to a more proximal position.

As a PTCRA procedure progresses, appearance of new pseudolesions may cause some concerns regarding the possibility of new thrombus, occult lesions, or dissections. Withdrawing the wire so that the flexible spring tip is in the area of the pseudolesion or changing to a soft PTCA wire is sometimes necessary to determine whether it is only a pseudolesion, a new dissection, or a thrombus.

**Selection of burr size: The maximum burr size is generally 60–85% of the reference diameter and the initial burr is at least 0.5 mm smaller than the target anticipated burr. An example would be a vessel of 2.8 mm – approximately 75% is 2.1 mm and therefore the final burr size would be between 2.25 mm (closer to 80%) or 2.0 mm (closer to 70%). A smaller initial burr size is chosen for long lesions, severe calcification, large plaque mass, total occlusions, or any situation where a trial with a small burr is needed to assess the lesion response to PTCRA.

Undersized burrs of 0.25–0.50 mm less than would conventionally be used, had this been a straight segment, are suggested in the following scenarios in Table 19-1.

**Failure to advance the burr: Difficulty in advancing a burr may be found with distal lesions, in vessels with proximal tortuosity or angiographically occult lesions, and in heavily calcified or longer lesions. If a burr fails to advance on a Rotawire Floppy, changing to a stiffer type C wire may help to advance the burr.

In some cases, better guide support will solve the problem.

**Visual assessment during ablation run: Rotational ablation is a dynamic process. During burr activation, intermittent visual assessment with contrast injection provides important information.

If there is burr deceleration, visualization of the burr location can explain whether the drop in speed is due to overaggressive advancement into the lesion or vessel tortuosity. In the case of vessel tortuosity, contrast will flow unimpeded around the burr.

In the case of wire bias, visualization of the burr as it advances may demonstrate the preferential orientation of the burr to one side of the vessel or lesion. This orientation may affect the results achieved with the burr and influence subsequent sizing.

Table 19-1
Factors suggesting initial undersized burr

1. Vessels with proximal tortuosity making it difficult to advance the burr
2. Vessels with angulated segments of more than 60°, because of higher risk of perforation
3. Vessels with pseudolesions and severe guide bias in the proximal segment
4. Excessive plaque burden (long, heavy calcification, total occlusion)

In long, heavily calcified, and diffuse lesions, contrast injection during runs can help monitor progress through the lesion and provide identification of anatomic landmarks for subsequent ablations.

Obstructive burrs: When ablating a lesion, the flow should not be totally obstructed for more than a few seconds. If there is no antegrade flow around the burr during contrast injection, retract the device until complete clearance of contrast occurs. This is needed to ensure that particulates created by the ablation can be cleared in small increments.

If there is vasospasm or attenuated distal flow, these are warning signs or harbingers of the slow flow or no-re-flow phenomenon.

**Blood pressure during ablation runs: Low blood pressure secondary to transient bradycardia may indirectly indicate hypovolemia. Since diastolic pressure and, consequently, coronary perfusion pressure are reduced during bradycardia, particulate clearance may be diminished. The ablation times should be reduced during bradycardia. Atropine and theophylline can be given prior to the ablation runs. The use of pressor infusion or small boluses of an alpha agonist should be used liberally to maintain a decent blood pressure.

**Ablation strategies: After optimal position of the wire and burr, a first ablation run is to create a pilot channel. An angiogram is done to check the results of the first ablation. Flexibility after analyzing the results after each burr is essential throughout the procedure to modify subsequent burr selection and ablation strategy. Small burr increments are used if the distal lumen is poorly defined and the exact size of the reference segment is not known. Also, the amount of tissue removed and the rate of removal are important in maintaining the level of debris to be absorbed by the microcirculation. As the burr passes through the lesion, one should be careful not to let it jump when exiting the distal part of the plaque. Just as when sawing wood, a jagged edge results when one moves forcibly at the completion of the cut.[9]

**Prevention of vasospasm: Distal vasospasm is frequently caused by rotablation. It may be due to vibration of the wire secondary to spinning of the burr. To prevent spasm, a flush solution containing nitroglycerin and vera-pamil "cocktail" is infused under pressure through the driveshaft (Table 19-2).[10] There appears to be a diminished tendency for vessel spasm during rotational atherectomy procedures when the cocktail is used. Some operators prefer ionic contrast during PTCRA procedures to prevent

Table 19-2
The flush cocktail

1. 0.9% NS 1000 cc
2. Heparin 10,000 units (10 units/mL)
3. Verapamil 10 mg (10 mcg/mL)
4. Nitroglycerin 5 mg (5 mcg/mL)

vessel spasm and because of its strong antiplatelet effect. However, if the procedure is prolonged, with use of large contrast amount, the patient can suffer heart failure due to contrast overload. Glycoprotein 2b3a inhibitors can prevent platelet aggregation better than the high ionic contrast agent.

**Prevention of slow flow or no-reflow: It is rare (0.5% to 2%)[11] and usually transient but can be severe, resulting in extreme hemodynamic dysfunction. If the lesions are thrombotic, long, diffuse, or contain large amounts of fatty atheroma, they are more likely to cause no-reflow. Too aggressive an ablation technique with creation of large particles also compromises the distal microcirculation. The best technical methods for prevention of slow flow are listed in Table 19-3.

The prophylactic use of antiplatelet drugs may diminish the incidence of slow flow and no-reflow. Pretreatment with clopidogrel for more than 24 hours may have an effect similar to that reported by prophylactic glycoprotein 2b2a receptor blockade.[12]

**Balloon pump support: A balloon pump may be placed for support during the procedure in a high-risk patient. If no complications occur and right heart pressures remain acceptable, the pump may be removed in the laboratory at the conclusion of the procedure. The insertion of a prophylactic intra-aortic balloon pump is considered in patients listed in Table 19-4.

Table 19-3
Strategies for prevention of slow or no-reflow

1. Slower initial speeds of 140,000–160,000 rpm
2. Minimal deceleration during ablation runs
3. Multiple short runs of 30 seconds or less
4. Ample rest periods between runs
5. Liberal use of intracoronary nitroglycerin and calcium channel blocker

---

Table 19-4
Indication for intra-aortic balloon pump

---

1. Severe LV dysfunction
2. In cases where the target vessel has a complex lesion and supplies the majority of the myocardium[13]

**Management of slow flow or no-flow: Because the driving force for clearing the microparticles is systemic pressure, the main measures are to sustain coronary perfusion pressure such as forced injection of blood through the guide catheter, IABP, and the use of pressors. Slow flow is also caused by vascular spasm, so injection of small amounts of intracoronary calcium blockers (100 µg of verapamil or diltiazem) can relieve arterial spasm and increase flow. This is more effective than nitroglycerin.[14] There was no large report of detrimental hypotension. When administering intracoronary drugs for no-reflow, it is important to use a distal intracoronary end-hole catheter to allow injection of the drug past any side hole in the guide to ensure local delivery to the microcirculation. Platelet glycoprotein receptor antagonists are also suggested.[15] Some operators have had success with IC adenosine or nitroprusside.

**Perforation: Perforation is infrequent and occurs between 0.05% and 1%.[16] Most perforations are small and can be treated with partial reversal of heparin by protamine and a prolonged balloon inflation using a perfusion balloon when possible. Rare cases require pericardiocentesis and, even less frequently, surgical repair. Perforations are most likely to occur with ablation across extremely angulated obtuse marginal or diagonal branches. When such vessels are treated, a bend in the wire to facilitate passage of the burr around a sharp angle and very short ablation runs are sometimes helpful. A "pecking" motion at the lesion is an ideal approach. If the burr remains in contact with an angulated lesion for too long a time, it may drift into the wall of the vessel and result in perforation. Perforation may also occur with prolonged burr contact with the vessel wall under a myocardial bridge. This excessive contraction in systole against the burr can eliminate some of the differential cutting properties specific to rotational atherectomy. Perforation can happen because after fracture of the distal wire, the burr can jump forward freely, unrestrained by the wire, and cause perforation.[17]

**Dissection: Angiographically visible dissection occurs in 2–15% and is usually minor. Minute dissections are detected more by IVUS. One of the theories postulates that as the forward movement of the burr is intercepted by a hard lesion, its in-place rotation at a high speed will channel the rotational energy backward, causing rotational torsion of the whole shaft that grips the plaque and produces dissection. The treatment is low-pressure angioplasty. If the dissection is extensive, then a prolonged perfusion balloon inflation is preferred. In the current era of combined debulking and stent use, dissections are rarely of clinical importance.

**Entrapped burr: During rotablation of an ISR, or through a side branch for bifurcation PCI or due to undilatable stent, a burr can be advanced and trapped distal to the stent. Since there are no diamond chips on the proximal surface of the burr, there is no cutting ability upon pulling back and retrieving burr may be impossible.[18] A patient with a severe calcified lesion in the mid-LAD underwent rotational atherectomy. In a case report by Grise *et al.*, after the first passage of a 1.25-mm diameter burr, the burr could be advanced but not be withdrawn. A fixed balloon catheter (Ace Balloon, Scimed, Maple Grove, MN) was inserted at the lesion and inflated to break the plaque at the mid-LAD site. After successful dilation, the 1.25-mm burr could be easily removed. One of the theories postulates that a presumed ledge of calcium that had opened wide enough to allow passage of the burr but incomplete ablation may have prevented its withdrawal.[19]

PRACTICAL APPLICATIONS

Rotational atherectomy finds its greatest use in patients with smaller vessels, calcified lesions, and complex or long coronary artery disease. The low restenosis rates reported in stent trials have been achieved with relatively discrete lesions and reference diameters averaging 3.0 mm or larger. As many as three-quarters of coronary artery patients are not similar to those treated in the large stent trials and require a large armamentarium of devices and approaches to achieve optimal results. The ability to combine atherectomy, angioplasty, and stenting in these complex lesion subsets promises the best short-term results and the largest lumen diameters with least residual stenoses and the best potential for both good acute results and durable long-term results. The concept that bigger is better is clearly feasible in patients with arteries larger than 3 mm. Smaller arteries simply cannot be made "bigger" than their reference diameter. The use of atherectomy is an essential tool in the management of this large segment of the coronary artery disease population. When combined with PTCA and stenting, rotational atherectomy also offers many patients with complex coronary anatomy a chance to undergo percutaneous revascularization rather than bypass surgery.

REFERENCES

1. Reisman M, Rivera L, McDaniel M *et al*. Absence of recoil following percutaneous coronary rotational ablation: Analysis by quantitative coronary angiography. *Eur Heart J* 1992; **13**: 425.

2. Reisman M. *Guide to Rotational Atherectomy.* Physicians' Press, 1998.

3. Kaplan BM, Safian RD, Mojares JJ *et al*. Optimal burr and adjunctive balloon sizing reduces the need for target artery revascularization after coronary mechanical rotational atherectomy. *Am J Cardiol* 1996; **78** (11): 1224–9.

4. Safian RD, Freed M, Reddy V *et al*. Do excimer laser angioplasty and rotational atherectomy facilitate balloon angioplasty? Implications for lesion-specific coronary intervention. *J Am Coll Cardiol* 1996; **27**(3): 552–9.

5. Casterella P, Terstein P. Rotational coronary atherectomy. In: Grech ED, Ramsdale DR, eds. *Practical Interventional Cardiology.* Martin Dunitz, 1997.

6. Stuver TP, Ling FS. The "furrowing effect": Guidewire-induced "directional" lesion ablation in rotational atherectomy of angulated coronary artery lesions. *Cathet Cardiovasc Diagn* 1996; **39**: 385–95.

7. Reisman M, Harms V. Guidewire bias: Potential source of complications with rotational atherectomy. *Cathet Cardiovasc Diagn* 1996; (Suppl 3): 64–8.

8. Bowling LS, Guarneri E, Schatz RA, Teirstein PS. High-speed rotational atherectomy of tortuous coronary arteries with guidewire-associated pseudostenosis. *Cathet Cardiovasc Diagn* 1996; (Suppl 3): 82–84.

9. King SB, Douglas J. Rotational coronary ablation. In: King SB, Douglas J, eds. *Atlas of Heart Disease, Interventional Cardiology.* Mosby, 1997.

10. Cohen BM, Weber VJ, Blum RR *et al*. Cocktail Attenuation of Rotational Ablation Flow Effects (CARAFE) pilot study. *Cathet Cardiovasc Diagn* 1996; (Suppl 3): 69–72.

11. Sharma SK, Dangas G, Mehran R *et al*. Risk factors for the development of slow flow during rotational coronary atherectomy. *Am J Cardiol* 1997; **80** (2): 219–222.

12. Gregorini L, Marco J, Fajadet J *et al*. Ticlopidine and aspirin pretreatment reduces coagulation and platelet activation during coronary dilation procedures. *J Am Coll Cardiol* 1997; **29** (l): 13–20.

13. O'Murchu B, Foremean RD, Shaw RE *et al*. Role of IABP counterpulsation in high-risk coronary atherectomy. *J Am Coll Cardiol* 1995; **26** (5): 1270–5.

14. Piana RN, Paik GY, Mosucci M *et al.* Incidence and treatment of no-reflow after percutaneous coronary intervention. *Circulation* 1994; **89**: 2514–18.

15. Rawitscher D, Levin TN, Cohen L, Feldman T. Rapid reversal of no-reflow using abciximab after coronary device intervention. *Cathet Cardiovasc Diagn* 1997; **42**: 187–90.

16. Cohen BM, Weber VJ, Reisman M, Casale A, Dorros G. Coronary perforation complicating rotational ablation: The US multicenter experience. *Cathet Cardiovasc Diagn* 1996; (Suppl 3): 55–59.

17. Foster-Smith K, Garratt KN, Holmes DR Jr. Guide transection during rotational coronary atherectomy due to guide catheter dislodgment and wire kinking. *Cathet Cardiovasc Diagn* 1995; **35**: 224–7.

18. Feldman T. Rotational ablation of stent metal components: The intersection between coronary intervention and auto body repair. *Cathet Cardiovasc Interv* 2001; **52**: 212–13.

19. Grise M, Yeager M, Terstein P. A case of an entrapped rotational atherectomy burr. *Cathet Cardiovasc Interv* 2002; **57**: 31–3.

Chapter 20

Intravascular Ultrasound

Guy Weigold, Neil J Weissman

INTRODUCTION

Intravascular ultrasound (IVUS) is an exciting technology that allows *in vivo* visualization of vascular anatomy by using a miniature transducer at the end of a flexible catheter. The catheter is placed into the coronary artery by standard retrograde catheterization techniques. Because of the high quality cross-sectional images of the atherosclerotic plaque and surrounding vascular structures, IVUS is now clinically used to delineate plaque morphology and distribution, and to provide a rationale for guiding transcatheter coronary interventions.[1] Furthermore, IVUS technology has advanced our knowledge of atherogenesis, vascular remodeling, and mechanisms associated with coronary interventions and restenosis.

ANGIOGRAPHY VERSUS IVUS

IVUS provides a cross-sectional view of all layers of the coronary artery: the intima, media and adventitia. Working from the inside of the blood vessel out, the first layer encountered, adjacent to the lumen, is the intima. The intima is

---

*Basic; **Advanced; ***Rare, exotic, or investigational.

From: Nguyen T, Hu D, Saito S, Grines C, Palacios I (eds), *Practical Handbook of Advanced Interventional Cardiology*, 2nd edn. © 2003 Futura, an imprint of Blackwell Publishing.

normally 1–2 layers of cells thick but can greatly enlarge with the deposition of atherosclerotic plaque. The intima is immediately surrounded by the media, which is predominantly a layer of homogenous smooth muscle cells providing vascular tone to the artery. The adventitia surrounds the media and is composed of multiple bands of fibrous connective tissue providing additional external support for the vessel. The cross-sectional images of the vessel provided by IVUS precisely characterize the extent and location of plaque within the artery (Figure 20-1).

As demonstrated by the image in Figure 20-1, precise determination of plaque burden, morphology, and distribution of plaques is possible through IVUS.[2,3] The most notable difference between angiography and ultrasound measurement is the extensive amount of plaque seen by ultrasound measurement that is not detected by angiography. Angiography displays the luminal contour which allows measurements of only the luminal diameter, typically in two or three orthogonal views. Detection of the presence of plaque is then assessed by comparing the degree of narrowing with that of a segment that is not "narrowed," assuming that this segment is free of atherosclerosis. Unfortunately, the reference segment is often found to be diseased when it is assessed by IVUS measurement, with up to a third of its cross-sectional area filled with plaque. As a result, plaque burden is often underestimated by angiography and the degree of underestimation is substantial for diffusely diseased vessels.[4] The tomographic view of IVUS (with 180 potential diameters) provides the true minimal and maximal luminal diameters together with measurements of cross-sectional area. More importantly, IVUS allows visualization of the arterial (external elastic lamina) area as a reference of the size the artery would be if it were devoid of plaque.

IVUS provides greater insight into the composition of atherosclerotic plaques than angiography. Denser atherosclerotic material, such as calcium, will reflect more ultrasound

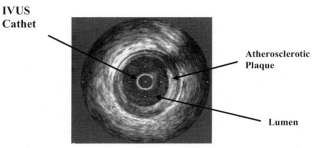

IVUS Cathet

Atherosclerotic Plaque

Lumen

Figure 20-1: Cross-sectional image of the artery with the three layers and the extent, location of the plaque.

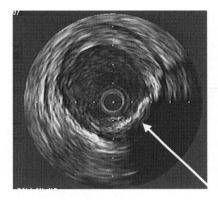

Calcified Lesion

Figure 20-2: Calcified lesion with acoustic shadow caused by minimal penetration of ultrasound to deeper tissues beyond the dense calcium deposit.

and appear very bright.[5] Since calcium is extremely dense, very little ultrasound penetrates to deeper tissues, producing an acoustic shadow beyond the very bright calcium deposit (Figure 20-2).

Although IVUS displays a cross-sectional image of the artery, it also provides location information within the coronary artery through the use of perivascular anatomic landmarks. Perivascular structures, such as the pericardium, myocardium and cardiac veins, have a characteristic appearance. Combining this information with the branching patterns of the arteries produces information for both axial position and tomographic orientation within the artery. For instance, identifying the pericardium from within the LAD provides the reference for anterior orientation, the diagonal branches for leftward orientation and for "downward" or posterior orientation, and septal branches. Pericardium appears as a bright, relatively thick structure. Typically, a small amount of pericardial fluid is enclosed, thereby providing a strong acoustic interface between itself and the pericardium. This enhances the IVUS appearance of pericardial reflections.[6]

TECHNIQUES OF IVUS

The risks are minimal, with very low reported complication rates, especially with the progressive miniaturization of transducers and IVUS catheters. The commonly used catheter is 3F, introduced through a guiding catheter over a standard intracoronary wire, imaging with a 40 MHz transducer. Most vessels can be imaged, but the diffusely severely diseased vessel remains a challenge, and an IVUS catheter may simply not pass through such a vessel.

After anticoagulation and predilation with intracoronary nitroglycerin (150–200 µg), the IVUS catheter is advanced as far down the artery as anatomy and equipment will allow. At this point, motorized pullback withdraws the catheter 0.5 mm per second. Standardization of this pullback is essential for "mapping" the coronary artery. As the catheter is withdrawn, side branches and perivascular landmarks identify the location of the image being viewed. Longitudinal reconstructions are also useful for vessel mapping, which becomes important when selecting stent or radiation source length. It is important to *complete* this pullback all the way back to the tip of the guiding catheter.

Vessel and lumen sizing during on-line IVUS analysis is used to assess lesion severity, select balloon/stent diameters for intervention and assess efficacy of the intervention. Physiologic studies have shown that the minimum lumen area (MLA) of a lesion predicts coronary flow reserve, fractional flow reserve, and perfusion scan results.[7–9] In general, MLAs (in proximal major epicardial arteries) less than 4.0 mm^2 are considered flow-limiting, though considerations of distance from the vessel ostium and size of a patient's vessels in general should be considered.

In determining stent and balloon size, assessment of the references is necessary. By definition, the *proximal* or *distal reference* site is that with the *largest lumen* proximal or distal to a stenosis but *within the same segment*, usually located within 10 mm of the stenosis with no major intervening branches.[10] IVUS often reveals more plaque than anticipated, and these reference sites may or may not be the sites with the least amount of plaque. The goal of the intervention, from the IVUS standpoint, is to obtain the best "match" between the reference lumen area and the final cross-sectional area of the stented segment. This ensures smooth "inflow" into and "outflow" out of the stented segment.

In addition to equipment sizing, IVUS can also be used to choose type of intervention and to alert operators to the potential for complications prior to proceeding with angioplasty. For example, finding significant concentric calcification at a lesion site may prompt use of rotational atherectomy to "break up" calcium prior to attempting vessel dilation, and this "plaque modification" of the vessel may help avoid what would otherwise become a dissection when the vessel is dilated.

Since the development of balloon angioplasty and, more recently, cutting balloons, it has become clear that the actual effect of the balloon is much more complex, involving tearing and displacement of the plaque and stretching of the arterial wall.[1] These factors vary from lesion to lesion and are unpredictable from angiographic appearance alone.[1] IVUS allows the visualization of these small splits, tears, fissures

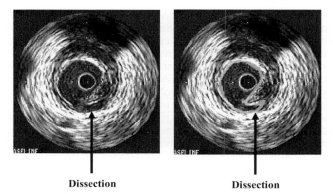

Dissection **Dissection**

Figure 20-3: The entry of the dissections appears at 6 o'clock at the shoulder (junction) between a calcified plaque and the normal intima.

or dissections that occur spontaneously or after a coronary intervention (Figure 20-3).

In addition to assessing plaque distribution, IVUS also allows for visualization of vessel injuries, such as intramural hematomas. Intramural hematomas are extravasations of blood localized in the arterial media. These can result from intimal fracture of an atherosclerotic plaque or bruising due to transcatheter interventions. Since intramural hematomas occur in the vessel wall, they may not be detectable through angiography. In one study, 30% of hematomas were not visualized by angiography. IVUS, on the other hand, allows visualization of all arterial layers, which greatly facilitates detection of intramural hematomas (Figure 20-4).

Calcified plaque   Calcified

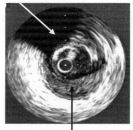 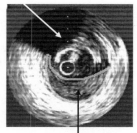

Hematoma   Hematoma

Figure 20-4: An intramural hematoma expands from 3 o'clock to 10 o'clock while a calcified plaque with an acoustic shadow covers the rest of the arterial wall.

Intramural hematoma production is associated with clinical vascular outcomes. Therefore it is important to be aware of this complication of PTCA if it occurs. IVUS can reliably identify it. In a study of 905 patients in native coronary arteries,[11] IVUS detected 72 hematomas out of 1025 PTCAs (7% of PTCAs), occurring in 68 (7.5%) of patients. Surprising, only a minority (18%) of hematomas occurred at the site of the lesion itself, while the remainder occurred in either the proximal (26 of 72) or distal (33 of 72) reference segment, which is defined as the segment with the largest lumen within 10 mm of the lesion. One-month target vessel revascularization was significantly higher in the patients who developed an intramural hematoma (6.3%) versus those who did not (1.9%, P=0.046).

ANEURYSMS: TRUE, FALSE, OR MISDIAGNOSIS?

IVUS can clarify the morphology of coronary abnormalities which appear to be aneurysms on angiography. What appear to be aneurysmal dilatations or "outpouchings" of a coronary vessel on angiography may actually be complex plaques, or even normal arteries adjacent to stenosed segments. In an intracoronary ultrasound study of 77 coronary aneurysms diagnosed by angiography,[12] 21 (27%) were true aneurysms (Figure 20-5) with an intact, three-layered vessel wall, but 41 (53%) were actually short normal segments flanked by stenotic portions. Three (4%) were actually pseudoaneurysms (Figure 20-6), in which vessel perforation had resulted in a disrupted vessel wall, leaving only a residual outward "bulging" monolayer. Twelve (16%) were not aneurysms at all, but complex plaques.

All of the pseudoaneurysms appeared as "saccular" types on angiography, while most (80%) of the normal segments flanked by stenoses had a "fusiform" appearance. True aneurysms and complex plaques appeared as either form equally, thus the angiographic shape of the aneurysm could not predict the true lesion anatomy.

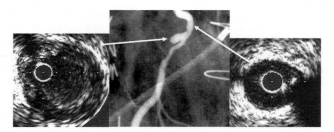

Figure 20-5: True aneurysm has intact, three-layered wall as seen from 1 o'clock to 6 o'clock position.

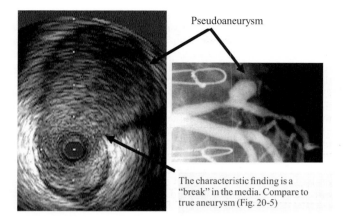

Pseudoaneurysm

The characteristic finding is a "break" in the media. Compare to true aneurysm (Fig. 20-5)

Figure 20-6: The pseudoaneurysm has only one layer in its wall which is the adventitia. The media was ruptured.

In summary, what appear to be coronary aneurysms on angiography may in many cases actually be pseudoaneurysms or not aneurysms at all. This can only be distinguished by IVUS analysis. Therapeutic and interventional decisions are likely to be heavily influenced by IVUS findings in these scenarios.

INTRAVASCULAR ULTRASOUND GUIDED INTERVENTIONS

IVUS can provide valuable insight prior to coronary intervention. Many lesions of various etiologies angiographically appear as areas of haziness. These hazy angiographic sites are often irregular plaques, distorted lumens, napkin-ring lesions, thrombi, or dissections. Also, because IVUS allows visualization beyond the lumen, vascular remodeling assessment or intervention planning in a remodeled vessel can be accomplished. Glagov et al.[13] have shown that coronary arteries will enlarge to accommodate focal deposition of plaque in an attempt to maintain luminal integrity. Since successful compensatory enlargement will preserve the luminal contour, there will be no angiographic stenosis despite the deposition of significant plaque. IVUS measurement can detect expansion of vessels (enlargements of media-to-media diameter) and the focal plaque burden, and allow the interventionalist to size the device appropriately.

Since many stents are difficult to visualize by angiography, complete assessment of adequate deployment is dependent upon IVUS. Angiographic assessment of stent apposition to the vessel wall is limited due to stent radiolucency, which may preclude radiographic identification of the stent silhouette and the propensity of the contrast media to flow outside of the stent borders.[14] In IVUS, stent metal is highly reflective and easy to visualize. As a result, IVUS is the only diagnostic technique that reliably visualizes the stent and adjacent vascular wall to ensure that the struts are well apposed against the wall (Figure 20-7). IVUS data from several clinical trials have indicated that stent deployment frequently results in inadequately expanded stents and unopposed struts, in up to 35% of cases, even after high pressure inflation.[15] In these studies, angiographic examination of the stented segments failed to identify the inadequate deployment that was evident on IVUS analysis.[16–18] There is emerging evidence that stents deployed with IVUS guidance have a lower restenosis rate than those deployed without IVUS.[15,19] This appears to be especially important for small vessel stenting, ostial lesions and patients with diabetes.

In addition to malapposition of stent struts immediately after angioplasty, malapposition may also occur later in the course after stenting. This has been reported after vascular brachytherapy[20] and in patients after implantation of drug coated stents.[21] In typical angioplasty and stenting with bare metal stents, late stent malapposition is seen as well. In one study[22] of 206 patients who had IVUS examinations at a six-month follow-up, nine (4.4%) demonstrated this problem, most commonly occurring at the stent edge. In these nine patients, the cross-sectional area of the vessel itself had grown by an average of 30%. Cross-sectional plaque expansion had occurred, but this accounted for only 75% of the change in vessel size. In other words positive remodeling of the vessel,

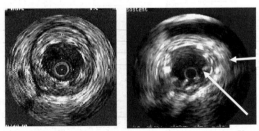

Well-apposed Stent   Unapposed Stent Struts

Vessel Wall

Figure 20-7: A stent with its struts well apposed in the wall. There is no space behind the struts. In contrast, in the second figure, the struts are well apposed in the arc from 9 o'clock to 2 o'clock while there is an empty space between the struts and the intima-media from 3 o'clock to 7 o'clock. The stent struts are not well apposed to the wall.

out of proportion to any change in plaque burden or intimal hyperplasia, accounted for the appearance of separation between stent strut and vessel wall.

Such late malapposition is problematic because it may form a nidus for thrombus formation: an area of altered blood flow (behind the stent struts) in contact with an altered and injured vessel wall. Malapposed stents should be postdilated to correct this problem and prevent subacute thrombosis.

IVUS is also currently being utilized in peripheral arteries, and in carotids. Figure 20-8 displays the cross-sectional images of the distal internal carotid with minimal plaque and the origin of the internal carotid with approximately 90° of calcified plaque. Similar to the coronaries, the tendency to minimize surgical procedures, or to abolish the necessity for operating, has led to an enormous increase in the use of interventional catheter-based therapeutic techniques for the treatment of peripheral vascular disease. Several vascular studies have demonstrated that real-time cross-sectional images may provide accurate information on vascular dynamics, on the composition and extent of atherosclerotic lesions and on the size and shape of the lumen.[23]

NEW ADVANCES IN IVUS UTILIZATION

3-D IVUS imaging: Many new advances have emerged in the area of intravascular ultrasound. Software programs 'stack' two-dimensional images to provide a three-dimensional reconstruction of the coronary and a longitudinal view,

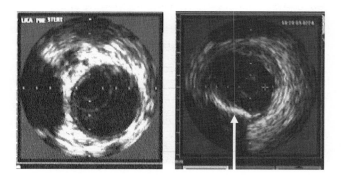

Normal Distal Internal Carotid   **Calcified Carotid Lesion**

Figure 20-8: Cross-sectional images of the distal internal carotid artery with minimal plaque and the origin of the internal carotid artery with calcified plaque.

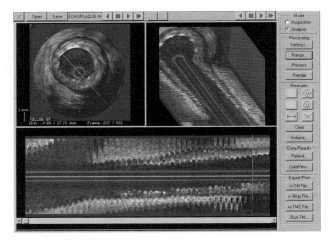

Figure 20-9: Two-dimensional images and three-dimensional reconstruction of the coronary artery giving a longitudinal view, similar to angiography.

similar to the orientation of angiography. These three-dimensional reconstructions facilitate our understanding about the extent and distribution of plaques. Longitudinal views are currently available on most IVUS machines (Figure 20-9).

Prevention of restenosis: Vascular brachytherapy: IVUS has been extensively utilized in clinical trials to evaluate the effectiveness of novel techniques to prevent in-stent restenosis. The use of IVUS allows a greater appreciation for the effectiveness of these new therapies. For example, preliminary results from irradiated stent trials have demonstrated little tissue re-growth within the body of the stent, but excessive tissue growth beginning at the edges of the stent and continuing into the vessel for several millimeters. It has been hypothesized that the radiation dose fall-off at the edges of the stent might be causing this hyperproliferation (Figure 20-10).

Preventing restenosis: Drug-eluting stents: IVUS has played a key role in the evaluation of early and long-term effects of drug-coated stents. IVUS is now considered the gold standard for assessing growth and severity of intimal hyperplasia. The drug-eluting stents (DES) have performed very well even under the intense scrutiny of IVUS interrogation. In a recently published two-year update on sirolimus-eluting stents implanted in 28 patients in Brazil, IVUS revealed that the accumulation of intimal hyperplasia (IH) within the entire length of the 18-mm stent amounted to only about 10 mm^3, an amount occupying only about 7% of the entire volume of the stent's lumen.[24] Late stent malapposition, however, has been recognized in these evaluations (see above). In an IVUS

Irradiated Stent at Index:

Proximal Stent Edge

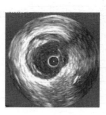

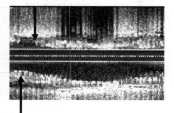

Normal Proximal Stent
Edge at Index

Longitudinal Display at Index

Displayed
Cross-section

Irradiated Stent at Six Month Follow-Up:

Proximal Stent Edge

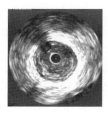

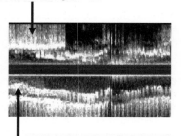

Tissue Proliferation at the
Proximal Edge

Longitudinal Display at Follow Up

Displayed
Cross-Section

Figure 20-10: Standard IVUS image and longitudinal re-constructed display of the proximal stent edge at the index brachytherapy session and at 6-month follow-up. There is geographic miss at the stent edge causing edge restenosis.

substudy of the RAVEL Trial, late stent malapposition was identified in 21% of DES patients, compared to 4% of patients receiving bare metal stents.[25] On a good note, at one year of follow-up, no adverse clinical events had been associated with this finding.

IVUS follow-up examinations of paclitaxel-coated stents has confirmed similar dramatic reductions in IH when compared to bare metal stents. On six-month follow-up of 56 patients receiving paclitaxel-coated stents in Asia, IH burden amounted to 13 to 18 mm^3, compared to 31 mm^3 in patients receiving bare metal stents.[26] This represented 13% to 17%

of the stent volume, compared to 30% in the control group. Minimum lumen area (the cross-sectional area of the "worst" part of the stent) remained above the flow-limiting threshold of 4 mm^2 on average for patients receiving the DES, but fell to an average of 3.1 mm^2 for patients receiving bare metal stents, even though both groups had had similar lumen cross-sectional areas (5.6–5.8 mm^2) immediately after stenting. Late malapposition was identified in this DES group, but occurred in only one patient.

Research into mechanisms of atherosclerosis in acute coronary syndromes: IVUS also plays a role in ongoing research into mechanisms of disease, especially the pathogenesis of plaque rupture and acute myocardial infarction (Figure 20-11). Morphologic studies of plaque rupture have included one study in which IVUS data of 300 ruptured plaques in 254 patients was analyzed for morphologic and angiographic correlates.[27] Twenty-two percent of these patients presented with *stable* angina or were asymptomatic (angiography indicated by noninvasive testing). On angiography, 265 of these 300 plaques were detected, in 223 patients: IVUS identified more ruptured plaques than angiography. By angiographic analysis (QCA), the recognized ruptured plaques predominantly appeared as ulcers (81% of plaques) and in 40% of angiograms a "flap" of intima, a clear indication of plaque disruption, was visualized. Thrombus was seen in only 7%. By IVUS, however, thrombus was visualized in association with 45% of the patients. This occurred more frequently in patients presenting with MI (58% of 83 patients) or unstable angina (42% of 116 patients), versus patients with stable angina (36% of 28 patients) or no symptoms (30% of 27 patients).

The rupture site was also the MLA site in only 28% of patients, while in 117 patients (46%) the narrowest portion of the artery was actually distal to the rupture site. In those cases,

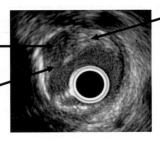

Plaque

Plaque core communicating with the lumen of the vessel

Site of plaque fibrous cap disruption

Figure 20-11: Plaque rupture causing acute coronary syndrome. Here the plaque is soft, without much calcification. There is empty space inside the plaque due to embolization of atherosclerotic material and this is the site for thrombus formation.

the rupture site and the most severe narrowing of the artery were separated by a mean of 4.2 ± 5.8 mm.

The rupture site in general had a larger vessel area associated with it (larger EEM) and larger lumen, and more frequently demonstrated remodeling (73% of rupture site vs 56% of MLA sites). Interestingly, multiple plaque ruptures were observed in 39 of the 254 patients (15%), and of the 33 patients in this retrospective study who had more than one vessel imaged by IVUS, three had multiple ruptured plaques in two separate coronary arteries. In fact, a prospective IVUS study[28] of all three vessels after coronary angiography in patients who were between 3 days and 4 weeks out from a first-ever ACS (STEMI treated with thrombolytics, or NSTEMI with elevated troponin I) revealed that 19 out of 24 patients (79%) had ruptured plaque by IVUS in a location other than the culprit angiographic lesion. Most (71%) of these other plaques were in a different vessel altogether. The majority of patients had one or two additional ruptured plaques, but some had up to five. In total, 50 ruptured plaques were revealed by IVUS (ranging from 0 to 6 per patient), of which 9 were at the site of the culprit angiographic lesion and 41 were elsewhere. This study represents the first to use IVUS comprehensively in all three main coronary arteries to assess atherosclerotic morphology in conjunction with the presentation of ACS. In conclusion, IVUS evidence of ruptured atherosclerotic plaque was seen in a variety of clinical settings, not just the setting of acute MI. Ruptured plaques as identified by IVUS correlated strongly with "complex" lesion morphology on angiography (with ulceration and flaps) and usually did not directly cause lesion compromise. Thrombus was seen more frequently in association with these lesions by IVUS than by angiography, and, perhaps most interesting, plaque destabilization and rupture may be found to occur at multiple sites within the coronary tree of the same patient. This last observation supports the growing concept of acute coronary syndromes as the manifestation of a systemic, probably inflammatory, process, as opposed to one confined to a single "vulnerable" plaque in a patient. Indeed, much work remains to be done regarding the actual triggers of myocardial infarctions.[29,30]

CONCLUSION

By providing *in vivo* cross-sectional visualization of vascular anatomy, intravascular ultrasound provides many advantages over traditional angiography. Through IVUS, plaque burden, distribution, and morphology in the coronary and peripheral vasculature can be determined. Also, IVUS provides an accurate illustration of coronary stents, thus playing a significant role in determining their optimal deployment. Recent advances in IVUS technology, such as those providing three-dimensional reconstruction of the artery, allow clinicians to obtain additional information regarding plaque distribution. Lastly, IVUS has proven to be an effective research tool, currently playing a tremendous role in determining the effectiveness of drug-eluting stents in preventing and treating restenosis.

REFERENCES

1. Yock P, Fitzgerald P, Popp R. Intravascular ultrasound. *Scientific Am Sci Med* 1995; **2**: 68–77.
2. Gussenhoven WJ, Essed CE, Lancee CT *et al.* Arterial wall characteristics determined by intravascular ultrasound imaging: an *in vitro* study. *J Am Coll Cardiol* 1989; **14**: 947–52.
3. Nishimura RA, Edwards WD, Warnes CA *et al.* Intravascular ultrasound imaging: *in vitro* validation and pathologic correlation. *J Am Coll Cardiol* 1990; **16**: 145–54.
4. Mintz GS, Painter JA, Pichard AD *et al.* Atherosclerosis in angiographically 'normal' coronary artery reference segments: an intravascular ultrasound study with clinical correlations. *J Am Coll Cardiol* 1995; **25**: 1479–85.
5. Tuzcu EM, Berkalp B, DeFranco AC *et al.* The dilemma of diagnosing coronary calcification: angiography versus intravascular ultrasound. *J Am Coll Cardiol* 1996; **27**: 832–8.
6. Kobayashi Y, Yock PG, Fitzgerald PJ. Perivascular IVUS landmarks. *Intravascular Imaging* 1998; **2**: 35–42.
7. Abizaid A, Mintz GS, Pichard AD *et al.* Clinical, intravascular ultrasound, and quantitative angiographic determinants of the coronary flow reserve before and after percutaneous transluminal coronary angioplasty. *Am J Cardiol* 1998; **82**(4): 423–8.
8. Takagi A, Tsurumi Y, Ishii Y, Suzuki K, Kawana M, Kasanuki H. Clinical potential of intravascular ultrasound for physiological assessment of coronary stenosis: relationship between quantitative ultrasound tomography and pressure-derived fractional flow reserve. *Circulation* 1999; **100**(3): 250–5.
9. Nishioka T, Amanullah AM, Luo H *et al.* Clinical validation of intravascular ultrasound imaging for assessment of coronary stenosis severity: comparison with stress myocardial perfusion imaging. *J Am Coll Cardiol* 1999; **33**(7): 1870–8.
10. Mintz GS, Nissen SE (Co-chairs). American College of Cardiology clinical expert consensus document on standards for acquisition, measurement and reporting of intravascular ultrasound studies (IVUS). *J Am Coll Cardiol* 2001; **37**(5): 1478–92.
11. Maehara A, Mintz GS, Bui AB *et al.* Incidence, morphology, angiographic findings, and outcomes of intramural hematomas after percutaneous coronary interventions: an intravascular ultrasound study. *Circulation* 2002; **105**: 2037–42.

12. Maehara A, Mintz GS, Ahmed JM *et al*. An intravascular ultrasound classification of angiographic coronary artery aneurysms. *Am J Cardiol* 2001; **88**: 365–70.

13. Glagov S, Weisenerg E, Zarins CK, Stankunavicius R, Kolettis GJ. Compensatory enlargement of human atherosclerotic coronary arteries. *N Engl J Med* 1987; **316**: 1371–5.

14. Ziada KM, Tuzcu M, Nissen SE. The role of intravascular ultrasound imaging in contemporary stenting. *Intravascular Imaging* 1997; **1**: 73–9.

15. Russo RJ, Nicosia A, Teirstein PS for AVID Investigators. Angiography versus intravascular ultrasound-directed stent placement [abstract]. *J Am Coll Cardiol* 1997; (suppl): 707–14.

16. Goldberg SL, Colombo A, Nakamura S *et al*. Benefit of intracoronary ultrasound in the deployment of Palmaz-Schatz stents. *J Am Coll Cardiol* 1994; **24**: 996–1003.

17. Nakamura S, Colombo A, Gaglione A *et al*. Intracoronary ultrasound observations during stent implantation. *Circulation* 1994; **89**: 2026–34.

18. Kiemeneij F, Laarman GJ, Slagboom T. Mode of deployment of coronary Palmaz-Schatz stents after implantation with the stent delivery system: an intravascular ultrasound study. *Am Heart J* 1995; **129**: 638–44.

19. Hayase M, Oshima A, Zidar JP *et al*. Comparison of ultrasound vs angiographic guidance for stenting in the CRUISE study [abstract]. *Circulation* 1996; **94** (suppl 1): 1228.

20. Mintz GS, Weissman NJ, Fitzgerald PJ. Intravascular ultrasound assessment of the mechanisms and results of brachytherapy. *Circulation* 2001; **104**: 1320–25.

21. Serruys PW, Degertekin M, Tanabe K *et al*. Intravascular ultrasound findings in the multicenter randomized double blind RAVEL (Randomized study with the sirolimus Velocity balloon-expandable stent in the treatment of patients with de novo native coronary artery Lesions) Trial. *Circulation* 2002; **106**: 798–803.

22. Shah VM, Mintz GS, Apple S, Weissman NJ. Background incidence of late malapposition after bare metal stent implantation. *Circulation* 2002; **106**: 1753–55.

23. Gussenhoven EJ, Hagenaars T, van Essen J, Honkoop J, van der Lugt A, van Lankeren W, van Overhagen H, Bom N. What has been learnt from 10 years of peripheral IVUS? *Intravascular Imaging* 1998; **2**: 43–50.

24. Sousa JE, Costa MA, Sousa AGMR *et al*. Two-year angiographic and intravascular ultrasound follow-up after implantation of sirolimus-eluting stents in human coronary arteries. *Circulation* 2003; **107**: 381–83.

25. Serruys PW, Degertekin M, Tanabe K *et al*. Intravascular ultrasound findings in the multicenter, randomized, double-blind RAVEL (Randomized study with the sirolimus-elucint Velocity balloon-expandable stent in the treatment of patients

with de novo native coronary artery Lesions) trial. *Circulation* 2002; **106**: 798–803.

26. Hong MK, Mintz GS, Lee CW *et al*. Paclitaxel coating reduces in-stent intimal hyperplasia in human coronary arteries: A serial volumetric intravascular ultrasound analysis from the Asian Paclitaxel-Eluting Stent Clinical Trial (ASPECT). *Circulation* 2003; **107**: 517–20.

27. Maehara A, Mintz GS, Bui AB *et al*. Morphologic and angiographic features of coronary plaque rupture detected by intravascular ultrasound. *J Am Coll Cardiol* 2002; **40**: 904–10.

28. Rioufol G, Finet G, Ginon I *et al*. Multiple atherosclerotic plaque rupture in acute coronary syndrome: A three-vessel intravascular ultrasound study. *Circulation* 2002; **106**: 804–8.

29. Weissman NJ. Intracoronary ultrasound. *Coronary Artery Disease* 1998; **9**: 435–41.

30. Weissman NJ. Update on intravascular ultrasound. *J Interv Cardiol* 1998; **11**: S83–S86.

—— *Chapter 21* ——

Percutaneous Ilio-femoral Revascularizations

Krishna Rocha Singh

GENERAL OVERVIEW

Percutaneous endovascular therapy of the ilio-femoral tree is the most frequently performed peripheral intervention and is an accepted first line of interventional care in selected patients with intermittent claudication (IC) in whom exercise treatment combined with pharmacologic therapy (i.e. cilostazol) has failed.[1] While the degree of a patient's disability is a prime consideration, the anticipated short- and long-term

*Basic; **Advanced; ***Rare, exotic, or investigational.

From: Nguyen T, Hu D, Saito S, Grines C, Palacios I (eds), *Practical Handbook of Advanced Interventional Cardiology*, 2nd edn. © 2003 Futura, an imprint of Blackwell Publishing.

clinical benefits are the major determinants of the role of catheter techniques in patients with ilio-femoral disease. Balloon angioplasty and metallic stents have made major technologic advances that have improved acute procedural results and increased the use of endovascular procedures in patients with more extensive, complex disease; however, the long-term clinical efficacy of endovascular procedures in complex lesion types has not been fully defined.

INDICATIONS

Management of these two lesion groups will vary according to local standards, individual physician experience, and available technology. The procedural and clinical success rates of iliac PTA in IC patients are generally high (80–100%) with 5-year patency rates approaching 60–80%.[2] The introduction of balloon-expandable metallic stents has improved procedural success and is indicated for the treatment of a suboptimal PTA result (dissection flaps, arterial recoil, residual pressure gradient). Clinical experience has evolved to include the following general recommendations: PTA restenosis, chronic occlusion, ostial disease, and symptomatic iliac artery ulceration. However, the usefulness and cost-effectiveness of multiple stent use is unknown.

EVIDENCE-BASED MEDICINE APPLICATIONS

The TransAtlantic Inter-Society Consensus for Iliac Disease: The TransAtlantic Inter-Society Consensus (TASC) document provides evidence-based recommendations for the treatment of IC patients.[1] Ilio-femoral lesions are classified into four categories: types A–D. The two extremes are type A lesions (i.e. stenosis <3 cm), in which an endovascular approach is the procedure of choice, and type D lesions (i.e. diffuse stenoses 5–10 cm or occlusions) in which surgery is preferred. There are no firm recommendations for the treatment of type B lesions (occlusion <3 cm/stenosis 3–5 cm) and type C lesions (occlusion >3 cm/stenosis 5–10 cm); however, endovascular treatment is more often used in type B lesions and surgery in type C lesions (Table 21-1).

EVIDENCE-BASED MEDICINE APPLICATIONS

The TransAtlantic Inter-Society Consensus for Femoropopliteal Disease: In contrast to the excellent procedural and clinical success of iliac PTA, results of superficial femoral artery (SFA) PTA have been less encouraging. SFA lesions have been categorized in a fashion similar to iliac circulation using lesion types A–D. Type A lesions (ste-

Table 21-1
The TASC recommendations for iliac artery disease

	Iliac lesions	Treatment of choice
TASC Type A	Single stenosis <3 cm of CIA/EIA (unilateral or bilateral)	Endovascular
TASC Type B	Single stenosis 3–10 cm not extending into CFA Total of 2 stenoses <5 cm in CIA and/or EIA and not into CFA Unilateral CIA occlusion	Uncertain
TASC Type C	Bilateral 5–10 cm stenosis of CIA and/or EIA, not into CFA Unilateral EIA occlusion not into CFA Unilateral EIA stenosis extending into CFA Bilateral CIA occlusions	Uncertain
TASC Type D	Diffuse, multiple unilateral stenoses involving CIA, EIA, CFA (usually > 10 cm) Unilateral occlusion involving both CIA and EIA Bilateral EIA occlusions Diffuse disease involving the aorta and both iliac arteries Iliac stenoses in a patient with an AAA	Surgery

CIA = common iliac artery; EIA = external iliac artery; CFA = common femoral artery; AAA = abdominal aortic aneurysm.

nosis <3 cm) are considered ideal for PTA, while long (>5 cm) occlusions are generally best treated surgically. Published experience in type B and C lesions is insufficient to make firm recommendations; however, several additional factors are important considerations in treating IC patients with SFA disease (Table 21-2).

First, these patients are generally older, with a higher incidence of symptomatic coronary artery disease, and the preservation of saphenous vein "capital" for future possible coronary artery bypass surgery should be considered. In this regard, treatment of long occlusive disease may be considered as it is claimed that once an occlusion has been recanalized, the long-term patency does not differ in comparison to a stenosis although the technical success rate is greater in treating a stenosis versus an occlusion (>90% vs 75–85%, respectively). Additionally, close attention must be paid to the number of patent infrapopliteal vessels as patients with poor run-off (0–1 vessels) consistently show poorer long-term outcomes than those with 2–3 vessel run-off.[1]

Table 21-2
The TASC recommendations for femoropopliteal disease

	Femoropopliteal lesion	Treatment of choice
TASC Type A	Single stenosis <3 cm (unilateral/ bilateral)	Endovascular
TASC Type B	Single stenosis 3–10 cm not involving distal popliteal	Uncertain
	Heavily calcified stenoses up to 3 cm	
	Multiple lesions, each <3 cm (stenosis or occlusion)	
	Single or multiple lesions in absence of continuous tibial run-off to improve inflow for distal surgical bypass	
TASC Type C	Single stenosis of occlusion > 5 cm	Uncertain
	Multiple stenoses/occlusion, each 3–5 cm, ± heavy calcification	Uncertain
TASC Type D	Complete CFA or SFA occlusion or complete popliteal and proximal trifurcation occlusions	Surgery

CFA = common femoral artery; SFA = superficial femoral artery.

> The routine use of stents as a primary intervention in treating SFA disease is not supported by available data. The intermediate and long-term patency rates are no different from PTA patency rates; however, stents may have a limited role in salvaging acute PTA failures or complications.[1,3]

DIAGNOSTIC ANGIOGRAPHY

Diagnostic contrast angiography represents the foundation of peripheral endovascular work; however, angiography should be performed in IC patients only after the decision to intervene has been made, if a suitable lesion is identified. While angiography carries a 0.1% risk of contrast reaction and a 0.7% complication risk severe enough to alter the patient's management,[4] use of nonionic contrast agents, limited views in patients with renal impairment, and magnetic resonance angiography (MRA) or color duplex imaging may be appropriate alternatives to angiography. In expert hands, both MRA and duplex Doppler are noninvasive and safe, and can provide essential anatomic information. Nevertheless, full angiography, with visualization from the renal arteries to the pedal arteries, remains the "gold standard."

Cardiologists are very familiar with angiographic techniques and have ready access to coronary imaging equipment; however, they may not have access to peripheral imaging equipment utilizing larger image intensifiers that incorporate larger fields (i.e. 15" image intensifier). Therefore, the ability to perform a peripheral angiogram using a smaller 9" intensifier is imperative. In most catheterization laboratory configurations, this can be done safely while minimizing excess contrast use via a single access site.

STANDARD TECHNIQUE

Peripheral angiogram on a 9" image intensifier: Elevate table height maximally and then bring the image intensifier down as close to the patient as possible to reduce magnification and to include as much anatomy as possible on 9" magnification. A radiopaque millimeter ruler or marker tape and a table-mounted injector are desirable. Recommended catheters and sheaths are listed in Table 21-3. If using cine angiography, contrast cannot be diluted. Use a pressure injector to create less streaming and good opacification (Table 21-3).

TECHNICAL TIP

**Optimal abdomino-femoral angiography: Use the racquet to inject the abdominal aorta, including the kidneys.
Protocol: 10 cc rate, 20 cc volume, no rate rise, and 1050 psi. The top of the racquet catheter should be placed at T-12; most renal arteries come off at L-2.
Bring the racquet catheter to the aortic bifurcation and inject at 25° RAO and LAO oblique views of the internal/external iliac arteries. Try to include the femoral necks of the femur so the SFA/profunda femoris bifurcation can be included without clipping the internal/external iliac artery bifurcation. Protocol: 10 cc rate, 20 cc volume at 1050 psi; use a 0.4-sec injection delay to allow for DSA masking.
Use the soft-angled Glidewire to place the crossover or LIMA catheter at the level of the contralateral distal external iliac artery to image the SFA. You may wish to extend the

Table 21-3
Recommended catheters and sheaths

5F sheath
5F racquet × 65 cm if via the common femoral artery approach
5F Crossover or LIMA catheter (to traverse the aortic bifurcation)
0.035 Soft × 260 cm angled Glidewire (Medi-Tech)
30" LV connector tube
5F Multipurpose catheter

wire further and exchange for a Multipurpose catheter. Do not use an end-hole catheter; a side-hole catheter is preferable. Start selective injections one leg at a time. Protocol: SFA: 8–10 cc rate and 8–10 cc volume. As you move into the infrapopliteal segments, larger volumes (10–20 cc) may be required to obtain good images. Pull back the Multipurpose catheter to the ipsilateral side at the level of the distal external iliac and image the ipsilateral SFA.

In the ilio-femoral tree, a diagnostic study includes straight anterior-posterior (AP) pelvic angiography with appropriate oblique views to define the ostia of the common iliac arteries, the bifurcation of the external and internal iliac arteries, and bifurcation of the superficial femoral and profunda femoral arteries. A "20/20 view" (20° contralateral angulation with 20° caudal angulation) is used to best define the relationship between the internal and the external iliac arteries. This view is particularly important as overlap of the internal and external iliac arteries may obscure significant disease.

PERIPHERAL ANGIOPLASTY AND STENTING

An experienced interventional cardiologist possesses many of the fundamental technical skills required to perform many basic peripheral interventional procedures. Indeed, many of the standard skills reviewed in Chapter 6 are applicable here; therefore, only important differences will be highlighted.

Arterial approach: Revascularization of any particular lesion in the ilio-femoral segment may be approached from one or more arterial access sites, either used solely or in combination. The decision to proceed with any particular access route must consider the ability to palpate and enter the access artery, the potential disease that may be encountered in reaching the desired arterial segment, equipment availability (i.e. long wires, sheaths, balloons, and stents), anticipated use of thrombolytic agents, and angiographic suite capabilities. In general, iliac stenoses are easily approached from the ipsilateral retrograde approach, while occlusive disease, depending on the proximity of the lesion to the common iliac ostium and the common femoral artery inlet, is easily approached from either the contralateral or the ipsilateral side. Frequently, particularly with occlusive disease, the brachial approach may be used because it allows for maximal coaxial manipulation of hydrophilic wires. The recommendations for vascular access are listed in Table 21-4.

TECHNICAL TIP

**Rationale for selection of vascular access: A short right external iliac occlusion may be approached: (1) Retrograde from the right common femoral artery. This approach

Table 21-4
Recommendations for vascular access

Location of lesions	Vascular access and arteries
Aortic bifurcation	Bilateral retrograde CFA
Common and external iliacs	Ipsilateral retrograde CFA
CFA, proximal SFA/PFA	Contralateral retrograde CFA
Mid/distal SFA/popliteal	Ipsilateral antegrade CFA

CFA = common femoral artery; SFA = superficial femoral artery; PFA = profunda femoral artery.

is most useful for all iliac artery lesions except those in the very distal external iliac artery. (2) Antegrade around the aortic bifurcation from the left common femoral artery. This approach is particularly useful in distal external iliac lesions or with lesions in the proximal internal iliac artery. It should be avoided for lesions in the very proximal common iliac because of the limited working area between the lesion and the aortic bifurcation. (3) From the right or left brachial artery. This approach may be useful in addressing long iliac occlusions where coaxial wire manipulation is desirable. Importantly, this approach should be avoided if thrombolytic therapy is anticipated.

Lesions that begin at the orifice of the common iliac artery impose a potential risk of "plaque shift" that may compromise the contralateral common iliac ostium. In this case, the "kissing balloon" technique protects the contralateral side, even in the absence of significant disease at the contralateral iliac ostium (see below).

SFA-popliteal segments are approached in an antegrade manner, either from the ipsilateral common femoral artery or from the contralateral side around the aortic bifurcation (see Chapter 1). Long occlusive SFA disease is best approached from the antegrade common femoral artery or retrograde from the popliteal artery as these two approaches allow for maximal coaxial manipulation of wires and pushing the catheters and balloons; the ability to torque/manipulate guidewires can be diminished when working from the contralateral side. Lesions in the proximal SFA, in bypass grafts, or in patients with high SFA/profunda femoral bifurcations are best treated by the contralateral approach.

Sheath selection: Appropriate sheath selection for the performance of peripheral interventions is akin to appropriate guiding catheter selection for the successful performance of coronary interventions. Appropriate sheath diameter, length, and flexibility allow for multiple wire and balloon exchanges, adequate contrast visualization of the lesion while minimizing contrast use, injecting vasodilators (i.e. nitroglycerin), and measuring pressure gradients while providing adequate support for delivery of devices (i.e. stents). Sheath length and flexibility are especially crucial for ipsilateral antegrade cannulation of the SFA and passage over the aortic bifurcation.

Balloon selection: A wide array of angioplasty balloons is commercially available. In selecting a given balloon, the following criteria should be considered: glidewire compatibility (0.014", 0.018", and 0.035"). The diameter of the balloon should be equivalent to the reference diameter. The general recommendations for the size of the balloons are listed in Table 21-5.

> **TECHNICAL TIP**
>
> ****The selection of balloon:** A balloon with a diameter equivalent to the reference segment should be selected. If the vessel diameter is in question, consider the use of intravascular ultrasound to better ascertain the true diameter. If in doubt, always underdilate the lesion to avoid rupture. Pay attention to the sheath size since larger diameter balloons, once inflated, may be difficult to retract. Compliant or semi-compliant balloon materials will permit oversizing while non-compliant, high-pressure balloon materials (i.e. Duralyn ST, Cordis) will avoid oversizing and the potential for vessel rupture.

Wire selection: The choice of a guidewire should take into consideration whether the diseased segment is stenotic or occluded, the vessel diameter and tortuosity, and device compatibility. In general, in larger vessels, a 0.035"−0.038" system (Wholey Wire or Magi-Torque Wire) is compatible; the TAD II wire system combines a 0.018" steerable, shapeable tip with a 0.035" shaft that makes crossing difficult lesions easier. In smaller vessels, 0.014" or 0.018" systems are best. Occluded vessels are best traversed using a hydrophilic glidewire; however, extreme care should be taken because these wires may pass easily into a subintimal course. Once the occlusion is traversed, the hydrophilic wire should be exchanged for a non-hydrophilic wire.

Table 21-5
General recommendations for selection of balloon size

Location	Recommended size
Common iliacs	8−10 mm
External iliacs	6−7 mm
Common femoral	5−6 mm
SFA	5−6 mm
Popliteal artery	4−5 mm

Traversing the aortic bifurcation: A preprocedure angiogram should be performed to make sure the common iliac arteries, aortic bifurcation is free of significant disease, aneurysmal, or occlusive disease. If significant disease is present, consider pretreatment (PTA, stenting) or an alternate approach (i.e. brachial approach). The angle of aortic bifurcation should be evaluated in detail. Consider the appropriate angle of the catheter to be used to traverse the bifurcation; the tighter the angle of the aortic bifurcation, the tighter the angle ("hook") of the catheter. In most circumstances, a 5F Crossover or IMA Catheter (Cordis) or Cobra 1 or 2 catheter will suffice.

TECHNICAL TIP

**The art of traversing the aortic bifurcation: Place the traversing catheter at the aortic bifurcation and "hook" the ostium of the contralateral common iliac artery. Make sure the catheter does not abrade the aortic wall and disrupt plaque. Advance a soft 0.035" wire (soft-angled Glidewire) through the catheter and advance the wire into either the profunda femoral or the SFA a sufficient distance to allow passage of the 5F catheter around the bifurcation and into the contralateral external iliac.

Remove the soft Glidewire and replace it with an Extra-Stiff J Amplatz Wire (Medi-Tech). Use an appropriately long flexible braided sheath (Arrow Sheath) with dilator in place. Carefully monitor the tip of the J wire to prevent distal migration during the passage of the braided sheath. Remove the sheath's dilator and maintain the J wire position. For most situations, a 7F sheath is sufficient to deliver self-expanding metallic stents and balloons. Balloons >10 mm diameter may require an 8F sheath. An appropriate sheath length advanced near the lesion site will simplify the procedure by minimizing fluoroscopy and contrast use.

When advancing or removing the Arrow Sheath, always replace the sheath dilator to prevent causing intimal dissection by the sheath's tip.

If catheter tracking over the aortic bifurcation angulation is inadequate due to severe angulation or tortuosity, use a shorter contralateral sheath that extends a relatively short distance into the contralateral common iliac.

Kissing balloons/stents technique: Disease that involves the distal aorta and/or orifice of either common iliac artery may require elevation of aortic bifurcation using the "kissing" balloon/stent technique. The sheaths are placed retrograde in both common femoral arteries and guidewires advanced into the distal aorta. Appropriately sized balloons of adequate length are passed over the glidewires and positioned in the distal aorta and common iliac arteries to cover the diseased segments. It is important to realize that simultaneously inflated balloons reach a diameter greater than their sum. Therefore, separate inflations of balloons of differing diameters may be required to treat disease in the distal aorta and proximal common iliac arteries.

The proximal radiopaque markers of each balloon should overlap slightly. Both balloons are inflated simultaneously using inflation devices or by hand using contrast-filled syringes. The angioplasty result is frequently inadequate due to elastic recoil and heavy calcification of this arterial segment and stenting is required.

TECHNICAL TIP

**The art of kissing stents deployment: 7F long sheaths, with dilators in place, are passed into the distal aorta over the indwelling glidewire. Appropriately sized balloon-expandable stents are crimped on balloons of desired diameter and length. The chosen diameter should be matched to the common iliac artery diameter, and the chosen length should be sufficient to cover the entire distal aortic and iliac lesions while being well anchored in the common iliac artery. The balloon-mounted stents are passed into the sheaths and positioned in the distal aorta such that the radiopaque balloon markers are "kissing" and not overlapping. The sheaths are withdrawn and stent position reconfirmed. Inflation devices are used to deploy the stents to ensure that balloon pressure is equal bilaterally. If needed, larger balloon diameters may be required to fully deploy the aortic portion of the stented segment. Care should be taken to avoid overdilating the iliac portion. This technique effectively elevates the aortic bifurcation several millimeters. Simultaneous peak-to-peak gradients from the distal aorta to the common femoral arteries should be <5 mm.

Management of total occlusive disease: Successful recanalization of a long occluded arterial segment represents a significant technical challenge that is associated with a complication rate twice that of revascularization of a stenotic arterial segment. Distal embolization, arterial rupture, or loss of collateral circulation associated with attempted recanalization can result in significant patient morbidity, potential mortality, and added expense. Procedural success is reduced with increased vessel tortuosity, lesion length, chronicity, and heavy calcification. Furthermore, the durability of a successful recanalization is predicted by these same factors. The recommended equipment is listed in Table 21-6.

TECHNICAL TIPS

**Preprocedural assessment and strategic planning: Assess the proximal and distal patent arteries angiographi-

Table 21-6
Recommended equipment for total occlusion

0.035" Glidewire (Wholey Wire or Magic Cross Wire)
0.035" Soft and Extra-Stiff hydrophilic J and angled wires
(Glidewire – MediTech)
0.018" hydrophilic glidewire (V-18 Wire – Medi-Tech)
5F hydrophilic end-hole catheters (Glide-Cath – Medi-Tech)
4F NYL Exchange Catheter (Medi-Tech)

cally (DSA is best) to determine the occlusion length, extent
of calcification, takeoff of collateral vessels, vessel tortuosity, and the vessel's embolic risk. These lesions include
those with visible thrombus, highly ulcerated plaque, aneurysmal lesions, and those located near the distal aorta.

Look specifically for the presence of a "nipple" at the
leading edge of the occlusion; this will facilitate glidewire
penetration into the occluded segment. Use a "road map"
angiogram to allow visualization of the entire occlusion
simultaneously. Use "road signs" (i.e. calcified segments,
position of collateral vessels) to construct a path in your
mind's eye.

**The art of crossing a total occlusive lesion: Advance
a 0.035" steerable glidewire into the lesion to assess its tex-
ture; if it contains significant thrombus, continue to advance
the wire. If the lesion is particularly calcified, consider use of
an extra-stiff angled hydrophilic wire. If the hydrophilic wire
buckles easily, advance a straight end-hole 5F catheter
(e.g. Glide Cath) to support the wire tip. However, do not
advance the straight catheter ahead of the wire because
this may result in arterial perforation.

Using a glidewire torque device, use a "drilling" motion
of the wire tip while slowly advancing and withdrawing the
wire. Pay attention to the "road signs" to guide you. Oblique
views are helpful to assure that you remain intraluminal. Inject small amounts of contrast through the sheath to assess
the exact position of the wire; if a subintimal course is suspected, withdraw the glidewire a short distance and redirect
its path. A new plane is often difficult to find; try a catheter
with a gentle bend at its tip (e.g. Berenstein catheter) to
direct the wire into another plane. If the guidewire will not
traverse the occlusion, leave the wire in place as a marker
and approach the occlusion from the opposite direction, if
possible. Use oblique views to assess the position of the two
wire tips. Balloon angioplasty should be considered only after the guidewire has traversed the entire occlusion. A subintimal glidewire course, though less desirable, is generally
unavoidable in large vessels. Primary stent deployment can
effectively resolve extensive arterial dissections.

**The "pull-through" technique: This technique is particularly useful in traversing a long occlusive iliac artery or in SFA disease and is an important adjunct technique when an ipsilateral retrograde or contralateral antegrade approach fails. On many occasions, this technique represents the final attempt at occlusive disease since it provides the opportunity to redirect a hydrophilic guidewire along a different intravascular path as it allows for improved "pushability" of wires.

1. Place a 5F sheath in the brachial artery. The presence of known supra-aortic disease and/or tortuosity and the quality of the radial pulse should be used to determine whether the right or the left brachial artery should be used.
2. A preprocedure angiogram should be performed to fully define the presence of distal aortic disease, the extent of occlusive disease, and the extent of bifurcation disease (Figure 21-1). In the illustrated case, occlusive disease involving the right common iliac and a high-grade stenosis involving the left common iliac are seen. This case will require both the pull-through technique and elevation of the aortic bifurcation.

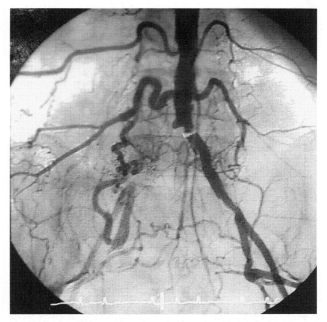

Figure 21-1: Preangioplasty angiogram with total occlusion of right iliac artery.

3. To allow imaging, a racket catheter is advanced via the left common femoral artery. Either a Multipurpose or an Amplatz L1 catheter is used because they provide excellent torqueability and "pushability." The tip of the catheter is imbedded in the "nipple" of the right iliac occlusion; using a 0.035" extra-stiff angled glidewire, the occlusion is gently probed (Figure 21-2).

4. Using a "drill" motion of the glidewire, the occlusion is traversed and the wire is placed in the external iliac (Figure 21-3).

5. The glidewire is extended through the right common femoral artery and into the SFA (Figure 21-4). Using the glidewire and femoral head as a landmark, a retrograde puncture of the right common femoral artery is performed and a 7F sheath is placed.

6. With the arterial sheath filled with contrast, the glidewire is maneuvered into the sheath (Figure 21-5) and

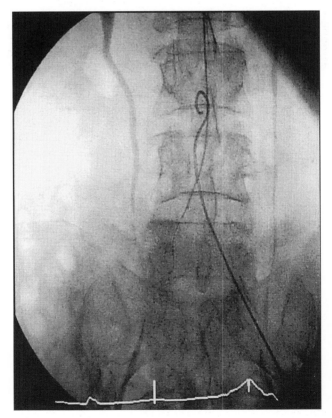

Figure 21-2

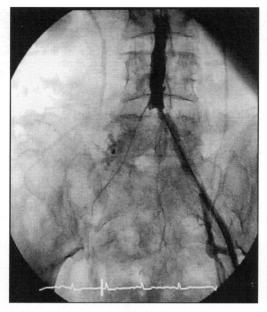

Figure 21-3

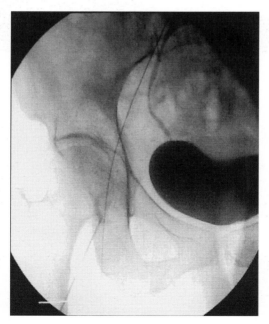

Figure 21-4

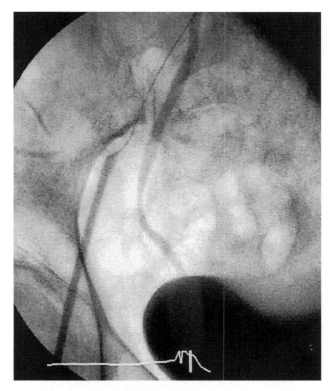

Figure 21-5

placed in the hub of the sheath. Using a vascular clamp, the external portion of the vascular sheath with the glidewire within the sheath is clamped and the wire is externalized as the vascular sheath with the attached wire is pulled through the right groin site (Figure 21-6).

7. A 7F sheath is placed on the externalized portion of the glidewire and the glidewire is pulled through the brachial arterial sheath to the level of the aortic bifurcation (Figures 21-7, 21-8).

8. Over the externalized glidewire, an angioplasty balloon is placed and advanced up through the occlusive lesion into the distal aorta. The glidewire is removed for a standard J wire and balloon angioplasty is performed (Figure 21-9).

9. A 0.035" Magic Torque wire is passed via the left common femoral artery, and balloon angioplasty of both the right and left common iliac arteries is performed (Figure 21-10); "kissing" stents are positioned (Figure 21-11).

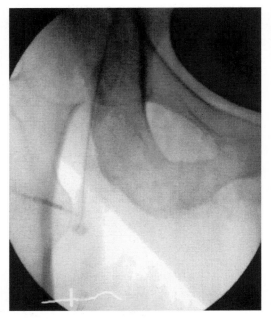

Figure 21-6

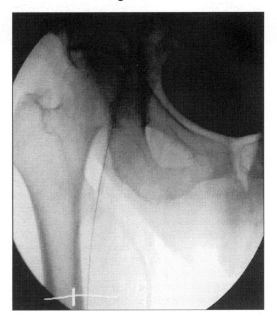

Figure 21-7

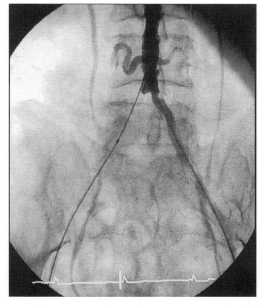

Figure 21-8

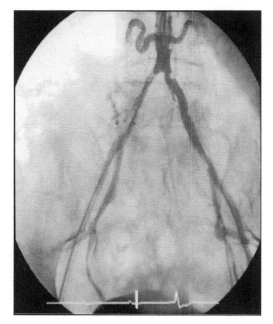

Figure 21-9

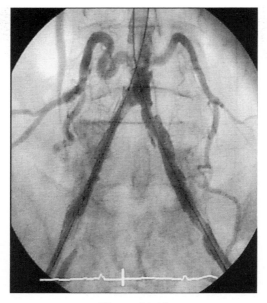

Figure 21-10

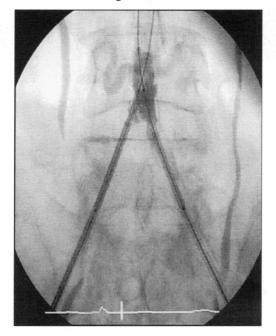

Figure 21-11

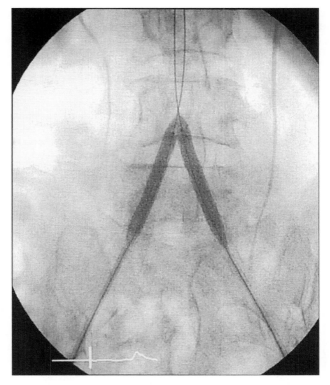

Figure 21-12

10. "Kissing" stents are deployed and an excellent final angiographic result with no significant pressure gradients between the distal aorta and common femoral arteries is achieved (Figure 21-12).

COMPLICATIONS

The rate of ilio-femoral endovascular complications requiring additional treatment or altering the patient's management is generally low (2.0–2.5%). However, the following complications may result in significant morbidity, risk of amputation, increased cost, and increased mortality.

Acute arterial occlusion: An acute arterial occlusion occurring after balloon angioplasty, most likely caused by arterial dissection, however, should be distinguished from arterial vasospasm. Deployment of a self-expanding Nitinol stent (i.e. SMART Stent) or braided metal stent (i.e. Wallstent) over the entire length of the dissection plane usually returns arterial patency.

Subacute arterial thrombosis may occur hours to days after the initial intervention and is associated with a heavy thrombus burden and risk for distal embolization. The recent withdrawal of urokinase from the US market has drawn attention to new thrombolytic strategies. The combined use of intravenous glycoprotein 2b3a receptor inhibitors (i.e. ReoPro, Lilly) with a low-dose of intra-arterial thrombolytic agent (i.e. Retavase, Centacor) is, in theory, attractive because it reduces the total dose of thrombolytic agent, which is associated with a higher rate of intracranial hemorrhage and reduced platelet activation, and may increase the rate of platelet-rich thrombus disaggregation. The protocol of ReoPro-Retavase infusion is shown in Table 21-7.

Arterial rupture: Arterial rupture may result in death and should be treated aggressively with surgical intervention. Do not stent a ruptured arterial segment with the hope that the stent will seal the rupture site; immediate balloon tamponade should be performed and reversal of heparin anticoagulation considered. The most common cause of angioplasty-associated arterial rupture is overdilatation.

TECHNICAL TIP

Arterial rupture: (1) Carefully consider the balloon diameter to be used; if in doubt, always use a smaller diameter balloon. Consider ultrasound to best assess luminal diameter. (2) Do not overdilate balloon-expandable stents; a simultaneous pressure gradient should be used to guide procedural completion and less attention paid to a perceived minor angiographic defect. (3) Accept an adequate result; know when to quit. Contained contrast extravasation or deep arterial wall straining should be closely observed. Prolonged, low-atmosphere balloon inflation may adequately seal these minor rupture sites; stenting should not be considered. Rupture of the SFA, popliteal, or tibial vessels is less likely to be life-threatening; however, it may result in arterial thrombosis or a compartment syndrome.

Table 21-7
ReoPro-Retavase protocol for acute arterial thrombosis

---

1. ReoPro (abciximab) 0.25 µg/kg bolus + 0.125 µg/kg/min intravenously × 12 hours or
2. Retavase (reteplase) 0.25–0.5 U/hr ± 3–5 U lace directly into the thrombus via a coaxial system × 24–48 hours.
3. Heparin 2000 U bolus and 500 U/hr; the heparin dose is not altered on the basis of the aPTT.

Close monitoring of distal pulses, tissue perfusion, and the neurovascular examination are important.

REFERENCES

1. TASC Working Group: Management of Peripheral Arterial Disease (PAD): TransAtlantic Inter-Society Consensus (TASC). *J Vasc Surg* 2000; **31**: S54–S126.

2. Brewster DC. Current controversies in the management of aortoiliac occlusive disease. *J Vasc Surg* 1997; **25**: 365–379.

3. Cejna M, Illiasch H, Waldenberg P *et al*. PTA versus Palmaz stent in femoropopliteal arterial occlusive disease: A prospective randomized trial – long-term results. *Radiology* 1998; **209**: 492.

4. Waugh JR, Sacharias N. Arteriographic complications in the DSA era. *Radiology* 1992; **182**: 243.

Chapter 22

Carotid Artery Interventions

Kasja Rabe, Herbert Cordero, Richard Heuser, L Nelson Hopkins, Horst Sievert

---

*Basic; **Advanced; ***Rare, exotic, or investigational.

From: Nguyen T, Hu D, Saito S, Grines C, Palacios I (eds), *Practical Handbook of Advanced Interventional Cardiology*, 2nd edn. © 2003 Futura, an imprint of Blackwell Publishing.

GENERAL OVERVIEW

Cerebrovascular strokes account for 500,000 deaths per year in the United States. Half of the patients that survive a stroke are permanently disabled.[1] Several epidemiologic studies have shown that ischemic events are four times more frequent than hemorrhagic events. The incidence of ischemic strokes increases with age (33% if <45 and 80% >50).[1] Carotid disease accounts for nearly one-third of all ischemic stroke cases. In patients with more severe and symptomatic disease, surgical intervention has been the main method of therapy.

After the introduction of carotid endarterectomy (CEA) as a therapy for the prevention of ischemic stroke due to carotid artery stenosis,[2,3] this treatment modality was widely used all over the world with more than 1 million procedures until 1985 although initial trials comparing surgery and medical treatment were negative.[4,5] Only in the early 1990s did several randomized trials show the superiority of surgery over medical treatment. After encouraging results obtained with angioplasty and stenting in the coronary,[6] renal, and peripheral vascular systems, applications of these new technologies were made to the cerebrovascular system. The first experience with balloon angioplasty of carotid bifurcation lesions was reported in 1979.[7,8] Elective stenting of carotid bifurcation lesions was performed for the first time in 1989.[9]

ADVANTAGES OF THE PERCUTANEOUS APPROACH

Carotid angioplasty and stenting has been of particular interest since it offers advantages over CEA that makes it attractive for the treatment of carotid disease (Table 22-1).

RESULTS OF SURGERY

Several randomized trials established the superiority of CEA over medical treatment in both symptomatic and asymptomatic carotid disease patients.

- **The NASCET trial:** The North American Symptomatic Carotid Endarterectomy Trial (NASCET)[12] was a multicenter randomized trial designed to determine if CEA reduced the risk of stroke in patients with recent nondisabling stroke and carotid stenosis. The patients were stratified in two groups based on carotid stenosis: 30% to 69% and 70% to 99%. The risk of any stroke at 2 years was 9% for CEA, 26% for medical therapy. The risk of major or fatal stroke at 2 years was 2.5% for CEA, 13.1% for medical therapy. The risk of stroke and perioperative death at 3 months was 5.8%.

Table 22-1

Advantages of the percutaneous approach in carotid interventions

1. It is performed with the patient fully alert, allowing close monitoring for neurologic complications during the procedure.
2. Since the majority of patients have coexistent coronary artery disease and other comorbidity, avoiding general anesthesia translates into a safer procedure for a population with a risk for myocardial infarction and cardiac death during general anesthesia (between 4% and 18%).[10]
3. It is less invasive and traumatic than CEA, thus avoiding local wound problems, medical complications, cranial nerve palsies, and scars.
4. Patients can expect to leave the hospital within 24 hours and return to work after 72 hours.[11]

- **The ECST trial:** The European Carotid Surgery Trial (ECST)[13] was a multicenter randomized trial designed to determine the role of CEA in patients after nondisabling stroke, transient ischemic attack, or retinal infarct who presented with a stenotic carotid lesion. The results showed that there was no benefit from CEA in patients with mild <30% stenosis. The benefit of CEA was uncertain in patients with stenosis between 30% and 69%. There was a 7.5% risk of stroke or death within 30 days of surgery in patients with severe >70% stenosis. At 3 years, an extra 2.8% risk was added for patients with CEA and 23.8% for patients treated with medical therapy. At 3 years, the risk of death or stroke was 12.3% for CEA and 21.9% for medical therapy.
- **The ACAS trial:** The Asymptomatic Carotid Atherosclerosis Study (ACAS)[14,15] was designed to determine if the addition of CEA to medical management reduced stroke in asymptomatic carotid disease in asymptomatic patients with NASCET-measured >60% stenosis. The 5 years risk of stroke or death was 5.1% for CEA and 11.0% for medical therapy. The risk of perioperative stroke at 30 days was 2.3%.
- **CASANOVA trial:** The Carotid Artery Surgery Asymptomatic Narrowing Operation Versus Aspirin (CASANOVA) trial randomized 410 patients including asymptomatic patients with ACI-stenosis of 50–90%. The trial showed no difference between the medical and medical + surgical group.[16]
- **VA trial:** The Veterans Affairs Asymptomatic Carotid Endarterectomy Trial included 444 asymptomatic patients with stenosis of the internal carotid artery of 50 to 99% treated either medically or surgically. When ipsilateral TIA and stroke were included as composite endpoints the results showed a reduction in the relative risk with surgery. When

ipsilateral stroke was considered alone, only a nonsignificant trend favoring surgery was noted. For the combined outcome of stroke and death, no significant differences were found between the two treatment arms.[17]

Of these trials, the reduction of risk for disabling stroke or death after CEA occurred in symptomatic patients with carotid stenosis exceeding ECST-measured 70% and NASCET-measured 50%; for asymptomatic patients, the surgical benefits occurred with stenosis exceeding NASCET-measured 70%.

Although these studies validated CEA, they also showed its limitations. If the surgical perioperative morbidity and mortality exceeded 3% in asymptomatic patients and 6% in symptomatic patients, the benefits of CEA were lost.[18] Therefore, according to the AHA guidelines[19] carotid endarterectomy should only be performed in institutions and by surgeons who are able to achieve a morbidity/mortality below these values. Also, patients in whom CEA was proven beneficial were very carefully selected and many were excluded as listed in Table 22-2. Despite these exclusion criteria, there was a high risk of stroke and perioperative deaths with CEA: 7.5% in ECST, 5.8% in NASCET and 2.3% in ACAS. In light of these limitations, carotid angioplasty and stenting evolved as an alternative in the therapy of carotid disease.[20–22]

Table 22-2
List of patients excluded from surgical trials

---

1. Age greater than 79 years
2. Heart, kidney, liver or lung failure
3. Cancer likely to cause death within 5 years
4. Cardiac valvular lesion or rhythm disorder likely to be associated with cardioembolic stroke
5. Previous ipsilateral CEA
6. Angina or myocardial infarction in the previous 6 months
7. Progressive neurologic signs
8. Contralateral CEA within 4 months
9. Major surgical procedure within 30 days
10. Severe comorbidity due to other surgical or medical illness
11. Cerebrovascular events in the distribution of the study carotid artery or in that of the vertebrobasilar arterial system with ongoing disabling symptoms
12. Symptoms referring to the contralateral side within the previous 45 days
13. More severe stenosis of an intracranial lesion than of the treated lesion

VALIDATION OF PERCUTANEOUS CAROTID INTERVENTIONS

Although low morbidity and mortality rates in the range 1%–7.2% were seen in the early clinical series of carotid angioplasty and stenting,[23-31] only a few rigorously controlled comparisons with CEA have been published. Randomized trials are needed for their validation as an alternative therapy to CEA. CAVATAS[32,33] was the first trial that has been completed. Brooks *et al.* published a small randomized study comparing surgery and stenting,[11] and recently first results of the SAPPHIRE trial comparing surgery and stenting under cerebral protection have been reported.[34,35] Several other projects (CAST,[29] CASET (the Carotid Artery Stenting versus Endarterectomy Trial),[36] ICSS=CAVATAS II,[37-39] Space,[40,41] EVA 3S,[42] Picasso, CARESS,[41,43] CREST[44]) are under way or in the planning stages.

The CAVATAS trial: The CAVATAS (Carotid and Vertebral Transluminal Angioplasty Study)[33] trial was a multicenter randomized trial designed to determine the risks and benefits of transluminal carotid and vertebral artery angioplasty and to compare them with CEA or medical treatment. It included a high-risk, symptomatic population with high-grade carotid stenosis.

The inclusion criteria were much broader than in the NASCET. Insofar the patient population resembled much more what is common in clinical practice than was the case in the randomized surgical versus medical treatment trials. However, the surgeons were experienced and the radiologists worked within their learning curve. At the beginning, stents were not available and later on they were mainly used in bail-out situations. Only one-third of patients received a stent. The stents and technical approach used were suboptimal and now considered outdated (i.e. stainless steel self-expanding stents, 0.035" wires, no carotid sheath). The results were similar for both early and late outcomes: the incidence for major stroke and death was 5% for both procedures. The incidence of all strokes (disabling and nondisabling) was close to 11% for both procedures and follow-up events were also similar.

The CAST trial: The CAST (Carotid Artery Stent Trial) trial[29] is a multicenter randomized trial designed to evaluate the safety of percutaneous carotid artery angioplasty and stenting. The entry criteria are: (1) symptomatic or asymptomatic patients >65 years of age, and (2) internal carotid artery stenosis of >70% and <2 cm long.

The CREST trial: The CREST (Carotid Revascularization Endarterectomy versus Stent Trial)[44] is an NIH-sponsored multicenter randomized trial designed to determine the risks of stroke, myocardial infarction, or death for carotid angioplasty and stenting and compare them with CEA. The trial has recruited till November 2002 272 high-risk patients at 58 centers with symptomatic carotid artery stenosis exceeding NASCET-measured 50%. The initial entry criteria are based on angiography or carotid duplex with stenosis of 70–99% severity. Follow-up will last 4 years. Newer stent technology (i.e. Nitinol self-expanding) is used.

The ICSS or Cavatas II study: The International Carotid Stenting Study[33] is a multicentered, randomized trial to compare the risks and benefits of primary carotid artery stenting to CEA in symptomatic patients with a severe (≥70%) stenosis. The trial started in November 2000 and will continue for 5 years. It is planned to enroll 2000 patients in 15 centers. Primary outcome measures the incidence of mortality and disabling stroke.

The Space study: The Space study (Stent protected Percutaneous Angioplasty vs Endarterectomy)[40,41] is a prospective, randomized trial including 1900 patients in 30 centers in Germany and Austria which started in March 2001. To February 2003 286 patients were included. Symptomatic patients with high grade stenosis can be recruited. Embolic protection is optional. Three coordinators (vascular surgery, neuroradiology, neurology) supervise this multidisciplinary trial.

The EVA 3S study: This evaluates carotid stenting vs endarterectomy in patients with severe carotid artery stenosis (≥70%). It is a randomized, prospective, multicenter trial with blinded judgement criteria. Radiologists, neuroradiologists and vascular surgeons participate in 30 centers with 900 patients in 2 years. The use of any CE marked stent is allowed. Embolic protection is optional.

The PICASSO study: This evaluates carotid artery stenting vs medical treatment. It is a randomized, prospective trial of 10 centers which include about 90% of all CAS done in Spain. One thousand symptomatic patients with a stenosis of 50–70% will participate. The Carotid Wallstent is currently the only stent to be used.

The CARESS study: In the Clopidogrel and Aspirin for Reduction of Emboli in Symptomatic Carotid Stenosis (CARESS) study, symptomatic and asymptomatic patients are included who are not eligible for the CREST study. It evaluates CAS vs CEA in a prospective trial recruiting all consecutive eligible patients. The doctor and patient choose the kind of treatment. In 20 to 30 US centers 2400 patients will be enrolled.

The SAPPHIRE trial: The Stenting and Angioplasty with Protection in Patients at High Risk for Endarcterectomy (SAPPHIRE) trial included 307 high-risk patients from 29 US centers with symptomatic (≥50%) and asymptomatic (≥80%) carotid disease. The definition "high-risk" is determined by congestive HF, chronic obstructive pulmonary disease, previous carotid endarterectomy, severe CAD, radical neck surgery, or radiation therapy. The patients where randomized to either CEA (151) or carotid artery angioplasty and stenting

(156). The stenting procedure combined Nitinol stent technology (Precise stent) with an embolic protection device, the Angioguard filter. Initial results with 30-day follow-up were reported at the AHA in November 2002. CAS patients had a 5.8% rate of death, stroke and MI compared with 12.6% in CEA patients (P=0.047).[34,35]

INDICATIONS AND CONTRAINDICATIONS OF CAROTID ARTERY INTERVENTIONS

There are no guidelines for percutaneous carotid angioplasty or stenting. The indications are evolving according to higher procedural success and a lower complication rate, which makes the benefits outweigh the risks. The list below includes the patients who are at high risk for surgical CEA and so will benefit the most from percutaneous carotid stenting. The contraindications are listed in Table 22-3. All these contraindications are of course relative and are less important if the patient needs treatment and has a high surgical risk and also if the operator has more experience. In the CAVATAS trial[33] it could clearly be shown that the results of stenting are strongly dependent on a steep learning curve. The clinical predictors of complications (death or CVA) are identified in Table 22-4. The anatomic factors with high success and low complication rates will help the inexperienced operators to select low-risk patients for the best success at the beginning of his or her learning curve.

1. **Patients with significant medical comorbidities:** Since this subgroup of patients was excluded from the CEA trials, the indications and results of surgery are not well estab-

---

Table 22-3
Contraindications for carotid interventions

1. Severely tortuous, calcified, and atheromatous aortic arch vessels that make access difficult.
2. Pedunculated thrombus at the lesion site. This type of thrombus is best seen using 15-frame-per-sec cine imaging.
3. Severe renal impairment precluding safe use of contrast agents.
4. Recent stroke (3 weeks). These patients are probably best stabilized on antiplatelet and possibly anticoagulant prior to stenting. Emergency carotid artery stenting is only indicated in patients with recurrent ischemia.
5. Patients unable to tolerate appropriate dose of antiplatelet agents.

Table 22-4
Classification of patients according to risk[57–59]

Higher risk	Lower risk
Clinical	**Clinical**
Clinical advanced age	Younger age
Prior CVA (large neurologic deficit)	No prior CVA
Cerebral atrophy/dementia	
Unstable neurologic symptoms	Neurologically intact
TIA, recent CVA	Asymptomatic
Diffuse severe peripheral vascular disease (involving aortic arch vessel)	No severe PVD
Anatomical	**Anatomical**
Severe tortuous, calcified and atherosclerotic arch vessels	Straight, noncalcified, "smooth" arch vessel
Coexistent proximal common carotid lesions	Noncommon carotid disease
High-grade and subtotal occlusion	Less severe stenosis
Severe concentric calcification	
Angiographic evidence of large amount of thrombi	No thrombus
Long, complex lesions extending into the distal internal carotid	Short lesions
Severe tortuosity just distal to the bifurcation	Nontortuous bifurcation

lished. Myocardial infarction was the leading long-term cause of death after CEA in patients with concomitant clinically important coronary artery disease.[45] Patients with significant carotid disease undergoing coronary artery bypass grafting (CABG) have a risk for stroke from hypotension during general anesthesia.[46] Published reports on combined CEA and CABG suggest that the risk of stroke or death ranges from 7.4% to 9.4%, 1.5 to 2.0 times the risk of each operation alone.[47]

2. **Carotid restenosis:** This is technically challenging because of scar tissue surrounding the carotid bifurcation. The complication rate of redo CEA approximates 10%.[48–50] Early results indicate that carotid angioplasty and stenting can be safely achieved and represent a valid alternative to carotid re-exploration in this high-risk group.[51–54]

3. **High-grade carotid stenosis with contralateral occlusion:** The perioperative risk of stroke or death in the presence of a contralateral carotid occlusion was 14.3% in NASCET.[55] There is no evidence that carotid shunting reduces the perioperative risk of stroke. Carotid angioplasty and stenting obviate the need for carotid occlusion in the presence of reduced cerebrovascular reserve.

4. **Radiation-induced carotid stenosis:** This is a surgical challenge because of both involvement of the distal common carotid artery and extensive scarring and fibrosis.[56] Infections and wound problems are increased by previous radiation.

5. **High cervical stenosis and tandem lesions:** High lesions in patients with short or thick necks are difficult to expose surgically. These high lesions are more likely to have less atherosclerosis and dense calcifications, and therefore are more suitable for the endovascular approach.[18] Patients with tandem lesions were excluded from the NASCET because of a high risk of postoperative occlusion from decreased flow velocity. Carotid angioplasty and stenting of tandem lesions can be done at the same time, so they represent a valid alternative to carotid surgery.

STANDARD PRE- AND POSTOPERATIVE PROCEDURES

These are listed in Table 22-5. As long as carotid stenting is not accepted as the new gold standard from all specialties it is strongly recommended that all these evaluations should be performed before doing the procedure. Of course it is essential that the diagnostic tests listed in Table 22-5 are repeated after the procedure.

CAROTID STENTING STEP BY STEP

Carotid intervention is a dynamic procedure that changes as progress is made.[60,61] The use and manipulation of guides, wires, sheaths, balloons, or stents evolves according to the experience of the operators to achieve higher procedural success and a lower complication rate. A generic step-by-step procedural approach for carotid intervention is suggested below.

1. **Vascular access:** The femoral access approach is the most commonly used. Femoral puncture is done with insertion of a standard 5F–9F 12-cm arterial sheath, a 23-cm sheath for a diseased iliac artery, and a 40-cm sheath in case of an abdominal aortic aneurysm. The patient is given heparin to obtain an activated clotting time of 200–250 sec.

2. **Cannulation of the common carotid artery (CCA):** A 5F diagnostic guide is advanced into the ascending aorta over a 0.035" wire. For a difficult or anomalous anatomy, an aortogram of the arch vessels can be done and used as a guide to selective cannulation. After angiography of the aortic arch and recognition of the anatomy, the diagnostic

---

Table 22-5
Pre- and postprocedural checklist for carotid procedures

---

1. Adequate medical and neurologic evaluation.
2. CT scan or MRI of the brain to document preprocedural anatomic deficits.
3. A formal neurologic assessment and completion of a National Institutes of Health (NIH) stroke scale pre- and post-procedure.
4. Explanation of benefits and potential complications of the procedure and informed consent.
5. Some operators still recommend a complete cerebral angiography in a separate examination or immediately before carotid angioplasty and stenting. However, in the days of MRI angiography this seems to be less important. In our center a 4-vessel angiography is rarely performed.
6. Duplex ultrasound is required pre- and post-stenting and is used as a baseline for follow-up.
7. Aspirin 300 or 325 mg and clopidogrel (Plavix) 75 mg once a day. Different from coronary interventions, the target is not so much to avoid thrombus formation after stent implantation as to avoid fresh thrombus prior to stent implantation. This fresh thrombus may embolize during the procedure. Therefore, the treatment with aspirin and clopidogrel should start at least one week before.

---

guide is advanced into the common carotid artery with the over-the-wire technique. Prior to cannulation of the common carotid, a careful flush of saline should be performed to clear any debris or thrombus.

3. **Road mapping and angiography of intracranial vessels:** Many investigators recommend road mapping to display the origin of the external carotid artery (ECA). To use bony landmarks, as we prefer, is an alternative. Perform angiography of intracranial vessels in two projections, lateral and AP-30° cranial. This angiogram will be very important for comparison and further intracranial rescue procedures in case embolization occurs during the intervention.
4. **Wire advancement:** Advance the wire into the ipsilateral ECA and follow with a 5F diagnostic guide.
5. **Carotid sheath placement:** Replace the current wire with an exchange length 0.035" wire. Generally, a stiff Amplatz-type wire should be used. An alternative is the TAD wire. This wire has a 0.018" distal tip and stiff proximal 0.035" shaft. The diagnostic guide is then exchanged over the wire for a 6F–10F 90-cm sheath that is then advanced into the common carotid artery below the bifurcation. Usually a 6F sheath is sufficient, though larger sheaths are required for some emboli protection devices. Gently

manipulate the sheath during engagement because it can cause a tear at the ostium of the common carotid artery or dislodge arteriosclerotic debris. Flush meticulously so there is no air inside.

6. **Landmark identification:** Remove the 0.035" wire for pressure measurement. "Back bleed" and flush carefully and take a "guiding" image lesion by injecting through sheath. An arteriography is performed to maximize the opening of the bifurcation and pinpoint the severity of the stenosis. Then, during the intervention, the most useful projection is not necessarily the one showing the maximum stenosis, but the one separating the internal and external carotid arteries and the one showing the bony landmarks.

7. **Emboli protection:** Distal embolization is the major cause of complications during carotid stenting. Therefore, we use emboli protection devices in all cases. They are described in more detail later in this chapter. Generally, the device has to be introduced and placed distal (filter or occlusion balloon) or proximal (occlusion balloon) of the lesion.

8. **Atropine:** Give atropine (1 mg intravenously) to prevent bradycardia 2 to 3 min before balloon inflation.

9. **Predilation:** This is in order to facilitate introduction of the stent delivery system. We use it only occasionally (for example if we failed with an attempt to introduce the stent without predilation) but some other operators recommend predilation in all cases. A 3 or 4-mm monorail or coaxial angioplasty balloon is advanced to the lesion over the 0.014" wire which is attached to the filter or distal occlusion balloon or over a separate 0.014" wire in case a proximal occlusion balloon is used for emboli protection. Usually stiff wires are preferred. For predilation the angioplasty balloon is inflated at low pressures 1 ATM above the disappearance of the waist. On very rare occasions (very tight and calcified lesions) predilation has to be performed even before introduction of an emboli protection device.

10. **Stent deployment:** Exchange the balloon system for a stent system. The diameter of the stent should be 1–2 mm larger than the largest segment to be covered. Most often stents with a diameter between 6 (if the stent is implanted into the ICA only) or 8 and 10 mm are used. Nitinol self-expanding stents are superior to both stainless steel balloon and self-expanding stents since they are more pliable to accommodate vessel tortuosities. Although the internal carotid artery is 2–3 mm smaller than the CCA, oversizing the stent in the internal carotid artery does not cause late problems. Covering the ECA is safe and rarely causes occlusion of the ECA. The stent should be long enough to cover the lesion completely. Most often we use stents 2–3 cm long.

11. **Post-stenting management:** Post-stent deployment dilatations should be done at nominal pressure to prevent

dissection. The balloon diameter should equal the diameter of the ICA distal of the stent. Post-stent dilatation of the stent segment in the CCA is not necessary and not recommended. If the external carotid artery becomes significantly stenosed or occluded after dilatation of the stent, this vessel can be approached through stent mesh and reopened. However, usually there is no need to do this. Remove the stent system to perform carotid angiography to identify further lesions, dissections, and embolic complications.

12. **Removal of the emboli protection device:** Almost all currently available filter devices are removed with a retrieval catheter. In case of an occlusion balloon, the debris in the ICA has to be aspirated before occlusion balloon deflation and retrieval. Perform carotid angiography including intracranial branches to document the final result and to exclude distal embolization.

General measures: Continuous monitoring of the heart rate, blood pressure, and neurologic status throughout and after intervention is mandatory. Good hydration and maintenance of an appropriate blood pressure are important in the recovery period. Usually, the systolic blood pressure after the procedure should be between 120 and 140 mmHg. A lower pressure is preferable in case of a very tight lesion before stenting, especially in case of a contralateral occlusion, because these patients have a higher risk of intracranial bleeding. The sheath is removed when the ACT is <180 sec. We often use vascular closure devices in carotid stenting especially if a large sheath has been used. The patient usually can be discharged after 6–8 hours if no complications are encountered and if blood pressure and heart rate are stable.

EMBOLIC PROTECTION DEVICES

Filter devices
Angioguard XP™ (Cordis): The Angioguard filter was the first filter which became available. The Angioguard XP™ (Figure 22-1) is the newest version of this filter. It consists of the filter itself, which is mounted on a 300 cm long 0.014" wire, a delivery catheter and a retrieval catheter. The filter comes in diameters between 4 and 8 mm.

The filter membrane is made of polyurethane. The pores in the filter have a diameter of 100 μm. The filter has eight Nitinol struts. Four of these struts have a radiopaque marker. The delivery catheter has a diameter of 3.2–3.9F. The retrieval catheter has a diameter of 5.1F.

E.P.I. FilterWire™ (Boston Scientific): This filter (Figure 22-2) is mounted to a 0.014" wire by means of an eccentric Nitinol wire loop. Due to this design, the entry of the particles

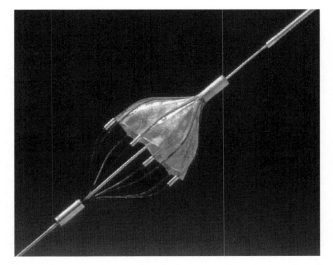

Figure 22-1: Angioguard embolic protection device (Cordis Corporation, Miami, FL, USA).

into the filter is not impeded by filter struts. The membrane of the filter is made of polyurethane and has pores with a diameter of 80 µm. The delivery catheter has an outer diameter of 3.8F. The filter comes in one size and adopts to vessel diameters between 3.5 and 6.0 mm in diameter. It can be withdrawn with a retrieval catheter or with any 0.018" compatible balloon catheter.

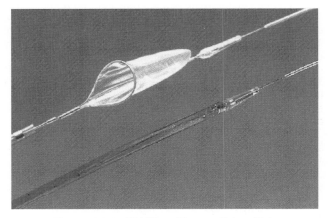

Figure 22-2: EPI Filter (Boston Scientific).

A new version of this device named FilterWire EZ will become available soon. It is expected that this will have a better vessel wall apposition than the current device.

MedNova NeuroShield™ Cerebral Protection System (Abbott): Currently the third generation of this device is available. It consists of a guidewire, a delivery catheter (3.7–3.9F), a filter basket (3–6 mm) and a retrieval catheter. Initially the lesion is crossed with the guidewire alone. Thereafter, the filter is loaded into the delivery catheter, which is advanced over the wire distal to the lesion. After angioplasty and stenting the retrieval catheter is advanced over the wire and the filter. The retrieval catheter has an expansile distal section which expands upon filter retrieval and allows full recapture of the filter. The fourth generation of this filter is currently under evaluation in clinical trials.

Microvena Spider™ Vascular Filtration System (ev3): The newest version of this filter is the Microvena Spider XLP™ Vascular Filtration System (Figure 22-3). This is a completely new design with a windsock-type filter basket. The design of this filter has some similarities with the EPI filter. However, it comes in different sizes between 4 and 7 mm. At the entrance of this filter there is a clasp to ensure a better vessel wall apposition of the opening of the filter. This filter is the only filter which allows usage of a wire of the operator's choice to cross the lesion. After crossing the lesion with the wire the delivery catheter of the system is introduced. The crossing profile of the delivery catheter is only 2.9F. The wire is removed and the filter is advanced through the delivery catheter and placed distal of the stenosis. After balloon angioplasty and stenting the retrieval catheter with a diameter of 5 or 6F is introduced over the wire.

The Distal Protection Device (Medtronic): This device consists of a Nitinol filter basket attached to a 0.014" guidewire. The basket diameter ranges between 3.5 and 6.0 mm. There are four entry ports in the proximal end of the filter. The size of the pores of the filter ranges between 75 and 125 μm. The filter may be retrieved with a retrieval catheter or with any over-the-wire balloon catheter.

AccuNet™ Embolic Protection Device (Guidant): This is a polyurethane filter with a diameter ranging from 4 to 8 mm. The pore size is 120 μm.

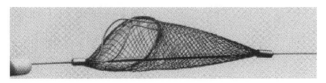

Figure 22-3: Microvena Spider vascular filtration system.

Occlusion devices

Percusurge GuardWire™ (Medtronic): This was the first occlusion device which was available commercially (Figure 22-4). An elastomeric balloon is fixed at the tip of a 0.014" or a 0.018" wire. The balloon can be filled through a lumen inside of the wire up to a diameter between 4 and 6 mm. This is done via a so-called MicroSeal™ adapter. With this adapter a MicroSeal in the wire can be opened and closed. When the MicroSeal is closed, the adapter can be removed from the wire without balloon deflation. After crossing the lesion with the GuardWire the distal balloon is inflated distal of the stenosis to occlude the internal carotid artery. The MicroSeal adapter is removed and the angioplasty balloon and the stent are introduced over the wire. After stent implantation an aspiration catheter is advanced over the wire into the internal carotid artery. The debris which may have been dislodged from the lesion is aspirated and removed. Thereafter, the distal occlusion balloon is deflated.

The advantage of this technique compared to filter techniques is that even very small particles can be captured. Furthermore, the crossing profile of the device is very low. However, some patients do not tolerate the balloon occlusion of the internal carotid artery.[62] It is possible in these patients to do the procedure stepwise with intermittent deflation of the balloon. Obviously this makes the procedure a little bit cumbersome. Another disadvantage is that angiography during the procedure is not possible.

Parodi AES (ArteriA Medical Science, San Francisco, CA): This device prevents distal embolization by establishing a retrograde flow in the internal carotid artery (Figure 22-5).

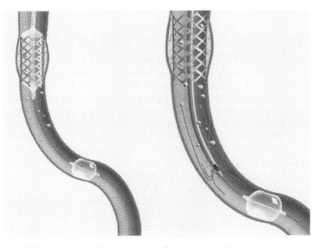

Figure 22-4: Percusurge Guardwire (Medtronic).

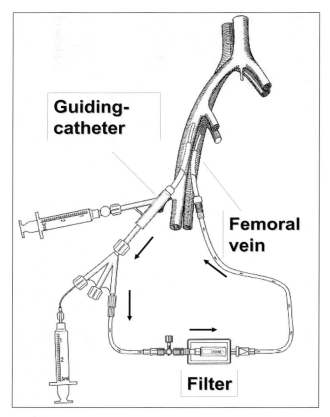

Figure 22-5: Parodi AES (Arteria Medical Science).

It consists of a 10F guiding catheter with a balloon at its distal tip. This balloon is inflated in the common carotid artery. To avoid blood flow from the external to the internal carotid artery, the external carotid artery is occluded with a separate balloon mounted on a wire which is introduced through the lumen of the guiding catheter. The proximal hub of the guiding catheter is connected with a venous sheath. Due to the pressure difference between the distal internal carotid artery and the venous system, a retrograde blood flow is established. A filter located in the arteriovenous shunt prevents embolization of the debris into the venous system.

The major advantage of this technique is that during the procedure emboli can not move towards the brain. This protection starts already before crossing the lesion. This is of special importance in lesions which contain fresh thrombus (Figure 22-6).

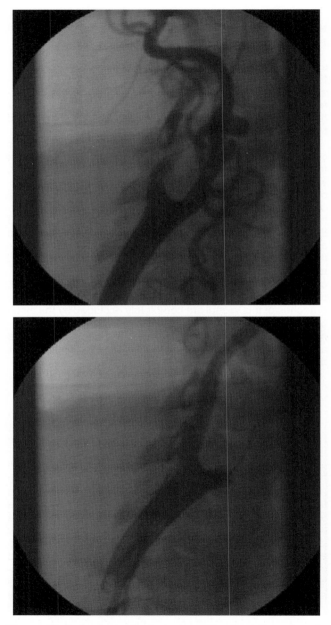

Figure 22-6: Angioplasty of a lesion with a fresh thrombus. In this situation a proximal occlusion system as embolic protection device should be used.

The operator may use the wire of his choice which helps to cross difficult lesions. There is no risk of distal problems in severely elongated vessels (Figs 22-7 and 22-8).

Disadvantages of this technique are the need for a 10F sheath and intolerance of balloon occlusion in some patients. In contrast to the distal balloon occlusion technique (Percusurge), angiography during the procedure is possible. To perform the procedure in a stepwise fashion is easier and faster than with the Percusurge technique, because there is no need for an aspiration catheter before deflating the balloon.

MO.MA (Invatec, Roncadelle, Italy): This device has some similarities with the Parodi AES. The occlusion balloon for the external carotid artery is fixed to the guiding catheter, which allows faster and more reliable placement. This obviously also implies that the external carotid artery has to be open and not severely stenosed and that the fixed distance between the balloon at the tip of the guiding catheter and the external occlusion balloon is suitable for the individual anatomy of the patient. Instead of a continuous retrograde flow to the venous system, an aspiration with a syringe is used to aspirate the debris between the different steps of the procedure or at the end of the procedure. It is mandatory that not only the external carotid artery itself but also all proximal side branches of this vessel are completely occluded by the distal occlusion balloon. As with the Parodi AES device, angiography during the procedure is possible. The operator may use any kind of wire to cross the lesion and in case of intolerance the procedure can be performed stepwise.

TECHNICAL TIPS

Cannulation of the brachiocephalic arteries: We usually start with a right Judkins catheter. Catheters with a similar shape are the head hunter H1 and the Bentson/Hannafee JB1 catheter (Cook, Bloomington, IN). This type of catheter is advanced over the aortic arch by keeping the tip pointed inferiorly or over a guidewire. This avoids trauma to the intima of the aortic arch and prevents the catheter tip from becoming trapped by vessel ostia. In the ascending aorta the catheter is turned around 180°, which places the tip in a vertical upright position. Thereafter, the catheter is gently pulled back. Usually this motion will bring the catheter tip into the brachiocephalic artery. If the left common carotid artery is the target, the catheter should be pulled further distally very slowly. During this period, the catheter should be turned 20° counterclockwise to make the tip point slightly anterior. This helps to engage the left common carotid artery. To stabilize the catheter in the left common carotid artery, it is necessary to rotate the catheter 20° clockwise to make the tip of the catheter point vertical or slightly posterior again.

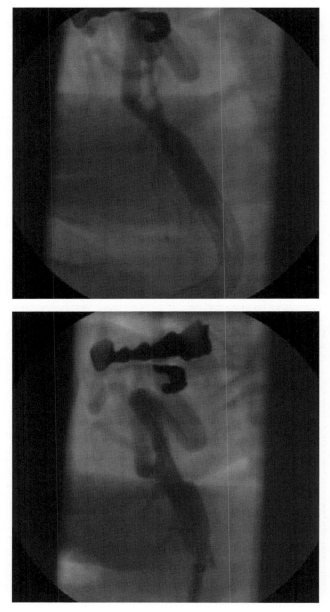

Figure 22-7: Angiogram of severely elongated vessel. As it might be difficult to place a distal protection system in the internal carotid artery we would suggest the use of a proximal occlusion system.

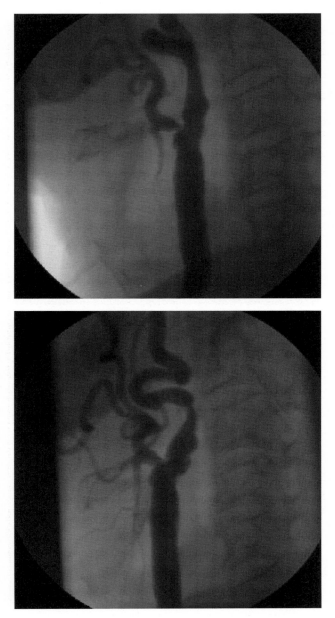

Figure 22-8: Angiogram of severely elongated vessel. As it might be difficult to place a distal protection system in the internal carotid artery we would suggest the use of a proximal occlusion system.

If we are not successful with one of these simple catheters, we usually switch to a Vitek catheter (Cook, Bloomington, IN). A catheter with a similar shape is the Mani catheter. This catheter forms a loop in the descending aorta. By pushing the catheter towards the ascending aorta, the tip engages the left subclavian artery, the left common carotid artery and finally the brachiocephalic trunk. In contrast, with the Simmons/Sidewinder catheters (AngioDynamic, Queensbury, NY) a loop is formed in the ascending aorta. By pulling back this type of catheter, again the tip engages the vessels of the aortic arch (brachiocephalic trunk first).

*Injection of contrast media: After the guide enters into the artery, slow hand injection is done to confirm the position of the guide, to make sure that good blood flow is maintained and that there is no subintimal entry of the contrast agent. Injections of contrast agent into all brachiocephalic arteries should be done by hand and with small amounts of contrast (no more then 6 cc per injection). Larger volumes create a mixture of arterial, intermediate, and venous phases, thus obscuring early filling veins and other pathologies.

**The need for diagnostic angiography of the brachiocephalic arteries: Some operators always perform a 4-vessel angiography to check collaterals for interventions and rescue when needed. We usually do not do this in order to avoid the additional risk, especially if we have an angio MRI. Of course, the angio MRI does not provide information about the functional capacity of the intracranial collaterals. If the internal carotid artery provides collaterals to the contralateral system, balloon inflation with transient occlusion of the ICA can cause seizure. On the other hand, this would not prevent us from doing angioplasty.

**Cautions prior to catheterization of the left vertebral artery: The left vertebral artery catheterization is begun by placing the catheter tip, under fluoroscopic control, into the proximal portion of the left subclavian artery. A small injection of contrast medium is used to demonstrate the origin and the proximal portion of the left vertebral artery. If the origin or the proximal portion of the left vertebral artery is stenotic, no attempt should be made to catheterize the artery. If there is no stenosis or extreme kinking of the origin of the vertebral artery, it is alright to proceed with the catheterization.[63]

Once a catheter has been placed into a vertebral artery, it is important to do two fluoroscopic observations of the opacification of the vertebral artery. These observations are made during and after a test injection of contrast medium.

First, observe that the vertebral artery does not end blindly in the posterior inferior cerebellar artery (PICA). This is a normal variation. Injection of 6–8 mL of contrast material into this type of vertebral artery may damage the small branches of the PICA or the brain tissue supplied by these vessels. The best way to know whether or not this anatomic variation exists is to make certain that you see opacification of the basilar artery when you do the test injection. Having the patient turn the chin to the right before the injection will help in the fluoroscopic visualization of the basilar artery. If the basilar artery is seen, a blind termination of the vertebral artery into the PICA cannot exist. If the basilar artery is not seen, however, this anatomic variation may well exist, or the distal portion of the vertebral artery or the proximal portion of the vertebral artery may be occluded. In cases of subarachnoid hemorrhage, when this anatomic variation is present, a small amount of contrast material (3–4 mL) can safely be injected to rule out aneurysm at the origin of the PICA. Otherwise, the catheter tip should be withdrawn from the left vertebral artery and the right one should be catheterized.

Second, observe that the contrast medium from the test injection passes out of the opacified vertebral artery freely. If the catheter size is not suitable for the artery, the catheter may partially or completely obstruct the vessel. This causes slow clearing of the contrast medium from the vertebral artery due to the decreased blood flow. On observing this phenomenon, the catheter should be withdrawn from the left vertebral artery orifice immediately and exchanged for a smaller, more suitable catheter, or the catheterization of right vertebral artery should begin. After making these observations, it is safe to proceed with vertebral angiography.

As soon as the injection is made, withdraw the catheter from the vertebral artery. This maneuver shortens the time in which the catheter tip is available to decrease blood flow through the vertebral artery and cause complications. Also, because the catheter is removed at the beginning of the film series, there is no overlapping of arterial, capillary, and venous angiographic phases because of poor vertebral artery blood flow. Preventing this type of overlapping makes the interpretation easier.

**Technique of engagement of the external carotid artery: The head of the patient is rotated to the contralateral side. This acts as a lateral projection and separates the internal and the external carotid arteries. If selective catheterization of the external carotid artery is desired, the neck of the patient is extended. This will cause the external carotid trunk to be aligned to the CCA. The tip of the catheter is then pointed anteriorly and the guidewire is inserted (Figs 22-9 and 22-10).

Two major reasons for failure of superselective catheterization in the external carotid system are tortuosity and

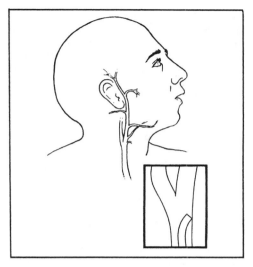

Figure 22-9: Catheterization of the external carotid artery. The neck is extended. This maneuver brings the ECA in line with the common carotid artery. Note the tip of the catheter, which is pointed anteriorly (inset). (Adapted from Gerlock AJ, Mirfakhraee M. Difficulty in catheterization of the internal and external carotid arteries. In: Gerlock AJ, Mirfakhraee M, eds. *Essentials of Diagnostic and Interventional Angiographic Techniques*. WB Saunders, 1985. With permission from the publisher.)

spasm. In most cases, these problems can be overcome by using smaller catheters and floppier guidewires and by manipulating the catheter and guidewires gently. If spasm occurs, no further manipulation is performed, and the catheter is flushed with heparinized saline solution for 10–15 min. The spasm usually will subside and catheterization is tried again.[56]

**Technique of engagement of the left carotid artery: If catheterization of the internal carotid artery is desired, the head is again turned to the contralateral side; however, the neck is flexed to align the internal carotid artery with the common carotid artery. The tip of the catheter is now pointed posteriorly and the guidewire is inserted. The catheter is advanced over the guidewire, and its tip is placed at the level of C2. It is important not to advance the catheter farther, since this may cause spasm. In cases of a cervical carotid loop, the catheter is placed below the loop (Figure 22-11).[56]

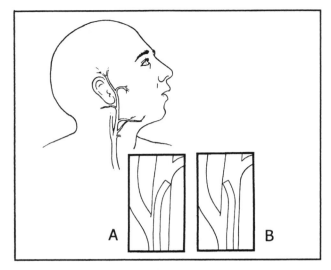

Figure 22-10: Technique of selective catheterization of the external carotid artery branches with catheter tip directed anteriorly (A) and posteriorly (B).[38] (Adapted from Gerlock AJ, Mirfakhraee M. Difficulty in catheterization of the internal and external carotid arteries. In: Gerlock AJ, Mirfakhraee M, eds. *Essentials of Diagnostic and Interventional Angiographic Techniques.* WB Saunders, 1985. With permission from the publisher.)

**The art of advancing the catheter: The clue is to advance the guide slowly over the wire while maintaining the wire deep inside the carotid artery. The left wall of the upper thoracic aorta can be used to support advancement of the guide into the carotid artery. One has to recognize "bad" and "good" curves of the guide within the aortic arch while advancing the guide. The guide is pushed over the wire slowly, also taking advantage of the pulsating blood flow. This maneuver, advancement of the guide, and withdrawal of the wire is made several times until the guide is securely placed in the artery. If there is a tortuosity of the proximal segment, the artery can be straightened with a wire. The guide can also be rotated while being advanced, clockwise or counterclockwise, depending on the curve formation in the aortic arch. Asking the patient to take a deep breath would help to elongate and thus straighten the great vessels. During that short window of opportunity, the guide is moved farther. Another important aspect is to gently "ease back" on the guide curve in the arch as successive wires are advanced. This reduces the curve in the arch and prevents

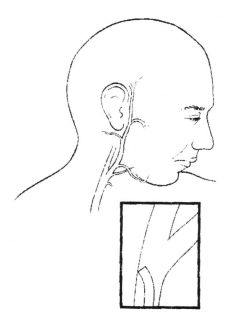

Figure 22-11: Catheterization of the internal carotid artery. The neck is flexed. This maneuver brings the ICA in line with the CCA. Note the position of the tip of the catheter, which is pointed posteriorly (inset). (Adapted from Gerlock AJ, Mirfakhraee M. Difficulty in catheterization of the internal and external carotid arteries. In: Gerlock AJ, Mirfakhraee M, eds. *Essentials of Diagnostic and Interventional Angiographic Techniques*. WB Saunders, 1985. With permission from the publisher.)

the successively stiffer wires from prolapsing the guide down into the ascending aorta.[60] Excessive manipulation of the guide in the arch may predispose to distal embolization.

**Difficult carotid access: With experience, 95% of bifurcations can be accessed using the current guide and wire systems. However, it may be difficult to access severely tortuous, calcified arteries using the standard approach. In those arteries in which the wire will not advance without "kicking" the guide back, alternative strategies have to be considered. If the common carotid artery is very atherosclerotic along its course, it may be prudent to refer the patient to surgery since the additional manipulation may produce embolic complications.[60]

***Alternative carotid access:** Access to the common carotid artery is possible via the brachial or radial artery. Furthermore, direct puncture of the common carotid artery is feasible.

Transbrachial and radial approach: Puncture (radial artery and brachial artery) or cut down (brachial artery) is performed according to standard techniques. We prefer the right arm for both carotid arteries (right and left side). A 5 or 6F sheath is introduced. Cannulation of the common carotid artery is usually possible with a right Judkins catheter or with a Mammaria catheter. If this turns out to be difficult, a Sidewinder catheter (Cordis, Miami Lakes, FL) can be used. After entering the ostium of the right or left common carotid artery with the catheter, a guidewire with hydrophilic coating (Terumo – Terumo, Tokyo, Japan) is advanced. Over this wire, a 6F long sheath is introduced.

In a patient without elongation of the aortic arch the angle between the right brachial artery and the right common carotid artery is not suitable for the transbrachial approach whereas in a patient with aortic arch elongation the angle is often more favorable. Figure 22-12 shows how to enter the left common carotid artery via the right brachial artery with a Sidewinder catheter together with a Terumo wire.

In our experience, in most patients both common carotid arteries can more easily be cannulated from the right arm. This is especially true in patients with an elongated aortic arch. Figure 22-13 shows an example of a transradial stent implantation of the right internal carotid artery.[64]

***Cervical approach via direct puncture:** The patient is placed on the table with a cushion under the shoulders. The head is turned away from the side which has to be punctured. Duplex ultrasound should be used to locate and mark the carotid bifurcation.

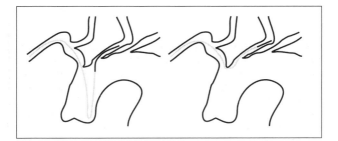

Figure 22-12: Entering the LCCA from the right brachial approach: the left common carotid artery can be entered via the right brachial artery using a Sidewinder catheter.

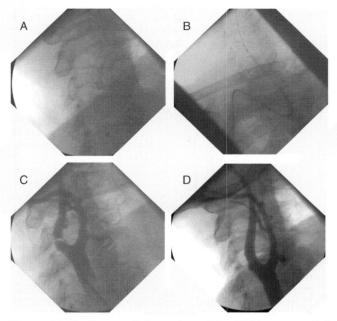

Figure 22-13: Transradial stenting of the RICA: transradial approach via the right arm for angioplasty and stenting of the right internal carotid artery.

The best puncture side is located approximately 1.5 to 2 cm above the clavicle. The position of the needle tip in relation to the carotid bifurcation has to be checked with a contrast injection before any further steps are taken. If the position is correct, the needle is exchanged for a 5 or 6F sheath over a 0.035" guidewire.

After the procedure the sheath is withdrawn and gentle pressure has to be applied for 10 to 15 minutes. Protamine should not be given. Needless to say, compression bandage cannot be applied.

**Why a guide fails to advance through tortuous artery: One major problem is the failure of advancing the catheter into the carotid artery. Persistent forward movement of the catheter will cause a loop to form in the aorta or the catheter tip flips back into the aorta (Figure 22-14). The physical and technical mechanisms of the above problems are discussed below (Table 22-6). These mechanisms and their solutions can be applied universally during instrumentation of any vascular bed including the coronary, carotid, or renal arteries or their anomalies. The example illustrations are based on the anomaly of the left common carotid artery.

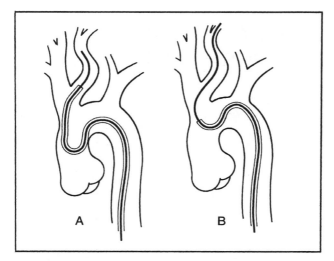

Figure 22-14: Difficulty in advancing the catheter over the guidewire. (A) The catheter forms a loop in the aorta. (B) The tip of the catheter flips back into the aorta. (Adapted from Gerlock AJ, Mirfakhraee M. Difficulty in catheterization of the internal and external carotid arteries. In: Gerlock AJ, Mirfakhraee M, eds. *Essentials of Diagnostic and Interventional Angiographic Techniques.* WB Saunders, 1985. With permission from the publisher.)

Table 22-6
Mechanisms of failure in advancing the catheter

---

1. The wire is not strong enough to support the catheter.
2. The angle of the origin of the carotid artery is too acute.
3. Too much friction exists between the guidewire and the internal surface of the catheter.
4. The curve of the distal end of the catheter prevents further advancement.

To solve the problem of a weak platform created by a floppy wire (mechanism 1), the wire has to be advanced further so the stiff segment is in the proper area. If the wire is not strong enough, it has to be exchanged to a stiffer one.[65]

To solve the problem of acute angle at the origin of the artery (mechanism 2), a stiff wire will straighten out the angle and help to advance the wire. To solve the problem created by mechanism 3 due to excessive friction between the wire and the internal surface of the catheter, the catheter should be advanced and the guidewire withdrawn

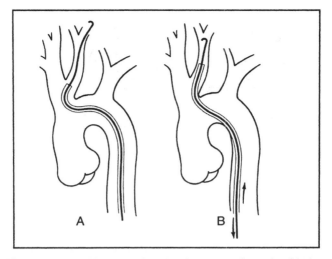

Figure 22-15: Diagram showing how to reduce the friction between the wire and the internal surface of the catheter. (A) The catheter tip is at the orifice of the left CCA and the tip of the wire is in the left ICA. (B) The catheter is advanced while the wire is withdrawn. (Adapted from Gerlock AJ, Mirfakhraee M. Difficulty in catheterization of the internal and external carotid arteries. In: Gerlock AJ, Mirfakhraee M, eds. *Essentials of Diagnostic and Interventional Angiographic Techniques.* WB Saunders, 1985. With permission from the publisher.)

simultaneously (Figure 22-15). This maneuver reduces significantly the friction between the wire and the internal surface of the catheter. Another way is to change the size of the wire to a smaller one, although this wire would not provide the same support as the previous wire; however, it would help to advance the catheter if the problem is related primarily to friction rather than support.[65]

To solve the problem of mechanism 4 (a sharp angle at the end of the catheter), while the wire is fixed, the catheter is advanced over it while rotating the catheter gently. The goal is to straighten the distal segment of the catheter by the wall of the artery so the catheter can adopt itself more to the angle and be advanced further (Figure 22-16). In difficult situations, two or three of the above-mentioned maneuvers may be required before the tip of the catheter can be advanced to the desired level.

***Carotid access in presence of occluded ECA, CCA lesion below bifurcation, or ostial CCA lesion: Placing the 7F 90-cm access sheath into the CCA may present

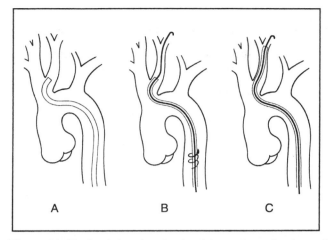

Figure 22-16: Straightening the tip of the catheter by the wall of the artery. (A) The tip of the catheter is at the orifice of the left CCA. (B) While the wire is fixed, the catheter is advanced over it using rotating forward movement. (C) The catheter has advanced over the wire into the vessel. (Adapted from Gerlock AJ, Mirfakhraee M. Difficulty in catheterization of the internal and external carotid arteries. In: Gerlock AJ, Mirfakhraee M, eds. *Essentials of Diagnostic and Interventional Angiographic Techniques.* WB Saunders, 1985. With permission from the publisher.)

special challenges when the ECA is occluded, a critical lesion is situated below the bifurcation, or there is a critical ostial common carotid lesion. If possible, avoid crossing the lesion with a stiff 0.038" wire since this is more likely to disrupt the necrotic plaque material and cause distal embolization. When possible, advance the 5F diagnostic guide over the 0.038" glidewire to be placed more distally. In this situation, the glidewire and 5F guide are first advanced through the lesion. This maneuver should be done only in patients considered at high risk from carotid surgery if the risk-benefit ratio still favors stenting.

In the presence of a carotid ostial lesion, the origin of the CCA should be first dilated to allow sheath access. The bifurcation should be stented first, and the ostium stented with a Palmaz stent on the "way out".

***Choice of balloon expandable or self-expandable stents:** The use of balloon expandable stents was abandoned with 3 exceptions listed in Table 22-7. Forcing the current high-profile delivery systems may break off plaque and cause distal embolization. In this situation, a short bal-

Table 22-7
Indications for use of balloon expandable stents

1. When the ostium of the common carotid artery is treated and the proximal end of the stent has to be placed with precision.
2. When the most distal segment of the internal carotid artery is treated (present delivery systems for a self-expanding stent cause dissections in the petrous portion of the internal carotid artery).
3. When the self-expanding stent delivery system will not pass through a calcified, recoiling lesion.

loon expandable stent may be placed to hold the lesion open before passing a definitive self-expanding stent.

**Postdilation: It is safer to underdilate than overdilate the oversized self-expanding stents. Overdilatation squeezes the atherosclerotic material through the stent mesh, causing emboli. A 10–15% remaining stenosis does not cause clinical problems. Importantly, it is not necessary to dilate the stent to obliterate segments of contrast-filled ulcerations external to the stent. This angiographic appearance is of no prognostic significance and follow-up angiography has documented complete fibrotic healing of these lesions over time. Importantly, it is not necessary to overexpand the stent to produce a 0% residual diameter narrowing. Covering the external carotid artery with a stent does not cause problems. Our follow-up arteriograms showed the external carotid artery to be patent with rare exceptions. If the external carotid artery becomes significantly stenosed with <TIMI-3 flow or occluded after postdilation of the stent, this vessel can be approached through the stent mesh, and reopened using coronary balloon techniques. A 0.014" wire is used to enter the external carotid artery, a 2-mm balloon to predilate, and a 4-mm balloon for final dilation. However there is almost never a clinical indication to do this.

COMPLICATIONS OF CAROTID INTERVENTIONS

Although major complications can be encountered during the learning curve of carotid angioplasty and stenting,[66] they are minimized by the use of meticulous techniques.

Thrombotic and embolic complications: A recent survey on carotid artery angioplasty and stenting[67] revealed a 30-day minor stroke rate of 2.72% and a major stroke rate of 1.49%. Advantages of the endovascular approach over CEA include the ability to immediately diagnose and treat these complications, and the patient can be awake, allowing close neurologic monitoring. For acute thrombosis, local intra-arterial thrombolysis can be carried out using mechanical as well as chemical disruption of the clot.[68] Extreme care must be exercised to avoid vessel perforation. Only very flexible microcatheters and soft wires may be used in the intracerebral circulation.

To prevent thrombotic complications, investigators have advocated the use of glycoprotein 2b3a platelet inhibition.[69] However, this encounters the risk of cerebral bleeding and therefore it should not be used routinely. Today, embolic protection devices are widely used although no randomized trials with versus without protection have been performed.[70] Atherosclerotic debris can be found in the filter in the majority of cases. Therefore, most investigators consider it to be unethical to conduct such a trial.

Carotid artery spasm: Guidewire-induced phenomena are minimized by the use of 0.014−0.018" wires. Carotid artery spasm can be successfully treated with papaverine[21] or nitroglycerin. Often they disappear spontaneously.

Transient bradyarrythmias and hypotension: Mediated by stretch of the carotid baroreceptors. This can usually be avoided by atropine given at least 2 to 3 minutes before balloon inflation.

Asystole is very rare, but if it occurs, it is transient and resolves with balloon deflation. A routine pacemaker is not necessary.

Post-stenting hypotension: Mediated by stretch of the carotid baroreceptors. Treat aggressively if the patient has severe distal or contralateral disease. Puncture site complications should be ruled out.[58]

External carotid artery occlusion: Acute occlusion of the ECA is well tolerated. In the absence of collateral circulation, patients may experience jaw muscle angina which is usually transient.

Stent restenosis: The restenosis rate for carotid stenting is less than 10%. It is treated with balloon dilatation.[71] A new stenosis may occur at the distal end of a stiff stent. This may require an additional stent.

Carotid perforation: This can be seen after excessive balloon sizing prior to or after stent placement. If encountered, try to seal it with a prolonged balloon inflation. Covered stents can be used if there is no compromise of major side branches.

Carotid dissection: This is seen mainly in areas of vessel tortuosity or calcification. Stented segments should not be overdilated in comparison to the reference vessel. Further stenting may be necessary to avoid flow disruption in the area of dissection.

Cerebral hemorrhage: Associated with a combination of excessive anticoagulation, uncontrolled hypertension, intracranial vessel manipulation, and stenting after a recent stroke (<3 weeks). Terminate the procedure, reverse the anticoagulation, and control the hypertension. An emergency brain CT scan should be performed. Operators should be familiar with the angiographic features of an intracranial mass effect. Sudden loss of consciousness preceded by a severe headache in the absence of intracranial vessel occlusion should alert the operator to this devastating event. Fortunately, with careful patient selection and compulsive attention to the above technical and anticoagulation issues, cerebral hemorrhage should be a very rare occurrence.

Jaw claudication: After carotid stenting, some patients complain of pain when masticating, especially if the ECA is jailed. Jaw claudication should slowly disappear in 1 to 2 weeks.

Problems and complications with embolic protection devices: Embolic protection devices may also cause problems. All devices placed distally in the internal carotid artery may cause spasm or dissection. Rarely additional balloon inflations and/or stent implantations have been necessary to solve the problem. It may be difficult to retrieve these devices through the implanted stent. It may happen that the filter is not fully apposed to the vessel wall. In contrast, the major disadvantage of the occlusion devices is intolerance in patients with occlusion or high-grade stenosis of the contralateral internal carotid artery or patients with poorly developed intracranial collaterals. A specific disadvantage of the MO.MA and the ArteriA device is the need for a large sheath, which may cause vascular access problems.

FUTURE DIRECTIONS

Future developments in the field of carotid percutaneous intervention will include new stents with higher flexibility which can be introduced through smaller sheaths (5F). We will have improved embolic protection devices with better wall apposition and without need for a retrieval catheter. All these new developments will help carotid stenting to become the new gold standard for treatment of carotid arteriosclerotic disease within the next few years.

REFERENCES

1. Wolf PA, Kannel WB, McGee PC. Epidemiology of strokes in North America. In: Barnet HJM, Stein BM, Mohr JP, Yatsu FM, eds. *Stroke: Pathology, Diagnosis and Management.* Vol 1. Churchill Livingstone, 1986: 1929.
2. Eastcott HHG, Pickering GW, Rob CG. Reconstruction of ICA in a patient with intermittent attacks of hemiplegia. *Lancet* 1954; **267**/II: 994–6.

3. DeBakey M. Carotid endarterectomy revisited. *J Endovasc Surg* 1996; **3**(1): 4.

4. Fields W, Maslenikov V, Meyer J *et al*. Joint study of extracranial arterial occlusion. *J Am Med Assoc* 1970; **211**: 1993–2003.

5. Shaw D, Venables G, Cartlidge N *et al*. Carotid endarterectomy in patients with transient cerebral ischemia. *J Neurol Sci* 1984; **64**: 45–53.

6. Yadav JS, Roubin GS, Iyer S *et al*. Application of lessons learned from cardiac interventional techniques to carotid angioplasty. *J Am Coll Cardiol* 1995; **25**: 392A.

7. Mathias K, Mittermayer C, Ensinger H *et al*. Perkutane Katheterdilatation von Karotisstenosen. *Rofo Fortschr Geb Rontgenstr Neuen Bildgeb Verfahr* 1980; **133**: 258–261.

8. Mathias K. Katheterbehandlung der arteriellen Verschlusskrankheit supraaortaler Gefässe. *Radiologie* 1987; **27**: 547–54.

9. Mathias K, Jäger H, Hennigs S *et al*. Endoluminal treatment of internal carotid artery stenosis. *World J Surg* 2001; **25**: 328–36.

10. Abrams J. Preoperative cardiac risk assessment and management. *Current Opinion Gen Surg* 1993; **13**: 8.

11. Brooks WH, McClure RR, Jones MR *et al*. Carotid angioplasty and stenting versus carotid endarterectomy: randomized trial in a community hospital. *J Am Coll Cardiol* 2001; **38**(6): 1589–95.

12. North American Symptomatic Carotid Endarterectomy Trial collaborators (NASCET collaborators): Beneficial effect of carotid endarterectomy in symptomatic patients with high-grade carotid stenosis. *N Engl J Med* 1991; **325**: 445–53.

13. European Carotid Surgery Trialists' Collaborative Group. MRC European Carotid Surgery Trial: Interim results for symptomatic patients with severe (70–99%) or with mild (0–29%) carotid stenosis. *Lancet* 1991; **337**: 1235–43.

14. Asymptomatic carotid atherosclerosis study group. (ACAS group): Carotid endarterectomy for patients with asymptomatic internal carotid artery stenosis. *J Am Med Assoc* 1995; **273**: 1421–8.

15. Asymptomatic Carotid Atherosclerosis Study. Clinical advisory: Carotid endarterectomy for patients with asymptomatic internal carotid artery stenosis. *Stroke* 1994; **25**: 2523–4.

16. CASANOVA Study Group. Carotid surgery versus medical therapy in asymptomatic carotid stenosis. *Stroke* 1991; **22**: 1229–35.

17. Hobson RW 2nd, Weiss DG, Fields WS *et al*. and the Veterans affairs cooperative study group (1993): Efficacy of carotid endarterectomy for asymptomatic carotid stenosis. *N Engl J Med* 1993; **328**: 221–7.

18. Grotta J. Elective stenting of extracranial carotid arteries (editorial). *Circulation* 1997; **95**: 303–5.

19. Guidelines for Carotid Endarterectomy. A multidisciplinary consensus statement for the ad hoc committee, American Heart Association. *Stroke* 1995; **26**: 188–201.

20. Joint Officers of the Congress of Neurological Surgeons and the American Association of Neurological Surgeons. Carotid angioplasty and stent: An alternative to carotid endarterectomy. *Neurosurgery* 1997; **40**: 344–5.

21. Diethrich EB. Indications for carotid artery stenting: A preview of the potential derived from early clinical experience. *J Endovasc Surg* 1996; **3**: 132–9.

22. New G, Roubin GS, Iyer SS *et al.* Carotid artery stenting: rationale, indications and results. *Comp Ther* 1999; **25**: 438–45.

23. Bergeron P. Carotid angioplasty and stenting: Is endovascular treatment for cerebrovascular disease justified? *J Endovasc Surg* 1996; **3**: 129–31.

24. Diethrich EB, Ndiaye M, Reid DB. Stenting in the carotid artery: Initial experience in 110 patients. *J Endovasc Surg* 1996; **3**: 42–62.

25. Henry M, Amor M, Masson I *et al.* Angioplasty and stenting of the extracranial carotid arteries. *J Endovasc Surg* 1998; **5**(4): 293–304.

26. Iyer SS, Roubin GS, Yadav S *et al.* Angioplasty and stenting for extracranial carotid stenosis: Multicenter experience. *Circulation* 1996; **94**(Suppl 1): I-58.

27. Yadav JS, Roubin GS, Iyer S *et al.* Elective stenting of the extracranial arteries. *Circulation* 1997; **95**: 376–81.

28. Yadav JS, Roubin GS, Vitek J *et al.* Late outcome after carotid angioplasty and stenting. *Circulation* 1996; **94**(Suppl I): I-58.

29. Bergeron P, Becquemin JP, Jausseran JM *et al.* Percutaneous stenting of the internal carotid artery: the European CAST I Study. Carotid Artery Stent Trial. *J Endovasc Surg* 1999; **6**(2): 155–9.

30. Wholey MH, Wholey MH, Tan WA *et al.* Management of neurological complications of carotid artery stenting. *J Endovasc Ther* 2001; **8**(4): 341–53.

31. Liu AY, Paulsen RD, Marcellus ML *et al.* Long-term outcomes after carotid stent placement treatment of carotid artery dissection. *Neurosurgery* 1999; **45**: 1368–74.

32. Sivaguru A, Venables GS, Beard JD *et al.* European Carotid Angioplasty Trial. *J Endovasc Surg* 1996; **3**(1): 23–30.

33. Endovascular versus surgical treatment in patients with carotid stenosis in the Carotid and Vertebral Artery Transluminal Angioplasty Study (CAVATAS): a randomised trial. *Lancet* 2001; **357**(9270): 1729–37.

34. **www.cardiologytoday.com/200212/frameset.asp?article=SAPPHIRE.asp**

35. Yadav J. SAPPHIRE: Stenting and Angioplasty with Protection in Patients at High Risk for Endarterectomy.

Presented at the American Heart Association Scientific Sessions 2002. Nov. 17–20, 2002. Chicago.

36. Clagett GP, Barnett HJ, Easton JD. The carotid artery stenting versus endarterectomy trial (CASET). *Cardiovasc Surg* 1997; **5** (5): 454–6.

37. Presented at the 25th International Stroke Conference (February 2000). *Stroke* 2000; **31**: 2536.

38. Presented at the 28th International Stroke Conference (February 2002).

39. ICCS Trial Website.

40. **www.strokeconference.org/abstracts/ongoing28/CTP6.pdf**

41. The American Stroke Association 28th International Stroke Conference, February 13–15, 2003, Phoenix, Arizona.

42. **www.strokecenter.org**

43. **www.strokeconference.org**

44. Hobson RW 2nd, Brott T, Ferguson R *et al.* CREST: Carotid revascularization endarterectomy versus stent trial. *Cardiovasc Surg* 1997; **5**: 457–8.

45. Yashon D, Jane JA, Javid H. Long-term results of carotid bifurcation endarterectomy. *Surg Gynecol Obstet* 1966; **122**: 517–23.

46. Faggioli GL, Curl R, Ricotta JJ. The role of carotid screening before coronary artery bypass. *J Vasc Surg* 1990; **12**: 724–31.

47. Loftus CM, Biller J, Hart MN *et al.* Management of radiation-induced accelerated carotid atherosclerosis. *Arch Neurol* 1987; **44**: 711–14.

48. Bergeron P, Chambran P, Benichou H *et al.* Recurrent carotid artery disease: Will stents be an alternative to surgery? *J Endovasc Surg* 1996; **3**: 76–9.

49. Gray WA, DuBroff RJ, White HJ. A common clinical conundrum. *N Engl J Med* 1997; **336**: 1008–11.

50. Meyer FB, Piepgras DG, Fode NC. Surgical treatment of recurrent carotid artery stenosis. *J Neurosurg* 1994; **80**: 781–7.

51. Lanzino G, Mericle RA, Guterman LR *et al.* Angioplasty and stenting of recurrent carotid stenosis. Presented at the Annual Meeting of the Neurosurgical Society of the Virginias. Richmond, VA, January 23–27, 1998.

52. Theron J, Raymond J, Casasco A *et al.* Percutaneous angioplasty of atherosclerotic and postsurgical stenosis of carotid arteries. *Am J Neuroradiol* 1987; **8** (Suppl 3): 495–500.

53. Yadav SS, Roubin GS, King P *et al.* Angioplasty and stenting for restenosis after carotid endarterectomy: Initial experience. *Stroke* 1996; **27**: 2075–9.

54. Vitek JJ, Roubin GS, New G *et al.* Carotid angioplasty with stenting in post-carotid endarterectomy restenosis. *J Invasive Cardiol* 2001; **13** (2): 123–5.

55. Gasecki AP, Eliasziw M, Ferguson GG *et al.*, for the North American Symptomatic Carotid Endarterectomy Trial (NASCET) Group. Long-term prognosis and effect of endarterectomy in patients with symptomatic severe carotid stenosis and contralateral carotid stenosis or occlusion: Results from NASCET. *J Neurosurg* 1995; **83**: 778–782.
56. Gerlock A, Mirfakhraee M. Difficulty in catheterization of the left common carotid arteries. In: Gerlock A, Mirfakhraee M, eds. *Essentials of Diagnostic and Interventional Angiographic Techniques.* WB Saunders, 1985: 106–19.
57. Qureshi AI, Luft AR, Janardhan V *et al.* Identification of patients at risk for periprocedural neurological deficits associated with carotid angioplasty and stenting. *Stroke* 2000; **31**: 376–82.
58. Qureshi AI, Luft AR, Sharma M *et al.* Frequency and determinants of postprocedural hemodynamic instability after carotid angioplasty and stenting. *Stroke* 1999; **30**: 2086–93.
59. Roubin GS, Iyer SS, Vitek JJ. Carotid artery stenting: Rationale, indications, technique and results. In: Heuser RR, ed. *Peripheral Vascular Stenting for Cardiologists*. Martin Dunitz, 1999: 67–117.
60. Gerlock A, Mirfakhraee M, eds. *Essentials of Diagnostic and Interventional Angiographic Techniques*. WB Saunders, 1985.
61. Guterman LR, Wakhloo AK, Mericle RA *et al.* Treatment of cervical carotid bifurcation stenosis with angioplasty and stent assisted revascularization. Presented at the 35th Annual Meeting of the American Society of Neuroradiology. Toronto, Canada, May 18–22, 1997.
62. Theron JG, Payelle GG, Coskun O *et al.* Carotid artery stenosis: Treatment with protected balloon angioplasty and stent placement. *Radiology* 1996; **201**: 627–36.
63. Gerlock A, Mirfakhraee M. Difficulty in catheterization of the internal and external carotid arteries. In: Gerlock A, Mirfakhraee M, eds. *Essentials of Diagnostic and Interventional Angiographic Techniques*. WB Saunders, 1985: 120–3.
64. Sievert H, Ensslen R, Fach A *et al.* Brachial artery approach for transluminal angioplasty of the internal carotid artery. *Cathet Cardiovasc Diagn* 1996; **39**: 421–3.
65. Mathur A, Roubin GS, Iyer SS *et al.* Predictors of stroke complicating carotid artery stenting. *Circulation* 1998; **97**: 1239–45.
66. Dorros G. Complications associated with extracranial carotid artery interventions. *J Endovasc Surg* 1996; **3**: 236–70.
67. Wholey MH, Wholey M, Mathias K *et al.* Global experience in cervical carotid artery stent placement. *Cathet Cardiovasc Interv* 2000; **50** (2): 168–9.
68. Wechsler LR, Jungreis CA. Intra-arterial thrombolysis for carotid circulation ischemia. *Crit Care Clin* 1999; **15**: 701–18.

69. Coller BS. GPIIb/IIIa antagonists: Pathophysiologic and therapeutic insights from studies of c7E3 Fab. *Thromb Haemost* 1997; **78**: 730–5.
70. Kastrup A, Groschel K, Krapf H *et al.* Early outcome of carotid angioplasty and stenting with and without cerebral protection devices: a systematic review of the literature. *Stroke* 2003; **34** (3): 813–19.
71. Chakhtoura EY, Hobson RW, Goldstein J *et al.* In-stent restenosis after carotid angioplasty-stenting: incidence and management. *J Vasc Surg* 2001; **33** (2): 220–5.

Chapter 23

Endovascular Abdominal Aortic Aneurysm Exclusion

Edward B Diethrich

General clinical overview
Indications for the procedure
Standard procedure
Complications
Clinical trials

GENERAL CLINICAL OVERVIEW

The early work of Dr Juan Parodi paved the way for endoluminal graft (ELG) exclusion of abdominal aortic aneurysms (AAAs),[1] and further investigation in clinical centers all over the world has advanced ELG technology considerably since its inception. While initial study demonstrated that the prototype straight tube graft designs without distal stent fixation were unsatisfactory, a number of ELG designs are now available and have been used to treat thousands of AAAs in a variety of patients.

The Mintec device was the first commercially available bifurcated ELG and was sold originally in Europe. Boston Scientific Corporation purchased the Mintec graft, design changes were made, and the device was reintroduced in Europe under the name Stentor, and later as Vanguard. In the United States, the first two commercial products approved were the Ancure device by Guidant (Menlo Park, CA) and the AneuRx device by Medtronic (Sunnyvale, CA). More recently, other devices, such as the Talent graft by World Medical/Medtronic (Sunrise, FL), the Zenith graft (Cook, Bloomington, IN), the Endologix graft (Endologix, Irvine, CA), the Lifepath graft (Edwards, Irvine, CA), the Excluder graft (WL Gore, Flagstaff, AZ), and

*Basic; **Advanced; ***Rare, exotic, or investigational.

From: Nguyen T, Hu D, Saito S, Grines C, Palacios I (eds), *Practical Handbook of Advanced Interventional Cardiology*, 2nd edn. © 2003 Futura, an imprint of Blackwell Publishing.

the Teramed graft (Cordis Endovascular, Warren, NJ) have been introduced. Most of these designs have received a CE mark (European Commission approval) and are being sold in Europe. Although results from a number of studies with 1st, 2nd, and even 3rd generation devices have been reported, there are no long-term ELG outcome data available, and intermediate-term success must be evaluated separately for each specific device. Recently, a collaborative evaluation of endovascular aneurysm repair has been undertaken as part of the Lifeline Registry.[2] The aim of the registry is to collect data that will eventually provide a large body of information regarding the safety and effectiveness of ELGs in the United States and Canada.

INDICATIONS FOR THE PROCEDURE

The indications for endovascular AAA exclusion have changed since the introduction of the technique. Originally, patients with hostile abdomens, cutaneous fistulas such as colostomies and ureterostomies, critical cardiac and pulmonary pathologies, and severe comorbidities were the primary recipients of endovascular treatment. Later, as results from worldwide investigations were evaluated, protocols were designed to include patients with less severe comorbidities, smaller aneurysms, and those with lesions <5 cm who would not normally have been considered even for an open procedure.[3] Indeed, it appears that endovascular AAA repair has augmented treatment options rather than replacing the conventional procedure.[4] However, offering endovascular procedures to those with serious comorbidities can yield poor results unless other factors are carefully evaluated. In one study, the cumulative 1-year survival rates for patients considered to be unfit for open surgery or general anesthesia were less than 25% after ELG implantation.[5]

Overall, early evidence suggests that the most important determinant of a successful ELG procedure is vascular anatomy.[6–9] Research indicates that patients with less tortuous arteries are often the best candidates, and men tend to have larger, straighter vessels that are better suited to ELG procedures.[6] In one study,[7] women were shown to be more likely than men to require readmission for correction of complications following endovascular repair. Length of stay for these women was also significantly longer than that of men who were readmitted following ELG placement.

While vascular anatomy certainly contributes to the ease of device placement, the contour, length, and diameter of the aneurysm neck itself have been linked to the risk of endoleaks.[8] If the contour of the aneurysm neck changes by >3 mm (P=0.003), or the neck length is <20 mm long (P=0.045), the risk of proximal endoleak is significantly increased. Recent

Table 23-1
Anatomic characteristics that predict successful endovascular intervention in abdominal aortic aneurysms*

1. Cephalad neck length ≥2 cm
2. Cephalad neck diameter < 26 mm
3. Absence of cephalad neck calcium or thrombosis
4. Zero angulation of the proximal neck between the renal arteries and the origin of the AAA
5. Normal renal artery orifices at the same aortic level
6. Absence of accessory renal arteries below principal renal arteries
7. A straight 10-cm aorta between the renal arteries and the aortic bifurcation
8. Patent celiac axis and superior mesenteric arteries
9. Occluded inferior mesenteric artery at its origin
10. Absence of occlusive disease of the common and external iliac arteries and the common femoral artery
11. Absence of tortuosity and calcification of the above arteries with a minimum internal diameter of 8 mm
12. Common iliac arteries 4 cm in length between their origin and the bifurcation into the external and internal arteries
13. Absence of patent lumbar arteries within the aneurysm
14. Normal renal function
15. Normal coagulation profile
16. Lack of obesity, particularly at arterial access sites

*As the number of these favorable characteristics decreases, so does the chance of successful intervention

data do indicate, however, that complications are not related to aneurysm size, and that while endovascular repair of large aneurysms may be "challenging," a short proximal aortic neck is the major significant anatomic risk factor for intra- and postoperative complications.[9] At the Arizona Heart Institute, we select patients for endovascular AAA procedures on the basis of favorable anatomy rather than relying solely on surgical risk status. Table 23-1 lists anatomic characteristics associated with positive outcomes of endovascular intervention for AAAs.

STANDARD PROCEDURE

While the AAA procedure is fairly standardized, there are certainly device-dependent variations. For this procedure description, placement of the Endologix graft (Figure 23-1) is detailed since it has the potential for percutaneous delivery, an aspect that is attractive to interventional cardiologists.

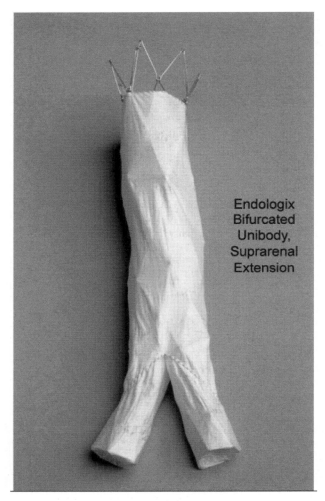

Endologix
Bifurcated
Unibody,
Suprarenal
Extension

Figure 23-1: The Endologix graft.

If the common femoral artery (CFA) is to be exposed an oblique incision is made just below the inguinal ligament. If the CFA is small, the external iliac artery is exposed beneath the inguinal ligament and used for entry of the delivery device. Alternatively, a 12.5F peel-away sheath (Safe Sheath, Pressure Products, Inc., Rancho Palos Verdes, CA) is inserted after selection of an appropriate closure device, and the opposite CFA is cannulated with a 9F sheath (Figure 23-2), and heparin (5000 units) is injected. Contrast is injected bilaterally to

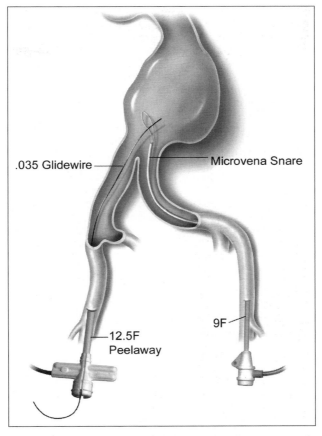

.035 Glidewire

Microvena Snare

12.5F
Peelaway

9F

Figure 23-2: A 12.5F peel-away sheath is inserted after selection of an appropriate closure device, and the opposite common femoral artery is cannulated with a 9F sheath. Bilateral 0.035" angled Glidewires are passed into the lower abdominal aorta, and a Microvena snare is used to pull one of the Glidewires (does not matter which) to the appropriate sheath where it exits.

evaluate the iliac arteries, the origin and nature of the internal iliac arteries, and the degree of iliac tortuosity. Bilateral 0.035" angled Glidewires (MediTech/Boston Scientific, Natick, MA) are passed into the lower abdominal aorta, and a Microvena snare (Microvena Corp., White Bear Lake, MN) is used to pull one of the Glidewires (does not matter which) to the appropriate sheath where it exits (Figure 23-2).

An aortogram is performed using a pigtail catheter, and the image intensifier is positioned so that the renal arteries are seen at the top of the fluoroscopic screen, and the crossover wire is visible below them. A needle is then placed transversely on the skin to identify the level of the renal arteries (optional). Once the image is obtained, the image intensifier is not moved, thereby eliminating the problem of parallax. A crossover catheter is passed from the left (contralateral) to the right (ipsilateral) side. The catheter is positioned on the fluoroscopic screen so that the radiopaque beads are located at about the eleven o'clock position. This ensures that the stiff wire (Nitinol Guidewire, Microvena Corp., White Bear Lake, MN) used to deliver the prosthesis will pass into the suprarenal position through the hole in the crossover catheter marked by the beads.

The AAA device (in this case the Endologix graft) is placed on the table and prepared for delivery. The stiff delivery wire is passed through the device, and the contralateral pullwire is loaded into the crossover catheter and pulled through until it appears on the opposite side (Figure 23-3). The crossover catheter is removed while the crossover wire is firmly held at its junction on the delivery sheet; this prevents premature disconnection of the wire and contralateral limb. The prosthesis is then advanced to the CFA sheath. The sheath is withdrawn, and the CFA is squeezed between the thumb and index finger to prevent bleeding while the peel-away sheath is removed. The prosthesis is advanced into the CFA as the contralateral pullwire is pulled gently.

In order to ensure proper alignment from the contralateral sheath and avoid wire twist, the orientation is always pullwire-medial and guidewire-lateral at the groin level. Additionally, the irrigation port on the delivery sheath should always point towards the contralateral side. The prosthesis is delivered under fluoroscopic control above the aortic bifurcation. The contralateral pullwire is withdrawn into the left groin in order to remove excess "slack." The contralateral limb is freed by retracting its retaining sheath while the contralateral pullwire is gently pulled from the groin (Figure 23-4). The main body of the prosthesis is re-sheathed (Figure 23-5). The cephalad end of the graft is lowered and positioned at the renal artery level (Figure 23-6). The body of the graft is deployed up to the last cephalad stent. This deployment is caudad to cephalad.

Until the body is completely deployed by releasing the most cephalad stent, the graft can be moved in relation to the renal arteries. The prosthesis is held in position as the contralateral pullwire is pulled to release the contralateral limb (Figs 23-7 and 23-8), and the last stent is released to complete the deployment of the main body (Figure 23-9). The pusher rod is further advanced until it encapsulates the nose cone. The nose cone is withdrawn through the body of the graft down to

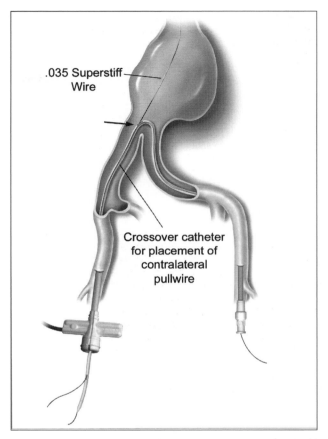

.035 Superstiff
Wire

Crossover catheter
for placement of
contralateral
pullwire

Figure 23-3: The stiff delivery wire is placed, and the contralateral pullwire is loaded into the crossover catheter and pulled
through until it appears on the opposite side.

the ipsilateral limb still covered by the sheath (Figure 23-10).
The ipsilateral limb is deployed (Figure 23-11), and the nose
cone is withdrawn into the sheath; the entire assembly is removed (Figure 23-12). A 9F sheath is inserted into the right
common femoral artery, and a control angiogram is obtained.
Bilateral femoral sheath angiograms are performed to confirm
the absence of a distal endoleak. The right CF artery is closed
with a closure device or using a simple purse-string suture
through the fascia. The patient is returned to the recovery
unit; the left CFA sheath is removed when the ACT returns to
normal range.

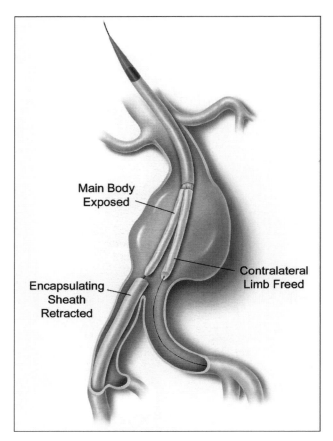

Figure 23-4: The contralateral limb is freed by retracting its retaining sheath while the contralateral pullwire is gently pulled from the groin.

TECHNICAL TIP

Techniques for success: As indicated in Table 23-1, it is important not to overstep the accepted or recommended patient selection criteria on the device labeling material. Each deviation from the accepted criteria multiplies the potential for failure not only acutely, but also during the follow-up period. Three major complications related to deviations from these criteria have been identified: (1) migration, (2) endoleak, and (3) rupture. Careful adherence to the protocol can, in most cases, prevent these complications.

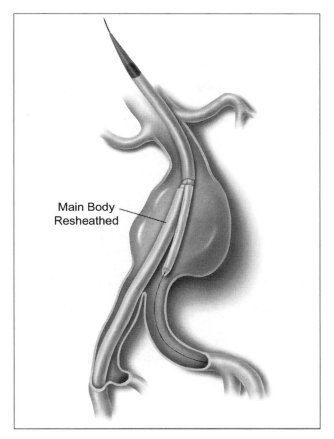

Figure 23-5: The main body of the prosthesis is re-sheathed.

In short, whenever possible, remain in the "perfect world" for the device.

In spite of such an admonition, the "perfect" patient is seldom seen, or may not be a candidate for the AAA graft procedure. One example is the female patient with small, calcified or tortuous arteries. None of the devices currently available can be delivered through a 6.5 mm external iliac artery. Refrain from trying unless rupture is a condition the endovascular team does not fear. It is prudent to approach such a case with a vascular surgeon colleague, who will expose the common iliac artery using a retroperitoneal approach and prepare a conduit for ELG delivery.

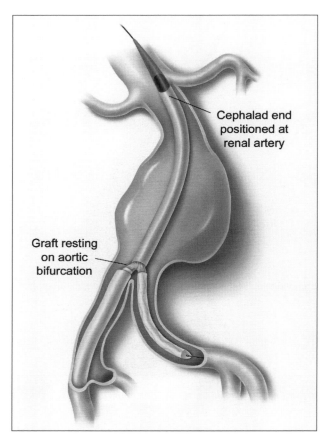

Figure 23-6: The cephalad end of the graft is lowered and positioned at the renal artery level.

COMPLICATIONS

The most common complication associated with endoluminal grafting is the endoleak. Endoleaks have been categorized as follows: type I – related to graft attachment; type II – retrograde flow from collateral branches (called a "retroleak"); type III – fabric tears, graft disconnection, or disintegration; and type IV – flow through graft wall due to porosity.[10] Recent improvements in ELG prostheses have virtually eliminated type IV endoleaks.

Research indicates that the potential for endoleaks may be predicted in some cases. In a group of patients treated with AneuRx grafts, Cox proportional hazards regression

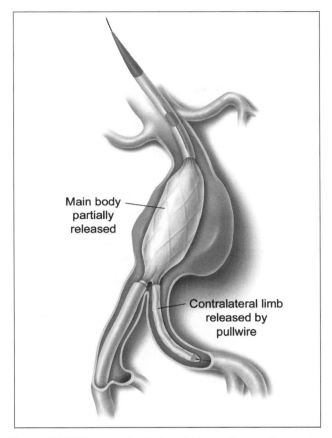

Figure 23-7: The prosthesis is held in position as the contralateral pullwire is pulled to release the contralateral limb. *(Continued in Fig. 3.28)*

analysis demonstrated that both patent internal mesenteric arteries (P<0.01) and patent lumbar arteries (P<0.0001) were independent risk factors for persistent endoleaks.[11] The researchers also concluded that persistent type II endoleaks were associated with an increase in AAA size and no significant change in the infrarenal neck diameter. As described in "Indications for the procedure" above, patient selection that is based on careful evaluation of vascular anatomy is extremely important in the overall success of the endovascular AAA procedure.

Endoleaks are treated by a variety of means, including conversion to surgical repair, or insertion of a new stent or

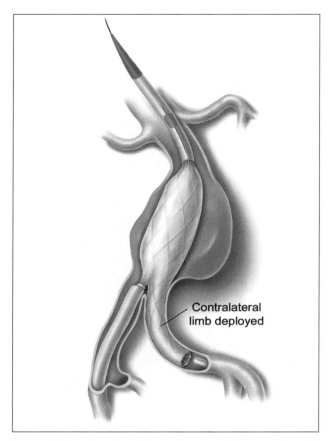

Figure 23-8: *(Continued from Fig. 23.7)* The prosthesis is held in position as the contralateral pullwire is pulled to release the contralateral limb.

graft. Unfortunately, both primary and secondary conversion carry a high operative mortality rate.[12] Recently, type II endoleaks have been treated with a liquid embolic agent containing an ethylene-vinyl-alcohol copolymer.[13] The liquid is injected in the endoleak sac, and early experience indicates it may be a viable treatment alternative. While further study is required, injecting the copolymer may reduce procedure time and achieve a complete, durable occlusion in many cases.

Other less frequent although potentially more serious complications are also associated with ELGs and appear to be somewhat device dependent. The Ancure graft (Guidant,

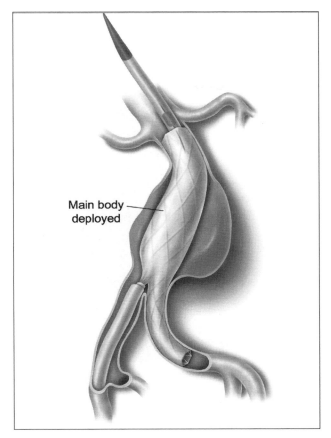

Main body
deployed

Figure 23-9: The last stent is released to complete the deployment of the main body.

Menlo Park, CA) has been linked with a high occlusion rate of the bifurcated limb, and conversion rates with these stent-grafts have been higher than those associated with other devices.[12] Although late (2-year) type II endoleaks have been a problem and multicenter trials of the tube and bifurcated devices indicate evidence of proximal neck dilatation at 1–3 years,[14] the incidence of aneurysm rupture following successful deployment of the Ancure prosthesis has been extremely low.[15] In contrast, rupture has been more frequently associated with the AneuRx stent-graft (Medtronic, Santa Rosa, CA), and the FDA issued a Public Health Notification of the problem in April 2001.[16] Migration of the device has also

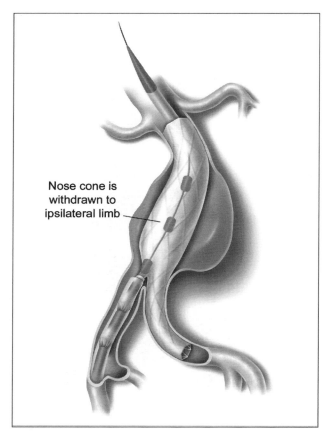

Nose cone is
withdrawn to
ipsilateral limb

Figure 23-10: The nose cone is withdrawn through the body of the graft down to the ipsilateral limb still covered by the sheath.

been reported.[17] It is worth noting that complications with the AneuRx graft have been reduced significantly since a more flexible prosthesis was introduced.[18]

CLINICAL TRIALS

Although more than a decade has passed since the first published account of endoluminal grafting of an AAA,[1] we are still at a relatively early stage in ELG technology. Our understanding of patient selection and the prevention and management of complications has improved, and ELG designs have advanced considerably. While there are those who will argue

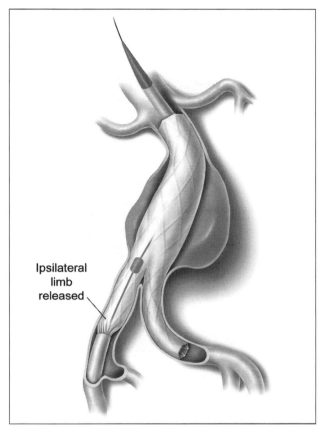

Figure 23-11: The ipsilateral limb is deployed.

that the open surgical procedure offers a more dependable long-term solution and is the procedure of choice for AAA exclusion,[19] endoluminal grafting compares very favorably with surgical intervention.[20–23] Indeed, the minimally invasive procedure reduces operating time and the need for blood transfusions and yields lower infection rates and shorter ICU and hospital stays as compared with open surgery.[20] In another study, survival curves favored the endoluminal graft group (P = 0.004), and a Kaplan-Meier curve for graft failure revealed 3-year success probabilities were similar (82% versus 85% in the endoluminal graft and open repair group, respectively).[21] Following elective repair of infrarenal abdominal aortic aneurysms, significantly more patients went home (rather than to a rehabilitation facility) after an endovascular procedure than after open surgery.[22] In addition, patients who have had

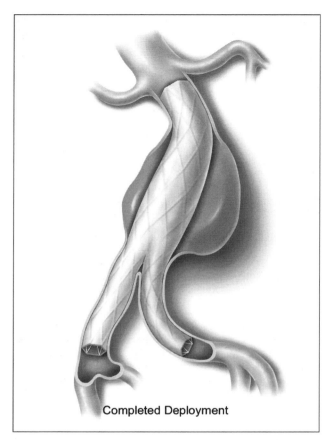

Completed Deployment

Figure 23-12: Completed deployment of the Endologix graft.

surgical AAA repair report substantial functional impairment; a third of the patients in one trial stated they had not fully recovered at a mean follow-up of 34 months, and nearly 20% of patients said they would not undergo AAA repair again given the required recovery.[23] Overall, it certainly appears that despite the acknowledged durability of open repair, endoluminal grafting is an attractive alternative for treatment of AAAs.

REFERENCES

1. Parodi JC, Palmaz JC, Barone HD. Transfemoral intraluminal graft implantation for abdominal aortic aneurysms. *Ann Vasc Surg* 1991; **5**: 491–9.

2. Lifeline Registry Committee. Lifeline registry: collaborative evaluation of endovascular aneurysm repair. *J Vasc Surg* 2001; **34**: 1139–46.

3. May J, White G, Yu W, Waugh R, Stephen MS, Harris J. Concurrent comparison of endoluminal repair versus no treatment for small abdominal aortic aneurysms. *Eur J Vasc Endovasc Surg* 1997; **13**: 472–6.

4. Wolf YG, Fogarty TJ, Olcott C IV *et al*. Endovascular repair of abdominal aortic aneurysms: eligibility rate and impact on the rate of open repair. *J Vasc Surg* 2000; **32**: 519–23.

5. Laheij RJ, van Marrewijk CJ. Endovascular stenting of abdominal aortic aneurysms in patients unfit for elective open surgery. Eurostar group. *Lancet* 2000; **356**: 832.

6. Velazquez OC, Larson RA, Baum RA *et al*. Gender-related differences in infrarenal aortic aneurysm morphologic features: Issues relevant to Ancure and Talent endografts. *J Vasc Surg* 2001; **33**: S77–84.

7. Carpenter JP, Baum RA, Barker CF *et al*. Durability of benefits of endovascular versus conventional abdominal aortic aneurysm repair. *J Vasc Surg* 2002; **35**: 222–8.

8. Stanley BM, Semmens JB, Mai Q *et al*. Evaluation of patient selection guidelines for endoluminal AAA repair with the Zenith Stent-Graft: the Australasian experience. *J Endovasc Ther* 2001; **8**: 457–64.

9. Hovsepian DM, Hein AN, Pilgram TK *et al*. Endovascular abdominal aortic repair in 144 patients: correlation of aneurysm size, proximal aortic neck length, and procedure-related complications. *J Vasc Interv Radiol* 2001; **12**: 1373–82.

10. May J, White GH, Waugh R *et al*. Adverse events after endoluminal repair of abdominal aortic aneurysms: a comparison during two successive periods of time. *J Vasc Surg* 1999; **29**: 32–7.

11. Arko FR, Rubin GD, Johnson BL, Hill BB, Fogarty TJ, Zarins CK. Type II endoleaks following endovascular repair: preoperative predictors and long-term effects. *J Endovasc Ther* 2001; **8**: 503–10.

12. Cuypers PW, Laheij RJ, Buth J. Which factors increase the risk of conversion to open surgery following endovascular abdominal aortic aneurysm repair? The EUROSTAR collaborators. *Eur J Vasc Endovasc Surg* 2000; **20**: 183–9.

13. Martin ML, Dolmatch BL, Fry PD, Machan LS. Treatment of type II endoleaks with Onyx. *J Vasc Interv Radiol* 2001; **12**: 629–32.

14. Makaroun MS, Deaton DH for the Endovascular Technologies Investigators. Is proximal aortic neck dilatation after endovascular aneurysm exclusion a cause for concern? *J Vasc Surg* 2001; **33**: S39–45.

15. Makaroun MS. The Ancure endografting system: An update. *J Vasc Surg* 2001; **33**: S129–34.

16. Feigal DW. FDA Public Health Notification: Problems with Endovascular Grafts for Treatment of Abdominal Aortic Aneurysm (AAA). **www.fdagov/cdrh/safety.html**

17. Tutein Nolthenius RP, van Herwaarden JA, van den Berg JC, van Marrewijk C, Teijink JA, Moll FL. Three-year single centre experience with the AneuRx aortic stent graft. *Eur J Vasc Endovasc Surg* 2001; **22**: 257–64.

18. Arko FR, Lee WA, Hill BB, Cipriano P, Fogarty TJ, Zarins CK. Increased flexibility of AneuRx stent-graft reduces the need for secondary intervention following endovascular aneurysm repair. *J Endovasc Ther* 2001; **8**: 583–91.

19. Biancari F, Ylonen K, Anttila V *et al.* Durability of open repair of infrarenal abdominal aortic aneurysm: a 15-year follow-up study. *J Vasc Surg* 2002; **35**: 87–93.

20. Treiman GS, Lawrence PF, Edwards WH, Galt SW, Kraiss LW, Bhirangi K. An assessment of the current applicability of the EVT endograft for the treatment of patients with an infrarenal abdominal aortic aneurysm. *J Vasc Surg* 1999; **30**, 68–75.

21. May J, White GH, Waugh R *et al.* Improved survival after endoluminal repair with second-generation prostheses compared with open repair in the treatment of abdominal aortic aneurysms: A 5-year concurrent comparison using life table method. *J Vasc Surg* 2001; **33**: S21–6.

22. Bosch JL, Beinfeld MT, Halpern EF, Lester JS, Gazelle GS. Endovascular versus open surgical elective repair of infrarenal abdominal aortic aneurysm: predictors of patient discharge destination. *Radiology* 2001; **220**: 576–80.

23. Williamson WK, Nicoloff AD, Taylor LM Jr, Moneta GL, Landry GJ, Porter JM. Functional outcome after open repair of abdominal aortic aneurysm. *J Vasc Surg* 2001; **33**: 913–20.

Chapter 24

Inoue Balloon Mitral Valvuloplasty

Jui-Sung Hung, Nguyen Quang Tuan, Pham Manh Hung, Moo Hyun Kim, Kean Wah Lau

General overview
Location of transseptal access
    **Variances of the mid-line
    **Appropriateness of the Inoue method
Septal puncture
    **Exact positioning of the tip of the catheter/needle
    **Exact positioning of the tip of the needle/catheter in giant left atrium
    **Repositioning the tip of the needle/catheter after failed first try
    **Needle tip reshaping
    **How to puncture a thick septum
    **How to avoid puncturing the right atrium
    **How to avoid puncturing the aorta, tricuspid valve, and coronary sinus
    **How to avoid puncture medial to the "mid-line"
Selection of balloon catheter
    **Pretesting for balloon-syringe mismatch
Advancement of the balloon catheter
    ** Resistance at groin access site
    **Septal resistance
    **Deep catheter placement in left atrium
Crossing the mitral valve
    **Optimal position of the stylet
    **Stylet reshaping
Balloon inflation
    **If the balloon strays among the chordae
    **Severe subvalvular disease undetected by echocardiography

---

*Basic; **Advanced; ***Rare, exotic, or investigational.

From: Nguyen T, Hu D, Saito S, Grines C, Palacios I (eds), *Practical Handbook of Advanced Interventional Cardiology*, 2nd edn. © 2003 Futura, an imprint of Blackwell Publishing.

**Balloon sizing in patients with pliable, noncalcified valves
**Balloon sizing in patients with calcified valves and/or with severe subvalvular disease
**Balloon sizing in case of "balloon impasse"
**Balloon "popping" to the left atrium
**Subsequent valve crossings and dilations
**Catheter entrapment at the atrial septum
**Avoiding the left atrial appendage
**Withdrawing the catheter from the ventricle
**Subsequent crossings
**Avoiding entry into the left atrial appendage
**Minimizing atrial septal injury
**Bent balloon tip
Indications
Contraindications

GENERAL OVERVIEW

Percutaneous balloon mitral valvuloplasty (BMV) introduced in 1984 by Inoue et al.[1] has opened a new dimension in the treatment of patients with mitral stenosis. Extensive clinical studies have established this invasive, nonsurgical procedure to be a safe and effective therapeutic modality in selected patients with mitral stenosis.[2–8]

With successful balloon valve enlargement, there is generally a 2-fold increase in the mitral valve area[2–8] and an associated dramatic fall in transmitral valve gradient, left atrial pressure, and pulmonary artery pressure. These hemodynamic benefits are mirrored in clinical improvements in the patients' symptoms and improved exercise tolerance after BMV.[9] The long-term results of BMV are excellent, especially when the acute results are optimal and in the presence of good valve morphology.[9–13] Hernandez and associates[14] found that survival free of major events (cardiac death, mitral surgery, repeat BMV, or functional impairment) was 69% at 7 years, ranging from 88% to 40% in different subgroups of patients. Mitral area loss, though mild (0.13 ± 0.21 cm^2), increased with time and was ≥ 0.3 cm^2 in 12%, 22%, and 27% of patients at 3, 5, and 7 years, respectively.

Besides the original Inoue technique using size-adjustable, self-positioning balloon catheters, various other techniques using fixed-sized balloon catheters have been developed for performing BMV. These include the antegrade (transvenous) approaches with one or two balloon catheters through one or two interatrial septal punctures[15,16] or the retrograde (transarterial) approaches with transseptal wiring or without transseptal access.[17] However, the Inoue balloon catheter system via the transvenous approach has remained the principal BMV technique used today.

Our extensive experience in Inoue BMV has demonstrated that incremental operator experience and ongoing technical refinements in BMV techniques have resulted in a nearly 100% technical success rate and a significant diminution in complications despite the presence of a significant number of technically demanding scenarios and high-risk comorbid conditions.[4] This is attributable to operator experience and continuously evolving Inoue BMV technique.[9,18–20] The present chapter discusses the pitfalls and tricks in Inoue balloon BMV to facilitate success and minimize complications of the BMV. We hope that this chapter will be beneficial to all Inoue BMV operators at different levels of experience. The instrumentation of the Inoue balloon catheter system has been extensively described in previous publications,[1–3] and is thus not included in this chapter.

LOCATION OF TRANSSEPTAL ACCESS

Transseptal catheterization is a vital component of BMV. Transseptal puncture must not only be executed safely to avoid cardiac perforation, but also made at an appropriate septal site to facilitate balloon crossing of the stenosed mitral valve. To avert cardiac perforation during transseptal catheterization, some operators have resorted to routine intraprocedural transesophageal echocardiography to facilitate optimal transseptal needle placement; however, even with the echocardiographic guidance, cardiac perforation may still occur.[21] Therefore, acquisition of basic transseptal skill is essential. To perform transseptal procedure, biplane fluoroscopic equipment is preferable, but single-plane fluoroscopy is usually sufficient. The needed instruments are listed in Table 24-1.

The use of the sheath is optional, but its utility is recommended, especially for inexperienced operators, for two reasons: (1) to prevent inadvertent perforation of the dilator by the needle during its insertion, and (2) to prevent left atrial perforation during insertion of the catheter/needle into the left atrium because the sheath tip works as a safety stopper at the septum.

Catheter/needle fitting exercise: A catheter/needle fitting (Figure 24-1) should be performed before its insertion into the patient. First, fully insert the transseptal needle until its tip extends beyond the catheter. Then withdraw the needle

---

Table 24-1 **Instruments for septal puncture**

1. A Brockenbrough needle
2. A 7F or 8F dilator catheter
3. An outer sheath catheter

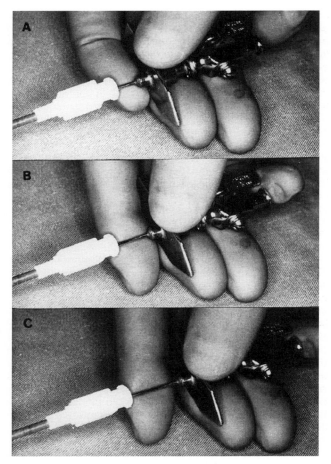

Figure 24-1: Catheter/needle fitting exercise. (A) First, fully insert the transseptal needle until its tip extends beyond the dilator tip. (B) The needle is then withdrawn until its tip is aligned with the dilator tip. (C) It is pulled back farther, thus the needle tip is concealed slightly (2–3 mm) from the dilator tip. The index finger is fixed as a stopper on the needle between the direction indicator and the catheter hub to prevent the needle from moving forward and protruding from the dilator tip. This is of vital importance during *in vivo* manipulation of the catheter/needle. The depth and the angle of the stopper-finger (C) are adjusted according to the distance between the direction indicator and the catheter hub in each catheter/needle set. Each side of the direction indicator is held by the thumb and the index finger, respectively. This makes rotation of the indicator easier, and also allows the blunt part of the direction indicator visible to the operator and the tutor (if any). (From *Cathet Cardiovasc Diagn* 1992; **26**: 275–84.)

until its tip is concealed slightly (2–3 mm) within the tip of the catheter. The operator should fix his/her right index finger as a stopper on the needle between the direction indicator and the catheter hub to prevent the needle from moving forward and protruding from the catheter tip. This is of vital importance during *in vivo* manipulation of the catheter/needle. Each side of the direction indicator is held by the thumb and the index finger, respectively.

Landmarks for optimal puncture site: The target site is usually located in its latitude on the vertical "mid-line," and in its altitude on the horizontal M-line. The vertical "mid-line" is a conceptual line dividing the intra-atrial septum into anterior and posterior halves. The M-line is a horizontal line crossing the center of the mitral annulus or valve. In individual cases, however, the puncture latitude may have to be adjusted. For example, in patients with a more vertically oriented left ventricle, the puncture site is chosen slightly above the M-line. In patients with giant left atria, the operator is often forced to make septal puncture more caudal to the M-line.

1. Definition of the vertical "mid-line" – Inoue's angiographic method: Inoue has devised a specific trans-septal puncture technique designed for the Inoue BMV, incorporating the concept of a vertical "mid-line," a line assumed to divide the intra-atrial septum into anterior and posterior halves.[22] This line is defined based on the landmarks obtained from frontal plane right atrial angiography during normal respiration, as shown in Figure 24-2.

2. Definition of the vertical "mid-line" – Hung's modified fluoroscopic method: Because in most cases of mitral stenosis the left atrial silhouette is visible under fluoroscopy, Hung has modified Inoue's method of defining the "mid-line." In this method, the aortic valve is used to substitute the tricuspid valve because the two valves are in close proximity to each other. Therefore, point T is substituted with the tip of a pigtail catheter (Figure 24-2, right panel, point A) touching the aortic valve (usually the noncoronary sinus of Valsalva) in the frontal view. A horizontal line is drawn from point A to L_2, where the line intersects the right lateral edge of the left atrium. The "mid-line" thus derived is usually identical to that from Inoue's angiographic method (Figure 24-2, right panel).

TECHNICAL TIP

**Variances of the mid-line: The septum lies within the superimposed area between the two atria, and therefore there is no septum outside this area. The lateral (or posterior) limit is the lateral border of the medial atrium, usually the left atrium. Infrequently (such as in patients with giant left atria), the lateral border of the right atrium is medial to that of the left atrium, and thus point L should be on the right atrial border because there is no septum laterally beyond

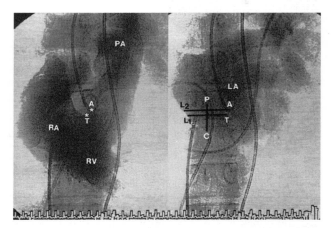

Figure 24-2: The "mid-line." The upper end of the tricuspid valve at systole (T) is determined on a stop-frame frontal right atrial angiographic image (left panel) and translated to a stop-frame left atrial image (right panel). On the latter image, an imaginary horizontal line is drawn from point T to point L_1, where the line intersects the lateral border of the atrium encountered first (usually the left atrium, as in this case). Point L_1 is assumed to be the posterior limit of the septum. The vertical line crossing at the mid-point between T and L_1 is the "mid-line" (Line PC). LA = left atrium; PA = pulmonary artery; RA = right atrium.(From *Cathet Cardiovasc Diagn* 1992; **26**: 275–84.)

this point. BMV can be performed with the patient in a semi-recumbent position in an urgent situation. In this setting, the "mid-line" can be defined in frontal view with appropriate caudal tilting.[23] The frontal image intensifier needs to be tilted in a caudal angle corresponding to the degree of semi-recumbency to negate the patient's tilt and "normalize" the positional relationship of the various intrathoracic structures. For example, if the patient is lying at 30° to the horizontal, the frontal image intensifier should be rotated to 30° caudally.

3. Definition of the horizontal "M-line": The "M-line" is a horizontal line crossing the center of the mitral annulus (point M). It is derived from a diastolic stop frame of diagnostic left ventriculography obtained in 30° RAO projection (Figure 24-3 A). The latter is identical to the projection used when manipulating the catheter balloon across the mitral valve. This line is memorized in relation to the vertebral body. The stop frame angiogram is also used as a road map during transseptal puncture and balloon catheter manipulation. The above landmarks can be drawn in the mind, and, therefore, actual plotting and drawings on the image monitor are not necessary.

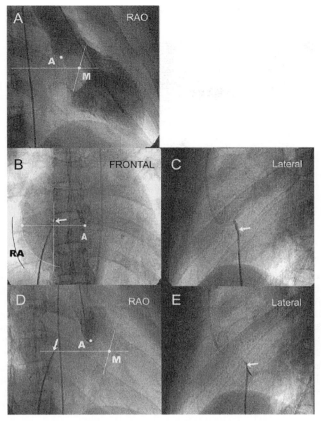

Figure 24-3: Catheter/needle manipulation. (A) Stop-frame left ventriculogram in 30° RAO view shows a horizintal line, M-line, crossing the center of the mitral annulus. (B) Under frontal fluoroscopic view, the needle-fitted transseptal catheter is slowly withdrawn downward (caudally) from the superior vena cava to align the catheter/needle on the vertical mid-line. The catheter/needle is further withdrawn until its tip reaches the level of the pigtail tip touching the aortic valve (point A). (C) Under lateral view, the catheter/needle is further withdrawn caudally while contrast medium is being injected (septal flush method) to outline the right atrial margin of the septum. (D) The catheter/needle is further withdrawn to set its tip at the curvilinear portion of the septum at the altitude of the M-line. At this point, the catheter/needle is observed to be pointed dorsally. (E) Subsequently, the catheter/needle tip position is viewed under 30° RAO projection, contrasted with the left ventriculogram road map (A), to confirm optimal septal puncture site as well as to avoid puncture of other structures (the aorta, the coronary sinus and the tricuspid valve). The catheter/needle tip is now seen on the M-line, usually just anterior to the vertebra.

TECHNICAL TIP

**Appropriateness of the Inoue method: The Inoue angiographic method is suitable in the following situations: (1) for operators inexperienced with the transseptal puncture technique; (2) in cases in which atrial silhouettes are not well visualized under fluoroscopy; (3) in extremely difficult cases of transseptal puncture, e.g. in the presence of a giant left atrium;[22] (4) and if there is kyphoscoliosis.[24] In these cases, it may be necessary to perform biplane (frontal and lateral) right atrial angiography to properly visualize the atrial septal orientation and relative anatomic relationships of both atria, the tricuspid valve, and the aorta.

SEPTAL PUNCTURE

Placement of transseptal catheter/needle: The catheter/sheath is inserted via the right femoral vein over a guidewire into the superior vena cava to the level of the carina. The catheter is aspirated and flushed after removal of the wire. Then, the Brockenbrough needle, attached to a 5-cc plastic syringe containing pure contrast medium, is inserted into the catheter and carefully advanced under fluoroscopic view until its tip reaches the predetermined position (refer to "Catheter/ needle fitting exercise" above). The needle is allowed to rotate freely during its passage. The right-hand stopper-finger is now firmly kept between the catheter hub and the direction indicator of the needle to prevent the needle from moving forward (Figure 24-1). Extreme care should be taken not to let the needle slip forward during subsequent manipulation of the catheter/needle.

Catheter/needle manipulation: Under frontal fluoroscopic view, the needle-fitted transseptal catheter with its direction indicator pointing about 4 o'clock is slowly withdrawn downwards (caudally) from the superior vena cava. A clockwise rotation is applied to the direction indicator to align the catheter/needle on the "mid-line." The catheter/needle is further withdrawn until its tip reaches the level of the pigtail tip touching the aortic valve (Figure 24-3 B).

Under lateral view, the catheter/needle is further withdrawn caudally while contrast medium is injected (septal flush method),[22] by an assistant or using the operator's right hand while fixing the catheter hub and the direction indicator using the left hand to outline the right atrial margin of the septum (Figure 24-3 C,D). The catheter tip is finally set at the curvilinear portion of the septum at the altitude of the M-line (Figure 24-3 E).

Subsequently, the catheter needle/needle tip position is viewed under 30° RAO projection, contrasted with the left ventriculogram road map, to confirm optimal septal puncture site as well as to avoid puncture of other structures (Figure 24-3 D). The catheter/needle tip is now seen on the M-line, usually just anterior to the vertebra, and away from the ascending aorta, the coronary sinus and the tricuspid valve. While frontal and lateral views are sufficient for experienced operators, the RAO view is especially vital for inexperienced operators.

TECHNICAL TIPS

**Exact positioning of the tip of the catheter/needle: In most cases of mitral stenosis, a sudden sharp movement of the catheter/needle toward the left is not observed when the tip of the transseptal assembly falls over the limbic ledge and enters the fossa ovalis. This is because the atrial septum bulges markedly toward the right atrium, making the fossa ovalis more shallow.

When the septal bulge begins in the upper septum, the catheter/needle being withdrawn from the superior vena cava takes a lateral course to the "mid-line." In this case, turning the needle to the 3 o'clock direction may lead the catheter/needle to a medial position. If not, the needle alone can be withdrawn slightly, and the floppy tip of the catheter should tend to flip medially. Then the needle is advanced slowly and carefully to bring its tip back to the original position while keeping the catheter tip in the medial position. If the above means also fail to place the catheter/needle medially, the latter is withdrawn further downward and close to the lower edge of the left atrium (passing the caudal end of the bulge). With the needle pointing toward the left (about 3 o'clock), the catheter tip is allowed to shift medial to the "mid-line" and then carefully advanced cephalad. A clockwise twist is made to the needle and the catheter tip is steered to or near the target point.

**Exact positioning of the tip of the needle/catheter in giant left atrium: If the atrial septum bulges markedly toward the right atrium, especially in cases of a giant left atrium, it is difficult to align the catheter tip with the "mid-line" and perpendicular to the septum. The catheter tip faces a strong resistance at 4 o'clock when it touches the bulged septal surface. As the needle is being rotated clockwise, the catheter/needle will give way suddenly. In effect, the needle tip flips over the crest of the bulge and toward the right side of the patient pointing to 9 o'clock. To prevent this, the catheter should be pressed slightly against the septum as the needle is being rotated clockwise to 6 to 7 o'clock. At the same time, a slight counterclockwise twist is applied to the catheter with the left hand to counter any excessive clockwise rotation of the needle. If the crest of the bulge happens to be at the "mid-line," it is not possible to make a puncture on the line. In this case, the puncture site is settled in the region slightly lateral to the "mid-line."

**Repositioning the tip of the needle/catheter after failed first try: If the initial pass of the transseptal catheter/ needle is not successful in engaging it at an appropriate puncture site, the needle is removed from the catheter and the second attempt is begun by repositioning the catheter in the superior vena cava over a guidewire. The alternative is to reposition the catheter/needle high in the right atrium. This is done by setting the needle in the 12 o'clock direction (ventrally) and carefully moving the catheter/needle upward (cephalad), while slightly rotating the direction indicator of the needle clockwise and counterclockwise to make certain that the catheter tip is free and not caught against the right atrial appendage or its free wall.

**Needle tip reshaping: Reshaping of the distal needle to make it more curved may be necessary in the following situations: (1) when the catheter/needle tip tends to take a more lateral course to the "mid-line" despite counterclockwise rotation of the direction indicator to 3 o'clock direction; and (2) at the intended puncture site, there is a sharp angle between the direction of the catheter/needle and septum, therefore making the septal penetration impossible or causing septal dissection when the needle is advanced forward.

The technique of septal puncture: When the operator is satisfied with the intended puncture site, the catheter/ needle is pressed firmly against the septum. Usually, cardiac pulsations (so-called septal bounce) are felt by the right hand holding the catheter/needle. While keeping the catheter firmly against the septum to prevent it from slipping away from the puncture site, the operator releases the stopper-finger and advances the needle forward. The needle is aspirated and contrast medium is injected to confirm its entry into the left atrium. If no blood is aspirated, the needle either has dissected the high septum or is caught in the thickened septum. Staining of the septum with injection of a small amount of contrast medium (septal stain method)[22] easily distinguishes between the two (Figure 24-4). This type of septal staining is of no consequence since contrast medium is absorbed rapidly. When the high septum is dissected, it is stained in more vertical fashion. In this situation, the needle is withdrawn and septal puncture is made at a slightly more caudal site.

TECHNICAL TIPS

**How to puncture a thick septum: When the needle is caught in the thick septum (usually, in the muscular sep-

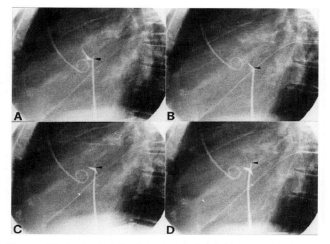

Figure 24-4: Septal flush/stain method illustrated in lateral views. (A) As the catheter/needle assembly is withdrawn caudally it is flushed with contrast medium which outlines the right atrial margin of the septum. The tip of the catheter/needle (black arrow) is at the high anterior septum. (B) The catheter/needle is withdrawn to set its tip at the puncture target site, and the needle is advanced. (C) Since the puncture is made in the thickened muscular septum, the needle is caught in the septum as demonstrated by oblique septal stain. When the catheter/needle is advanced, a "tenting" of the septum is observed. (D) The needle is carefully forced through the septum. (From *Cathet Cardiovasc Diagn* 1992; **26**: 275–84.)

tum), the stain takes more oblique orientation (Figure 24-4 C,D). In this case, the catheter/needle is carefully forced across the septum as described below or the puncture is attempted at another site. When the catheter/needle is being advanced, a "tenting" of the septum is observed before the septum is entirely pierced by the catheter/needle. With pressure monitoring, it is not possible to differentiate dissection of the high septum from entrapment of the needle in the thick septum. This is another reason why the authors perform the transseptal puncture without constant pressure monitoring.

When marked resistance is encountered during septal puncture, a sustained force is applied to the catheter/needle. After several cardiac beats, not infrequently a "give" is felt or seen under fluoroscopy when the catheter/needle finds its way into the left atrium. If this means fails to place the catheter/needle across the septum, a Bing stylet, which has a blunt tip, is inserted and extended beyond the needle. The catheter/needle is carefully forced through the tough septum by a forward push with the right hand while applying counter-resistance with the left hand. During the process, the operator must be prepared to withdraw the needle as soon as the catheter enters the left atrium, so that the excessive forward momentum does not carry the needle forward and perforate the left atrial wall, causing cardiac tamponade.

**How to avoid puncturing the right atrium: To avoid injury of the right atrium, the catheter/needle should be carefully manipulated and the needle tip always kept inside the catheter tip. When right atrial puncture or perforation is detected by contrast opacification of the pericardial space, do not advance the catheter and withdraw the needle/catheter immediately. Usually cardiac tamponade does not ensue, and the operator may proceed with puncture attempt at the optimal site. It is important to note that there may not be a septum in an area near the inferior (caudal) border of the left atrium caudal to the M-line because the atrium often bulges caudally beyond the true septal boundary. This is especially true in patients with a large left atrium. If this region is punctured, the catheter/needle may perforate through the right atrial wall and then enter the left atrium (the so-called "stitching" phenomenon).[22] After the guidewire is placed in the left atrium and the catheter is withdrawn, cardiac tamponade ensues.

**How to avoid puncturing the aorta, tricuspid valve, and coronary sinus: When the catheter/needle is set on the "mid-line," puncture of these structures can be avoided. Being confirmed in the RAO projection, the intended puncture site is clearly separated from the aorta, the tricuspid valve, and the coronary sinus (Figure 24-2). Inadvertent puncture of the aorta, as confirmed by contrast injection or pressure recording, is usually uneventful if the needle is withdrawn immediately; however, if the operator unknowingly advances the catheter into the aorta, it should not be withdrawn. The patient should be sent for emergency surgery with the catheter left in the aorta.

**How to avoid puncture medial to the "mid-line": When a puncture is made medial to the line, there is a risk of puncturing the aorta, tricuspid valve, or coronary sinus. More importantly, the puncture site thus made is too close to the mitral valve, and this makes balloon crossing of the mitral valve difficult or even impossible, unless the posterior loop method (refer to "Crossing the mitral valve") is employed. Slight lateral deviation of the puncture site to the "mid-line" is permissible, especially in patients with relatively small left atria.

Confirmation of left atrial entry: After entry of the needle in the left atrium is confirmed, first by contrast medium injection followed by pressure recording and blood oximetry, the needle direction is set toward 3 o'clock (left side of the patient). If there is no or little resistance, the catheter/needle is advanced forward about 2 cm into the left atrium. Then, the catheter alone is advanced another 2 cm (or until the tip of the sheath meets a resistance at the septum), while the needle is being withdrawn.

Heparinization: Upon removing the needle after the catheter is placed in the left atrium, heparin, 100 units/kg body weight, should be given immediately through the catheter. After baseline hemodynamic studies, including simultaneous measurement of cardiac output, BMV is performed. If the patient has been on warfarin prior to BMV, the drug is discontinued 2–3 days before the procedure and substituted with intravenous unfractionated or subcutaneous low-molecular weight heparin until just before the procedure.

SELECTION OF BALLOON CATHETER

Selection of an appropriate-sized balloon catheter for the controlled stepwise dilatation technique is extremely important in order to avoid creating severe mitral regurgitation during BMV. Our balloon catheter selection methods have evolved from our continuing efforts to minimize this complication (Table 24-2).[4,9,18–20]

Selection guidelines are based on balloon reference size derived from patient height, transthoracic echocardiographic findings of the mitral valve, and fluoroscopic presence of valvular calcification. The reference size (RS) is calculated according to the simple formula:[9,18] patient height (in cm) is rounded to the nearest zero and divided by 10, and 10 is added to the ratio to yield the RS (in mm); e.g. if height = 147 cm, then RS = 150/10 + 10 = 25 mm. In patients with pliable, noncalcified valves, as determined by echocardiography, a catheter with a nominal balloon size at least that of the RS (an RS-matched catheter) is used. In contrast, in patients at high risk for creating severe mitral regurgitation (valvular calcification and/or severe subvalvular lesions), a balloon catheter 1 size smaller than an RS-match is selected. Therefore, in the above example with an RS of 25 mm, a PTMC-26 catheter would be selected for a pliable, noncalcified valve, and a PTMC-24 catheter for a calcified valve and/or a valve with severe subvalvular disease.

TECHNICAL TIP

**Pretesting for balloon-syringe mismatch: Although the volume predefined by red marks on the syringe and

Table 24-2
Catheter selection and balloon sizing based on patient height and valvular status

---

Reference size (RS) (mm)

Height (cm) (rounded to nearest 0) × 1/10 plus 10
e.g., height = 147 cm
RS = 150 × 1/10 + 10 = 25 mm

Catheter selection

Valvular status	Balloon catheter
Pliable	RS-matched (e.g., PTMC-26 for RS = 25 mm)
Calcified/SL	One size < RS-matched (e.g., PTMC-24 for RS = 25 mm)

Balloon sizing

Valvular status	Initial	Increments
Pliable	(RS - 2) mm	1 mm or 0.5 mm in high-pressure zone** (if MR or unilateral commissural split)
Calcified/SL	(RS - 4) mm	1 mm (low-pressure zone*) 0.5 mm (high-pressure zone**)

MR = mitral regurgitation, pre-existing or increased; RS-matched = catheter with its nominal balloon size ≥ RS; SL = severe subvalvular lesions.
Low-pressure zone* = balloon diameter <2 mm of nominal balloon size.
High-pressure zone** = balloon diameter within 2 mm of nominal balloon size.

its corresponding balloon size at full inflation have been tested by the manufacturer, balloon-syringe mismatch may occur. While this mismatch is usually mild, gross mismatch may take place when the catheter and the syringe are from different packagings or are reused after sterilization. The mismatch, if undetected, may result in either underinflation or overinflation of the balloon. The former may result in suboptimal valvular dilatation, and the latter in severe mitral regurgitation. Therefore, before inserting the balloon catheter into each patient, the balloon diameters should be confirmed using a 2-step test. First, the syringe should be filled with diluted contrast to the mark corresponding to the balloon diameter chosen for the first inflation (see "Balloon sizing" below). The balloon should then be fully inflated, and its diameter measured with a caliper. If there is a mismatch, the difference should be noted and adjusted during the second step of testing when the balloon is inflated to its nominal diameter.

After the pretesting exercise, the syringe is disconnected from the balloon catheter for two reasons. One is to purge the syringe of any remaining air, and the other to avoid any inadvertent overinflation of the balloon at its nominal size. After the catheter has been inserted into the left atrium, the air-free syringe filled with diluted contrast corresponding to the predetermined initial balloon diameter is reconnected to the catheter.

ADVANCEMENT OF THE BALLOON CATHETER

Insertion of the stretched Inoue balloon catheter over the 0.025" stainless steel coiled-tip guidewire into the right femoral vein goes smoothly in the majority of patients. Occasionally, difficulties arise from resistance to the catheter at the entry site, at the interatrial septum, or from migration of the balloon catheter in the left atrium.

TECHNICAL TIPS

**Resistance at groin access site: To avoid creating a long subcutaneous tunnel that may pose some resistance during insertion of the balloon catheter, the puncture needle is angled more vertically than usual during the initial vascular access (at about 60° to the skin surface instead of 45°). After transseptal puncture and insertion of the coiled-tip guidewire into the left atrium, the shorter subcutaneous track is then well stretched with an artery forceps along the guidewire. This is followed by use of the 12F dilator (enclosed with the Inoue balloon assembly), which is also used to dilate the atrial septum. Finally, when inserting the stretched balloon catheter, firm compression with the flat of the fingertips cephalad to the puncture site and over the subcutaneous track may be needed to aid catheter entry.

If significant resistance is encountered during insertion of the stretched balloon catheter, it is inserted into the vein at a more obtuse angle of about 90° until its tip touches the posterior venous wall. The catheter is then tilted more horizontally and advanced over the wire. During the latter process, to facilitate catheter insertion and avoid bending the guidewire, firm compression should be applied cephalad to the puncture site and over the subcutaneous track (as described above), and the guidewire should be held taut by an assistant. If this technique fails, the subcutaneous track and the vein should be redilated with a 14F dilator. If these precautionary measures are exercised, the need for a 14F intravascular sheath for insertion of the balloon catheter is rare in our experience, even in patients with the right groin scarred from previous catheterization. However, one should not hesitate to use a 14F vascular sheath to avoid bending the guidewire or metal tube, when a difficulty is encountered during the catheter insertion process.

It is also important to note that during insertion of the catheter into the femoral vein, the catheter should never be twisted, lest the metal tube be bent. If the tube is inadvertently bent, it should be replaced with a new one. On the other hand, if the guidewire is bent, a 12F dilator is reinserted over the wire and carefully left into the left atrium. The wire is then replaced.

**Septal resistance: After atrial septal puncture and placement of the coiled-tip guidewire in the left atrium, there may be some difficulty at times in advancing the balloon catheter across the septum, particularly when the latter is markedly thickened at the puncture site. When this occurs, forceful action is to be avoided as the catheter may curve excessively in the inferior vena cava, resulting in abdominal discomfort for the patient. Rather, the balloon catheter should be turned slightly, usually in a clockwise direction as it is pushed forward (screwdriver maneuver) to overcome septal resistance. In the rare instances when this method also fails, the septum is redilated with the dilator. After passage across the septum, it is also important not to push the catheter tip up against the left atrial roof, or the guidewire may be bent into an acute angle, making subsequent catheter manipulation difficult.

**Deep catheter placement in left atrium: The balloon catheter is introduced under frontal fluoroscopic view into the atrium over the coiled-tip guidewire to form a large loop with the tip medial to the mitral orifice, pointing in a 6 to 7 o'clock direction (Figure 24-5, upper panel 1). This placement has the following advantages: (1) the catheter thus positioned is less likely to flip to the left atrial appendage area when the stylet is inserted to the catheter tip; (2) the catheter will not enter the pulmonary veins; and (3) in subsequent manipulations to cross the mitral valve, because the catheter has already been advanced deep into the atrium, it will need only to be withdrawn. Thus, potential entrapment by a tough septum, which is encountered only during catheter advancement, is avoided (see "Catheter entrapment at the atrial septum" below).

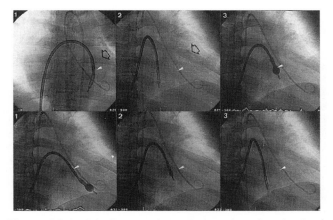

Figure 24-5: A balloon catheter is introduced under frontal fluoroscopic view into the left atrium over the coiled-tip guidewire to form a large loop with the tip medial to the mitral orifice, pointing in the 6 to 7 o'clock direction (upper panel 1). After the deep catheter placement, the projection is changed to a 30° right anterior oblique view (upper panel 2), and with the stylet inserted into the catheter tip, the partially inflated distal balloon is directed toward the anteriorly located mitral orifice. The catheter is then withdrawn gradually, to direct the balloon to the mitral valve (white arrowhead) (upper panel 3) and to cross the mitral valve (lower panel 1). After the balloon inflation procedure, the catheter balloon is then withdrawn to the left atrium. In subsequent crossing of the mitral valve with the stepwise dilation technique, the stylet is inserted on the catheter tip (bottom panel 2) and the catheter is advanced to deep-seat the balloon (bottom panel 3). During balloon catheter manipulation under a 30° right anterior oblique fluoroscopic view, the catheter tip should always be kept to the left of the pigtail catheter preplaced in the left ventricle to avoid trespassing on the left atrial appendage area (open arrowhead).

CROSSING THE MITRAL VALVE

After deep catheter placement in the left atrium, the fluoroscopic projection is changed from a frontal to a 30° right anterior oblique view (Figure 24-5, upper panel 2) that displays the left ventricular long axis in profile. In patients with giant left atria, additional use of lateral fluoroscopic view may be needed to facilitate crossing of the valve.

Methods of crossing

With the stylet inserted to the catheter tip, the partially inflated distal balloon is directed toward the anteriorly located mitral orifice. The balloon is directed anteriorly by applying a counterclockwise twist (usually 180°) to the stylet with the right hand (in a right-handed operator). The catheter is then withdrawn gradually, using the left hand, until a horizontal bobbing motion of the balloon is noted, indicating close proximity of the balloon to the mitral valve. Mitral valve crossing is then attempted using four methods in order of: (1) the vertical, (2) the direct, (3) the sliding, and (4) the posterior loop method. The vertical method employed first is the most frequently successful crossing method (in about 70% of cases).

1. The vertical method: Upon further slight retraction of the catheter, the balloon is observed to move in (during diastole) (Figure 24-6 A,C) and out (during systole) of the left ventricle (Figure 24-2 B,D) even though the catheter is not aligned with the orifice-apex axis. Coincident with diastole, only the stylet is withdrawn. To accomplish this, the operator must carefully watch the rhythmic motion of the heart. This al-

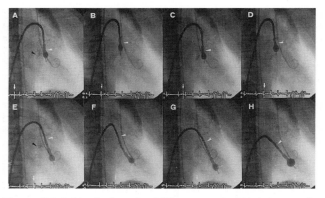

Figure 24-6: Vertical method. Fluoroscopic 30° right anterior oblique views during manipulations of Inoue balloon catheter to cross mitral valve. (A–D) During diastole ((A) and (C)), the catheter balloon crosses calcified mitral valve (black arrowhead) into left ventricle while during systole ((B) and (D)), it pops back into left atrium. (E) During diastole of the same cardiac cycle in (D), only the stylet is withdrawn and the distal catheter thus adopts a more horizontal orientation, permitting the balloon to enter into the left ventricle. (F–H) The catheter is retracted to align along the left ventricular long axis. White arrowheads indicate the stylet tip position. White arrows at bottom of each frame depict timing of the cardiac cycle on the electrocardiogram (see text for discussion). (From *J Invasive Cardiol* 1998; **10**: 548–50.)

lows the distal segment of the catheter to take on a more horizontal orientation to cross the valve and enter deep in the left ventricle (Figure 24-6 E–G). If the distal portion of the catheter is still vertically oriented and points to the inferior wall of the left ventricle (Figure 24-6 G), the catheter is carefully withdrawn to align it with the orifice-apex axis (Figure 24-6 H). During the process, the distal balloon may need to be inflated further to prevent it from popping out of the ventricle.

This vertical approach keeps the catheter from inadvertent flipping into the appendage, thus minimizing the risk of catheter encroachment into the left atrial appendage in cases with thrombi confined to the appendage.[25]

2. The direct method: When the vertical method fails, the balloon catheter is further withdrawn until the catheter balloon is near the valve and the catheter is well aligned with the orifice-apex axis. At this time, a "woodpecking" sign is observed as the balloon moves away from the mitral orifice in systole, and toward it in diastole along the axis between the mitral orifice and the left ventricular apex (the orifice-apex axis). Once this sign is evident, the balloon is in position to cross the mitral orifice. With careful attention to the rhythmic motion, the operator jerks the stylet back slightly (4–5 cm) as the balloon approaches the orifice, and simultaneously advances the catheter with the left hand to drive the balloon across the valve deep into the left ventricle. Since hand-eye coordination is vital, the beginner may choose to conduct these movements in two steps: while holding the catheter still, the stylet is withdrawn to allow the balloon to flow across the valve, and then the catheter is pushed. Because timing is critical, in an operator's early experiences with BMV, selection of patients with sinus rhythm is recommended, as it is then easier to make use of the regular cardiac cycle to advance the balloon across the mitral orifice.

TECHNICAL TIP

**Optimal position of the stylet: In the vertical and direct methods, it is important to insert the spring-wire stylet all the way to the balloon catheter tip to straighten the latter. Occasionally, however, the stylet may be too short to reach the catheter tip, thus making a slight bend in the catheter tip. If this occurs, the rubber grip at the proximal end of the stylet can be pulled further back to lengthen the exposed segment of the stylet or, failing that, the rubber grip is cut at 1–2 mm from its distal end and removed. To maintain the anterior orientation of the balloon (toward the mitral valve), the stylet must be kept twisted at all times. An extra counterclockwise twist is occasionally needed to direct the catheter tip anteriorly, especially in cases with giant left atria. In these cases, the septum is displaced markedly to the anterior, and thus the balloon catheter tends to point more posteriorly. An added lateral fluoroscopic view will facilitate manipulation of the catheter/stylet for balloon crossing of the mitral valve in these instances.

3. The catheter sliding method: When the vertical or direct method fails, another technique that may be useful for crossing the mitral valve is the catheter sliding method.[18] This method has proven to be effective in cases when the septal puncture is made too caudally and/or the left ventricle takes a more horizontal orientation (Figure 24-7 A). The balloon is still directed toward the mitral valve by keeping the stylet twisted counterclockwise. The distal catheter segment is then made more flexible by withdrawing the stylet clear out of the balloon segment (Figure 24-7 B). Once the slightly inflated balloon is at the mitral orifice, cardiac contractions will cause the balloon segment to tilt upward during systole (Figure 24-7 C). In diastole, the balloon segment aligns with the catheter shaft (Figure 24-7 D). With the operator carefully watching the rhythmic motion of the cardiac cycle, only the catheter is advanced forward (with the stylet kept fixed) during diastole to cross the valve (Figure 24-7 E). The stylet is then advanced to help align the catheter with the orifice-apex axis (Figure 24-7 F).

4. The posterior loop method: Crossing the valve with the balloon catheter may be difficult with the above-mentioned methods in patients with giant left atria, or when the atrial septal puncture has been made inappropriately either too cephalad or too anterior in relation to the mitral valve. In such circumstances, the loop approach may be used. This method, which has been well described previously,[2,3] is infrequently used in the authors' experience.

TECHNICAL TIP

**Stylet reshaping: The J-tipped stylet with its original curve will, in most instances, steer the balloon toward and across the mitral orifice; however, when it is difficult to direct the balloon toward the mitral orifice by aligning the catheter with the orifice-apex axis, the stylet should be reshaped according to the positional relationship between the septal puncture site and the valve orifice. For example, in patients with a giant left atrium where the puncture site is often made more caudally and laterally in relation to the mitral orifice, the distal segment of the stylet can be shaped into a larger smooth curve to facilitate passage of the balloon across the mitral valve. Conversely, in those with a relatively small left atrium, when the puncture site is made suboptimally, either too medially or anteriorly (in relation to the mitral valve), the stylet can be reshaped into a tighter loop (or the posterior loop method described above can be employed).

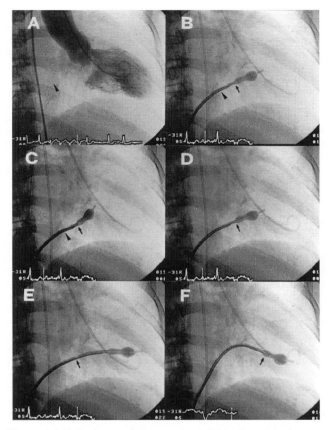

Figure 24-7: Catheter sliding method. (A) Left ventriculogram in a 30° right anterior oblique view, showing position of the transseptal puncture site (arrowhead), quite caudal to the mitral orifice; the left ventricle is more horizontally oriented. (B) The stylet (arrow) is slightly withdrawn from the balloon segment. (C,D) During a cardiac cycle, the balloon segment bobs up and down in systole and diastole, respectively, indicating proper positioning of the catheter tip at the mitral orifice. (E) During diastole, when the balloon bobs down and is aligned with the distal catheter (as in D), only the catheter is advanced forward (with the stylet kept fixed) to place the balloon into the left ventricle. (F) Thereafter, the stylet is carefully advanced to align the catheter with the mitral orifice/ventricular apex axis before initiating the balloon inflation procedure. (From *Cathet Cardiovasc Diagn* 1996; **37**: 188–99.)

BALLOON INFLATION

Assuring free movement of the balloon in the left ventricle: One of the most dreaded complications of BMV is the development of severe mitral regurgitation requiring surgery. Once the mitral valve has been crossed, the free movements of the partially inflated distal balloon in the left ventricle should be ascertained to prevent the disastrous consequences, i.e. rupture of chordae, papillary muscles, or leaflets, stemming from its subsequent full inflation between the chordae. This is done by simultaneously pushing the catheter and pulling the stylet slightly in opposite directions ("accordion" maneuver)[18] to ensure that the partially inflated distal balloon slides freely along the orifice-apex axis.

TECHNICAL TIP

**If the balloon strays among the chordae: After crossing the mitral valve, the catheter balloon may point more vertically and deviate away from the orifice-apex axis. This suggests that the catheter has strayed among the chordae. To correct this situation, the catheter is carefully pulled back to allow the balloon segment to assume a more horizontal orientation. After satisfactory alignment of the catheter with the orifice-apex axis, the catheter is advanced toward the apex, and the previously described accordion maneuver is performed before initiating the inflation procedure. Similarly, a twist in the balloon during the inflation process may also indicate that the catheter has tethered among the chordae. In this case, the inflation should be promptly aborted and the balloon repositioned.

Reassessment of subvalvular status: Before BMV, mitral valvular status is determined by preprocedural transthoracic echocardiography and fluoroscopy (for the presence of valvular calcification), and an appropriate balloon catheter is then chosen accordingly (see "Selection of balloon catheter" above). Extensive subvalvular disease has been found by various investigators to be a predictor for significant mitral regurgitation. Because echocardiography (either transthoracic or transesophageal) often underestimates the severity of subvalvular disease,[18] severe mitral regurgitation may be created during BMV despite the presence of an apparently favorable valve morphology. Therefore, during the actual balloon dilatations, vigilance is required to identify the presence of previously undetected severe subvalvular disease. We and others have found other more reliable signs of significant subvalvular involvement.[9,20,26] Even in patients in whom no severe subvalvular disease is demonstrated by preprocedural echocardiography, when any of these signs are observed, the balloon dilatation protocol is altered accordingly as described below (see "Balloon sizing" below).

TECHNICAL TIPS

**Severe subvalvular disease undetected by echocardiography: The following signs suggest or indicate the presence of severe subvalvular disease.

1. Difficulty in performing the accordion maneuver. This occurs because of resistance at the subvalvular level. If this difficulty is not appreciated, subsequent full inflation will be within the left ventricle as the balloon is not anchored at the mitral valve. Hence, it is the subvalvular apparatus and not the mitral valve that is dilated. Although severe mitral regurgitation may result from such an accidental subvalvular dilatation,[26] the inflation is usually harmless. However, it should be promptly recognized and the balloon quickly deflated. The size of the distal balloon is then reduced during subsequent attempts to anchor the balloon at the mitral valve.

2. Gross indentation of the inflated distal balloon (balloon compression sign). This indicates severe subvalvular disease (Figure 24-8).[9,20] As soon as compression is observed on the distal balloon, the inflation procedure is aborted and the inflation strategy reassessed.

3. "Balloon impasse" (Figure 24-8 F). In cases of tight mitral stenosis, valve crossing may be difficult even when the catheter, with its distal balloon partially inflated, is properly aligned with the long axis of the left ventricle. If this occurs, the balloon size is gradually reduced until it is accommodated by the mitral orifice. In rare and extreme instances, even when the balloon is not inflated, the catheter is checked (or entrapped) at the mitral valve. This finding, which we have termed "balloon impasse," reflects resistance caused by severe obstructive subvalvular lesions.[20] In the presence of this sign, BMV performed with the usual catheter selection and balloon sizing is likely to tear the mitral leaflets and/or chordae and thus create severe mitral regurgitation. Our experience in a limited number of patients suggests that in addition to stepwise dilatations previously emphasized, the use of smaller balloon catheters may prevent severe regurgitation.[20]

4. Cogwheel resistance. Rarely, while withdrawing the partially inflated balloon to anchor it at the mitral valve, cogwheel resistance may be encountered. This suggests the presence of subvalvular disease.

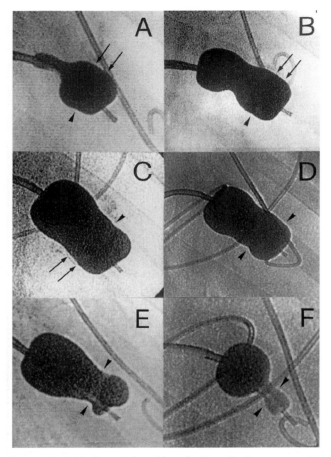

Figure 24-8: Various deformities of inflated balloon caused by severe subvalvular disease. (A–E) Indentation (arrowheads) and compression (arrows) are observed on the distal balloon segment. (F) During in-situ test inflation of balloon at the mitral valve, the proximal but not the distal segment is inflated as the latter is compressed (arrowheads) by severe subvalvular disease (see text for discussion). (From *Cathet Cardiovasc Diagn* 1996; **37**: 188–99.)

Controlled stepwise dilatations

In order to avoid or minimize the complication of severe mitral regurgitation, the selection of an appropriate balloon catheter (discussed above) and the controlled stepwise dilatation technique are mandatory. In addition, one should be familiar with the pressure-volume relationship and inflation limit of the less compliant balloon of the second-generation catheter now in use.[19]

Pressure-volume relationship: The intraballoon pressure transits from the "low-pressure" to the "high-pressure" zone as the balloon is inflated to within 2 mm of its nominal size, e.g. the 24–26 mm zone in a 26-mm balloon catheter. Each catheter can be safely inflated to a maximal diameter of 1 mm above the nominal size because of the built-in safety margin. Initial balloon inflation is never to be performed with balloon diameter in the high-pressure zone regardless of the valvular morphology.

Balloon sizing: Balloon sizing for the stepwise dilatation technique is crucial in avoiding the complication of severe mitral regurgitation (Table 24-2). Our balloon sizing methods have evolved through our continuing efforts to minimize this complication. By adhering to the cautionary methods outlined below, especially in patients with severe subvalvular disease, creation of significant mitral regurgitation (increase of ≥2 angiographically) can be minimized.[4]

TECHNICAL TIPS

**Balloon sizing in patients with pliable, noncalcified valves: In patients with pliable, noncalcified valves and no severe subvalvular lesions, as determined by the subvalvular reassessment outlined above, an RS-matched balloon catheter is selected as stated previously. The initial inflated balloon diameter is RS minus 2 mm. In subsequent dilatations, the balloon size is increased by 1 mm. When there is preexisting mitral regurgitation or any question of increase in the degree of mitral regurgitation, the increment should be 0.5 mm in the high-pressure zone. This approach also applies when unilateral commissural splitting occurs during the previous dilatation, as observed by asymmetrical balloon waisting on fluoroscopy. The final diameter is best kept within 1 mm above the RS to avoid oversizing: our previous study[9] showed that oversizing of the balloon is a risk factor for creating severe mitral regurgitation in this group of patients.

**Balloon sizing in patients with calcified valves and/or with severe subvalvular disease: In patients with either fluoroscopically visible valvular calcification, or severe subvalvular lesions as observed by transthoracic echocardiography, instead of an RS-match, a balloon catheter 1 size smaller than the RS-match is selected at the outset. For those whose subvalvular lesions are not detected by preprocedural echocardiography, the RS-matched catheter already placed in the patient may still be used if the dilatation procedures are carried out with extra care. Ideally, the catheter should be exchanged for a smaller one, but this is quite costly.

For the first dilatation, a balloon diameter 4 mm less than the RS is used. For subsequent dilatations, the balloon size is increased by 1 mm in the low-pressure zone and by 0.5 mm in the high-pressure zone until satisfactory results are obtained or until mitral regurgitation develops. In cases where the gradient has already been reduced to one-half and several more dilatation attempts have failed to reduce it further, the procedure is terminated to avoid creating severe mitral regurgitation.[19] Reducing the mitral valve gradient by one-half should result in a 41% increase in the mitral valve area, as calculated by the Gorlin formula, provided that heart rate and cardiac output remain the same. Our previous study[19] suggests that a 40% improvement is sufficient for symptomatic improvements in patients with a more sedentary lifestyle.

**Balloon sizing in case of "balloon impasse": If balloon impasse (Figure 24-8 F) is encountered, the initial catheter is exchanged for a smaller PTMC-18 or -20 catheter to predilate the valve and the subvalvular structures, regardless of the echocardiographic findings of the mitral valve.[20] We no longer force the usual-sized balloon through the valve to the left ventricle by slenderizing and stretching the deflated balloon segment, as previously recommended;[2] nor do we recommend advancing the balloon across the mitral valve over a guidewire preplaced in the left ventricle. Both maneuvers may cause the catheter to stray among the chordae, and with larger-sized balloon catheters, it is difficult or impossible for the operator to execute the precautionary "accordion" maneuver to ensure that the catheter is not tethered among the chordae.

However, if a smaller PTMC-18 or -20 catheter also fails to cross the mitral valve with the catheter uninflated, the balloon segment of this small balloon catheter is slenderized and stretched for crossing the mitral valve into the left ventricle. Before the balloon inflation procedure, it is mandatory to exercise the "accordion" maneuver with the distal balloon slightly inflated to ensure that the balloon catheter is free in the left ventricle. This maneuver would not have been possible with larger-sized catheters. The initial inflation is then performed with the balloon diameter at its nominal size. If further dilatations are required, the catheter is exchanged for one a size larger, and stepwise dilatations are done according to the sizing method in patients with severe subvalvular lesions, as discussed above.

Exchange for different-sized balloon catheters: Exchange of balloon catheters is carried out for two reasons. The first, as alluded to above, is to downsize the catheter because of the "impasse" posed by severe subvalvular distortions.

The second reason occurs in the rare instance when there is a need to upsize the balloon catheter to one that is one size larger because of inadequate hemodynamic improvement. In such a situation, before exchanging for a larger catheter, it is vital that the initial catheter's final balloon diameter be remeasured and reverified after its complete removal from the patient, particularly when it has been inflated beyond its nominal size. This precautionary exercise is essential because, not uncommonly, despite pretesting, the balloon size is smaller than what it is supposed to be after *in vivo* usage. When this occurs, the original balloon catheter is retested to determine the actual volume of diluted contrast in the syringe necessary to achieve maximum balloon size (as mentioned above, the Inoue balloon tolerates about 1 mm in excess of its nominal size before rupturing), the original balloon catheter is reintroduced into the patient, and the dilatation process is repeated. However, if the balloon matches its predefined size, an exchange for a larger-sized catheter is made and dilatations with the larger balloon are performed. Failing to reverify maximum balloon size before inflating a much larger balloon creates the risk of severe mitral regurgitation.

TECHNICAL TIPS

**Balloon "popping" to the left atrium: When the mitral valve has already been enlarged by dilatations, the balloon may occasionally slip into the left atrium during subsequent inflations with larger balloon diameters. To prevent the latter from occurring, the stylet is advanced far into the balloon segment to stiffen the catheter, and before the catheter is retracted to anchor the balloon at the orifice, the distal balloon is inflated to a diameter slightly larger than the previous one. As soon as the balloon assumes an hourglass configuration, the catheter is advanced slightly to prevent it from jerking out into the left atrium, and full balloon expansion is then executed. With this extra dilatation, although the mitral gradient may be unchanged, further shortening of the A_2-opening snap interval and enhanced splitting of the commissures, as assessed by echocardiography, are often observed.

The balloon "popping" signals enlargement of the mitral orifice with wide splitting of the commissures. It is usually encountered in patients with pliable, noncalcified valves and foretells excellent BMV results; however, suboptimal hemodynamic results are occasionally observed despite the balloon "popping" sign, especially in the presence of atrial fibrillation. In these cases, although the mitral valve with split commissures can be forced to accommodate the fully inflated balloon, the effective mitral valve area is, in reality, limited by the thickened and stiff leaflets, and by ineffective atrial contractions in the beating heart.

**Subsequent valve crossings and dilations: After the initial balloon inflation procedure, the catheter balloon is then withdrawn to the left atrium, while keeping the catheter tip to the left of the pigtail catheter (Figure 24-5, lower panel 2). The effects of the balloon dilation are assessed by observing the left atrial pressure waveforms and measuring the transmitral gradient and also by auscultation. If mitral regurgitation is suspected by the advent of a large V wave and by a new or worsening systolic murmur, echocardiography or left ventriculography may be performed. In subsequent crossings of the mitral valve with the stepwise dilation technique, the stylet is inserted into the catheter tip and the catheter is advanced to deep-seat the balloon (Figure 24-3, bottom panel 3). Then the above manipulations are repeated to cross the mitral valve for valve dilations.

**Catheter entrapment at the atrial septum: When the septal puncture site is thick and tough, the catheter may be entrapped by the septum, thereby making manipulations difficult during subsequent attempts at crossing the mitral valve. The operator should be alert to the possibility of this entrapment when marked resistance is encountered at the septum during septal puncture. This vexing problem usually does not occur during the first crossing of the valve because, as alluded to earlier, the catheter is already deeply placed and coiled in the left atrium. However, entrapment may occur during subsequent crossings, when it becomes necessary to advance the catheter, which has been inadvertently withdrawn too far back into the atrium after valvular dilatation and caught at the thick septum. If the catheter cannot be advanced with the stylet inserted all the way to the catheter tip, a clockwise twist is applied to the stylet, directing the catheter tip posterolaterally to align it more or less perpendicular to the septal plane. The catheter may then be advanced forward together with the stylet. If even this approach fails, the coiled-tip guidewire should be reinserted to facilitate deep placement of the catheter in the left atrium (Figure 24-9).

**Avoiding the left atrial appendage: Left atrial appendage thrombus may be unsuspected when BMV candidates are screened only with insensitive transthoracic echocardiography. To minimize the risk of inadvertent thrombus dislodgment and systemic embolism, the anterolateral appendage region must be avoided. During balloon catheter manipulation performed under 30° right anterior oblique fluoroscopic view, the catheter tip should always be kept to the left of the pigtail catheter preplaced in the left ventricle (Figs 24-5, upper panel 2 and 24-3, lower panel). After the precautions detailed below have become rote, it may be possible to perform BMV safely even in the presence of left

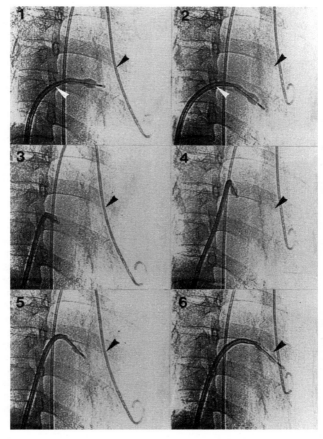

Figure 24-9: Sequence of steps to disengage a catheter entrapped in a thick septum. (1) Balloon catheter with stylet inserted at the tip is entrapped at the atrial septum (white arrowhead). (2) When the catheter is pushed, it does not advance forward, but rather turns downward. (3) Slight clockwise twist is made to the stylet to direct the catheter tip posteriorly. (4) The catheter, now aligned more or less perpendicular to the septal plane, can be effectively advanced farther into the left atrium. (5) Counterclockwise twist is now made to the stylet to direct the catheter tip anteriorly. (6) The catheter is carefully withdrawn to bring its tip toward the mitral orifice (black arrowhead).

atrial appendage thrombi.[27,28] The alternatives are either to subject patients with appendage thrombi to mitral valve surgery or to defer BMV for stable patients until resolution of the thrombi after warfarin treatment.[28]

**Withdrawing the catheter from the ventricle: After each balloon inflation procedure, in order to exert better control over the catheter tip and to prevent it from encroaching on the left atrial appendage, the stylet is advanced halfway into the balloon segment, and a slight clockwise twist to the stylet is applied as the catheter is withdrawn back to the left atrium. The balloon catheter, with its tip thus directed posteriorly, can then be safely pulled to the atrium by cautiously withdrawing the catheter and the stylet in steps. The catheter, however, should not be withdrawn too far during the process (see "Catheter entrapment at the atrial septum" above). The stylet is then removed entirely from the catheter for left atrial pressure measurement, leaving the deflated balloon segment pointing vertically. Again, during hemodynamic measurements, care should be exercised to avoid accidentally pushing the catheter forward into the appendage (Figure 24-5, lower panel 2).

**Subsequent crossings: The catheter, after having been withdrawn from the left ventricle, stands fairly straight up without looping. Thus, for the next crossings of the mitral valve, extra care is needed to keep the catheter to the left of the pigtail catheter. The stylet is carefully inserted to the catheter tip to bend the catheter downward into a generous arch with the distal catheter segment oriented more vertically (Figure 24-5, lower panel 3). Then a counterclockwise twist to the stylet is made, and the catheter is slowly withdrawn to direct the partially inflated balloon toward the mitral valve.

**Avoiding entry into the left atrial appendage: It should be noted that the catheter has a propensity to enter the left atrial appendage if the catheter is more horizontally oriented and the stylet is pulled back too vigorously during a failed crossing attempt. To avoid this, a catheter loop should be made after reinserting the stylet as noted above, and the stylet should not be withdrawn too much during any manipulation in the left atrium, including during withdrawal of the catheter from the ventricle after each balloon inflation-deflation cycle.

**Minimizing atrial septal injury: Inherent in the antegrade BMV approach is the creation of an atrial septal defect. Fortunately, most of these defects are small and of no clinical consequence and they tend to close spontaneously with time.

To minimize the occurrence of these defects and to avoid septal avulsion, a number of precautionary steps should be adopted. First, prior to full balloon inflation, i.e. after the balloon has attained its hourglass configuration and is securely anchored at the mitral valve, the distal segment of the catheter shaft (between the septal puncture site and the balloon) should be allowed to take on a gentle curve by releasing the tension exerted on the balloon catheter during its placement across the mitral valve. Second, it is mandatory to adhere to the standard practice of balloon slenderization during balloon passage across the septum (on both entry into and withdrawal from the left atrium). Third, before removing the stretched balloon catheter from the left atrium to the right atrium, the guidewire should be withdrawn, leaving only its soft distal floppy segment exposed. This may avoid "slicing" the septum by the stiff portion of the wire during withdrawal of the catheter/wire assembly.

**Bent balloon tip: Kinking of the stretched balloon occurs during placement of the catheter in the left atrium if the guidewire is withdrawn before releasing the inner tube from its locked position. The balloon segment, unsupported by either the metal tube or the guidewire, may also be inadvertently bent by advancing the inner tube alone. Once the tip is bent, subsequent attempts at crossing the mitral valve with the catheter may be extremely difficult, if not impossible. In addition, it may be impossible to reinsert the guidewire to retrieve the balloon catheter from the left atrium. This problem may be overcome by (1) pulling the inner tube to its limit to shorten the balloon segment, (2) carefully inflating the entire balloon in the left atrium to sufficiently straighten the kinked inner tube, and (3) passing the guidewire through the deflated balloon to reestablish its natural shape (Figure 24-10).

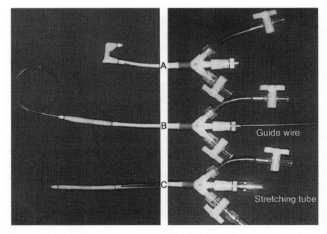

Figure 24-10: Kinked balloon. (A) Kinking of unsupported balloon segment occurs when inner tube is pushed to stretch the catheter balloon. (B) Balloon segment is supported by guide. (C) Balloon segment is supported by stretching tube.

INDICATIONS

The selection of patients for BMV procedure is a complex decision involving the consideration of multiple variables, including the clinical profile, valve morphology, and the operator's skill.

BMV procedure is best applied to symptomatic patients with moderate-to-severe mitral stenosis (mitral valve area <1.5 cm^2) and favorable mitral valve morphology (pliable, non-calcified valve without significant subvalvular disease). In this subset of patients, BMV predictably yields excellent results and a low risk of resultant severe mitral regurgitation. BMV can be performed in asymptomatic patients with favorable valve anatomy prior to noncardiac surgery or planned pregnancy.

Patients with moderate (angiographic grade 2+) mitral regurgitation but with otherwise favorable valve characteristics should be given a trial of Inoue balloon BMV where controlled stepwise dilation is possible, and the risk of severe mitral regurgitation in experienced hands is minimal. Should this procedure fail to provide sustained improvement, surgery in the form of valve replacement remains a viable option without exposing the patient to any additional risk.

Inoue BMV is technically less demanding and clearly more simple to perform than the double-balloon approach, thereby engendering a shorter procedural and irradiation time.[29] This advantage is vital in pregnant patients where the hazards of irradiation to the fetus are of paramount importance, and for patients with pulmonary edema in whom swift and expeditious BMV is clearly desirable.[23] However, to minimize the hazards of fetal irradiation, it should be performed after the mid-second trimester, with adequate total abdominal and pelvic shielding, minimal use of fluoroscopy (by omitting diagnostic right heart catheterization and left ventriculography), and only by interventional cardiologists skilled in the transseptal and valvuloplasty techniques.

The utility of BMV in patients with adverse valve morphology (calcified mitral valves and/or severe subvalvular disease) is unclear and controversial.[29] Most operators contend that these types of patients are better served with surgery, which often means mitral valve replacement, because BMV in this setting is associated with an increased risk of complications and inferior long-term results.[9,30,31] In patients who pose a prohibitively high risk for valve surgery, BMV may be a better option than surgery, and may occasionally be the only therapeutic modality available for some of these patients. On the other hand, some experienced operators[32,33] advocate more liberal use of the procedure because of a low risk of major complications, in particular, resultant severe mitral regurgitation, and the procedure continues to offer sustained functional benefits in a substantial number of patients. Notwithstanding, it cannot be overemphasized that BMV in these patients can be technically demanding, and does require a higher level of technical skill and extra caution in executing the procedure.

CONTRAINDICATIONS

There exist two absolute contraindications in BMV: (1) severe (≥ grade 3+) angiographic mitral regurgitation, and (2) the presence of left atrial cavity thrombus. The treatment for patients with ≥3+ mitral regurgitation is clearly that of mitral valve replacement. Patients with left atrial thrombus are subjected to open mitral commissurotomy or valve replacement, depending on the mitral valve status. Those patients with mobile thrombi in the left atrium are at a high risk of systemic embolism, and require urgent mitral valve surgery.

However, one may elect to administer long-term (3–12 months) warfarin therapy in patients with non-mobile thrombi in the left atrial cavity if their clinical and hemodynamic status does not warrant immediate surgery and the mitral valves are deemed suitable for BMV. Transesophageal echocardiography is deferred until thrombi resolution is observed by transthoracic echocardiography performed at 3-month intervals.[28] When transesophageal echo confirms the absence of left atrial cavity thrombus, BMV can then be performed safely.[18,27,28,34] In our centers, the presence of thrombi confined to the left atrial appendage (without protruding into the left atrial cavity) is not a contraindication. BMV can be performed safely in this setting when performed with extra care using the Inoue balloon technique.[18,27] The risk of cardioembolism is low in this setting when Inoue balloon PTMC is performed by experts.[4]

Patients with lytic-resistant thrombi after 12 months of warfarin treatment should be considered for open surgical commissurotomy with direct visual clot removal.

TECHNICAL TIP

Inoue balloon mitral valvuloplasty in double-orifice mitral stenosis (incomplete bridge-type): Double-orifice mitral valve (DOMV) is a rare congenital anomaly characterized by the presence of two mitral orifices, each possessing an independent chordal attachment to a papillary muscle.[35,36] DOMV may occur as an isolated anomaly or, more often, in association with other congenital anomalies like endocardial cushion defect, bicuspid aortic valve and coarctation of the aorta.[35,36] Echocardiographically, DOMV is classified into three types: complete bridge-, incomplete bridge- and hole-type.[37] The complete bridge-type is characterized by the presence of a fibrous tissue visible from the leaflet edge through the valve ring. In the incomplete form, however, the fibrous connection occurs only at the leaflet edge. In the hole-type, the secondary orifice with its sub-valvular apparatus occurs in the lateral commissure and is visible only at the mid-leaflet level.

The isolated form of DOMV is more frequently observed in the bridge-type,[35,36] and is usually associated with no significant hemodynamic abnormality. However, we have encountered seven moderately symptomatic, middle-aged patients with stenotic DOMV of incomplete bridge-type.[38,39] Their clinical presentations and physical findings were indistinguishable from those in rheumatic mitral stenosis. However, vigilance acquired from the experience in the first case[40] contributed to expeditious echocardiographic identification of the incomplete bridge-type DOMV in the subsequent patients (Figure 24-11). All patients underwent Inoue balloon mitral valvuloplasty successfully.

Based on the experience in the seven patients, several important technical tips and guidelines have evolved as follows.

1. Transseptal catheterization and left atrial placement of the balloon catheter can be performed in the usual manner.

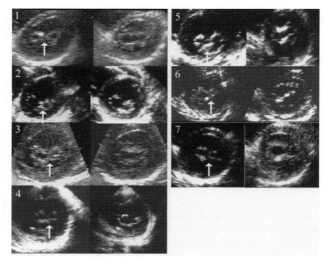

Figure 24-11: Transthoracic 2-dimensional echocardiograms of mitral valves before (left panels) and after (right panels) balloon mitral valvuloplasty in seven cases. In each case, two stenotic orifices are separated by a fibrous bridge tissue (arrow) (left panels). Balloon splitting of the fibrous septation results in a single, enlarged mitral orifice (right panels).

2. Balloon crossing of posteromedial orifice is simple and stepwise dilations of the latter orifice alone are sufficient to split the fibrous bridge between the two leaflets. Crossing attempts of the anterolateral orifice are futile because the orifice is located more cranially, making it impossible to align the distal balloon catheter with the orifice/apex (ventricular) axis.
3. Balloon catheter selection can be based on the height-derived reference size as in ordinary cases of mitral stenosis.
4. Stepwise dilations can be initiated at a balloon diameter of 4 mm less than the reference size. The procedure is terminated when the waist of the inflated balloon suddenly disappears, and echocardiography confirmed separation of the mitral valve septation resulting in a single enlarged orifice (Figure 24-11).
5. Application of the described Inoue balloon valvuloplasty should only be limited to patients with the incomplete bridge-type of DOMV.

REFERENCES

1. Inoue K, Owaki T, Nakamura T *et al*. Clinical application of transvenous mitral commissurotomy by a new balloon catheter. *J Thorac Cardiovasc Surg* 1984; **87**: 394–402.
2. Inoue K, Hung JS. Percutaneous transvenous mitral commissurotomy (BMV): The Far East experience. In: Topol EJ, ed. *Textbook of Interventional Cardiology.* WB Saunders, 1990: 887–99.
3. Inoue K, Hung JS, Chen CR *et al*. Mitral stenosis: Inoue balloon catheter technique. In: Cheng TO, ed. *Percutaneous Balloon Valvuloplasty,* 1st edn. Igaku-Shoin Medical Publishers, Inc, 1992: 237–79.
4. Hung JS, Lau KW, Lo PH *et al*. Complications of Inoue balloon mitral commissurotomy: Impact of operator experience and evolving technique. *Am Heart J* 1999; **138**; 114–21.
5. Arora R, Kalra GS, Murty GSR *et al*. Percutaneous trans-atrial mitral commissurotomy: Immediate and intermediate results. *J Am Coll Cardiol* l994; **23**: 1327–32.
6. Ruiz EC, Zhang HP, Macaya C *et al*. Comparison of Inoue single-balloon versus double-balloon technique for percutaneous mitral valvotomy. *Am Heart J* 1992; **123**: 942–7.
7. Iung B, Cormier B, Ducimetiere P *et al*. Immediate results of percutaneous mitral commissurotomy. *Circulation* 1996; **94**: 2124–30.
8. A report from the National Heart, Lung, and Blood Institute Balloon Valvuloplasty Registry. Complications and mortality of percutaneous balloon mitral commissurotomy. *Circulation* 1992; **85**: 2014–24.

9. Hung JS, Chern MS, Wu JJ *et al*. Short- and long-term results of catheter balloon percutaneous transvenous mitral commissurotomy. *Am J Cardiol* 1991; **67**: 854–62.

10. Pan M, Medina A, de Lezo JS *et al*. Factors determining late success after mitral balloon valvulotomy. *Am J Cardiol* 1993; **71**: 1181–1185.

11. Iung B, Cormier B, Ducimetiere P *et al*. Functional results 5 years after successful percutaneous mitral commissurotomy in a series of 528 patients and analysis of predictive factors. *J Am Coll Cardiol* 1996; **27**: 407–14.

12. Dean LS, Mickel M, Bonan R *et al*. Four-year follow-up of patients undergoing percutaneous balloon mitral commissurotomy. *J Am Coll Cardiol* 1996; **28**: 1452–7.

13. Meneveau N, Schiele F, Seronde MF. Predictors of event-free survival after percutaneous mitral commissurotomy. Heart 1988; **4**: 359–64.

14. Hernandez R, Banuelos C, Alfonso F *et al*. Long-term clinical and echocardiographic follow-up after percutaneous mitral valvuloplasty with the Inoue balloon. *Circulation* 1999; **99**: 1580–6.

15. Lock JE, Khalilullah M, Shrivastava S *et al*. Percutaneous catheter commissurotomy in rheumatic mitral stenosis. *N Engl J Med* 1985; **313**: 1515–18.

16. Al Zaibag M, Ribeiro PA, Al Kasab S *et al*. Percutaneous double-balloon mitral valvotomy for rheumatic mitral valve stenosis. *Lancet* 1986; **1**: 757–61.

17. Stefanadis C, Toutouzas P. Retrograde nontransseptal mitral valvuloplasty. In: Topol EJ, ed. *Textbook of Interventional Cardiology*, 2nd edition. WB Saunders, 1994: 1253–67.

18. Hung JS, Lau KW. Pitfalls and tips in Inoue-balloon mitral commissurotomy. *Cathet Cardiovasc Diagn* 1996; **37**: 188–199.

19. Lau KW, Hung JS. A simple balloon-sizing method in Inoue balloon percutaneous transvenous mitral commissurotomy. *Cathet Cardiovasc Diagn* 1994; **33**: 120–9.

20. Lau KW, Hung JS. "Balloon impasse": A marker for severe mitral subvalvular disease and a predictor of mitral regurgitation in Inoue balloon percutaneous transvenous mitral commissurotomy. *Cathet Cardiovasc Diagn* 1995; **35**: 310–19.

21. Goldstein SA, Campbell A, Mintz GS *et al*. Feasibility of on-line transesophageal echocardiography during balloon mitral valvulotomy: Experience with 93 patients. *J Heart Valve Dis* 1994; **3**: 136–48.

22. Hung JS. Atrial septal puncture technique in percutaneous transvenous mitral commissurotomy: Mitral valvuloplasty using the Inoue balloon catheter technique. *Cathet Cardiovasc Diagn* 1992; **26**: 275–84.

23. Wu JJ, Chern MS, Yeh KH *et al*. Urgent/emergent percutaneous transvenous mitral commissurotomy. *Cathet Cardiovasc Diagn* 1994; **31**: 18–22.

24. Ramasamy D, Zambahari R, Fu M, Yeh KH, Hung JS. Percutaneous transvenous mitral commissurotomy in patients with severe kyphoscoliosis. *Cathet Cardiovasc Diagn* 1993; **30**: 40–4.

25. Hung JS, Lau KW. Vertical approach: A modified method in balloon crossing of mitral valve in Inoue balloon mitral valvuloplasty. *J Invasive Cardiol* 1998; **10**: 548–50.

26. Hernandez R, Macaya C, Banuelos C *et al.* Predictors, mechanisms and outcome of severe mitral regurgitation complicating percutaneous mitral valvotomy with the Inoue balloon. *Am J Cardiol* 1992; **70**: 1169–74.

27. Yeh KH, Hung JS, Wu JJ *et al.* Safety of Inoue balloon mitral commissurotomy in patients with left atrial appendage thrombi. *Am J Cardiol* 1995; **75**: 302–4.

28. Hung JS. Mitral stenosis with left atrial thrombi: Inoue balloon catheter technique. In: Cheng To, ed. *Percutaneous Balloon Valvuloplasty.* Igaku-Shoin Medical Publishers, Inc., 1992: 280–293.

29. Lau KW, Hung JS, Ding ZP *et al.* Controversies in balloon mitral valvuloplasty: The when (timing for intervention), what (choice of valve), and how (selection of technique). *Cathet Cardiovasc Diagn* 1995; **35**: 91–100.

30. Dean LS, Mickel M, Bonan R *et al.* Four-year follow-up of patients undergoing percutaneous balloon mitral commissurotomy. *J Am Coll Cardiol* 1996; **28**: 1452–7.

31. Yoshida Y, Kubo S, Tamaki S *et al.* Percutaneous transvenous mitral commissurotomy for mitral stenosis patients with markedly severe mitral valve deformity: Immediate results and long-term clinical outcome. *Am J Cardiol* 1995; **76**: 406–8.

32. Hung JS, Lau KW. Percutaneous transvenous mitral commissurotomy is an acceptable therapeutic alternative in patients with calcified mitral valve. *J Invasive Cardiol* 1999; **11**: 362–3.

33. Wahl A, Meier B. Percutaneous mitral balloon valvuloplasty in non-ideal patients: Go for it without expecting too much. *J Invasive Cardiol* 1999; **11**: 359–61.

34. Hung JS, Lin FC, Chiang CW. Successful percutaneous transvenous catheter balloon mitral commissurotomy after warfarin therapy and resolution of left atrial thrombus. *Am J Cardiol* 1989; **64**: 126–8.

35. Rosenberg J, Roberts WC. Double orifice mitral valve: study of the anomaly in two calves and a summary of the literature in humans. *Arch Pathol* 1968; **86**: 77–80.

36. Bano-Rodrigo A, Praagh SV, Trowitzsch E, Praagh RV. Double orifice mitral valve: A study of 27 postmortem cases with developmental, diagnostic and surgical consideration. *Am J Cardiol* 1988; **61**: 152–60.

37. Warnes C, Somerville J. Double mitral valve orifice in atrioventricular defects. *Br Heart J* 1983; **49**: 59–64.

38. Trowitzsch E, Bano-Rodrigo A, Burger BM *et al*. Two-dimensional echocardiographic findings in double orifice mitral valve. *J Am Coll Cardiol* 1985; **6**: 383–7.

39. Kim MH, Cha KS, Kim JS *et al*. Successful Inoue-balloon mitral commissurotomy in double-orifice mitral stenosis. *Cathet Cardiovasc Interv* 2000; **49**: 200–203.

40. Lo PH, Kim MH, Hung JS. Inoue-balloon mitral valvuloplasty in double-orifice mitral stenosis. *J Invasive Cardiol* (in press).

Chapter 25

Percutaneous Mechanical Mitral Commissurotomy

Alain Cribier, Helene Eltchaninoff

GENERAL OVERVIEW

Balloon mitral valvuloplasty has become an accepted alternative to surgical commissurotomy in selected patients, offering comparable immediate and long-term results.[1–6] However, the cost of the balloon catheters does limit its application in developing countries where the incidence of mitral stenosis remains the highest. Consequently, the disposable balloon catheters are reused several times, with the subsequent hazards due to imperfect sterilization and decreasing performance.

Over the last 5 years, we have developed a percutaneous metallic valvulotome.[7,8] The main goal was to provide a

*Basic; **Advanced; ***Rare, exotic, or investigational.

From: Nguyen T, Hu D, Saito S, Grines C, Palacios I (eds), *Practical Handbook of Advanced Interventional Cardiology*, 2nd edn. © 2003 Futura, an imprint of Blackwell Publishing.

device that could be reused several times without any loss of performance after proper resterilization, thus decreasing the procedural cost. Other goals were to improve the efficacy and tolerance of the technique resulting from the device's mechanical properties, which are aimed at acting principally on the mitral commissures.

The technical aspects of the procedure and the results of an international multicenter registry including 1087 patients will be presented here.

DESCRIPTION OF THE DEVICE

The device (Medicorp Inc, Nancy, France) consists of a metallic dilator screwed on the distal end of a disposable catheter. The entire system consists of four components (Figs 25-1 and 25-2):

- **The stainless steel metallic dilator** is a cylinder 5 cm long and 5 mm wide with a slightly tapered tip (Figure 25-1). Its distal half comprises 2 bars, 20 mm in length, that can be opened in parallel up to a maximum length of 40 mm using a lever arms system (Figure 25-2). An internal lumen allows the passage of a guidewire and the recording of the distal pressures. The metallic head is screwed on the distal end of the catheter and is detachable.
- **The catheter** has a diameter of 13F (4.3 mm) and a length of 170 cm. Its proximal end has a connector for recording

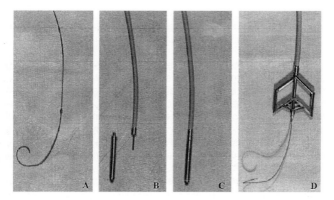

Figure 25-1: (A) Distal part of the 0.035" guidewire. Note the metallic bead soldered at the junction of the stiff proximal and flexible and pigtail curved distal segments of the wire. (B) Distal end of the catheter and metallic dilator before connection. (C) The dilator screwed at the extremity of the catheter. (D) The dilator in the opened (40 mm) position.

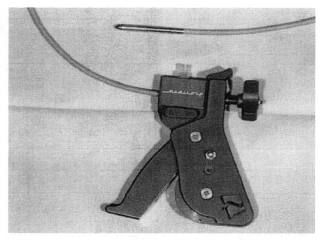

Figure 25-2: Proximal end of the catheter and activating pliers.

the distal pressures, and it enables the connection of the activating pliers. Its distal end enables the fastening of the dilator.

- **The metallic guidewire** has a length of 270 cm and a diameter of 0.035". A metallic bead of 2 mm in diameter is soldered at the junction of the stiff core and the 10-cm-long floppy distal end (Figure 25-3). The wire is used as a guidewire to drive the catheter across the valve, and then as a traction system that enables the opening of the dilator. For that, the metallic bead is positioned in contact with the distal end of the dilator and the guidewire is locked into the commissurotome using a threaded fastener located on the activating pliers. Squeezing the arms of the pliers causes a backward traction of the guidewire and the metallic bead, which is transmitted to the distal end of the dilator, thus forcing the distal bars to spread apart.

- **The activating pliers** are comprised of several elements: (1) A caliper used to program the degree of bars opening (30, 35, 37, or 40 mm). (2) A safety lock that prevents the complete closure of the dilator after the release of pressure exerted on the pliers (it holds the dilator open at 20 mm). To obtain a complete closure of the dilator after withdrawal from the mitral valve, the lock must be activated manually. This security system has been designed to avoid any accidental extraction of valvular tissue. (3) A threaded fastener that is designed to block the metallic guidewire into the commissurotome at the time of opening.

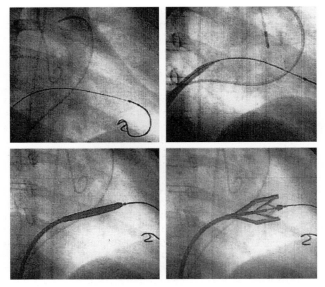

Figure 25-3: Upper left: position of the guidewire in the left ventricle. Upper right: 18F polyethylene dilator during the septum dilatation phase. Lower left: the commissurotome in position across the mitral valve before opening; the metallic bead of the guidewire has been placed against the tip of the dilator, and the pigtail catheter faces the proximal third of the dilator. Lower right: the dilator in the opened (40 mm) position during the commissurotomy phase.

After dilatation, the metallic dilator is unscrewed from the catheter and sterilized by autoclave for reuse. The activating pliers and the guidewire can also be resterilized.

TECHNIQUES OF MECHANICAL MITRAL COMMISSUROTOMY

Transseptal catheterization: Transseptal catheterization constitutes an essential step because the transseptal puncture site greatly influences both the safety and the effectiveness of the procedure. The puncture site is ideally situated 1–2 cm below the spot usually recommended for the Inoue technique. The approach described here seems particularly recommended. This technique helps to prevent punctures that are too high, too low, or too posterior.

In the anteroposterior view, the Mullins sheath with the Brockenbrough needle is pulled back from the superior vena cava until its distal tip is positioned midway between the tip of the pigtail (lying just above the aortic valve in the ascending aorta) and the top of the right hemidiaphragm (Figure 25-4 A). At this stage, it is not necessary to get a contact of the needle with the septum.

While carefully maintaining the position of the assembly, the image intensifier is moved to the 90° lateral position. The needle is then rotated in such a way that the distal tip of the dilator points upward (in as straight a vertical line as possible) and makes contact with the septum. Ideally, the contact will be made at a point two-thirds of the way down from the pigtail to the posterior border of the heart (Figure 25-4 B). The needle is deployed and the transseptal puncture performed. Left atrial pressure should now be seen through the needle. In no case should the septum be punctured high and anterior (Figure 25-4 C) or low and posterior (Figure 25-4 D).

Crossing the mitral valve: In the 30° RAO position, the Mullins catheter is advanced into the left atrium gently and the needle is withdrawn from inside the catheter. When the sheath is situated inside the left atrium, the dilator is withdrawn. The Mullins sheath should now appear with its distal curvature directed toward the mitral orifice, lying in a plane close to horizontal, and entirely below the pigtail catheter (Figure 25-4 E). If the two catheters appear on the screen to cross over each other, then the septal puncture is too high and will render subsequent crossing of the mitral valve with the commissurotome difficult if not impossible (Figure 25-4 F). In this setting, it is recommended that the transseptal puncture be repeated at a slightly lower site. At this point, 2000 IU of heparin is given intravenously.

Using the Mullins sheath in the left atrium and the pigtail catheter advanced into the left ventricle, the transmitral pressure gradient is recorded. The mitral valve area can also be evaluated using the Gorlin formula.[9] The pigtail catheter is then withdrawn into the ascending aorta to a point just in contact with the aortic valve; this position is important because it serves as a marker for the subsequent positioning of the commissurotome.

Through the Mullins sheath, a 7F Critikon-type balloon catheter is advanced, the balloon is inflated, and the valve is crossed. As far as possible, the balloon is advanced all the way to the apex (Figure 25-5 A). The Mullins sheath is then advanced until it contacts the tip of the balloon (Figure 25-5 B), the balloon is deflated, and the catheter is withdrawn. The Mullins sheath is left free in the left ventricle (Figure 25-5 C).

The commissurotomy guidewire is advanced through the Mullins sheath into the left ventricle. Its flexible distal tip is left in place in the apex of the left ventricle. The Mullins sheath is pulled back when its tip reaches the tip of the guidewire (Figure 25-5 D). Ideally, the bead on the guidewire is maintained in the center of the ventricular cavity. During the dilatation maneuvers, the bead should never move all the way to the apex to avoid the risk of laceration of the wall of the heart by

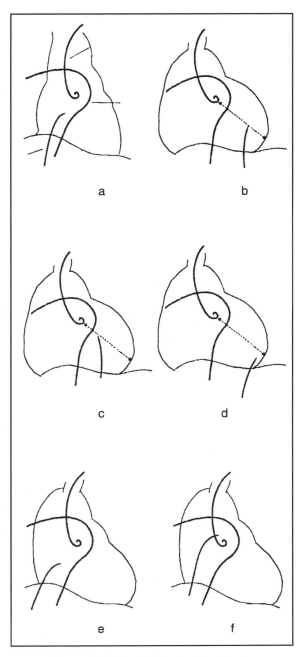

Figure 25-4(A–F): See text for details.

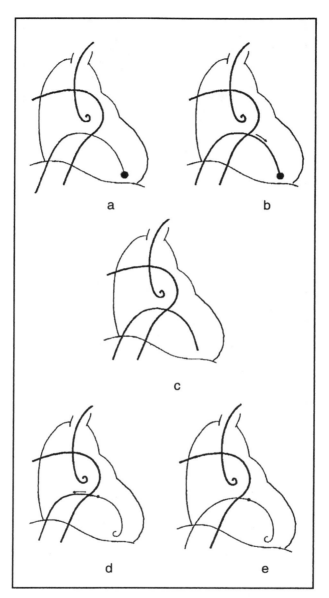

a   b

c

d   e

Figure 25-5(A–E): See text for details.

the rigid portion of the guidewire. The Mullins sheath is withdrawn, and the guidewire is maintained in the same position (Figure 25-5 E).

Dilatation of the interatrial septum: A 14F polyethylene dilator is pushed over the guidewire, advanced 2–3 cm across the interatrial septum, and left in place for approximately 30 sec (Figure 25-6 A). The same procedure is performed using an 18F dilator. This dilator should be left in place across the septum for approximately 60 sec (Figure 25-6 B).

Before completely withdrawing the 18F dilator, it should be passed back and forth through the femoral venous puncture site several times. This step is very important because it greatly facilitates the introduction of the metal commissurotome into the femoral vein. At this point, additional intravenous heparin (50 IU/kg) should be administered.

Mechanical mitral commissurotomy: The commissurotome should have been assembled and flushed and the degree of opening selected with the aid of the calibration device. The tightening screw is relaxed in order to permit the advance of the catheter over the guidewire. A pressure line is connected to the proximal port of the catheter and an active flushing of heparinized saline should be maintained throughout the procedure. The safety latch is confirmed to be raised into the locked position. Technical tips during the different steps of the procedure, also shown in Figure 25-3, are as follows.

TECHNICAL TIPS

**Introduction and advancement of the guidewire: During introduction into the distal tip of the commissurotome and advancement to the site of the femoral puncture,

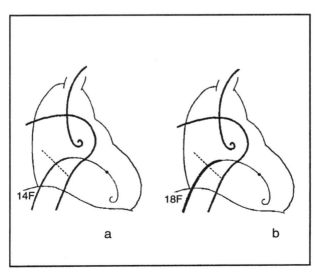

Figure 25-6(A, B): See text for details.

the second operator must maintain traction on the device handle and the guidewire and maintain a straight line along the shaft of the catheter.

**Introduction of the metal head: In order to introduce the metal head into the femoral vein at an approximately 45° angle, it is recommended that the catheter be held at the point where the metallic head is attached to the rest of the catheter, and that any rotational motion once it is introduced be avoided. The position of the guidewire in the left ventricle is monitored by fluoroscopy during this maneuver as well as during the advancement of the device up to the mitral valve.

**Advancement of the catheter: During advancement of the catheter to the interatrial septum and across the septum, the traction on the guidewire may be exerted by the second operator, or better yet by the principal operator himself, in order to optimally coordinate the pushing of the catheter and the traction on the wire in such a way as to maintain the metallic ball at the center of the left ventricular cavity.

**Crossing of the mitral orifice: The same maneuver is used to pass the metal head through the mitral orifice. The metal head is advanced across the mitral orifice until its proximal third is situated roughly along a vertical line from the pigtail that was left in place above the aortic valve (Figure 25-7 A). It is inadvisable to push the device further forward into the left ventricle because the bars opening will then be at the level of the subvalvular apparatus.

**Positioning of the ball: In this position, traction is placed on the guidewire and the ball is brought into firm contact with the distal extremity of the metal head (Figure 25-7 B). The screw at the back end of the device must now be tightened around the guidewire to lock the ball in place.

**Opening of the commissurotome and valvular dilatation: Opening of the commissurotome must be performed slowly and in two phases. The commissurotome is opened partially to allow for the metal struts to position themselves along the lines of least resistance, which in the majority of cases is along the commissural lines. One can observe on the fluoroscopy screen that the struts separate along a slightly oblique line. The dilator is then totally opened and maintained open during a 3- to 5-sec period (Figure 25-7 C), and then closed. In reality, the relaxation of pressure on the handle leads to a partial closure of the metal struts, maintaining a half-open position thanks to the position of the security latch (Figure 25-7 D).

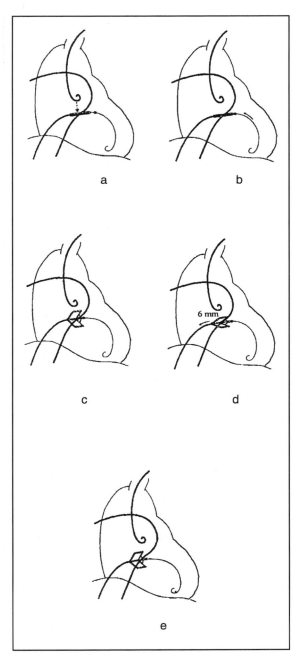

Figure 25-7(A–E): See text for details.

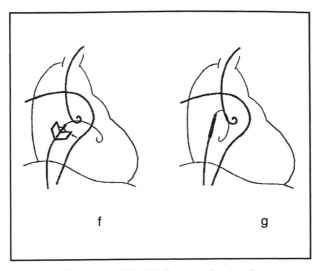

f

g

Figure 25-7(F, G): See text for details.

Three or four additional openings of the valvulotome are then performed in sequential fashion, separated each time by pulling back the head of the device approximately 5 mm (Figure 25-7 E). It is important to never push the commissurotome forward in a semi-open position (Figure 25-7 F). If additional dilation is required with the head placed more distally, the metal head must be retracted into the left atrium, closed completely, and then readvanced to the chosen position. The operator should feel progressive diminution in the resistance to opening of the commissurotome after repeated dilatations; this confirms the success of the commissurotomy. The withdrawal of the metal head into the left atrium will appear on the screen as a vertical rocking motion (Figure 25-7 G). At this stage, if the maximal degree of opening calibrated on the handle has already been achieved (40 mm), the dilatation procedure is finished.

**Withdrawal of the commissurotome: The metal head in its semi-opened position in the left atrium is closed totally by repositioning the security latch (the lever is pulled backward). The metallic head is pulled back to the edge of the septum and the guidewire is withdrawn from the left ventricle and maintained in position in the left atrium. Left atrial pressure can be recorded through the line attached to the proximal portion of the catheter. At this stage, a first evaluation of the transmitral pressure gradient may be obtained by simultaneously recording the left atrial pressure and the left ventricular pressure, the latter using the catheter that was left in the aorta. An echocardiographic and Doppler evaluation of the results can also be performed. In a closed position, the commissurotome is withdrawn, the guidewire being maintained in the left atrium.

EVALUATION OF THE PERCUTANEOUS MECHANICAL MITRAL COMMISSUROTOMY (PMMC) RESULTS

1. **Final verification of the left atrial pressure using the Mullins catheter placed back into the left atrium:** It is preferable to confirm the left atrial pressure previously obtained using the lumen in the commissurotome, given the possibility of artifact caused by pooling of blood in the lumen (the likelihood of which is increased if flushing is not maintained throughout the procedure). The gradient can also be measured. In addition, pulmonary artery pressure and, subsequently, the cardiac output can be determined to calculate the post-commissurotomy mitral valve area using the Gorlin formula.
2. **Immediate post-commissurotomy evaluation:** To the extent possible, immediate post-commissurotomy results should be obtained by echocardiographic and Doppler methods.
3. **In case the results are judged to be inadequate** (mitral valve area <1.5 cm^2 or unilateral opening of the commissures) and in the absence of significant mitral valve regurgitation (>grade 2), repeat dilatation can be performed after recrossing of the mitral valve by the commissurotome. This is particularly the case when the initial setting for opening of the commissurotome was less than maximal (40 mm). Before reusing the commissurotome, it is advisable to unscrew the metal head and rinse it thoroughly with heparinized saline while opening it manually. After screwing the metal head back on the catheter, the commissurotome is carefully flushed before reuse.
4. **At the end of the procedure, left ventricular angiography is performed** to evaluate the degree of post-commissurotomy mitral insufficiency, if any. Withdrawal of the catheters is followed by manual compression of the puncture sites.

THE MULTICENTER REGISTRY

Study population: From November 1995 to August 1999, PMMC was performed at 66 centers in 15 countries, with a majority of patients being recruited in India, Egypt, and France.

Table 25-1
Baseline clinical characteristics of the population

- 1087 patients: 728 females, 359 males
- Mean age: 35 ± 14 years (12 to 86)
- NYHA Class III/IV: 630 patients (58%)
- Sinus rhythm: 859 patients (79%)
- Previous commissurotomy 155 patients (15%)

The series included 1087 patients with mitral stenosis considered suitable for percutaneous valvotomy. The demographic data are shown in Table 25-1. Contraindications to the procedure were: no commissural fusion, MR Sellers' grade >2, recent embolic event, left atrial thrombus on transesophageal echocardiography that was performed within 2 weeks before the procedure in the vast majority of cases.

Results: PMMC could be achieved in 1066 out of the 1087 patients (98%). In 7 patients, it was not possible to cross the mitral valve with either the Critikon balloon catheter or the commissurotome. A crossover to the Inoue technique was performed in 5 cases and was successful in 3, while a direct crossover to surgery was performed in the other patients.

Maximum extent of bars opening was 40 mm in 87%, 37 mm in 12%, and 35 mm in 1%. The mean number of openings was 3.3 ± 1.7.[1–10]

A successful result was defined as a final valve area >1.5 cm^2 on planimetry, with no MR > grade 2. It was obtained in 93% of the patients. The technique resulted in a significantly decreased transmitral gradient and increased valve area as shown in Figure 25-8. At day 1, the mitral valve area had increased from 0.93 ± 0.2 cm^2 to 2.10 ± 0.4 cm^2 (P<0.001). Bilateral splitting of the commissures was noted in 86% of

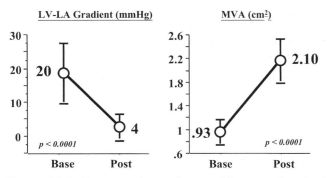

Figure 25-8: Decrease in gradient and increase in mitral valve area after PMMC in the overall population.

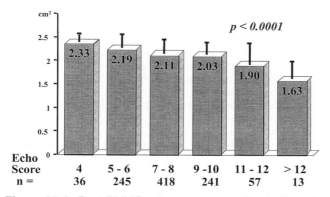

Figure 25-9: Post-PMMC valve areas according to the echo score.

the patients. According to the echocardiographic score, the mean post-PMMC mitral valve area was 2.18 ± 0.4, 2.09 ± 0.3, and 1.91 ± 0.1 in patients with a score <8 (385 patients), 8 and 9 (229 patients), and above 9 (105 patients), respectively. Detailed results according to the echo score are shown in Figure 25-9. The success rate in these subsets of patients was respectively 96%, 94%, and 89%. The mean duration of the procedure from the time the septal puncture was completed to the withdrawal of the catheters (which was recorded in the last 108 patients) was 28 ± 14 min.

Complications: Severe complications occurred in 44/1087 patients (4%). There were 14 pericardial tamponades (1.3%), 9 requiring surgery, and 1 leading to death. The incidence of MR > grade 2 was 2.4%, including 6 grade 4 (surgical) and 21 grade 3 (nonsurgical) MR. Finally, 3 patients had a transient stroke with no neurologic sequel. On transthoracic color flow Doppler, transseptal shunting was not detected or was trivial after the procedure. In the subgroup of 45 patients who also had transesophageal color flow Doppler, transseptal shunting was detected in 32 patients, trivial in 29, and small in 3. There were no other complications. The patients were discharged on an average of 2 days after the procedure.

Balloon mitral valvuloplasty is associated with 1.4% to 7.5% severe MR in the literature[11–17] and the incidence of tamponade is reported to be 1% to 9%.[14,17,18]

The role of the learning curve in the occurrence of complications has been clearly demonstrated. When two subgroups are compared according to the investigator's experience of <20 patients (n = 599) or >20 patients (n = 488), the incidence of complication is, respectively, 5.3% versus 2.4% (P<0.001). This is particularly confirmed as per the incidence of pericardial tamponades (1.7% vs 0.5%) and > grade 2 MR (3.3% vs 1.4%).

Mechanism of action: It has been demonstrated by 2D echocardiography that the device enlarges the stenotic orifice primarily by separating the fused commissures. Actually, the two bars start to open in the way of less resistance, i.e. on the commissures line. No hand rotation of the catheter is necessary. Stretching and separation of the commissures are obtained without injury to the leaflets or the chordae, thus decreasing the risk of MR.

Economical aspects: An important potential advantage of the metallic dilator is the expected decrease in procedural cost. The detachable metallic head allows multiple safe reuse after sterilization using autoclave. Some investigators have performed over 40 procedures with a single device without any deterioration of the dilator components. Consequently, in India, the cost per procedure has been recently evaluated to be about US $100. Thus, it is expected that the final cost per patient will be confirmed to be markedly lowered and this should be considered as a major advantage in countries with low financial resources.

FUTURE PERSPECTIVES

The multicenter international registry is still ongoing and will definitely determine the benefits, limitations, and cost-effectiveness of the procedure. A French prospective study started in January 1998 with the goal of assessing the immediate as well as the long-term results of the technique; these results are under evaluation by independent core laboratories. Finally, the results of a first randomized study from Egypt comparing this technique with the current balloon techniques will be reported this year.

Furthermore, a small (9F) device, similar otherwise to the present dilator, has been designed, and the clinical experience with it should start in the coming months. This smaller device should in the near future widen the indications of this technique to children under 12 years of age with mitral stenosis, and to some other indications such as congenital or rheumatic aortic stenosis.

REFERENCES

1. Inoue K, Owaki T, Nakanura T, Kitamura F, Miyamoto N. Clinical application of transvenous mitral commissurotomy by a new balloon catheter. *J Thorac Cardiovasc Surg* 1984; **87**: 394–402.
2. Arora R, Nair M, Kalra GS, Nigam M, Khalilullah M. Immediate and long-term results of balloon and surgical closed

mitral valvotomy: A randomized comparative study. *Am Heart J* 1993; **125**: 1091–4.

3. Reyes VP, Raju BS, Wynne J *et al*. Percutaneous balloon valvuloplasty compared with open surgical commissurotomy for mitral stenosis. *N Engl J Med* 1994; **331**: 961–7.

4. Iung B, Cormier B, Ducimetiere P *et al*. Functional results 5 years after successful percutaneous commissurotomy in a series of 528 patients and analysis of predictive factors. *J Am Coll Cardiol* 1996; **27**: 407–14.

5. Orrange SE, Kawanishi DT, Lopez BM, Curry SM, Rahimtoola SH. Actuarial outcome after catheter balloon commissurotomy in patients with mitral stenosis. *Circulation* 1997; **95**: 382–9.

6. Palacios IF, Tuzcu ME, Weyman AE, Newell JB, Block PC. Clinical follow-up of patients undergoing percutaneous mitral balloon valvotomy. *Circulation* 1995; **91**: 671–6.

7. Cribier A, Rath PC, Letac B. Percutaneous mitral valvotomy with a metal dilator. *Lancet* 1997; **349**: 1667–8.

8. Cribier A, Eltchaninoff H, Koning R *et al*. Percutaneous mechanical mitral commissurotomy with a newly designed metallic valvulotome: Immediate results of the initial experience in 153 patients. *Circulation* 1999; **99**: 793–9.

9. Wilkins GT, Weyman AE, Abascal VM, Block PC, Palacios IF. Percutaneous mitral valvotomy: An analysis of echocardiographic variables related to outcome and the mechanism of dilatation. *Br Heart J* 1988; **60**: 299–308.

10. Arora R, Kalra GS, Murty GSR *et al*. Percutaneous transatrial mitral commissurotomy: Immediate and intermediate results. *J Am Coll Cardiol* 1994; **23**: 1327–32.

11. Ben Farhat M, Betbout F, Gamra H *et al*. Results of percutaneous double-balloon mitral commissurotomy in one medical center in Tunisia. *Am J Cardiol* 1995; **76**: 1266–70.

12. Vahanian A, Cormier B, Iung B. Percutaneous transvenous mitral commissurotomy using the Inoue balloon: International experience. *Cathet Cardiovasc Diagn* 1994; **2**: 8–15.

13. Chen CR, Cheng TO. Percutaneous balloon mitral valvuloplasty by the Inoue technique: A multicenter study of 4832 patients in China. *Am Heart J* 1995; **129**: 1197–203.

14. A report from the National Heart, Lung, and Blood Institute balloon valvuloplasty Registry. Complications and mortality of percutaneous balloon mitral commissurotomy. *Circulation* 1992; **85**: 2014–24.

15. Hernandez R, Macaya C, Banuelos C *et al*. Predictors, mechanisms and outcome of severe mitral regurgitation complicating percutaneous mitral valvotomy with the Inoue balloon. *Am J Cardiol* 1992; **70**: 1169–74.

16. Herrmann HC, Lima JA, Feldman T, Chisholm R, Isner J, O'Neill W, Ramaswamy K, for the North American Inoue Balloon investigators. Mechanisms and outcome of severe mitral regurgitation after Inoue balloon valvuloplasty. *J Am Coll Cardiol* 1993; **22**: 783–9.

17. Feldman T. Hemodynamic results, clinical outcome, and complications of Inoue balloon mitral valvotomy. *Cathet Cardiovasc Diagn* 1994; **2** (Suppl): 2–7.
18. Nobuyoshi M, Hamasaki N, Kimura T *et al.* Indications, complications, and short-term clinical outcome of percutaneous transvenous mitral commissurotomy in 200 patients. *Circulation* 1989; **80**: 782–92.

Chapter 26

Retrograde Balloon Percutaneous Aortic Valvuloplasty

Ted Feldman

General overview
Standard technique
    **Necessity of temporary pacemaker
    **Vascular access
    **Preparatory installation of closure device suture
    **Local pain management with lidocaine
    **Dobutamine for low cardiac output
    **Manipulating the catheter
    **Wiring
    **Balloon inflation
    **Balloon preparation
    **Set-up for balloon inflation
    **Balloon deflation
    CAVEAT: Differential diagnoses of hypotension
    **Hypotension caused by the wire
Post-procedure management

GENERAL OVERVIEW

Although not commonly performed in many catheterization laboratories, balloon aortic valvuloplasty (BAV) has an important role in the management of patients who do not have an option for surgery with aortic valve replacement. BAV is a palliative procedure, and can be applied in appropriately selected patients with excellent relief from the symptoms of congestive heart failure associated with aortic valve stenosis. The AHA-ACC guidelines[1] recognize BAV as a Class 1 treatment for children and young adults with aortic stenosis under the age of 21 years (Tables 26-1, 26-2), and as a Class 2B

*Basic; **Advanced; ***Rare, exotic, or investigational.

From: Nguyen T, Hu D, Saito S, Grines C, Palacios I (eds), *Practical Handbook of Advanced Interventional Cardiology*, 2nd edn. © 2003 Futura, an imprint of Blackwell Publishing.

Table 26-1
Indications for diagnostic and therapeutic procedures

Definition	Class
General agreement procedure is useful/effective	I
Conflict evidence/divergent opinion	II
Weight of evidence/opinion in favor	IIa
Less well established	IIb
Evidence/agreement that procedure is not useful/ harmful	III

Table 26-2
Balloon valvuloplasty in the young adult (<21 years) with aortic stenosis and normal cardiac output

Indication	Class
Angina, syncope, DOE with peak gradient >50 mmHg	I
Cath peak gradient >60 mmHg	I
New onset ECG changes at rest or with exercise with gradient >50 mm	I
Gradient >50 mm, patient desires competitive sports or pregnancy	IIa
Cath gradient <50 mm, no symptoms or ECG changes	III

indication among older patients with multiple comorbid conditions that preclude aortic valve replacement surgery (Table 26-3). In my own practice, one-third of these patients are nonagenarians, and half are octogenarians. Many have had prior coronary bypass or mitral valve replacement, or have comorbid conditions such as chronic lung disease or multi-organ compromise. These patients typically obtain about 1 year of improved symptoms, with diminished need for re-hospitalization for their symptoms.[2] It is clear that no overall survival benefit is conferred by this procedure in studies of groups of

Table 26-3
Balloon valvuloplasty in adults with aortic stenosis

Indication	Class
Bridge to surgery in hemodynamically unstable high-risk patients for AVR	IIa
Palliation in patients with serious comorbid conditions	IIb
Prior to urgent non-cardiac surgery	IIb
Alternative to AVR	III

patients, though for individual patients it seems likely that some may derive this benefit.[3,4,5]

STANDARD TECHNIQUE

The basic technique of retrograde BAV involves passing a catheter via the femoral arterial route retrograde across the aortic valve, placing a wire in the LV apex, and then via the femoral sheath passing a balloon into the aortic valve. Numerous special tips and tricks are critical to make this procedure successful.

TECHNICAL TIPS

**Necessity of temporary pacemaker: The pre-procedural electrocardiogram has great bearing on planning for the procedure. Patients with pre-existing bundle branch block or IVCD should have a temporary pacemaker placed for the procedure, or at very least have a venous sheath for pacemaker access. Complete heart block occurs infrequently but can be difficult to manage when it does occur in this group of patients. Since a right heart catheter is used, and the left ventricle is instrumented significantly by the balloon, both sides of the septum may be abraded with resultant loss of AV conduction. In addition, among patients with pre-existing conduction abnormalities, the displacement of aortic annular calcification by the balloon may impinge on the atrioventricular conducting system, with exacerbation of heart block or pre-existing conduction delays. When complete heart block does occur, it usually resolves within 12 to 24 hours, but may be permanent. Infrequently, these patients need permanent pacemakers following the procedure, and I find it useful to warn most patients and families pre-procedure that permanent pacing is an occasional consequence of the effort.

**Vascular access: One of the most critical elements of the BAV procedure is assessment of the femoral artery. Fluoroscopic guidance of the initial puncture is critical, so that the common femoral artery is entered rather than the superficial femoral or the profunda femoris. Large sheaths needed for the balloons require the puncture to be above the femoral bifurcation. In between two-thirds and three-quarters of patients, the common femoral artery will be entered if the puncture is made at the level of the mid femoral head. Since the procedure is used principally in elderly patients, the location of the femoral crease is an unreliable landmark to guide the femoral puncture. Heavier patients may have two creases, and many thin elderly patients have lost the battle with gravity, and the crease has moved substantially caudal to the femoral head. Angiographic assessment of the femoral artery after the sheath is placed is also critical. I like to start with a 6F long sheath. If femoral angiography demonstrates too much atherosclerotic disease, a left internal mammary diagnostic catheter can be used to shoot over the top of the iliac bifurcation into the left iliac and femoral system to see if they are suitable for the large valvuloplasty sheath. In addition, if the puncture is below the femoral bifurcation a sheath may be placed above the existing sheath on the right, or the left side might be used with angiographic guidance for the puncture.

**Preparatory installation of closure device suture: Pre-closure of the puncture is important at this juncture within the order of the procedure.[6,7] The 6F sheath can be exchanged for a 10F Perclose device and sutures delivered into the artery. The sutures are of course not tied at this point. A wire is reintroduced into the Perclose delivery device, the delivery device backed out of the artery, and a 12F or 14F sheath passed back over the wire. It is especially helpful to use an extra stiff wire to allow passage of the large arterial sheath. It is my own preference to use a 30-centimeter long sheath. Sometimes this is not possible due to calcification or tortuosity of the iliac vessels, in which case a shorter sheath will suffice.

**Local pain management with lidocaine: The liberal use of lidocaine for local anesthesia is important to make passage of these large sheaths tolerable for the patient. At the same time, in the very elderly, especially among those with a history of prior stroke or seizure disorder, care must be taken not to create lidocaine toxicity. Changes in consciousness during the procedure may represent a variety of complications, but it is important to remember that lidocaine toxicity is among them and that lidocaine levels should be obtained any time there is a change in consciousness during a valvuloplasty procedure.[8]

**Dobutamine for low cardiac output: After right heart catheterization and baseline pressure measurements, special consideration should be given for the cardiac output. Among patients with cardiac output less than 3 liters per minute, and certainly less than 2.5 liters per minute it is useful to use dobutamine support. The decrease in blood pressure associated with balloon inflation may not be tolerated by patients with a low baseline cardiac output. It is my own practice to use a dobutamine infusion to improve cardiac output in those patients with low baseline pre-procedure, and to reassess valve area after the dobutamine infusion is started, for a new baseline measure.[9]

Crossing the aortic valve: Crossing the aortic valve is an important challenge in this procedure. My preference is to use a catheter I have designed specially for this purpose.[10] There are two catheter shapes: the first with an angled design [type B] and the second a curve design [type A]. Each is constructed in small (A, B), medium (A1, B2) curve lengths. The displacement from the shaft to the catheter tip, or the "reaching distance" of the catheter, measures 4 cm, 5 cm, and 6 cm for the small, medium, and large curves, respectively. A moveable core straight wire can be used to change the angle of the catheter. When the aortic root is very small in diameter, the catheter can be straightened with the wire and formed into shape similar to a right Judkins curve. The angled design catheter can reach the center of the aortic root in most patients unless the left ventricle and aortic root meet at an extremely acute angle. The curve catheter is designed to reach a more acutely angled left ventricular chamber but is slightly more difficult to maneuver into the left ventricle in some patients.[10]

TECHNICAL TIPS

**Manipulating the catheter: The catheter is selected based on the fluoroscopic appearance of the width of the aortic root. It is inserted into the aortic root with a straight wire and rotated clockwise to direct the tip of the catheter toward the center of the aortic root. A moveable core straight wire can be used to change the angle of the catheter, allowing the operator to scan the surface of the aortic valve. Wires with a tapered moveable core are not stiff enough for this purpose. The wire is initially made extremely soft by withdrawal of 3–4 inches of moveable core, which allows the tip to assume its formed curve completely. The catheter tip is positioned over the center of the aortic valve as determined from the appearance of the heavily calcified leaflets on fluoroscopy. The straight wire is passed back and forth until it crosses into the aortic valve. Occasionally, a hand injection above the valve will help define the central area of the commissures. Of course, the wire may cross at some distance away from the commissures, but the central point represents the best chance for success. The catheter is advanced over the wire into the left ventricle and the wire withdrawn. In all patients, a small or medium length catheter is selected initially. Based on the direction of the wire, subsequent catheter choices are made. It should be noted that both catheters can be passed into the left ventricle with much greater ease than most coronary artery catheters.

**Wiring: After the left ventricle has been entered and hemodynamic measurements confirm the severity of aortic stenosis,[11] a 260-centimeter long 0.038" exchange wire must be used to allow exchange or a valvuloplasty balloon.

The wire must be as stiff as possible, but with the tip curled to make it less dangerous for left ventricular apical perforation. It is helpful to grasp the wire over the end of a hemostat and "Christmas ribbon" the end into a ram's horn shape with multiple concentric coils to protect the LV apex from wire trauma or perforations. The stiffest possible wire available is the best wire. It is critical to have a firm rail to allow the balloon to traverse tortuous anatomy in the aorta, and to have the support to keep the balloon in position in the aortic valve during balloon inflations. The assistant helping maintain wire position is as critical to the success of the procedure as the principal operator is.

Balloon manipulation: Once a balloon has been passed into the aortic valve orifice, maintaining its position is challenging. In patients with poor left ventricular function there is less of a tendency for the balloon to be ejected by the ventricle. When left ventricular systolic performance is preserved, the balloon "watermelon seeds" back and forth during inflations.

TECHNICAL TIPS

**Balloon inflation: It is useful to partially inflate the balloon in the ascending aorta above the valve prior to trying to engage the valve, so that less inflation is needed to achieve adequate inflation within the valve orifice. If the balloon is fully inflated in the valve orifice and continues to move back and forth, it may be undersized. The balloon "locks" in the valve when it is fully inflated and delivers adequate dilating force to displace the leaflets. If a first balloon is too small, it is often necessary to size up the sheath. A 20-millimeter diameter balloon catheter will require a 12F or 13F sheath. It is my own practice to use a 12.5F sheath for this purpose. A 23-millimeter balloon requires a 14F sheath.

**Balloon preparation: Careful preparation of the balloon is necessary, because it is common for the balloon to rupture during inflations in the calcified aortic valve. Great care to remove all the air during the preparation process is essential. Preparation and balloon inflation is easiest if the contrast is diluted as much as possible. A ratio of 7:1 will allow the balloon to be visualized fluoroscopically, but inflated and deflated with the least difficulty. The contrast is ideally an old-fashioned ionic contrast, since these agents are less viscous than low osmolarity contrast. It is my approach to use a 50-cc bottle of Hypaque diluted with an additional 350 cc of saline to a total volume of 400 cc. Many of the basins used on the cath lab back table are graduated. There is thus no need to use a syringe to top off the total volume, since the graduated basin allows one simply to pour saline in to the 400 cc mark after the contrast has been placed in the bowl.

**Set-up for balloon inflation: The set-up for balloon preparation includes a short pressure tube to the inflate lumen, connected to a high-pressure stopcock. A 60-cc syringe is attached to one arm of the stopcock, and a 10-cc to the other arm. If the 60-cc syringe is used to inflate the balloon, it is not possible to deliver adequate force to fully inflate the balloon.[12] Once the balloon has been inflated as much as possible with the 60-cc syringe, the stopcock can be switched to allow the 10-cc to finish the inflation, or "boost" the total inflation volume. If this is done on the back table, you will note that the balloon clearly increases in inflation volume when the booster syringe is used to fully inflate it. Thus, *in vivo* the balloon is passed across the valve and inflated as much as possible with the 60-cc syringe and then the stopcock is flipped and the 10 cc additional inflation used to maximize the balloon diameter.

**Balloon deflation: The strategy of balloon deflation is as important as the inflation. Once the balloon is fully inflated in the valve there is a precipitous decrease in systemic blood pressure, and usually significant ventricular ectopy. Rather than waiting for the balloon to deflate to withdraw it from the valve, it can be pulled back from the valve orifice into the aortic root while it is still inflated, or just as the process of deflation begins. This allows a restoration of antegrade blood flow before balloon deflation is even initiated. It is easier for patients to tolerate this very brief effective cross-clamping of the aorta than if the entire inflate-deflate cycle were performed within the valve orifice. When the balloon is withdrawn into the aortic root it is possible for the arch vessels to be obstructed, so care must be taken to avoid covering the carotid origins.

Management of hypotension: The management of hypotension during the procedure is one of the greater challenges.[13,14] The blood pressure inevitably falls during balloon inflations. In most cases there is a steady recovery of systolic pressure immediately following balloon deflation, and when the valve is successfully opened there is a rebound or increase in aortic peak systolic pressure above the baseline. Pressure can be monitored via the sidearm of the 12F sheath. If the pressure does not recover rapidly after a balloon inflation, it is unwise to proceed with further inflations. This represents left ventricular depression that may require support with pressors, sometimes for as long as a day or two.

CAVEAT: Differential diagnoses of hypotension: Other causes of hypotension must be considered. Since the arterial sheath is large, femoral hematoma, retroperitoneal bleeding, or even venous bleeding from the venous access site must be considered. Patients with significant anemia prior to the procedure should be considered for transfusion so that they have a "full tank" before the procedure begins. If they are borderline, or there is some relative contraindication to transfusion, consider obtaining a type-and-screen or type-and-cross match so that blood will be readily available if needed. Vagal reactions from insertion of the large sheath may occur though they are rare. This should be considered only after bleeding has been carefully evaluated and excluded. During the balloon inflations, the guidewire is forced into the left ventricular apex, and the tip of the balloon may also impact on the apex with considerable force. Ventricular perforation is another important consideration for hypotension. Echocardiography should be used liberally in the catheterization lab to exclude this possibility when hypotension is persistent. In the worst cases, the aortic annulus may be ruptured, or a valve leaflet avulsed with catastrophic results. Hypotension associated with these latter complications is usually fatal, and cannot be reversed.

TECHNICAL TIP

**Hypotension caused by the wire: In some cases, the ventricular ectopy produced by the wire in the ventricle for a prolonged period of time is not tolerated, and is another source of hypotension. Reshaping the wire or repositioning the wire may give some relief from persistent ventricular ectopy. In some cases the procedure cannot be performed due to ectopy. I have encountered a patient who had ventricular fibrillation requiring DC countershock each time the wire was introduced into the left ventricle. After two attempts it became clear that it was not feasible to perform aortic valvuloplasty for this patient.

Sheath removal: Sheath removal is an important challenge in the management of these patients. The large caliber femoral artery sheath has been associated with transfusion rates in about one-quarter of patients in the past, and the need for vascular surgical repair in 5% to 10%. Recently, the use of percutaneous suture closure has been described as an adjunct to sheath removal. Pre-closure using a 10F Perclose (Abbotts Vascular, Redwood City, CA) device prior to insertion of the 12F or 14F sheath has been successful in almost 90% of patients with an almost complete elimination of the need for blood transfusion following this procedure. For those patients in whom pre-closure is unsuccessful, or in whom femoral anatomy does not allow its use, it is critical to use a pneumatic compression device such as the RADI FemoStop (Femostop, Radi Medical Systems AB, Sweden). Manual compression by itself is extremely difficult, since prolonged compression for this large sheath size is necessary. The rigid clamp devices cannot be monitored adequately and may result in either inadequate hemostasis or over-compression of the vessel with the potential for thrombosis. The FemoStop device can be applied with a graded pressure, so that initially it is inflated to about the level of systolic pressure. Since the device is transparent, hemostasis can be visualized directly. The pressure can be decreased 10 mm to 20 mm every 10–30 minutes depending on the activated clotting time, until hemostasis is achieved. Another benefit of the FemoStop device is that it helps keep the patient immobile during the period of vascular compression.

POST-PROCEDURE MANAGEMENT

Other than management of the punctures, the major issue is whether left ventricular depression has been engendered by the balloon inflations. Patients who develop pulmonary congestion during the valvuloplasty procedure require special monitoring, and may need inotropic support and intensive heart failure management for 1 to 2 days post-procedure, until their left ventricular performance recovers.

Long-term follow-up requires no more than surveillance for recurrent symptoms, and periodic echocardiographic examinations to monitor the transaortic valve pressure gradient. An important consideration in follow-up is the status of other valve lesions. When the aortic valve is successfully opened, afterload reduction will often result in improvement in the associated mitral regurgitation that these late-stage aortic stenosis patients often have.

Among patients who have recurrence of the stenosis, repeat valvuloplasty may be accomplished with a high expectation for success.[15] I rarely offer repeat procedures to patients who re-stenose quickly, within 6 to 8 months following the initial procedure. For those who achieve a year or more of clinical benefit, repeat procedures can be performed even 3 or 4 times, though the resultant valve areas are usually no better than the first procedure.

REFERENCES

1. ACC/AHA guidelines for the management of patients with valvular heart disease. A report of the American College of Cardiology/American Heart Association. Task Force on Practice Guidelines (Committee on Management of Patients with Valvular Heart Disease). *J Am Coll Cardiol* 1998; **32**: 1486–588.

2. Levinson JR, Akins CW, Buckley MJ *et al.* Octogenarians with aortic stenosis. Outcome after aortic valve replacement. *Circulation* 1989; **80** (3 Pt 1): I49–56.

3. Safian RD, Berman AD, Diver DJ *et al.* Balloon aortic valvuloplasty in 170 consecutive patients. *N Engl J Med* 1988; **319**: 125–30.

4. Otto CM, Mickel MC, Kennedy JW *et al.* Three-year outcome after balloon aortic valvuloplasty. Insights into prognosis of valvular aortic stenosis. *Circulation* 1994; **89**: 642–50.

5. The NHLBI Registrty Participants. Percutaneous balloon aortic valvuloplasty. Acute and 30-day follow-up results in 674 patients from the NHLBI Balloon Valvuloplasty Registry. *Circulation* 1991; **84**: 2383–97.

6. Feldman T. Percutaneous suture closure for management of large French size arterial and venous puncture. *J Intervent Cardiol* 2000; **13**: 237–42.

7. Solomon LW, Fusman B, Jolly N, Kim A, Feldman T. Percutaneous suture closure for management of large French size arterial puncture in aortic valvuloplasty. *J Invasive Cardiol* 2001; **13**: 592–6.

8. Guth A, Hennen B, Kramer T, Stoll HP, Bohm M. Plasma lidocaine concentrations after local anesthesia of the groin for cardiac catheterization. *Cathet Cardiovasc Interv* 2002; **57**: 342–5.

9. Feldman T, Ford LE, Chiu YC, Carroll JC. Changes in valvular resistance, power dissipation, and myocardial reserve with aortic valvuloplasty. *J Heart Valve Dis* 1992; **1**: 55–64.

10. Feldman T, Carroll JD, Chiu YC. An improved catheter for crossing stenosed aortic valves. *Cathet Cardiovasc Diagn* 1989; **16**: 279-83.

11. Fusman B, Faxon D, Feldman T. Hemodynamic rounds: Transvalvular pressure gradient measurement. *Cathet Cardiovasc Interv* 2001; **53**: 553–61.

12. Feldman T, Chiu YC, Carroll JD. Single balloon aortic valvuloplasty: increased valve areas with improved technique. *J Invasive Cardiol* 1989; **1**: 295–300.

13. Feldman, TE. Balloon valvuloplasty. In: Nissen SE, Popma JJ, Kern MJ, Dehmer GJ, Carroll JD, eds. *CathSAP II*. American College of Cardiology, 2001.

14. Feldman T. Inoue balloon mitral commissurotomy and aortic valvuloplasty. In: Kern MJ, ed. *Interventional Cardiac Catheterization Handbook*, 2nd edn. Mosby Year Book (in press).

15. Feldman T, Glagov S, Carroll JD. Restenosis following successful balloon valvuloplasty: bone formation in aortic valve leaflets. *Cathet Cardiovasc Diagn* 1993; **29**: 1–7.

Chapter 27

Percutaneous Implantation of Aortic Valve Prosthesis

Alain Cribier, Helene Eltchaninoff, Christophe Tron

General overview
Equipment: prosthetic valve and delivery system
Technique
    **Advantages of the antegrade transseptal route
Future directions

GENERAL OVERVIEW

In acquired aortic stenosis, aortic valve replacement (AVR) is the treatment of choice, offering symptomatic relief and improving survival.[1–3] Whereas the rate of operative mortality ranges from 2 to 8% in the majority of patients, the risk is much higher for emergency operations, elderly patients, patients with advanced heart failure, associated coronary artery disease and/or severely reduced left ventricular function.[4–10] Balloon aortic valvuloplasty (BAV), introduced in 1986,[11,12] has been proposed as an alternative treatment for high surgical risk patients or patients with contraindications to surgery (see Chapter 26). However, BAV has been shown to provide a temporary improvement of valvular function and relief of symptoms[13–15] resulting from a small increase in valve area and a high mid-term restenosis rate (>60% at 6 months and 100% at 2 years). Given the limited therapeutic options in patients with very high surgical risk and the poor long-term efficacy of BAV, there has been interest in the development of a percutaneous delivered aortic heart valve. Andersen *et al.* in 1992[16] reported an animal trial in which a prosthetic valve

---

*Basic; **Advanced; ***Rare, exotic, or investigational.

From: Nguyen T, Hu D, Saito S, Grines C, Palacios I (eds), *Practical Handbook of Advanced Interventional Cardiology*, 2nd edn. © 2003 Futura, an imprint of Blackwell Publishing.

consisting of a porcine bioprosthesis attached in a wire-based stent frame could be successfully deployed at various aortic sites. More recently, Bonhoeffer *et al.*[17,18] reported the results obtained in animals with a percutaneous implantable prosthetic valve harvested from bovine jugular vein and mounted in a stent, and published the first successful clinical cases of trans-catheter valve placement in right ventricle to pulmonary artery conduits previously implanted for pulmonary atresia.[19,20] In April 2002, after extensive *ex vivo* testing and animal implantation studies,[21] the first successful implantation of a new percutaneous aortic valve was performed on a patient with end stage aortic stenosis.[22] The technical aspects of this procedure are discussed in this chapter.

EQUIPMENT: PROSTHETIC VALVE AND DELIVERY SYSTEM

The percutaneous heart valve (PHV) is a bioprosthetic valve designed for implantation via a transluminal approach. Implantation of the PHV must be preceded by dilatation of the stenotic aortic valve by BAV. The device consists of a PHV, a crimping tool, and a commercially available Z-MED II (NuMED, Inc., Hopkinton, NY) balloon valvuloplasty catheter. The balloon is 30 mm in length, with a maximal diameter of 23 mm.

The PHV (Percutaneous Valve Technologies, Inc., Fort Lee, NJ) is a radiopaque tubular, slotted, stainless steel balloon expandable stent, 14 mm in length, with an integrated, trileaflet, tissue valve made of three equal sections of bovine pericardium firmly sutured to the stent frame (Figure 27-1). The stent is designed to achieve a diameter of 21 to 23 mm. The crimping tool is a compression device that symmetrically reduces the overall diameter of the PHV from its expanded size to its collapsed size over the balloon delivery catheter (Figure 27-2). The PHV/balloon assembly can be introduced into the vessels via a 24F sheath. In *ex-vivo* pulse duplicator models, the PHV durability passed 100 million cycles (2 years and 6 months).

TECHNIQUE

The procedure requires mild sedation and local anesthesia. A bolus of 10 000 IU of heparin is administered after transseptal catheterization.

1. **Basic preparations:** Through a 5F catheter from the left femoral artery used for blood pressure monitoring, two supra-aortic angiograms (50° LAO and 40° RAO views) are performed and saved on the screen. These angiograms

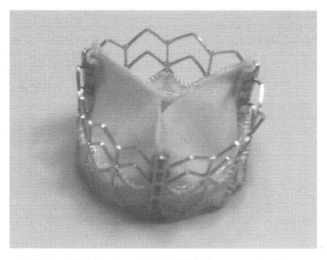

Figure 27-1: Aspect of the PHV in the open position.

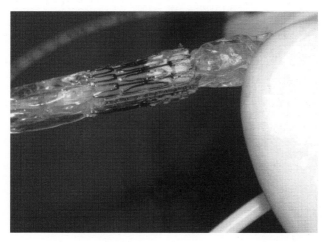

Figure 27-2: The PHV crimped over the NuMED balloon catheter.

are used to accurately locate the position of the coronary ostia. Through the left femoral vein, a 5F pacing wire is placed in the right ventricle (RV) apex, connected to a pulse generator and set on stand-by for any possibility of advanced AV block.

2. **Transseptal catheterization:** The technique is similar to the one used for percutaneous mitral commissurotomy,

details of which are extensively given in Chapters 24 and 25. Using an 8F Mullins sheath from the right femoral vein, the transatrial septum is crossed in the 90° lateral view. In the 40° RAO view, a 7F Swan-Ganz or Pulmonary artery (PA) catheter (Edwards Lifesciences, Irvine, CA) is advanced through the Mullins sheath and used to cross the mitral valve (Figure 27-3 A). The transvalvular gradient across the aortic valve is recorded using the PA catheter in the left ventricle and 5F pigtail catheter in the ascending aorta.

3. **Crossing the aortic valve:** The Mullins sheath is then advanced over the PA catheter with its tip positioned about 2 cm beyond the mitral valve (Figure 27-3 B). The PA catheter (with its balloon inflated) is then pushed in such a way that its distal tip faces the aortic orifice (Figure 27-3 C). A 0.035" straight wire is advanced inside the PA catheter and used to cross the aortic valve (Figure 27-3 D). The PA catheter is pushed over the wire, across the valve (with its balloon deflated), and advanced into the descending aorta.

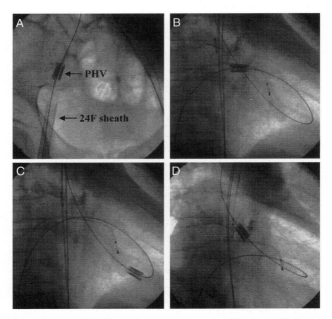

Figure 27-3: (A) The mitral valve crossed by the 7F Swan-Ganz catheter advanced through the 8F Mullins sheath. (B) The Mullins sheath is advanced over the Swan-Ganz catheter beyond the mitral valve. (C) The Swan-Ganz catheter is pushed in the left ventricle and the inflated balloon positioned in front of the aortic valve. (D) The aortic valve is crossed with a 0.035" straight guidewire advanced through the Swan-Ganz catheter.

4. **Stiff 260-cm wire placement:** The straight wire is then removed and replaced by a stiff 260-cm long wire (Amplatz, Cook Inc, Bloomington, IN) which is advanced in the descending aorta to below the renal arteries level (Figure 27-4 A). Through a large 8F left femoral arterial sheath, a snare (Amplatz Goose Neck, Microvena, Minneapolis, MN) is advanced to the descending aorta, manipulated to catch the tip of the 260-cm stiff wire and externalize it via the femoral sheath (Figure 27-4 B).

5. **Interatrial septum dilatation:** Through a 14F sheath introduced into the right femoral vein, a 10-mm diameter septostomy balloon catheter (Owens, Scimed, Boston, MA) is advanced over the 260-cm stiff wire, inflated twice across the interatrial septum (Figure 27-4 C), deflated and removed.

6. **Balloon aortic predilation:** Via the 14F sheath in the right femoral vein, a 23-mm diameter NuMED balloon catheter is advanced over the 260-cm wire through the interatrial septum, the mitral valve, the left ventricle and the aortic valve and fully inflated at the level of the calcific native valve using a 20 mL hand-held syringe with 1:9 mixture of contrast media and saline, then deflated and removed.

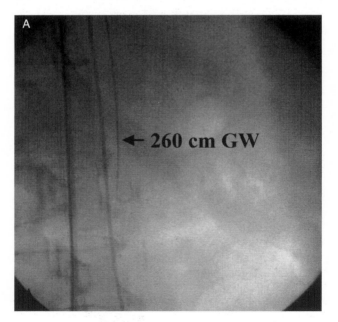

Figure 27-4: (A) The 260-cm, 0.035", stiff wire is advanced through the Swan-Ganz catheter and placed beyond the renal arteries. (*Continued*)

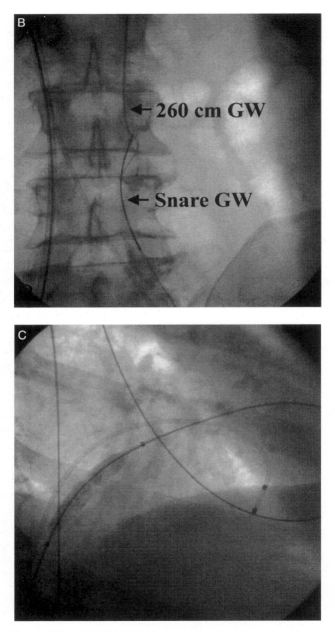

Figure 27-4: (B) This wire is snared and externalized to the left femoral artery. (C) Dilatation of the interatrial septum with a 10-mm diameter balloon catheter.

7. **PHV implantation:** The 14F sheath is removed from the right femoral vein and exchanged with a 24F sheath (Cook Inc, Bloomington, IN). The PHV is crimped over the delivery balloon catheter and the PHV/balloon assembly is introduced into the 24F sheath over the 260-cm stiff wire (Figure 27-5 A) and easily advanced across the interatrial septum (Figure 27-5 B), the left ventricle (Figure 27-5 C) and the native aortic valve. Using the valvular calcifications as a marker, the PHV is positioned at mid-part of the aortic valve (Figure 27-5 D). The balloon is then rapidly and fully inflated using a 20 mL hand-held syringe with the same solution as for aortic predilation, and rapidly deflated and withdrawn (Figure 27-6 A–C).

8. **Post-implantation hemodynamic and echocardiographic measurements:** The 260-cm stiff wire is then removed from the right femoral vein, with its distal end left inside the left ventricle. A 6F pigtail catheter is pushed over this wire from the right femoral vein to the left ventricle. The following hemodynamic and angiographic controls are to be obtained:

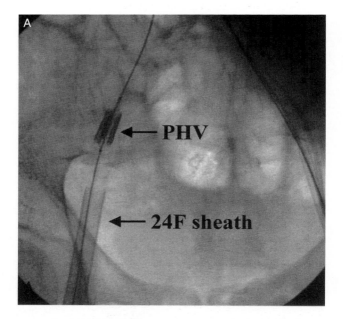

Figure 27-5: The PHV is advanced into the 24F sheath over the stiff wire through (A) the femoral vein, (B) the trans-atrial septum, (C) the left ventricle and (D) positioned at the mid-part of the native aortic valve. *(Continued)*

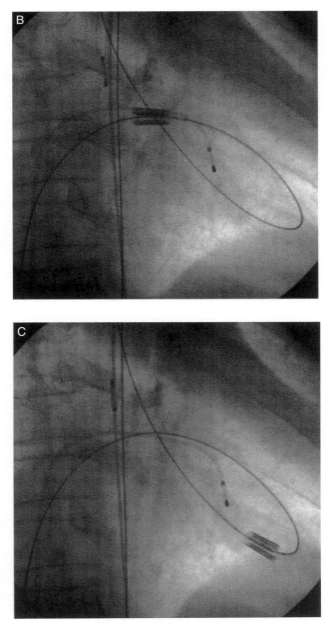

Figure 27-5 B,C *(Continued)*

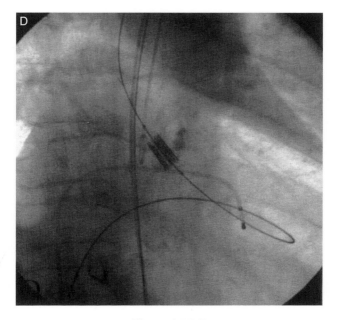

Figure 27-5 D

1. measurement of the trans-PHV gradient (using the pigtail in the left ventricle and a 6F pigtail placed in the ascending aorta from the left femoral artery);
2. measurement of the aortic valve area using the Gorlin formula, the cardiac output being obtained from a PA catheter placed in the pulmonary artery from the left femoral vein;
3. selective left ventricular angiogram to assess the left ventricular function and the degree of any mitral regurgitation;
4. supra-aortic angiogram to assess the degree of any aortic regurgitation and the patency of the coronary arteries. 2D (TTE) and trans-esophageal (TEE) echocardiographies are also obtained.

At the end of the procedure, the venous and arterial introducers are removed and manual compression is applied on the venous entry sites and right femoral artery site. A percutaneous occluder is used to close the left femoral arterial site.

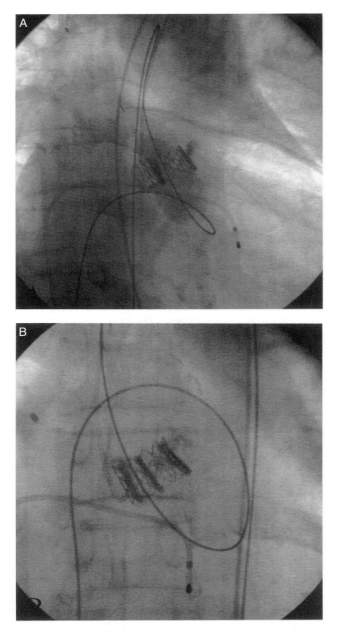

Figure 27-6: (A) The PHV is delivered across the native valve by full balloon inflation. (B) The balloon is rapidly deflated and removed. *(Continued)*

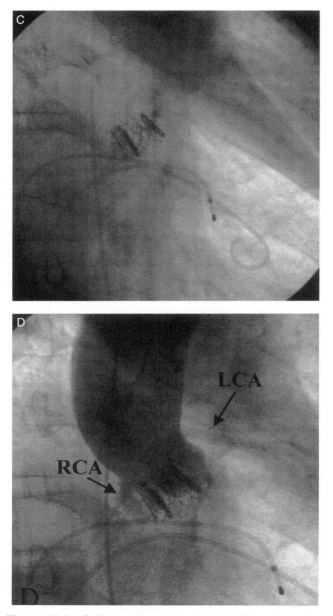

Figure 27-6: (C) The guidewire is removed. (D) A supra-aortic angiogram shows the lack of significant aortic regurgitation and the coronary ostia away from the superior limits of the stent (LCA: left coronary artery, RCA: right coronary artery).

TECHNICAL TIP

**Advantages of the antegrade transseptal route: The antegrade septal route was chosen because of the possibility of percutaneous insertion of the 24F sheath, with excellent support obtained from the 260-cm wire exiting the left femoral artery. These technical arrangements help the precise and predictable placement of the PHV, which moves in concert with the heart during left ventricular contraction.

Case report

The first patient was a 57-year-old man for whom aortic valve replacement had been declined by several cardiac surgeons. Besides a very severely calcific aortic stenosis, he had a history of peripheral vascular disease with aorto-bifemoral bypass in 1996, silicosis, lung cancer with lobectomy in 1999, and chronic pancreatitis. He presented in cardiogenic shock and with a subacute ischemia of the right leg due to the recent occlusion of the right bypass limb. On TTE and TEE, the valve was bicuspid, with a gradient of 30 mmHg and a valve area of 0.6 cm^2. Left ventricular function was severely depressed with an ejection fraction of 14%. Dobutamine stress-echocardiography showed no myocardial contractility reserve. In the first intervention, BAV was performed with 20-mm-diameter balloon inflations, using the antegrade transseptal approach due to the severe bilateral peripheral artery disease. The gradient was reduced to 13 mmHg and the valve area increased to 1.06 cm^2. The patient sustained marked clinical improvement during the ensuing 4 days but his condition deteriorated thereafter with recurrence of cardiogenic shock and impending death. Under these circumstances, a week after BAV, PHV implantation appeared to be the only possible life-saving option for this patient. The patient successfully underwent implantation of the PHV.

Cardiac standstill occurred in the last 20 seconds of PHV deployment. After that, the aortic pressure increased to normal (120/60 mmHg). The transvalvular gradient was 6 mmHg and the aortic valve area 1.9 cm^2 by the Gorlin formula (Figure 27-7). On angiographies, the flow was normal across the PHV, there was a minimal paravalvular regurgitation and the coronary arteries were away from the upper edge of the prosthesis (Figure 27-6 D). On TEE, there was a mild paravalvular regurgitation, the native valve was completely excluded, the stent diameter was 21 mm and the valve area was 1.6 cm^2 by planimetry (Figure 27-8). The post-procedural treatment included anticoagulation with heparin and aspirin and administration of vasopressors at decreasing doses over 4 weeks. A dramatic clinical improvement was observed after PHV implantation with re-

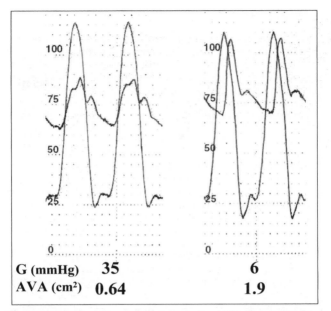

| G (mmHg) | 35 | 6 |
| AVA (cm²) | 0.64 | 1.9 |

Figure 27-7: Mean transvalvular gradient (G) and aortic valve area (AVA) before and after PHV implantation.

duced signs of congestive heart failure. During the 4-month follow-up, the valve function remained satisfactory and unchanged on TEE performed every 2 weeks. However, the ejection fraction remained in the range of 13 to 20% in this patient with no contractility reserve.

FUTURE DIRECTIONS

The first implantation of the PHV was performed in emergency after the device was successfully tried on animal models. Further improvements in design include a stent of higher resistance to external compression and a tissue valve made of equine pericardium. This new PHV, in which durability passed 200 million cycles in duplicator models, was first tested in animals before being successfully used in two additional patients. At the present time, PHV implantation can only be used in "compassionate cases", i.e. end-stage patients with contraindication to surgery. In the near future, a randomized multicenter trial would help in determining the potential role of this promising technique which might become a revolutionary lifesaving alternative in the high-risk patient.

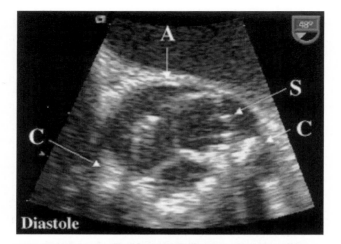

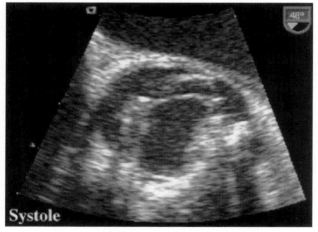

Figure 27-8: TEE in the short axis view showing the PHV function in systole and diastole, 10 weeks after implantation (A: aortic annulus, C: calcification on the native valve, S: stent frame of the PHV. The valve area was 1.6 cm² by planimetry).

REFERENCES

1. Schwarz F, Baumann P, Manthey J *et al*. The effect of aortic valve replacement on survival. *Circulation* 1982; **66**: 1105–10.
2. Bessell JR, Gower G, Craddock DR, Stubberfield J, Maddern GJ. Thirty years experience with heart valve surgery:

isolated aortic valve replacement. *Aust NZ J Surg* 1996; **66**: 799–805.

3. Vejlsted H, Skagen K, Hansen PF, Halkier E. Immediate and long-term results in aortic valve replacement. *Scand J Thorac Cardiovasc Surg* 1984; **18**: 41–4.

4. Korfer R, Schutt U, Minami K, Hartmann D, Kortke H, Luth JU. Left ventricular function in heart valve surgery: a multi-disciplinary challenge. *J Heart Valve Dis* 1995; **4** (Suppl 2): S194–7.

5. Mortasawi A, Gehle S, Schroder T *et al*. Aortic valve replacement in 80- and over 80-year-old patients. Short-term and long-term results. *Z Gerontol Geriatr* 2000 **33**: 438–46.

6. Mullany CJ. Aortic valve surgery in the elderly. *Cardiol Rev* 2000; **8**: 333–9.

7. Connolly HM, Oh JK, Schaff HV *et al*. Severe aortic stenosis with low transvalvular gradient and severe left ventricular dysfunction: result of aortic valve replacement in 52 patients. *Circulation* 2000; **101**: 1940–6.

8. Brogan WC 3rd, Grayburn PA, Lange RA, Hillis LD. Prognosis after valve replacement in patients with severe aortic stenosis and a low transvalvular pressure gradient. *J Am Coll Cardiol* 1993; **21**: 1657–60.

9. Powell DE, Tunick PA, Rosenzweig BP *et al*. Aortic valve replacement in patients with aortic stenosis and severe left ventricular dysfunction. *Arch Intern Med* 2000; **160** (9): 1337–41.

10. Pereira JJ, Lauer MS, Bashir M *et al*. Survival after aortic valve replacement for severe aortic stenosis with low transvalvular gradients and severe left ventricular dysfunction. *J Am Coll Cardiol* 2002; **39**: 1356–63.

11. Cribier A, Savin T, Saoudi N *et al*. Percutaneous transluminal valvuloplasty of acquired aortic stenosis in elderly patients: an alternative to valve replacement? *Lancet* 1986; **1**: 63–7.

12. McKay RG, Safian RD, Lock JE *et al*. Balloon dilatation of calcific aortic stenosis in elderly patients: post-mortem, intra-operative, and percutaneous valvuloplasty studies. *Circulation* 1986; **74**: 119–25.

13. Letac B, Cribier A, Koning R *et al*. Results of percutaneous transluminal valvuloplasty in 218 adults with valvular aortic stenosis. *Am J Cardiol* 1988; **6**: 598–605.

14. O'Neill WW, Mansfield Scientific Aortic Valvuloplasty Registry Investigators: Predictors of long-term survival after percutaneous aortic valvuloplasty: report of the Mansfield Scientific Aortic Valvuloplasty Registry. *J Am Coll Cardiol* 1991; **17**: 909–13.

15. Eltchaninoff H, Cribier A, Tron C *et al*. Balloon aortic valvuloplasty in elderly patients at high risk for surgery, or inoperable: immediate and mid-term results. *Eur Heart J* 1995; **16**: 1079–84.

16. Andersen HR, Knudsen LL, Hasemkam JM. Transluminal implantation of artificial heart valves. Description of a new expandable aortic valve and initial results with implantation by catheter technique in closed chest pigs. *Eur Heart J* 1992; **13**: 704–8.

17. Bonhoeffer P, Boudjemline Y, Saliba Z *et al*. Transcatheter implantation of a bovine valve in pulmonary position. *Circulation* 2000; **102**: 813–16.

18. Boudjemline Y, Bonhoeffer P. Steps toward percutaneous aortic valve replacement. *Circulation* 2002; **105**: 775–8.

19. Bonhoeffer P, Boudjemline Y, Saliba Z *et al*. Percutaneous replacement of pulmonary valve in a right-ventricle to pulmonary-artery prosthetic conduit with valve dysfunction. *Lancet* 2000; **356**: 1403–5.

20. Bonhoeffer P, Boudjemline Y, Qureshi SA *et al*. Percutaneous insertion of the pulmonary valve. *J Am Coll Cardiol* 2002; **39** (10): 1664–9.

21. Cribier A, Eltchaninoff H, Borenstein N *et al*. Transcatheter implantation of balloon-expandable prosthetic heart valves: early results in animal models. *Circulation* 2001; **104** (suppl II): II-552.

22. Cribier A, Eltchaninoff H, Bash A *et al*. Percutaneous transcatheter implantation of an aortic valve prosthesis for calcific aortic stenosis: first human case description. *Circulation* 2002; **106**: 3006–8.

Chapter 28

Interventions in Intracranial Arteries

Jay U Howington, Elad I Levy, Lee R Guterman, L Nelson Hopkins

INTRODUCTION

Intracranial atherosclerotic disease accounts for transient ischemic attacks (TIAs) and strokes in approximately 5% of the patients who present with these symptoms.[1] The disease most commonly affects the brain through thromboembolism, although the reduction in luminal diameter that results can also lead to flow-related ischemia. Patients with symptomatic intracranial atherosclerosis are at an increased risk for subsequent neurologic events, and anticoagulation therapy offers only a modest risk reduction.[2,3] The increasing experience with different endovascular therapies has shown that angioplasty, with or without the assistance of a stent, can be performed safely and decreases the risk of future strokes. The purpose of this chapter is to review the experience to date, define the appropriate population for treatment, describe the

*Basic; **Advanced; ***Rare, exotic, or investigational.

From: Nguyen T, Hu D, Saito S, Grines C, Palacios I (eds), *Practical Handbook of Advanced Interventional Cardiology*, 2nd edn. © 2003 Futura, an imprint of Blackwell Publishing.

techniques used in stent-assisted angioplasty (SAA) for intracranial atherosclerotic disease (IAD), as well as review the periprocedural management of these patients.

Grüntzig *et al.*[4] reported the first use of percutaneous transluminal angioplasty with a balloon (POBA) for the treatment of coronary artery stenosis in 1979. This new technique quickly gained favor throughout the medical community; and the following year, Sundt *et al.*[5] reported the first POBA for intracranial cerebrovascular occlusive disease. In that report, these authors described the successful treatment of basilar artery atherosclerotic stenosis using "transluminal balloon-catheter dilation." Since that report, Courtheoux *et al.*,[6] Theron *et al.*,[7] Higashida *et al.*,[8–10] Ahuja *et al.*,[11] Purdy *et al.*,[12] and others[13–23] have reported patient series in which these techniques have been used successfully to treat lesions in both the anterior and posterior circulations.

The use of intravascular stents for the treatment of atherosclerotic disease followed POBA by almost a decade, but efforts to design such a device had begun in the 1960s. Intravascular stenting was first proposed by Dotter and Judkins in 1964[24] and performed experimentally in canine popliteal arteries by Dotter in 1969.[25] Dotter was able to demonstrate that the lumen of a vessel in which a coilspring tube graft had been placed could remain patent. In 1983, he and his colleagues[26] reported the use of a stent in a dog, but this time the stent was made of Nitinol (a nickel-titanium alloy). Animal testing was continued; and in 1987, Rousseau *et al.*[27] reported the placement of the first human coronary stent. As with POBA, the use of this new technique broadened to include vessels throughout the body. In 1997, Higashida *et al.*[28] reported the first use of a stent in the intracranial circulation but did so as an adjunct to coil embolization of a fusiform aneurysm of the basilar artery.[28] Although Dorros *et al.*[29] and others[30,31] reported the use of a stent for the treatment of "intracranial" atherosclerotic disease, none of the lesions were present within the subarachnoid circulation. This distinction is important as the histology of the carotid artery before it enters the subarachnoid space differs significantly from that of the vessels within the subarachnoid space.[32] The protective environment of the intracranial cavity combined with the buffering action of the cerebrospinal fluid obviates the need for an external elastic lamina (EEL) or extensive adventitial layer. As a result, the walls of the subarachnoid vessels are thinner and more delicate than the extracranial ones. These vessels can also be extremely difficult to access owing to the tortuosity often present in the cavernous section of the carotid artery. The combination of access difficulty and lack of EEL increases the risk of dissection or rupture. Two years after Higashida and the UCSF group reported stent-assisted aneurysm coiling,[28] they described the first successful percutaneous endovascular deployment of a coronary stent for the treatment of an acute atherothrombotic occlusion of the basilar artery.[33] Since that report, several case reports and retrospective series dealing with SAA for IAD have been published.[33–45]

Technologic advances have focused on two areas: improvement in the devices used to access the intracranial circulation and coating of stents with drugs that improve their safety and effectiveness. Improvements in the design of wires, catheters, and stents have helped reduce the morbidity and mortality associated with the procedure. Levy et al. [28] recently published the results of a canine model in which they prospectively analyzed the effects of heparin-coated stents versus noncoated stents placed in the basilar artery. Other types of coating stents are being tried with promising results.

PERCUTANEOUS INTERVENTIONS OF INTRACRANIAL VESSELS

The standard for success in POBA has been defined in the coronary circulation as a 20% relative improvement in luminal diameter, with less than 30% residual stenosis.[46] The vessels of the intracranial circulation are smaller and, on the basis of Poiseuille's law, are more affected by smaller changes in luminal diameter than the coronary arteries. Therefore, the question is whether the same standards for successful coronary POBA can be applied to the intracranial lesions. Until further studies are done, the standard set for coronary POBA will have to be extrapolated to the intracranial circulation.

In their retrospective review of angiographic studies of intracranial atherosclerotic lesions, Mori et al.[14,16] found that certain lesion morphologic characteristics are predictive of both procedural morbidity and later restenosis. They divided lesions into three separate groups on the basis of length and location of the lesion, degree of stenosis and eccentricity, and level of calcification present. They are listed in Table 28-1.

After POBA, the patients with type C lesions, however, had a cumulative occurrence of ipsilateral stroke, ipsilateral bypass surgery, and repeat POBA of 100% at 1 year. Mori et al. suggested that POBA only benefits type A lesions and should not be attempted for type C lesions because of the low success rate and increased rate of restenosis. The benefit for POBA in type B lesions was limited to those lesions associated with crescendo TIAs and located in the posterior circulation (Table 28-2).

The histology of stenotic lesions has also been correlated with the rate of symptom development. Stary et al.[47] described the histologic features of unstable plaques (Grades IV–VI on a I–VI scale) in the coronary circulation; and those lesions with surface disruptions, hematoma, or thrombosis were associated with a greater risk of ischemic events. The type IV lesion, also known as an atheroma, has a dense accumulation

Table 28-1
Classification of lesions in the intracranial circulation[14]

Type A

- Discrete, <5 mm
- Little or no calcification
- Concentric
- Less than totally occlusive
- Eccentric (>70%, <90% diameter stenosis)
- No major branch involvement
- Absence of thrombus
- Readily accessible
- No angulated segment <45°
- Smooth contour

Type B

- Tubular, 5–10 mm
- Moderate or heavy calcification
- Eccentric (>90% diameter stenosis)
- Total occlusion <3 months
- Moderate tortuosity of proximal segment
- No major branch involvement
- Some thrombi present
- Moderate angulated segment >45° and <90°
- Irregular contour
- Bifurcation lesions requiring double wire technique

Type C

- Diffuse >10 mm
- Total occlusion > 3 months
- Excessive tortuosity of proximal segment
- Extreme angulated segment >90°

Table 28-2
Success and restenosis according to lesion type

	Type A	*Type B*	*Type C*
Degree of success	92%	86%	33%
1 year restenosis	0%	33%	56%

of extracellular lipid within the intima known as "the lipid core," whereas the type V lesion, or fibroatheroma, is one in which prominent new fibrous connective tissue has formed in association with the lipid core. These latter lesions tend to be thicker than the type IV lesions because of the fibrocellular response intermixed with calcium and lipid content. Both types IV and V lesions are considered dangerous because they are prone to fissures in the intimal surface. When this occurs, the lesions are then labeled as type VI lesions, or complicated plaques; and the majority of lesions in symptomatic patients fall within this category. Such disruptions in the intima expose the underlying proteoglycans, macrophage foam cells, and smooth muscle cells to circulating blood and that exposure initiates the coagulation cascade, resulting in thrombus formation. If we assume that similar lesion progression occurs in the intracranial circulation, one can begin to see a correlation between the classification described by Mori et al.[14,16] and the more advanced atherosclerotic lesions described by Stary et al.[47]

As previously mentioned, Mori et al.[14,16] demonstrated great success with intracranial POBA in type A lesions and lower success rate with longer and more complex lesions. Levy et al.[38] suggest that aggressive POBA in these advanced lesions causes immediate disruption of the intima, which increases the risk of progression to type VI lesions. Once such a progression occurs, the risk of an ischemic event secondary to thrombosis, embolic shower, or dissection increases dramatically. POBA technique has been shown to have an effect on intimal damage. Connors and Wojak[13] reported their experience over a 9-year period in which they performed POBA for intracranial atherosclerotic lesions and found that a slow, submaximal inflation of the balloon resulted in a decrease in intimal damage, acute thrombotic formation and abrupt occlusion of the vessel when compared with a technique in which the balloon was rapidly inflated. Using the latter approach, they reported a dissection rate of 50%; whereas the slow and submaximal technique was associated with a 14% rate of dissection and a good clinical outcome in 49 (98%) of 50 patients. Although more than 50% residual stenosis was seen in 8 (16%) patients treated with the gradual inflation technique, this method proved to achieve the clinical goal of revascularization safely.

In addition to the immediate intimal damage caused by the procedure, balloon POBA instigates smooth muscle proliferation and intimal healing, both of which remain active for up to 30 days following the procedure.[48–50] Wainwright et al.[50] described a three-phase remodeling process that begins with the release of biologically active mediators by platelets, thrombin, and leukocytes, followed by the proliferation and migration of smooth muscle cells to the subintimal region, and concludes with a chronic phase of remodeling by the production of an extracellular matrix. During the 30 days in which this remodeling process occurs, the lesion is fragile; and crossing it with a wire or other device could easily lead to an ischemic event. Because of the morphologic and histologic characteristics of IAD, the treatment of these lesions by POBA alone has often been accompanied by severe complications or death. In comparison to vascular territories in other parts of the body, the arteries within the subarachnoid space are more delicate, thin-walled, and prone to injury and, as such, present a technical challenge for the operator.

Higashida et al.[10] in a series of posterior cerebral circulation interventions reported the results of POBA in five distal vertebral and three basilar arteries. Three (38%) of the eight patients suffered strokes (two ischemic and one hemorrhagic) at the time of the procedure, and one (13%) other patient suffered a TIA. No occurrence of restenosis was reported, although it is not clear whether these patients underwent follow-up angiographic, ultrasound, or magnetic resonance angiographic evaluation. Clark et al.[23] reported their experience with intracranial POBA in a retrospective review of 17 patients with 22 total vessels treated. During the procedure, strokes occurred in two patients (30-day morbidity rate, 12%); and vessel dissections occurred in 3 (14%) of 22 vessels. The acute post-POBA residual stenosis was 51±10%. Among the 10 patients who underwent follow-up angiography (at approximately 6 months), five demonstrated progression of the post-POBA stenosis. Marks et al.[15] reported their long-term experience with intracranial POBA for symptomatic IAD in 23 patients with a mean follow-up of 35.4 months. One patient suffered a middle cerebral artery rupture at the time of POBA and died (mortality rate, 4%), and one other patient suffered a stroke months later referable to the vascular territory supplied by the treated artery (stroke rate, 5%). One other patient in the series suffered an acute occlusion 1 hour after the procedure, and the thrombus was successfully lysed without sequelae. In this series, the follow-up focused on the clinical examination, without routine performance of an angiogram. In other studies, all of which are single-center and retrospective, the composite rate of stroke and death during POBA varies from 4% to 40%.[17,22,51,52]

The initial results of POBA alone for CAD were also suboptimal owing to procedural complications and high restenosis. Stents were soon evaluated and shown to be superior to POBA alone. In every vascular bed in which they have been tried, stents have improved acute and long-term patency as well as decreased the risks of acute occlusion.[53-59] The prospective Stent Restenosis Study demonstrated a significantly larger postprocedural lumen diameter that was maintained at 6 months in those vessels treated with SAA, compared with those treated with POBA alone.[53] A restenosis rate of 50% or more occurred in 55% of the POBA group, compared with only an average of 34% in the SAA group. The 1-year event-free survival rate also differed in the two groups. In those patients receiving stents, 78% were symptom-free at 1 year, whereas 67% of those receiving POBA alone experienced no symptoms. However, this study focused on lesions in vessels that were at least 3 mm in diameter, which is larger than most intracranial vessels. The Stenting in Small Coronary Arteries trial, reported by Moer *et al.*, randomized 145 patients to receive either POBA alone or coupled with the placement of a heparin-coated stent.[54] All patients underwent follow-up angiography at 6 months. Event-free survival was significantly higher in the stent group, and both the minimal luminal diameter and restenosis rate were significantly improved in the stent group. Although the histologic composition of intracranial vessels differs from that of coronary arteries, the results of these studies suggest that SAA for IAD lesions might be superior to POBA alone.

INTRACRANIAL STENTING

The available literature on the safety and efficacy of intracranial SAA is relatively sparse and limited to either case reports or small case series.[33–45] The UCSF group[33] was the first to report a case of SAA in basilar artery atherothrombotic occlusion. The patient made a very good neurologic recovery but unfortunately died as a result of non-neurologic causes, and the postmortem examination revealed no evidence of perforator vessel occlusion. Gomez *et al.*[41] reported the first series of patients with symptomatic basilar artery stenosis treated with elective SAA. Twelve patients with symptoms of vertebrobasilar ischemia received successful stent placement, with a decrease of stenosis from 71.4% to 10.3%. Clinical follow-up reported only one TIA. Mori *et al.*[40] assessed the effectiveness and safety of SAA for vertebrobasilar and distal internal carotid atherosclerotic lesions in eight patients. The pretreatment stenosis was acutely reduced from $80\pm17\%$ to $7\pm7\%$ and to $19\pm9\%$ at 3 months follow-up. No morbidity or mortality was encountered. Lylyk *et al.*[34] reported their results with endovascular reconstruction of intracranial arteries using stents in 123 patients for a variety of reasons. SAA was performed in 36 patients. Twenty-seven (75%) of these patients had lesions that were classified as either type B or C lesions and a reduction of stenosis to less than 50% without neurologic sequelae was achieved in 32 (89%) of the patients. Levy *et al.*[38] reported their experience with staged SAA for symptomatic intracranial vertebrobasilar artery stenosis in eight patients. These patients underwent POBA to approximately 50 to 75% of the parent vessel lumen, which was followed by SAA approximately 1 month later. This interval was chosen to allow any intimal damage resulting from the initial POBA to heal prior to stent placement. The mean pretreatment stenosis was 77%, and this was reduced to 54% after POBA and to 30% after stent placement. There was no permanent neurologic morbidity. The above studies demonstrate that SAA decreases the risk of arterial injury, dissection, and thrombosis and can be performed safely in most individuals. Tortuous anatomy continues to be a major problem of intracranial stenting, and future innovations are needed to enhance the trackability of the stents.

Patient selection: The ideal candidates for intracranial SAA are the patients with hemodynamic-based cerebrovascular ischemia that are refractory to conventional antiplatelet and standard anticoagulant therapy (Table 28-3).

However, clinical findings and radiographic evidence of stenosis alone are insufficient to determine whether a patient with such a lesion is at increased risk for future neurologic events. Derdeyn et al.[21,60] reported that angiographic assessment alone could not assist in the treatment decision-making process. Until recently, however, cerebral angiography was the only readily accessible method of evaluating cerebral perfusion. The International Cooperative Study of Extracranial-to-Intracranial Arterial Anastomosis (EC-IC bypass study) showed no benefit for EC-IC bypass in patients with intracranial stenosis.[61] The major disagreement concerned selection bias: many patients were excluded from the study if the treating physician felt that they would greatly benefit from a bypass procedure.[62] At the time of the EC-IC bypass study, no objective method of measuring cerebral hypoperfusion was widely available. Therefore, patients with intracranial stenotic lesions and adequate cerebrovascular reserve were subjected to the sizable risk of an EC-IC bypass. An adequate reserve would decrease the risk of a hemodynamically-based stroke as the cerebral vasculature has compensated for the lesion by way of an intact and extensive collateral system from the contralateral hemisphere. Such patients randomized in the study would have skewed the results away from showing the benefit of an EC-IC bypass.

Currently several imaging modalities are available that can qualify or quantitate cerebral perfusion. These techniques are proving to be worthwhile, if not essential, adjuncts to cerebral angiography for the evaluation of patients with symptomatic intracranial stenosis. Further investigation with provocative testing will often provide the necessary confirmation of inadequate vascular reserve. Patients with symptomatic intracranial stenosis will usually have a subnormal vasodilatory response to the administration of acetazolamide on perfusion imaging (single photon emission

---

Table 28-3
Intracranial vessels suitable for stent-assisted angioplasty

1. Distal internal carotid artery
2. Distal vertebral artery, portion of the distal vertebral artery that extends into the basilar artery
3. Basilar artery

computed tomography (SPECT), CT perfusion imaging, or positron emission tomography (PET)). Such a lack of cerebral perfusion reserve has been correlated with treatment success in both surgical and endovascular series,[12,14,22,63-68] but at present, perfusion imaging is not required as a part of the periprocedural evaluation. Investigators at Washington University[68-70] have divided the compensatory responses made by the brain to progressive reductions in cerebral perfusion pressure into different stages as shown in Table 28-4.

With this classification of cerebral perfusion reserve, Grubb et al.[68] found that stage II hemodynamic failure conferred an age-adjusted relative risk of 7.3 for ipsilateral stroke in patients with internal carotid occlusion. In a prospective study of patients with carotid artery occlusions, 11 (28%) strokes occurred in 39 patients who demonstrated increased ipsilateral OEF to an occluded artery whereas only 2 (5%) strokes occurred in the 42 patients who demonstrated a normal OEF response. Although this study did not involve high-grade stenotic lesions, the correlation between occluded lesions and hemodynamically significant stenotic lesions is one that seems logical. Nemoto et al. added a further division to the brain's response to a lack of perfusion in which both cerebral blood volume and OEF decline.[71] They postulate that in stage III hemodynamic failure the area of the brain involved has suffered one or more ischemic events and as such has a lower overall metabolic rate and OEF. Stage III as a predictor of future ischemic events has yet to be evaluated in a clinical setting, but one can easily imagine that patients with this level of cerebral hemodynamic failure would be at significant risk for a stroke. A therapeutic option that carried with it less risk than the natural history of those lesions associated with a maximal compensatory response would stand to greatly

Table 28-4
Stages of cerebral perfusion reserve

- **Stage 0:** When the cerebral perfusion pressure is normal, the cerebral blood flow is closely matched to the resting metabolic rate of neuronal tissue, and the oxygen extraction fraction (OEF) varies little throughout the brain.
- **Stage I:** As the cerebral perfusion pressure begins to drop, the cerebrovascular autoregulation is activated and the brain arterioles become dilated to maintain perfusion. Little regional variation in OEF exists.
- **Stage II:** As the cerebral perfusion pressure continues to drop further as in cerebral hemodynamic failure, the arterioles are maximally dilated, and the OEF rises in an effort to maintain cerebral oxygen metabolism and neuronal function.

benefit this subgroup of patients. Those patients with IAD who are asymptomatic and have a normal vasodilatory response to acetazolamide will likely not benefit from a stent-assisted revascularization procedure.

Crucial to the evaluation of IAD is a thorough understanding of the symptoms referable to such lesions. Unlike embolic disease, which often affects different vascular territories, hemodynamic disease tends to target the same area of the brain with each repeating event. The anterior circulation lesions tend to have symptoms that involve the contralateral limbs or face in a consistent manner. These symptoms may take the form of transient weakness, numbness, tremors, and may or may not include dysphasia. While the anterior circulation lesions tend to produce lateralized findings, the posterior circulation lesions cause bilateral symptoms (Table 28-5).

Because SAA as a therapeutic option in the management of intracranial stenosis has yet to be proven by a large, prospective study and because it carries with it a significant risk, patients being considered for this procedure are usually those for whom medical therapy has failed to remedy their condition. The definition of failure in this setting is the occurrence of at least one neurologic deficit attributable to the stenotic lesion while the patient is receiving medical therapy. The standard for medical therapy is anticoagulation with warfarin to maintain the prothrombin time at 1.2 to 1.6 times the control value. The Warfarin-Aspirin Symptomatic Intracranial Disease (WASID) study demonstrated a reduction in the stroke risk for

---

Table 28-5
Signs and symptoms by major arterial territories

---

1. **The middle cerebral artery** lesions tend to affect the face and upper extremity
2. **The anterior cerebral artery** preferentially involves the lower extremity
3. **The internal carotid artery** lesions usually cause symptoms similar to middle cerebral artery lesions because of the protection afforded by the anterior communicating artery to the ipsilateral anterior cerebral artery
4. **The vertebral and basilar arteries:**
   a. Bilateral long tract signs (motor and sensory)
   b. Cross motor and sensory signs (facial weakness or numbness with contralateral extremities weakness and numbness)
   c. Cerebellar signs
   d. Cranial nerves signs (diplopia, dysarthria, facial numbness)
   e. Alterations of state of consciousness
   f. Disconjugate eye movement

those patients who received warfarin instead of aspirin.[2,3] In that study, patients receiving aspirin therapy had a stroke rate of 10.4 per 100 patient years, whereas those who received warfarin were found to have a stroke rate of 3.6 per 100 patient years. The patients in the warfarin group also had a higher rate of bleeding complications than did the aspirin group, but this increase did not counteract the decrease in stroke rate. Ironically, warfarin therapy was highly effective in reducing the rate of stroke in vascular territory beyond but not within that of the stenotic vessel. As our understanding of intracranial stenosis and its effect on cerebral perfusion matures, we are beginning to see a discrepancy between those lesions that have stimulated adequate reserve and those that have not. Neurologic symptoms that are hemodynamic in origin and not ameliorated with an adequate cerebrovascular reserve may respond to standard anticoagulation therapy but are likely to recur. Patients with such symptoms may comprise one subgroup that should be considered for SAA before failure occurs. Until an adequate study has been performed to analyze first, the role of perfusion testing, and second, the benefit of revascularization for these patients, the need for such testing and the timing of an intervention remain at the discretion of the treating physician.

PERIPROCEDURAL MEDICAL MANAGEMENT

Anticoagulation therapy should be discontinued before patients undergo SAA, but antiplatelet therapy should be maintained before, during, and after treatment with aspirin and clopidogrel.[72,73] Clopidogrel inhibits 55% of platelet aggregation within 1 hour and 80% within 5 hours after a loading dose of 375 mg followed by 75 mg daily, in combination with aspirin 325 mg.[74] Alternatively, a 10-day preprocedural regimen of clopidogrel (75 mg) and aspirin (325 mg) will achieve the same level of platelet inhibition.[75] After SAA, patients are maintained on clopidogrel and aspirin for 1 month. Thereafter, the patient remains on aspirin (325 mg, daily) indefinitely. The two drugs are given together for 1 month to prevent platelet-induced thrombosis until an endothelial layer has formed over the stent.[76,77] In addition to antiplatelet agents, the pre-treatment medical regimen should also include a lowering-cholesterol drug. Callahan et al.[78,79] have demonstrated the stabilization, and even improvement, of intracranial stenosis on serial angiography with the use of statins. For this reason, a statin is prescribed before and after intracranial SAA.

Some evidence exists showing the benefit of glycoprotein 2b3a inhibitor use during intracranial stenting.[72,73] When abciximab is given as a 0.25 mg/kg intravenous bolus before the procedure, followed with a 12-hour infusion of 10 μg/min, abciximab has been shown to affect a likely reduction in stroke risk. However, this potential benefit must be weighed against the inability to immediately reverse the drug's effect on coagulation. Unlike heparin, which can be reversed rapidly with protamine, abciximab requires the transfusion of platelets to restore normal coagulation parameters. Qureshi *et al.*[72,73] report that chronically ischemic neural tissue may be at an increased risk of hemorrhage following the use of glycoprotein 2b3a inhibitors. Such a hemorrhage is likely to be fatal because of the poor reversibility of the drug. For this reason, the authors do not advocate the use of glycoprotein 2b3a inhibitors during SAA of IAD.

TECHNIQUES: STENT-ASSISTED INTRACRANIAL ANGIOPLASTY

Local anesthesia in conjunction with adequate sedation is preferred instead of general anesthesia. This method obviates the risks inherent to general anesthesia and also allows for scrutiny of the patient's neurologic condition. The femoral approach is also preferred because it enables greater flexibility in the selection of the size of the guide. The transradial approach, which is common for coronary interventions, is used as an alternative route for patients with contraindicated or complicated femoral access. The standard Seldinger technique[80] is used to place a 6F sheath in the right common femoral artery. After a diagnostic angiogram is performed and the dimensions of the cerebral vessels measured, IV heparin bolus (50–70 U/kg) is given to achieve an activated coagulation time (ACT) of 250 to 300 seconds.

Advancement and positioning of guide: After adequate heparinization has been achieved, a guide connected to a continuous flush is positioned in the vertebral or internal carotid artery. In the case of anterior circulation lesions, the guide is positioned over an exchange-length guidewire that has been positioned in the distal external carotid circulation. Once the guide is secure in the common carotid artery, the wire is redirected into the internal carotid artery, and the guide is then advanced over the wire. The guide is advanced to a secure position prior to the removal of the wire. For those lesions located in the posterior circulation, the selection of the appropriate vertebral artery depends on whether the lesion involves the vertebral artery or which vertebral artery is more accessible. A lesion that incorporates the distal right vertebral artery must be accessed through that artery.

TECHNICAL TIP

**Optimal view: After the guide is adequately positioned, a diagnostic angiogram is obtained to ensure that no vessel injury occurred during the exchange process. The optimal view is then chosen that incorporates both the lesion and the distal tip of the guide. The tip of the guide is included in the field of view because the guide may be pushed down when any interventional device (balloon, stent, etc.) is advanced.

Advancement and manipulation of wire: With the aid of digital road mapping, a 0.014" microwire is placed coaxially within an appropriately sized microcatheter and advanced across the lesion to a normal distal branch of the stenotic lesion. The microcatheter is then passed over the microwire and positioned in this distal branch. A 300-cm medium-weight balance coronary exchange wire (Guidant, Menlo Park, CA) is then inserted through the microcatheter and advanced to the tip of the microcatheter, after which the microcatheter is removed. The exchange wire supplies the support needed to deliver either an angioplasty balloon or a stent.

Balloon angioplasty: For the initial treatment of an intra-cranial stenosis, only POBA is performed. The shortest balloon that will completely span the lesion is chosen, because shorter balloons are easier to navigate through the tortuous intracranial circulation than longer ones. The diameter of the balloon is chosen such that the nominal inflation diameter is less than that of the non-diseased artery immediately adjacent to the stenosis, which is felt to represent the actual diameter of the diseased segment.

TECHNICAL TIP

**Gradual pressure inflation: Once in place, the balloon is inflated slowly until the nominal pressure is reached. The purpose of the slow inflation is to avoid intimal damage and plaque rupture often seen with rapid inflation. The balloon is deflated and removed. An angiogram is immediately performed. If the vessel has been dilated sufficiently without evidence of arterial injury, the guide and exchange wire are removed.

Management of balloon angioplasty related complications: If there is angiographic evidence of arterial complication (thrombus or dissection), additional measures are taken to ensure vessel patency and perfusion.

TECHNICAL TIP

**Medical and mechanical thrombectomy: If there is a thromboembolic event, a microcatheter is advanced over the exchange wire and thrombolytic therapy is begun. It is the authors' practice to begin by administering 2 U of reteplase over the course of 10 minutes. A repeat angiogram is obtained. If the thrombus persists, attempts with mechanical thrombectomy are made. Such means take the form of a snare (Microvena Co, White Bear Lake, MN), wire manipulation using a microwire, or angioplasty. If after these measures the thrombus persists, 2 more units of reteplase are given followed by a second attempt at mechanical thrombectomy if needed. The rationale for this strategy to thromboembolic events is to dissolve the thrombus by first creating a lytic state and then attempting mechanical thrombectomy. The authors have found that reteplase, when given in a total dose of no more than 4 U, results in fewer hemorrhagic complications.[81]

**Bail-out stenting for dissection: If an arterial dissection is seen during the post-POBA angiogram, stents are used to tackle the dissecting segment to the arterial wall. By leaving the exchange wire in place until the angiogram is performed, there is no question as to whether the stent is being deployed within the true lumen or within the dissection. The heparin is not reversed, and the sheath in the femoral artery is removed once the ACT is within the normal range. Alternatively, a closure device is applied to the access site for the patient's comfort and to increase postprocedural mobilization.

Elective stenting: When using the staged approach to SAA, an interval of 4 to 6 weeks is allowed to pass between the initial POBA and stent deployment. During this time, the patient continues to receive both clopidogrel (75 mg) and aspirin (325 mg) on a daily basis. The same steps used before POBA are again used for stent placement. The stent is chosen so that it will cover the lesion entirely as well as match the diameter of the vessel. The stents used are balloon-mounted coronary stents. As a general rule, the smaller and shorter the stent is, the easier it is to navigate through the tortuous intracranial vessel. With digital road mapping, the stent is advanced over the exchange-length microwire to the lesion. Once the stent is positioned adequately, it is deployed by inflation of the balloon to 6 to 8 atmospheres. After the stent is deployed, the balloon is removed. The wire is left in place until procedural success is confirmed by repeat angiography (Figure 28-1). As with the initial POBA, the guide is removed; and, if possible, a closure device is used at the access site.

**CAVEAT: Optimal guide position: It cannot be emphasized enough that the guide be advanced as high as safely possible to provide the much needed support while the stent is pushed through the intracranial vessels. Resistance to stent delivery can result in the backing down of the guide to the level of the aortic arch if the guide tip is not in the field of view. This loss of guide position inevitably means that the case must begin again. Such a delay is frustrating for the operator but, more importantly, it carries with it the increased risk of crossing and recrossing the lesion with wires and catheters.

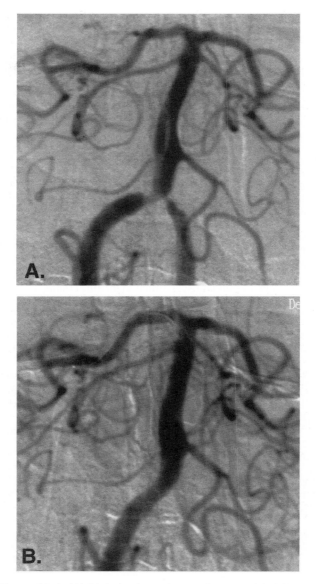

Figure 28-1: (A) Digital subtraction angiogram of a right vertebral artery injection demonstrates bilateral vertebrobasilar junction high-grade stenosis with reflux of contrast down the left vertebral artery. (B) Angiogram following stent placement in the distal right vertebral artery demonstrates excellent resolution of the stenotic segment. Reflux of contrast into the left vertebral artery is no longer seen.

FUTURE DIRECTIONS

Restenosis remains the major limitation of catheter-based intervention for IAD lesions. Neointimal hyperplasia is the main cause, and significant research has focused on devices or drugs that inhibit the endothelial response to SAA. Several trials and single-center studies have been conducted with stents that are coated with such chemicals.[82–85] The multicenter RAndomized double-blind study with the sirolimus (rapamycin) eluting Bx VELocity balloon-expandable stent (RAVEL) demonstrated that rapamycin-coated stents decrease minimal restenosis after PCI at 30 days and at the 6-month angiographic follow-up.[84–86] The results with these drug-coated stents in the coronary circulation suggest that similar products will prove useful in the cerebrovascular circulation.

The technique of SAA for symptomatic IAD has evolved over the past decade. Along with this evolution, advances have been made in the evaluation of cerebral hypoperfusion that have enabled treating physicians to better select patients for cerebral revascularization. As a result of these advances, endoluminal vascular reconstruction for intracranial stenosis is rapidly becoming a safe and efficacious treatment modality for IAD.

REFERENCES

1. Sacco RL, Kargman DE, Gu Q, Zamanillo MC. Race-ethnicity and determinants of intracranial atherosclerotic cerebral infarction. The Northern Manhattan Stroke Study. *Stroke* 1995; **26**: 14–20.

2. Chimowitz MI, Kokkinos J, Strong J *et al.* The Warfarin-Aspirin Symptomatic Intracranial Disease Study. *Neurology* 1995; **45**: 1488–93.

3. Prognosis of patients with symptomatic vertebral or basilar artery stenosis. The Warfarin-Aspirin Symptomatic Intracranial Disease (WASID) Study Group. *Stroke* 1998; **29**: 1389–92.

4. Gruntzig AR, Senning A, Siegenthaler WE. Nonoperative dilatation of coronary-artery stenosis: percutaneous transluminal coronary angioplasty. *N Engl J Med* 1979; **301**: 61–8.

5. Sundt TM, Jr, Smith HC, Campbell JK, Vlietstra RE, Cucchiara RF, Stanson AW. Transluminal angioplasty for basilar artery stenosis. *Mayo Clin Proc* 1980; **55**: 673–80.

6. Courtheoux P, Tournade A, Theron J *et al.* Transcutaneous angioplasty of vertebral artery atheromatous ostial stricture. *Neuroradiology* 1985; **27**: 259–64.

7. Theron J, Courtheoux P, Henriet JP, Pelouze G, Derlon JM, Maiza D. Angioplasty of supraaortic arteries. *J Neuroradiol* 1984; **11**: 187–200.

8. Higashida RT, Hieshima GB, Tsai FY, Bentson JR, Halbach VV. Percutaneous transluminal angioplasty of the subclavian and vertebral arteries. *Acta Radiol Suppl* 1986; **369**: 124–6.

9. Higashida RT, Hieshima GB, Tsai FY, Halbach VV, Norman D, Newton TH. Transluminal angioplasty of the vertebral and basilar artery. *Am J Neuroradiol* 1987; **8**: 745–9.

10. Higashida RT, Tsai FY, Halbach VV *et al*. Transluminal angioplasty for atherosclerotic disease of the vertebral and basilar arteries. *J Neurosurg* 1993; **78**: 192–8.

11. Ahuja A, Guterman LR, Hopkins LN. Angioplasty for basilar artery atherosclerosis. Case report. *J Neurosurg* 1992; **77**: 941–4.

12. Purdy PD, Devous MD, Sr., Unwin DH, Giller CA, Batjer HH. Angioplasty of an atherosclerotic middle cerebral artery associated with improvement in regional cerebral blood flow. *Am J Neuroradiol* 1990; **11**: 878–80.

13. Connors JJ 3rd, Wojak JC. Percutaneous transluminal angioplasty for intracranial atherosclerotic lesions: evolution of technique and short-term results. *J Neurosurg* 1999; **91**: 415–23.

14. Mori T, Fukuoka M, Kazita K, Mori K. Follow-up study after intracranial percutaneous transluminal cerebral balloon angioplasty. *Am J Neuroradiol* 1998; **19**: 1525–33.

15. Marks MP, Marcellus M, Norbash AM, Steinberg GK, Tong D, Albers GW. Outcome of angioplasty for atherosclerotic intracranial stenosis. *Stroke* 1999; **30**: 1065–9.

16. Mori T, Mori K, Fukuoka M, Arisawa M, Honda S. Percutaneous transluminal cerebral angioplasty: serial angiographic follow-up after successful dilatation. *Neuroradiology* 1997; **39**: 111–6.

17. Takis C, Kwan ES, Pessin MS, Jacobs DH, Caplan LR. Intracranial angioplasty: experience and complications. *Am J Neuroradiol* 1997; **18**: 1661–8.

18. Terada T, Higashida RT, Halbach VV *et al*. Transluminal angioplasty for arteriosclerotic disease of the distal vertebral and basilar arteries. *J Neurol Neurosurg Psychiatry* 1996; **60**: 377–81.

19. Yokote H, Terada T, Ryujin K *et al*. Percutaneous transluminal angioplasty for intracranial arteriosclerotic lesions. *Neuroradiology* 1998; **40**: 590–6.

20. Callahan AS, 3rd, Berger BL. Balloon angioplasty of intracranial arteries for stroke prevention. *J Neuroimaging* 1997; **7**: 232–5.

21. Derdeyn CP, Cross DT 3rd, Moran CJ, Dacey RG, Jr. Reversal of focal misery perfusion after intracranial angioplasty: case report. *Neurosurgery* 2001; **48**: 436–40.

22. Touho H. Percutaneous transluminal angioplasty in the treatment of atherosclerotic disease of the anterior cerebral circulation and hemodynamic evaluation. *J Neurosurg* 1995; **82**: 953–60.

23. Clark WM, Barnwell SL, Nesbit G, O'Neill OR, Wynn ML, Coull BM. Safety and efficacy of percutaneous transluminal angioplasty for intracranial atherosclerotic stenosis. *Stroke* 1995; **26**: 1200–4.

24. Dotter CT, Judkins MP. Transluminal treatment of arteriosclerotic obstruction. Description of a new technic and a preliminary report of its application. *Circulation* 1964; **30**: 654–70.

25. Dotter C. Transluminally-placed coilspring endarterial tube grafts. Long-term patency in canine popliteal artery. *Invest Radiol* 1969; **4**: 329–32.

26. Dotter CT, Buschmann RW, McKinney MK, Rosch J. Transluminal expandable Nitinol coil stent grafting: preliminary report. *Radiology* 1983; **147**: 259–60.

27. Rousseau H, Puel J, Joffre F *et al*. Self-expanding endovascular prosthesis: an experimental study. *Radiology* 1987; **164**: 709–14.

28. Higashida RT, Smith W, Gress D *et al*. Intravascular stent and endovascular coil placement for a ruptured fusiform aneurysm of the basilar artery. Case report and review of the literature. *J Neurosurg* 1997; **87**: 944–9.

29. Dorros G, Cohn JM, Palmer LE. Stent deployment resolves a petrous carotid artery angioplasty dissection. *Am J Neuroradiol* 1998; **19**: 392–4.

30. Emery DJ, Ferguson RD, Williams JS. Pulsatile tinnitus cured by angioplasty and stenting of petrous carotid artery stenosis. *Arch Otolaryngol Head Neck Surg* 1998; **124**: 460–1.

31. Feldman RL, Trigg L, Gaudier J, Galat J. Use of coronary Palmaz-Schatz stent in the percutaneous treatment of an intracranial carotid artery stenosis. *Cathet Cardiovasc Diagn* 1996; **38**: 316–9.

32. Lang J, Kageyama I. Clinical anatomy of the blood spaces and blood vessels surrounding the siphon of the internal carotid artery. *Acta Anat (Basel)* 1990; **139**: 320–5.

33. Phatouros CC, Higashida RT, Malek AM *et al*. Endovascular stenting of an acutely thrombosed basilar artery: technical case report and review of the literature. *Neurosurgery* 1999; **44**: 667–73.

34. Lylyk P, Cohen JE, Ceratto R, Ferrario A, Miranda C. Endovascular reconstruction of intracranial arteries by stent placement and combined techniques. *J Neurosurg* 2002; **97**: 1306–13.

35. Rasmussen PA, Perl J, 2nd, Barr JD *et al*. Stent-assisted angioplasty of intracranial vertebrobasilar atherosclerosis: an initial experience. *J Neurosurg* 2000; **92**: 771–8.

36. Levy EI, Boulos AS, Guterman LR. Stent-assisted endoluminal revascularization for the treatment of intracranial atherosclerotic disease. *Neurol Res* 2002; **24**: 337–46.

37. Levy EI, Horowitz MB, Koebbe CJ *et al*. Transluminal stent-assisted angioplasty of the intracranial vertebrobasilar system for medically refractory, posterior circulation ischemia: early results. *Neurosurgery* 2001; **48**: 1215–21; discussion 1221–3.

38. Levy EI, Hanel RA, Bendok BR *et al*. Staged stent-assisted angioplasty for symptomatic intracranial vertebrobasilar artery stenosis. *J Neurosurg* 2002; **97**: 1294–301.

39. Mori T, Kazita K, Mori K. Cerebral angioplasty and stenting for intracranial vertebral atherosclerotic stenosis. *Am J Neuroradiol* 1999; **20**: 787–9.

40. Mori T, Kazita K, Chokyu K, Mima T, Mori K. Short-term arteriographic and clinical outcome after cerebral angioplasty and stenting for intracranial vertebrobasilar and carotid atherosclerotic occlusive disease. *Am J Neuroradiol* 2000; **21**: 249–254.

41. Gomez CR, Misra VK, Liu MW *et al*. Elective stenting of symptomatic basilar artery stenosis. *Stroke* 2000; **31**: 95–99.

42. Nakahara T, Sakamoto S, Hamasaki O, Sakoda K. Stent-assisted angioplasty for intracranial atherosclerosis. *Neuroradiology* 2002; **44**: 706–10.

43. Ramee SR, Dawson R, McKinley KL *et al*. Provisional stenting for symptomatic intracranial stenosis using a multidisciplinary approach: acute results, unexpected benefit, and one-year outcome. *Cathet Cardiovasc Interv* 2001; **52**: 457–67.

44. Gomez CR, Misra VK, Campbell MS, Soto RD. Elective stenting of symptomatic middle cerebral artery stenosis. *Am J Neuroradiol* 2000; **21**: 971–3.

45. Morris PP, Martin EM, Regan J, Braden G. Intracranial deployment of coronary stents for symptomatic atherosclerotic disease. *Am J Neuroradiol* 1999; **20**: 1688–94.

46. Ryan TJ, Bauman WB, Kennedy JW *et al*. Guidelines for percutaneous transluminal coronary angioplasty. A report of the American Heart Association/American College of Cardiology Task Force on Assessment of Diagnostic and Therapeutic Cardiovascular Procedures (Committee on Percutaneous Transluminal Coronary Angioplasty). *Circulation* 1993; **88**: 2987–3007.

47. Stary HC, Chandler AB, Dinsmore RE *et al*. A definition of advanced types of atherosclerotic lesions and a histological

classification of atherosclerosis. A report from the Committee on Vascular Lesions of the Council on Arteriosclerosis, American Heart Association. *Circulation* 1995; **92**: 1355–74.

48. Tanaka H, Sukhova GK, Swanson SJ *et al.* Sustained activation of vascular cells and leukocytes in the rabbit aorta after balloon injury. *Circulation* 1993; **88**: 1788–803.

49. Anderson PG, Boerth NJ, Liu M, McNamara DB, Cornwell TL, Lincoln TM. Cyclic GMP-dependent protein kinase _expression in coronary arterial smooth muscle in response to balloon catheter injury. *Arterioscler Thromb Vasc Biol* 2000; **20**: 2192–7.

50. Wainwright CL, Miller AM, Wadsworth RM. Inflammation as a key event in the development of neointima following vascular balloon injury. *Clin Exp Pharmacol Physiol* 2001; **28**: 891–5.

51. Alazzaz A, Thornton J, Aletich VA, Debrun GM, Ausman JI, Charbel F. Intracranial percutaneous transluminal angioplasty for arteriosclerotic stenosis. *Arch Neurol* 2000; **57**: 1625–30.

52. Nahser HC, Henkes H, Weber W, Berg-Dammer E, Yousry TA, Kuhne D. Intracranial vertebrobasilar stenosis: angioplasty and follow-up. *Am J Neuroradiol* 2000; **21**: 1293–301.

53. George CJ, Baim DS, Brinker JA, Fischman DL, Goldberg S, Holubkov R, Kennard ED, Veltri L, Detre KM. One-year follow-up of the Stent Restenosis (STRESS I) Study. *Am J Cardiol* 1998; **81**: 860–5.

54. Moer R, Myreng Y, Molstad P, Albertsson P, Gunnes P, Lindvall B, Wiseth R, Ytre-Arne K, Kjekshus J, Golf S. Stenting in small coronary arteries (SISCA) trial. A randomized comparison between balloon angioplasty and the heparin-coated beStent. *J Am Coll Cardiol* 2001; **38**: 1598–603.

55. Morice M, Serruys P, Sousa J, Fajadet J, Perin M, Ban Hayashi E, Colombo A, Schuler G, Barragain P, Bode C. The Ravel Trial. In: Transcatheter Therapeutics (**www.tctmd.com/expert-presentations**); 2001.

56. Huang P, Levin T, Kabour A, Feldman T. Acute and late outcome after use of 2.5-mm intracoronary stents in small (<2.5 mm) coronary arteries. *Cathet Cardiovasc Interv* 2000; **49**: 121–6.

57. Roubin GS, Yadav S, Iyer SS, Vitek J. Carotid stent-supported angioplasty: a neurovascular intervention to prevent stroke. *Am J Cardiol* 1996; **78**: 8–12.

58. Yadav JS, Roubin GS, King P, Iyer S, Vitek J. Angioplasty and stenting for restenosis after carotid endarterectomy. Initial experience. *Stroke* 1996; **27**: 2075–9.

59. Yadav JS, Roubin GS, Iyer S *et al.* Elective stenting of the extracranial carotid arteries. *Circulation* 1997; **95**: 376–81.

60. Derdeyn CP, Grubb RL, Jr, Powers WJ. Cerebral hemodynamic impairment: methods of measurement and association with stroke risk. *Neurology* 1999; **53**: 251–9.

61. The International Cooperative Study of Extracranial/Intracranial Arterial Anastomosis (EC/IC Bypass Study): methodology and entry characteristics. The EC/IC Bypass Study group. *Stroke* 1985; **16**: 397–406.

62. Sundt TM, Jr. Was the international randomized trial of extracranial-intracranial arterial bypass representative of the population at risk? *N Engl J Med* 1987; **316**: 814–16.

63. Baron JC, Bousser MG, Rey A, Guillard A, Comar D, Castaigne P. Reversal of focal "misery-perfusion syndrome" by extra-intracranial arterial bypass in hemodynamic cerebral ischemia. A case study with ^{15}O positron emission tomography. *Stroke* 1981; **12**: 454–9.

64. Touho H, Karasawa J. Hemodynamic evaluation of the effect of percutaneous transluminal angioplasty for atherosclerotic disease of the vertebrobasilar arterial system. *Neurol Med Chir (Tokyo)* 1998; **38**: 548–55; discussion 555–6.

65. Powers WJ, Grubb RL, Jr, Raichle ME. Physiological responses to focal cerebral ischemia in humans. *Ann Neurol* 1984; **16**: 546–52.

66. Powers WJ, Raichle ME. Positron emission tomography and its application to the study of cerebrovascular disease in man. *Stroke* 1985; **16**: 361–76.

67. Samson Y, Baron JC, Bousser MG *et al*. Effects of extra-intracranial arterial bypass on cerebral blood flow and oxygen metabolism in humans. *Stroke* 1985; **16**: 609–16.

68. Grubb RL, Jr, Derdeyn CP, Fritsch SM *et al*. Importance of hemodynamic factors in the prognosis of symptomatic carotid occlusion. *J Am Med Assoc* 1998; **280**: 1055–60.

69. Powers WJ. Cerebral hemodynamics in ischemic cerebrovascular disease. *Ann Neurol* 1991; **29**: 231–40.

70. Derdeyn CP, Videen TO, Yundt KD *et al*. Variability of cerebral blood volume and oxygen extraction: stages of cerebral haemodynamic impairment revisited. *Brain* 2002; **125**: 595–607.

71. Nemoto EM, Yonas H, Chang Y. Stages and thresholds of hemodynamic failure. *Stroke* 2003; **34**: 2–3.

72. Qureshi AI, Luft AR, Sharma M, Guterman LR, Hopkins LN. Prevention and treatment of thromboembolic and ischemic complications associated with endovascular procedures: Part I – Pathophysiological and pharmacological features. *Neurosurgery* 2000; **46**: 1344–59.

73. Qureshi AI, Suri MF, Khan J, Fessler RD, Guterman LR, Hopkins LN. Abciximab as an adjunct to high-risk carotid or vertebrobasilar angioplasty: preliminary experience. *Neurosurgery* 2000; **46**: 1316–25.

74. Savcic M, Hauert J, Bachmann F, Wyld PJ, Geudelin B, Cariou R. Clopidogrel loading dose regimens: kinetic profile of pharmacodynamic response in healthy subjects. *Semin Thromb Hemost* 1999; **25** (suppl 2): 15–19.

75. Moshfegh K, Redondo M, Julmy F *et al.* Antiplatelet effects of clopidogrel compared with aspirin after myocardial infarction: enhanced inhibitory effects of combination therapy. *J Am Coll Cardiol* 2000; **36**: 699–705.

76. Jauhar R, Bergman G, Savino S *et al.* Effectiveness of aspirin and clopidogrel combination therapy in coronary stenting. *Am J Cardiol* 1999; **84**: 726–8, A8.

77. Muller C, Buttner HJ, Petersen J, Roskamm H. A randomized comparison of clopidogrel and aspirin versus ticlopidine and aspirin after the placement of coronary-artery stents. *Circulation* 2000; **101**: 590–3.

78. Callahan A. Cerebrovascular disease and statins: a potential addition to the therapeutic armamentarium for stroke prevention. *Am J Cardiol* 2001; **88**: 33–7.

79. Callahan AS, 3rd, Berger BL, Beuter MJ, Devlin TG. Possible short-term amelioration of basilar plaque by high-dose atorvastatin: use of reductase inhibitors for intracranial plaque stabilization. *J Neuroimaging* 2001; **11**: 202–4.

80. Seldinger S. Catheter replacement of the needle in percutaneous angiography: a new technique. *Acta Radiol* 1953; **39**: 368–76.

81. Qureshi AI, Luft AR, Sharma M, Guterman LR, Hopkins LN. Prevention and treatment of thromboembolic and ischemic complications associated with endovascular procedures: Part II – Clinical aspects and recommendations. *Neurosurgery* 2000; **46**: 1360–75; discussion 1375–6.

82. Hong MK, Mintz GS, Lee CW, Song JM, Han KH, Kang DH, Song JK, Kim JJ, Weissman NJ, Fearnot NE, Park SW, Park SJ. Paclitaxel coating reduces in-stent intimal hyperplasia in human coronary arteries: a serial volumetric intravascular ultrasound analysis from the ASian Paclitaxel-Eluting Stent Clinical Trial (ASPECT). *Circulation* 2003; **107**: 517–20.

83. Levy EI, Boulos AS, Hanel RA, Tio FO, Alberico RA, Fronckowiak MD, Nemes B, Paciorek AM, Guterman LR, Hopkins LN. In vivo model of intracranial stent implantation: a pilot study to examine the histological response of cerebral vessels after randomized implantation of heparin-coated and uncoated endoluminal stents in a blinded fashion. *J Neurosurg* 2003; **98**: 544–53.

84. Regar E, Serruys PW, Bode C, Holubarsch C, Guermonprez JL, Wijns W, Bartorelli A, Constantini C, Degertekin M, Tanabe K, Disco C, Wuelfert E, Morice MC. Angiographic findings of the multicenter Randomized Study With the Sirolimus-Eluting Bx Velocity Balloon-Expandable Stent (RAVEL): sirolimus-eluting stents inhibit restenosis irrespective of the vessel size. *Circulation* 2002; **106**: 1949–56.

85. Morice MC, Serruys PW, Sousa JE, Fajadet J, Ban Hayashi E, Perin M, Colombo A, Schuler G, Barragan P,

Guagliumi G, Molnar F, Falotico R. A randomized comparison of a sirolimus-eluting stent with a standard stent for coronary revascularization. *N Engl J Med* 2002; **346**: 1773–80.

86. Marx SO, Marks AR. Bench to bedside: the development of rapamycin and its application to stent restenosis. *Circulation* 2001; **104**: 852–5.

Chapter 29

Percutaneous Interventions in Adults with Congenital Heart Diseases

Phillip Moore, Huynh Tuan Khanh, Zhang Shuang Chuan, Nguyen Lan Hieu, David Teitel

Patent foramen ovale
    **Shaping the tip of the catheter in order to enter the PFO
    **Backbleed and flush the sheath in order to avoid air embolism
    **Device positioning across a thick septum primum and a stiff tunnel defect
Atrial septal defect
    **Identification of different types of ASD
    **Reshaping the tip of the catheter to enter the ASD
    **Detecting additional defects
    **Selecting the size of the device
    **Sheath placement in fenestrated ASDs
    **How to position the sheath perpendicular to the atrial septum
    **Final check of device position
Patent ductus arteriosus
    **Misleading systolic flow mimicking PDA
    **Locating the point of minimal diameter of the PDA
    **Crossing the PDA from the aorta
    **Use less coils in PDA closure
    **Inserting the sheath into the RVOT
    **Avoiding first coil embolism while deploying the second coil

---

From: Nguyen T, Hu D, Saito S, Grines C, Palacios I (eds), *Practical Handbook of Advanced Interventional Cardiology*, 2nd edn. © 2003 Futura, an imprint of Blackwell Publishing.

　　　**Avoiding entangling the already deployed coil by directional wire
　　　**Checking position of device prior to deployment
　　　**Closing the PDA with occluder
Coarctation
　　　**A note of caution
　　　**Measuring the gradient across the coarctation
　　　**Sequential dilation of the coarctation
　　　**Advantage of MRI-compatible stents
　　　**Optimal wire position
　　　**No problem with subclavian jailing
　　　**Post-dilation with high pressure balloon
　　　**Accurate pressure gradient measurement
Pulmonary valve stenosis
　　　**How to track the balloon across the valve
Pulmonary artery stenosis
　　　**Stabilizing wire position in the pulmonary artery branch
　　　**Using a stiffer wire to track a stent
　　　**Reshaping the pigtail catheter

INTRODUCTION

Adult patients with congenital heart disease are an exponentially increasing population due to improved treatment strategies for children resulting in excellent long-term survival. Newer interventional techniques and tools developed over the last 20 years are now able to treat the majority of common congenital lesions in the catheterization laboratory instead of the operating suite. This chapter will detail percutaneous interventional techniques for treating the most common congenital cardiac lesions seen in adults including patent foramen ovale (PFO), atrial septal defect (ASD), patent ductus arteriosus (PDA), coarctation of the aorta, valvar pulmonary stenosis, and branch pulmonary artery stenosis.

PATENT FORAMEN OVALE

Device closure of PFO was first described in 1987[1] for the prevention of recurrent stroke associated with paradoxical embolus.[2] It has also been used to prevent right to left shunting causing desaturation in patients with orthodeoxia-platypnea syndrome.[3] The foramen ovale is a flap valve in the atrial septum created by overlap of the superior anterior septum secundum on the inferior posterior septum primum (Figure 29-1). It is present in all fetuses during development to direct oxygenated venous return from the placenta through the inferior vena cava (IVC) across the atrial septum, bypassing the right ventricle (RV) and unexpanded lungs, to fill the left

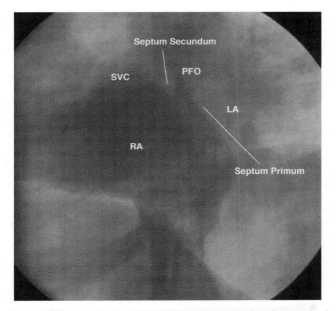

Figure 29-1: Lateral right atrial angiogram showing typical patent foramen ovale anatomy with a thin septum primum and thick septum secundum. LA, left atrium, PFO, patent foramen ovale, RA, right atrium, SVC, superior vena cava.

ventricle (LV) allowing optimal cerebral perfusion. After birth, with redistribution of flow due to lung expansion resulting in an increased left atrial (LA) pressure, the PFO closes and seals permanently in 65 to 80% of people, age dependant.[4] However, in 20–35% of the normal population the foramen ovale does not fibrous closed and remains patent allowing unidirectional flow from right to left if right atrial (RA) pressure exceeds LA pressure. This is physiologically insignificant for most people unless the amount of right to left shunting is significant causing orthodeoxia-platypnea syndrome or an embolus crosses right to left resulting in a cryptogenic transient ischemic attack (TIA) or stroke. Approximately 55% of patients who have had a stroke have a PFO,[5] suggesting it plays an important role in many of these patients.

Indications: Potential indications for PFO device closure include any patient who has had or has substantial risk for a cryptogenic stroke in the setting of a PFO. Absolute indications for PFO device closure remain controversial since there is limited controlled data comparing different treatment strategies and evaluating long-term follow-up. However, several clinical situations clearly warrant device closure, including: patients with active venous thrombus in the setting of a cryptogenic stroke; patients with recurrent cryptogenic stroke while on anticoagulation; patients with recurrent cryptogenic stroke and contraindications to anticoagulation; and scuba divers who have had significant decompression sickness but insist on continuing to dive. Based on current data PFO device closure is a reasonable therapeutic alternative for patients with an initial cryptogenic stroke and no additional risk factors.

Contraindications: There are no absolute contraindications for device PFO closure except for patients with active thrombus in the LA and those with a known allergy to the device implant materials, particularly the nickel in nitinol, an extremely rare condition. Patients who are hyper-coagulable, particularly those with disorders that predispose to arterial clots, should be considered very carefully as the post-placement risk of clot formation during the endocardialization process may be significantly increased. However, those patients who are predisposed to venous clots may be the very patients who benefit the most in the long term, albeit with a potentially increased thrombus risk during the first 6 months after implant. Patients who require anticoagulation long-term for other issues may get limited benefit from device closure.

The procedure: Over the last 14 years interventional device closure of PFO has become an attractive alternative therapeutic strategy to surgical PFO closure or lifelong anticoagulation for stroke prevention. No controlled comparative studies with these other treatment strategies exist for PFO closure although there are currently several active multi-center protocols in stroke patients comparing device closure with medical therapy. There is good comparative data from the ASD literature suggesting the efficacy of device closure of ASD is similar to surgical closure, with a significant reduction in complications, hospital stay, recovery time, and medical resource utilization.[6] Procedural success with PFO device closure is 98 to 100% with complete closure rates of 51 to 96% at 6 months if evaluated by saline contrast TEE[7–10]. Recurrent neurologic event risk following PFO device closure is 1–2% annually with a 96% 1-year and 90–94% 5-year event-free rate.[7–10] These results are significantly influenced by patient selection since some patients who undergo device closure may have recurrent strokes unrelated to either the PFO or device. More definitive information regarding recurrent stroke risk will be available from controlled randomized trials now under way comparing device closure with medical therapy. Procedural complications are uncommon, occurring in less than 2%, and include stroke, TIA, transient myocardial ischemia (the latter three due to air or clot embolism with the large delivery sheaths in the left atrium), device malposition or embolization, cardiac perforation with tamponade, and local femoral vein injury.[7] Late complications include atrial arrhythmias in 4%, although most are mild requiring no treatment,[11] and thrombus formation on the device.

There are currently six devices in use worldwide for PFO closure: the Amplatzer PFO Occluder (AGA Medical Corporation, Golden Valleys, MN); the Button device (Custom Medical Devices, Athens, Greece); the CardioSEAL STARFlex septal occluder (Nitinol Medical Technologies, Boston, MA); the Guardian Angel device (Microneva Inc, Minneapolis, MN); the Helix septal occluder (W.L. Gore Associates, Flagstaff, AZ); and the PFO Star (Cardia Star, Bunsville, MN). All these devices are similar in that they have all have a metal frame supporting two patches, left and right atrial patches, which are connected by a central core. These devices are folded or stretched into a loader to minimize their diameter for delivery through a 9F or 10F sheath positioned across the PFO. Once delivered from the sheath, the devices expand into position and immediately obstruct flow by mechanically by covering the flap valve. The final and complete seal comes from endocardial in-growth covering the patches completely within 8 to 12 weeks. Device implantation is most typically guided by both fluoroscopy and echocardiography (either transesophageal or intracardiac), although either alone will suffice.

Pre-procedure evaluation/management: Because most patients undergo PFO device closure for prevention of stroke recurrence it is essential to evaluate the patient's prior neurologic events and assure they were cryptogenic and likely related to the PFO. Stroke associated with paradoxical embolism is a diagnosis of exclusion so it is imperative to rule out other potential causes of stroke including cerebral aneurysm, carotid or vertebral vessel abnormalities, atrial arrhythmias, LA appendage thrombus, cardiomyopathy, or a hypercoagulable state. Standard pre-device closure evaluation includes head and neck MRI/MRA, carotid ultrasound, transesophageal echocardiogram with saline contrast, and hyper-coagulable screen including protein C and S, antithrombin III, factor V Leiden, prothrombin 20210, MTHFR, anticardiolipin antibody, and homocysteine. This latter workup is essential to help guide decisions regarding the appropriateness of implanting a device and the optimal medical strategy during the endocardialization process. Because of a small incidence of atrial arrhythmias after device placement, a baseline ECG should also be obtained. Standard protocols for anticoagulation, local anesthesia and antibiotic prophylaxis are listed in Table 29-1.

Defining the anatomy

A 9F or 10F sheath is placed in the femoral vein and right heart catheterization is performed using a Berman balloon-tipped or Multipurpose catheter with measurement of pressures and saturations in the SVC, RA, RV, and PAs to assure normal physiology and no evidence for significant left to right intracardiac shunt (to exclude additional pathology, especially an additional ASD or anomalous pulmonary vein). An angiogram is then performed in the low RA with the AP cam-

Table 29-1
Standard protocol for anticoagulant and antibiotic prophylaxis

1. If patients are on coumadin before the procedure, hold coumadin two days before and begin daily aspirin.
2. Give heparin to have ACT maintained at >250 seconds during the procedure.
3. Local anesthesia and mild to moderate sedation are used to maintain patient comfort.
4. A dose of antibiotics (cefazolin or clindamycin) is given IV prior to device implantation to protect against procedure-related sepsis/endocarditis.

era angled 20° RAO and 20° cranial and the lateral camera 70° LAO and 10° caudal. 24 cc of contrast is injected at a rate of 24 cc/sec. The lateral projection will profile the PFO nicely (Figure 29-1) and can be used as a road map for device delivery.

TECHNICAL TIP

**Shaping the tip of the catheter in order to enter the PFO: If the anatomy or size of the defect is in question cross the PFO with the Berman catheter by inserting the stiff end of a 0.035" straight wire shaped with a 45° angle at the distal 4 cm. This will give the end of the Berman catheter a "hockey stick" shape that can be easily directed slightly leftward and posterior to slip through the tunnel PFO. The balloon on the Berman catheter can then be inflated and the catheter withdrawn to the septum against the foramenal flap pulling it closed (Figure 29-2). Record an image of the balloon against the septum to create an additional road map for placement of the LA side of the device when appropriately positioned against the foramenal flap. If the inflated Berman balloon easily pulls through the defect, reassess the anatomy and consider a larger device.

Occasionally a pre-procedural echo will suggest a PFO with right to left shunting seen during saline contrast yet no PFO can be demonstrated by angiography or with catheter probing of the atrial septum. Consider the diagnosis of pulmonary arteriovenous malformations that are associated with paradoxical embolism and will have right to left contrast shunting on echo that can be mistaken for a PFO shunt. Perform selective right and left pulmonary artery angiography to make the diagnosis. If present these can be treated with coil embolization.

Choosing device size
In general, the smallest device which effectively covers the defect should be used to minimize foreign body mass and

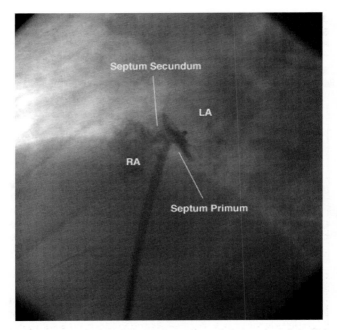

Figure 29-2: Lateral angiogram through long sheath in RA showing the LA side of an 18 mm AGA PFO occluder snug against the septum.

optimize closure rates. Most PFOs are 4 to 6 mm in diameter and stretch minimally in the left to right direction. Some operators use balloon stretch diameter to assist with device size choice. We have not found this helpful unless the anatomy is poorly defined on angiography and an ASD is suspected. For the Amplatzer device either the 18 mm or 25 mm devices suffice for most defects. If the right atrial side of the defect is quite large or a large atrial septal aneurysm is present then the larger 35 mm device can be used, assuming the total atrial size is adequate. For the STARFlex device (Nitinol Medical Technologies, Boston, MA) the 23 or 28 mm devices are adequate for most defects with the 33 mm device chosen for exceptionally large defects or those with large atrial septal aneurysms.

Sheath placement

The sheaths required for device closure are large but easily pass through the foramen ovale over a guidewire positioned in a left pulmonary vein, preferably the left upper. A multipurpose or directional end-hole catheter such as a JR4 can be used to direct a stiff 0.035" wire with a soft tip (Rosen or Amplatz) through the PFO and into the LUPV. The sheath and dilator are then advanced into the vein, wire and dilator removed and sheath cleared. It is imperative that these sheaths are cleared carefully because air embolism is directly into the systemic circulation and is by far the most common and serious side effect associated with this procedure.

> ### TECHNICAL TIP
>
> ****Backbleed and flush the sheath in order to avoid air embolism:** Flush the sheath continuously when advancing into the LA and during removal of the dilator and wire. Refrain from negative suction on these large sheaths. Allow passive bleed back and keep the end of the sheath significantly below the level of the patient's heart to facilitate bleed back. Be aware of the patient's breathing and be sure to time clearance of the sheath with exhalation to minimize the risk of air embolism. Give supplemental nasal cannula O_2 during sheath and device placement to minimize effects if air embolism occurs.

Device positioning

The device is soaked in heparinized saline and inspected for defects. It is compressed into the loader with constant flushing to remove any residual air and loaded into the sheath. Connect a large syringe with contrast to the side arm of the delivery sheath for hand angiography during device positioning. Withdraw the sheath tip to the middle of the left atrium and advance the distal patch of the device out of the sheath until it expands completely. Withdraw the sheath and device together until the device is in firm contact with the septum. You will feel the beat of the heart on the end of the sheath and can confirm position with your RA angiographic and balloon-sizing road maps. Perform a hand angiogram through the delivery sheath. This should outline the RA side of the septum and confirm the distal patch position on the left atrial side snug against the septum (Figure 29-2). If the angiogram shows marked filling of the left atrium, the device and sheath need to be pulled more tightly against the septum. Once appropriate LA patch position is confirmed the device is held firmly in place and the sheath withdrawn over the device, uncovering the right atrial patch. Once the right atrial patch is completely open, move the sheath and delivery cable to a neutral position and repeat a hand angiogram through the sheath to confirm optimal position. A small residual leak through the center or edge of the device is not atypical with this injection due to distortion of the device from the plane of the septum while connected to the delivery cable. If in appropriate position, the device is released and the delivery cable removed.

TECHNICAL TIP

**Device positioning across a thick septum primum and a stiff tunnel defect: Occasionally the septum primum is extremely thick and creates a rigid tunnel that cannot be displaced by exerting pull on the left atrial patch. This can be recognized prior to device release by an inability to position the center point of the device on the right atrial side of the septum because the entire device is held up in the left atrial side of the stiff tunnel. After release the device will not lie flat to the septum but the inferior portion of the left atrial patch and the superior portion of the right atrial patch will protrude from the septum due to malposition (Figure 29-3). This can be avoided by performing a transseptal puncture in the thick septum primum, just below the foramenal opening. TEE or ICE guidance is needed to assist with optimal puncture site location. The long sheath is passed through the transseptal puncture site and the device positioned in the transseptal defect, resulting in coverage of the foramen

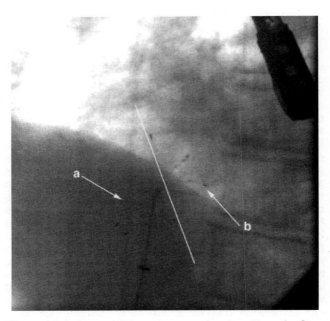

Figure 29-3: Lateral RA angiogram of malposition of a Starflex device in a PFO. Line denotes plane of the septum. Note that the superior right atrial arm (arrow a) and inferior left atrial arm (arrow b) are away from the septum indicating poor position due to a rigid septum primum maintaining the tunnel shape to the PFO.

without crossing it. This allows for excellent closure while avoiding device distortion due to the rigid foramenal tunnel.

Post-placement assessment

Repeat pressure and saturation measurements in the RA should be performed to assure hemodynamic stability post device. An angiogram at the SVC-RA junction consisting of 24 cc of contrast injected at 24 cc/sec should be performed to confirm device position and evaluate for residual right to left shunting. The cameras are positioned to evaluate the device in the AP plane (usually 15° RAO and 10° caudal) and on profile in the lateral plane (75° LAO and 5° caudal). If echocardiographic assessment is used then a saline contrast echo should be performed to evaluate right to left shunting.

ATRIAL SEPTAL DEFECT

Secundum ASDs are one of the more common congenital heart defects, making up 6–10% of all congenital anomalies, occurring in 1/1500 live births.[12] Anatomically, secundum ASDs are due to absence, perforation, or deficiency of the septum primum. This defect typically occurs sporadically but has been linked to genetic abnormalities such as Holt-Oram syndrome and mutations on chromosome 5p.

Device closure of an ASD was first performed in 1974 by King and Mills[13,14] using a 24-gauge surgically placed femoral sheath and a double-sided disk device. Technology and technique have been modified and refined over the years; however, the procedure remains conceptually identical. A collapsible double-sided disk device with a metal frame and fabric patches is positioned antegrade through a long femoral sheath across the secundum ASD. Upon extrusion from the sheath the device expands, creating a patch on both sides of the septum clamping the surrounding ASD tissue rim. The endocardium grows in to cover the device and create a permanent seal. Because of the need for surrounding rim tissue, device closure is limited to secundum type defects, not applicable to either primum (no inferior posterior rim) or venosus (no superior rim) ASDs. With recent technology, device closure has rapidly become the treatment of choice for secundum ASDs.

Concurrent controlled trials comparing surgical closure with device closure have shown efficacy rates of over 96% with significantly lower complications and hospital stay.[6] Most patients can be discharged the day of the procedure with return to full activity within 48–72 hours, significantly reducing costs and medical resources.[15] Early complications have been minor occurring in <9% of patients consisting primarily of transient arrhythmias, vascular injury, or asymptomatic device embolization. Serious complications have been quite rare but include thrombus formation on the device, heart block requiring pacing, and cardiac perforation.[16]

Indications: Indications for ASD device closure include any size secundum ASD with evidence on echocardiogram of RV volume overload. Patients with ASD and symptoms of exercise intolerance or history of cryptogenic stroke should also be closed. There is mounting evidence that ASD closure, even in the elderly, can improve maximal oxygen consumption.[17] ASDs have been closed by device in small children including infants; however, the optimal timing for elective closure appears to be between 2 and 4 years of age.

Contraindications: There are no absolute contraindications for device ASD closure except for patients with active thrombus in the LA and those with a known allergy to the device implant materials, particularly the nickel in nitinol, an extremely rare condition. Patients who are hypercoagulable, particularly those with disorders that predispose to arterial clots, should be considered very carefully as the post-placement risk of clot formation during the endocardialization process may be significantly increased. Patients with significant left ventricular dysfunction also must be monitored closely after the procedure due to the potential for the development of acute LA hypertension and resultant pulmonary edema. Diuretics immediately post closure may be very helpful in this subgroup of patients. Patients with pulmonary hypertension must be considered carefully but may benefit as long as there is a baseline left to right shunt.[18]

The procedure: There are currently four devices used recently for ASD closure including: the Amplatzer septal occluder (AGA Medical Corporation, Golden Valleys, MN); the Button device (Custom Medical Devices, Athens, Greece); and the CardioSEAL, STARFlex Helix (Nitinol Medical Technologies, Boston, MA). By far the most commonly used device and the one capable of closing the largest ASDs is the Amplatzer septal occluder. Unlike the others, this device has a central stenting mechanism that expands to the edges of the defect, filling it with frame and patch material, improving stability and complete closure rates in large ASDs. It is available in sizes up to 4 cm – capable of closing a 3.8 cm defect. The combined global experience of these devices for ASD closure is well over 30,000 patients with extremely high success and low complication rates.

Pre-procedure evaluation/management: A complete omniplane TEE if the patient is an older adolescent or adult, is necessary to define the atrial septal anatomy prior to the procedure. Secundum ASDs are rarely round, so attention to defect dimensions in multiple planes is essential for a complete anatomic understanding. Documentation of an adequate atrial septal rim circumferentially (>3 mm, especially at the posterior inferior inlet portion), and evaluation for additional defects, tissue strands, or septal aneurysms with perforations is essential (Figure 29-4 A–D).

TECHNICAL TIP

**Identification of different types of ASD: Identification of all pulmonary veins, particularly the right upper, is essential due to the association of partial anomalous pulmonary venous return with sinus venosus ASD. Sinus venosus defects can and should not be closed by device as this will only complicate surgical repair of the anomalously draining vein.

Because of a small incidence of atrial arrhythmias after device placement a baseline ECG should also be obtained. Usual protocols for anticoagulant, antiplatelet, anesthesia, and antibiotic prophylaxis are suggested (Table 29-1).

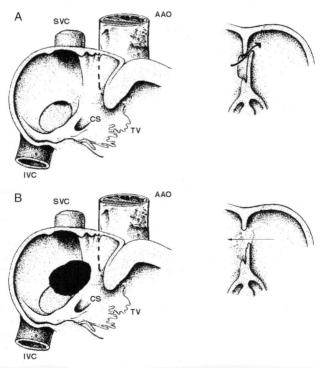

Figure 29-4: En faus and lateral view schematic drawing of the atrial septum: (A) patent foramen ovale; (B) isolated secundum ASD; (C) multiple defects; (D) fenestrated defects. AAO, ascending aorta; CS, coronary sinus; IVC, inferior vena cava; SVC, superior vena cava. *(Continued)*

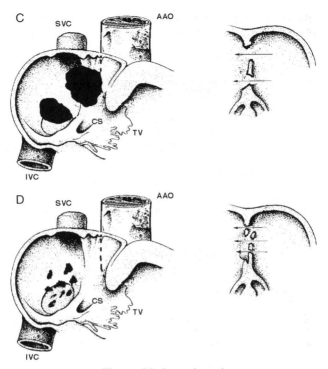

Figure 29-4 *continued.*

Defining the anatomy

An 8F or 10F sheath is placed in the femoral vein and right heart catheterization is performed using a Berman balloon-tipped or Multipurpose catheter with measurement of pressures and saturations in the SVC, RA, RV, and PAs to assess the degree of left to right intra-cardiac shunt and exclude pulmonary hypertension and additional pathology, especially anomalous pulmonary vein. An angiogram is then performed in the RUPV (this promotes contrast flow along the atrial septum to define the ASD optimally) with the AP camera angled 20° RAO and 20° cranial and the lateral camera 70° LAO and 10° caudal. 24 cc of contrast is injected at a rate of 24 cc/sec. The lateral projection will profile the ASD nicely while the AP camera will define LA free wall landmarks so that both can be used as road maps for device delivery (Figure 29-5). Echocardiographic evaluation of the ASD is performed using either TEE or ICE and will be used for device placement guidance as well as post-placement evaluation.

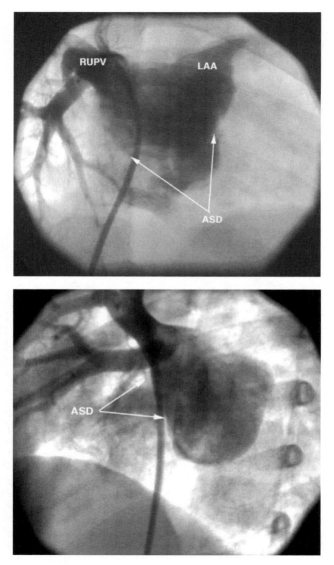

Figure 29-5: AP and lateral angiogram of a secundum ASD.

TECHNICAL TIP

**Reshaping the tip of the catheter to enter the ASD:
Cross the ASD with the Berman catheter by inserting the
stiff end of a 0.035" straight wire shaped with a 45° angle at

the distal 3 cm. This will give the end of the Berman catheter a "hockey stick" shape that can be easily directed slightly leftward and posterior to slip through the ASD. Clockwise rotation then turns the tip into the right upper pulmonary vein.

Balloon sizing of the defect is then performed. Exchange the Berman catheter for a directional, JR4 or Bentson tip to direct a 0.035" wire through the ASD into the left upper pulmonary vein. Position a compliant sizing balloon (both AGA Medical Corporation, and Nitinol Medical Technologies make ASD sizing balloon up to 3.5 cm in diameter) with reference markers across the defect and inflate until a discrete waist is detected. Measure the stretch diameter on AP and lateral angiogram as the echocardiographic measurement may not be as accurate or reliable.

TECHNICAL TIP

Detecting additional defects: It is essential to evaluate the defect with echocardiography while the defect is occluded with the balloon. This allows careful assessment of the septum for additional defects and assures accurate stretch diameter measurement by confirming complete occlusion of the defect with the balloon. We prefer ICE assessment due to improved patient comfort, reduced need for deep sedation and reduced need for echo personnel support. In general, ICE has been equivalent to TEE for assessing the atrial septum in experienced hands.

Choosing device size

In general, the smallest device that effectively covers the defect should be used to minimize foreign body mass and interference with intra-cardiac structures such as AV valves or pulmonary vein/SVC inflow. Total septal length should be measured both angiographically and by echo to determine the largest device that can safely fit in the patient's atrium. Specific sizing depends on the type of device being used. In general, for the CardioSEAL STARFlex, Button, and Helix devices the size should be chosen roughly two times the stretch diameter of the defect. The Amplatzer device, which is sized by the central stent diameter, should be 2 to 4 mm larger than the stretch diameter.

TECHNICAL TIP

Selecting the size of the device: The smaller the defect stretch diameter, the less you need to oversize devices, especially the Amplatzer device. For defects <16 mm we often use devices equal to the stretch diameter, for defects 17 to 32 mm we use the stretch diameter + 2 mm and for very large defects >32 mm we will oversize by 4 mm. If there is limited rim, particularly in the inferior portion, posterior portion, or the anterior superior portion (aortic region on echo short axis) of the defect, we will oversize by 3 or 4 mm from the stretch diameter. For the other devices the same concept holds; if there is limited rim in a region, choose a device closer to 2.5 times stretch diameter if total atrial chamber size will allow.

Sheath placement

The sheaths required for device closure range in size from 6F to 12F depending on device type and size. Because air embolus remains one of the major concerns and causes of significant complications, proper flushing of the sheath is imperative. Use of a curved tip sheath that can be manipulated directly from the RA to the LA without the use of a guidewire is preferred. The long sheath is placed in the RA over a wire, the wire and dilator removed and the sheath cleared of air and flushed. The sheath is then manipulated across the defect into the LA for placement of the device. For small defects the tip of the sheath can be positioned in the center of the LA, for large defects the tip should be positioned in the mouth of the right or left upper pulmonary vein.

TECHNICAL TIP

**Sheath placement in fenestrated ASDs: Sheath placement should be modified for fenestrated or multiple defect closure. In these cases proper placement of the sheath across the exact defect of interest is crucial to the success of the procedure. To assure the sheath crosses the same defect that was balloon-sized, a long 0.035" guidewire should be left across the defect of interest in the LUPV and the long sheath exchanged over the wire for the balloon sizing catheter. Flush the sheath continuously when advancing into the LA and during removal of the dilator and wire. Refrain from negative suction on these large sheaths. Allow passive bleed back and keep the end of the sheath significantly below the level of the patient's heart to facilitate bleed back. Be aware of the patient's breathing and be sure to time clearance of the sheath with exhalation to minimize the risk of air embolism. Give supplemental nasal cannula O_2 during sheath and device placement to minimize effects if air embolism occurs.

Device positioning

The device is soaked in heparinized saline and inspected for defects. It is compressed into the loader with constant flushing to remove any residual air and loaded into the sheath. The tip of the sheath is positioned in the mid LA and the distal disk of the device opened. Use angiographic and echocardiographic landmarks to assure the device is not opened in a pulmonary vein or pressed against the LA roof.

TECHNICAL TIP

**How to position the sheath perpendicular to the atrial septum: Often the angle of the sheath with the atrial septum is quite acute, making the approach of the device to the septum difficult, often resulting in device edge prolapse, particularly in the anterior superior region (especially if limited aortic knob rim) or superior SVC region (especially if a superiorly located defect). To improve the angle and bring the device more perpendicular to the atrial septum, rotate the sheath clockwise to drive the tip of the sheath posterior and superior. The sheath can be shaped with a posterior superior curve to improve device alignment (Cook Inc. currently has a commercial sheath available with this bend on the tip, called a Lock-Hausdorf sheath).

The LA side of the device is brought back toward the atrial septum but not snug as with PFO closure because this will promote device prolapse into the RA. For the CardioSEAL STARFlex type device the centerpin of the device should be kept slightly into the LA side of the septum for RA disk delivery. Both the Amplatzer and Helix devices can be kept centered on the atrial septum during RA disk delivery.

TECHNICAL TIP

**Final check of device position: The larger the defect, the further into the LA the device center should be kept during RA disk delivery to prevent LA disk prolapse into the RA.

After RA disk delivery but before device release, complete echocardiographic assessment of the device and the relationship to surrounding structures must be completed. Evaluation for new onset TR or MR, residual left to right ASD flow, and obstruction of SVC or right upper pulmonary vein flow all must be carefully assessed. For the STARFlex device all frame arms must be identified on the appropriate side of the septum. For the Amplatzer device atrial septum must be identified between the two disks circumferentially. Pulling and pushing slightly on the delivery cable to separate the two disks will facilitate this process and confirms device stability. If in appropriate position, the device is released and the delivery cable removed.

Post-placement assessment

Repeat pressure and saturation measurements throughout the right heart should be performed to assure hemodynamic stability post device and assess residual shunt. An angiogram at the MPA or RPA consisting of 24 cc of contrast injected at 24 cc/sec should be performed to confirm device position and evaluate for residual left to right shunting. The cameras can be positioned to evaluate the device on faux in the AP plane (usually 15° RAO and 10° caudal) and on profile in the lateral plane (75° LAO and 5° caudal). Echocardiographic assessment should be repeated following device release to assess final device position and residual shunt.

PATENT DUCTUS ARTERIOSUS

Patent ductus arteriosus (PDA) is the persistence of a normal fetal connection between the proximal descending aorta and proximal left pulmonary artery which allows the right ventricle to bypass the lungs and pump deoxygenated blood via the descending aorta to the placenta for oxygenation. Normal ductal closure occurs within the first 12 hours after birth by contraction and cellular migration of the medial smooth muscle in the wall of the ductus, resulting in protrusion of the thickened intima into the lumen, causing functional closure. Final closure and creation of the ligamentum arteriosum is completed by 3 weeks of age with permanent sealing of the duct by infolding of the endothelium, disruption of the internal elastic lamina, and hemorrhage and necrosis in the subintimal region leading to replacement of muscle fibers with fibrosis. This process of closure is incomplete in 1/2000 live births and accounts for up to 10% of all congenital heart disease.[19]

PDA closure was one of the first congenital heart lesions treated by interventional techniques, first reported by Dr Porstmann in 1968.[20,21] There have been substantial refinements in devices and techniques over the last 35 years but for the last 15 years interventional catheter treatment has been the preferred therapy in many large centers worldwide. It is a particularly attractive technique in adults, in whom surgical ligation and division can be problematic due to calcified ductal tissue and increased surgical risks. The technique is simple, consisting of placement of a device or vascular occlusion coil in the PDA either antegrade from the femoral vein or retrograde from the femoral artery. Once implanted, the device physically occludes ductal flow and over the first 6 to 8 weeks after implant endothelial overgrowth covers the device or coil from both the pulmonary artery and aorta, sealing the PDA permanently closed.

Indications: PDA closure is indicated in all patients with LA or LV enlargement due to left to right shunting or pulmonary artery pressure elevation. Small PDAs that do not result in hemodynamic effects are still at risk for the development of endocarditis. Controlled trials comparing antibiotic prophylaxis with device closure for the prevention of endocarditis have and will not be performed due to the limited number of patients and low incidence of endocarditis. There have been no late reports of endocarditis following interventional closure of the ductus although procedural infections have occurred rarely. Current clinical recommendations are for device or coil closure in small hemodynamically insignificant PDAs if they are audible on physical examination.

Contraindications: Patients with systemic pulmonary hypertension and right to left ductal shunting should not have their PDA closed. If pulmonary hypertension is noted during catheterization then an accurate assessment of the degree of hypertension and the reactivity of the pulmonary bed must be made during temporary occlusion of the ductus. A second venous sheath should be placed so that simultaneous PA pressure measurement and pulmonary vascular resistance calculations can be made while balloon occlusion of the PDA is performed. If there is baseline left to right shunt and a decrease in PA pressures with balloon occlusion then ductal closure is indicated.

The procedure: Several different closure devices are currently used due to the significant variability of ductal anatomy. The most common anatomic shape is conical, with a large aortic ampulla that narrows at the pulmonary artery end; however, other distinct anatomic forms exist including "tubular" without a narrowing at the pulmonary artery end, "complex" with narrowing at both the aortic and pulmonary end, and a short "window" which is an anatomy commonly found in adults.[22] Different closure tools and techniques may be needed to effectively address these less common PDA anatomic subtypes, but this section will focus on the two most common closure techniques for the conical shaped ductus. The most commonly used technique for closure of PDAs less than 4 mm is retrograde placement of embolization coils. For large ducts antegrade placement of an Amplatzer duct occluder device is the preferred method. These two techniques are described below.

Transcatheter ductal closure procedural success has been extremely high with rates of complete closure >96%.[23–28] The procedure takes approximately 2 hours with discharge within 6 hours. Full activity may resume within 48 hours of the procedure. No anticoagulation or antiplatelet therapy is recommended post coil closure procedure although most centers recommend daily aspirin for 4 to 6 months after Amplatzer duct occluder or device closure. Procedural complications are uncommon, occurring in less than 5%.[23,26] Hemolysis causing anemia may occur if a residual shunt is present after closure with either coils or device and requires repeat catheterization with placement of additional embolization coils. The major complication associated with coil closure of the PDA is coil embolization to the lungs. However, this is a technical issue that occurs at or immediately after implant, the incidence of which significantly decreases with operator experience. It is related to either undersizing of the coil or malposition upon placement.

In all but a very few patients, the coils can be snared from their embolized position in the pulmonary artery and removed from the body without sequela. Device embolization, thrombus, and ductal aneurysm have been reported in <1%.

Pre-procedure evaluation/management: A complete physical examination and surface echocardiogram is necessary prior to catheterization to make the diagnosis. Large PDAs will have a continuous murmur at the left infra-clavicular region, prominent pulses, and a widened pulse pressure. Small PDAs may only have a systolic ejection murmur with normal pulses and pulse pressure. Echo will show an abnormal systolic left to right color flow jet into the MPA or proximal LPA directed inferiorly and anteriorly. A CBC and type and screen is obtained for the procedure. Usual protocols for anticoagulant, antiplatelet, anesthesia, and antibiotic prophylaxis are suggested (Table 29-1).

| TECHNICAL TIP

Misleading systolic flow mimicking PDA: Be wary of a color flow jet seen on echo directed posteriorly from the anterior wall of the MPA associated with a systolic or continuous murmur. This most often represents a small coronary to pulmonary artery fistula but can easily be mistaken for a PDA.

Defining the anatomy

The procedure should be adjusted based on the size of the PDA and technique used for closure. Small PDAs can be addressed solely through a 5F or 6F femoral artery sheath with only retrograde catheterization. Larger PDAs require both femoral and venous access. The anatomy of the PDA is evaluated with a proximal descending thoracic aortic angiogram in straight lateral plane using a pigtail catheter to inject 35 cc of contrast at 35 cc/second (Figure 29-6). For small PDAs the pigtail catheter is then exchanged for a 5F or 6F directional catheter, either Bentson or JR4 shape, with a 0.038" lumen. The catheter is advanced to the proximal descending thoracic aorta and directed anteriorly and leftward. Often the catheter itself can be advanced across the PDA into the MPA, particularly if the catheter tip has been shaped by hand with an exaggerated anterior curve. If the catheter itself will not advance through the PDA then the soft end of a straight 0.035" wire can be advanced into the MPA and the catheter advanced over the wire. Pressure and saturation measurements should be obtained in the MPA and DAO to confirm catheter location and document left to right ductal shunting.

| TECHNICAL TIP

Locating the point of minimal diameter of the PDA: If the point of minimal diameter of the PDA is not well defined

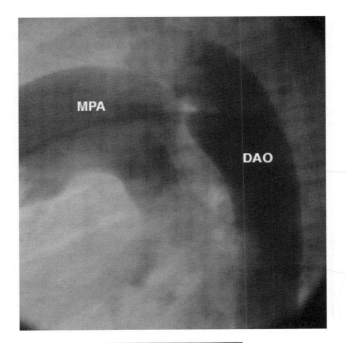

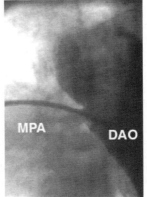

Figure 29-6: Lateral DAO angiogram showing a typical conical shaped PDA and a window type PDA.

angiographically, if can be located by correlating catheter tip position in relationship to bony and tracheal air column landmarks during pressure pullback from MPA to DAO through PDA. The point of acute pressure change from low MPA pressure to systemic DAO pressure will correspond to the minimal PDA diameter. This typically occurs at or just anterior to the anterior edge of the tracheal air column on straight lateral projection.

For larger PDAs a 7F balloon wedge or Multipurpose catheter can be manipulated through the right heart to the branch pulmonary arteries with measurement of pressures and saturations to determine the degree of ductal shunting. The catheter can be manipulated antegrade through the PDA by advancing with clockwise rotation in the distal MPA. If this does not track easily a floppy directional wire such as a 0.035" Terumo can be advanced across the PDA and the catheter advanced over the wire.

TECHNICAL TIP

**Crossing the PDA from the aorta: If you are having difficulty crossing the PDA from the MPA, cross retrograde from the DAO with a directional catheter. Place a 10 mm snare through the retrograde catheter that is now in the MPA and snare the soft end of a 0.035" straight wire protruding from the antegrade catheter in the MPA. The retrograde catheter can then be used to pull the antegrade catheter across the PDA for proper positioning.

Choosing device size

For small PDAs less than 4 mm in diameter Gianturco embolization coils (Cook Inc, Bloomington, IN) can be used for closure. They are available in a variety of wire diameters (0.018", 0.025", 0.035", 0.038" or 0.052"), loop diameters (3 through 15 mm) and total wire lengths (3 to 15 cm). For the most part 0.038" wire diameter coils are used, although 0.052" coils can be used for larger PDAs and 0.035" for very small ducts. Initial coil size is chosen based on minimal PDA diameter with the loop diameter ≥ 2 times the minimal PDA diameter. Coil length should allow for at least 4 loops of coil (one loop on PA side of PDA and the remainder in the aortic ampulla) so length $\geq 4 \times \pi \times$ loop diameter. For example, a 2.5 mm minimum diameter PDA can be closed with a 0.038", 7 cm long, 5 mm loop diameter coil which will provide a total of 4.4 loops.

For ducts 4 mm or greater the Amplatzer duct occluder device can be used. This Nitinol wire mesh self-expanding device has a wider aortic flange measuring 2 mm larger than the central ductal plug that ranges in length from 5 to 8 mm (Figure 29-7). Central ductal plug diameters range from 4 mm to 14 mm. The diameter of the ductal portion of the device should be 2 mm larger than the minimal diameter of the PDA so this device can close duct up to 14 or 15 mm in diameter. For example, a 5.7 mm minimal diameter ductus can be closed with a 10–8 mm diameter, 8 cm long Amplatzer ductal occluder.

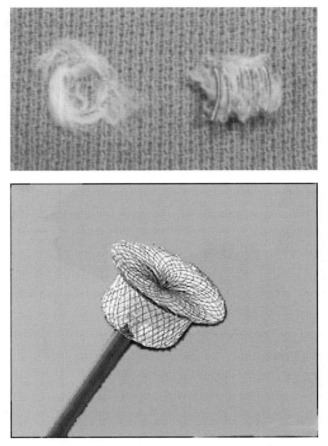

Figure 29-7: (A) Front and side view of 0.038" × 7 cm × 5 mm Gianturco coil. (B) Side view of Amplatzer 8–10mm duct occluder device.

TECHNICAL TIP

**Use fewer coils in PDA closure: You can reduce the ratio of minimal PDA diameter to coil loop diameter to 1.7 if you use the thicker stiffer 0.052" wire diameter embolization coils. In fact larger ducts, up to 7 mm in diameter, can be effectively closed with these 0.052" coils, particularly if simultaneous deployment of two 0.052" coils is performed antegrade through a long 7F sheath.

Sheath placement

For retrograde coil closure of the PDA a short 5F or 6F sheath in the femoral artery is all that is needed. For antegrade Amplatzer duct occlude PDA closure an appropriate 6F or 7F long sheath with a curved tip (180° transseptal shape) placed across the PDA into the DAO is needed. Once an end-hole catheter has been advanced antegrade across the PDA, advance it to the proximal abdominal aorta and place a 0.035" J-tipped exchange wire through the catheter. Remove both the catheter and short sheath and advance a long sheath from the femoral vein over the wire through the right heart into the DAO.

TECHNICAL TIP

**Inserting the sheath into the RVOT: To ease passage of the sheath through the RVOT and minimize ectopy, rotate the sheath clockwise as it moves into the RVOT to avoid getting caught on the moderator band. If difficult, passage of the sheath can be facilitated by either using a stiffer wire (such as a 0.038" or Amplatzer super stiff) or by snaring the tip of the wire in the DAO with the retrograde directional catheter and a 10 mm Nitinol snare loop.

Device positioning

For coil closure of the PDA retrograde the tip of the directional Bentson or JR4 with a 0.038" lumen is positioned across the PDA in the main PA. Lateral fluoroscopy is used to guide the procedure with a road map image from the lateral angiogram available to define ductal anatomy. A straight 0.035" wire is used to load the embolization coil into the catheter and advance or "push" the coil to the tip. One loop of coil is extruded from the tip of the catheter by advancing the 0.035" pushing wire and the entire catheter/coil/pushing wire is then brought back slowly together to position this extruded loop of coil against the PA end of the PDA. As the extruded end of the coil makes contact it will change shape by either rotating or opening slightly. The pushing wire is now held in position and the catheter is retracted over the pushing wire. This uncovers the proximal end of the coil in the aortic ampulla while maintaining the distal loop of coil on the PA side of the ductus. The catheter is brought back completely, uncovering the proximal end of the coil which will then spring from the tip of the catheter and coil up in the aortic ductal ampulla. Controlled release coils are available, allowing the pushing wire to be advanced once a secondary loop starts to form in the descending aorta for a more controlled release of the proximal end of the coil near the aortic ampulla.

TECHNICAL TIP

**Avoiding first coil embolism while deploying the second coil: Watch the PA loop of coil carefully while delivering the proximal portion of the coil. If additional coil loop is advancing forward into the PA as you deliver the proximal portion of the coil then the catheter and pushing wire must be pulled back more aggressively to avoid embolization of the entire coil into the PA. If the PA loop of coil is getting smaller and pulling into the aorta during delivery then the pushing wire must be held more stable or advanced to keep the distal loop in the PA and prevent embolization of the coil into the DAO.

Approximately 10 to 15 minutes after coil placement an angiogram should be performed by hand through the directional catheter, with the tip positioned at the inferior margin of the aortic ductal ampulla pointing anterior and leftward. If a significant residual leak exists through the initial coil then additional coils should be placed. A significant leak is contrast passing through the coil as a jet or contrast filling into the MPA 5 mm or more past the PA end of the existing coil. The second coil should be 2 mm smaller in loop coil diameter size and can have a length providing 3 to 4 loops. To cross the PDA with an existing coil in position the directional catheter is positioned at the inferior edge of the aortic ductal ampulla pointing toward the PA. The soft end of a 0.035" straight wire is advanced gently through the existing coil into the PA. This may take several attempts with slight angulation of the directional catheter on each attempt to find the residual defect.

TECHNICAL TIP

**Avoiding entangling the already deployed coil by directional wire: Be careful to use a non-steerable wire when you cross the initial coil. Directional wires with floppy ends that can be easily rotated can inadvertently have the tip spin in the existing coil. This will wrap fibers of the implanted coil around the directional wire, entangling the two and causing the implanted coil to dislodge.

Once the straight wire is through into the PA, advance the directional catheter over the wire. Delivery of the second smaller coil is performed similarly to delivery of the first coil. Occasionally a third coil may be necessary for complete closure.

For the Amplatzer PDA duct occluder device the long sheath should be positioned antegrade in the mid-thoracic DAO and kept there until the device is advanced to the tip of the sheath. This prevents the sheath from inadvertently being withdrawn through the duct into the MPA as the device advances. The entire system is then brought back until the tip of the sheath is just off the posterior wall of the DAO at the level of the ductal ampulla. The device is held in position and the sheath retracted to open the distal flange of the device only.

The entire system is withdrawn together and the aortic flange is pulled firmly against the aortic ampulla. A pigtail catheter is positioned from the femoral artery in the thoracic DAO for a lateral angiogram to confirm appropriate position of the aortic end of the device. Once position is confirmed the device cable is held in position and the sheath is retracted, opening the ductal plug within the PDA.

TECHNICAL TIP

**Checking position of device prior to deployment: A hand angiogram through the delivery sheath can be performed to assess the PA side of the device. If the PA end protrudes more than 3 mm or there is evidence of LPA obstruction the device should be recaptured and repositioned.

A repeat angiogram is performed in the DAO to confirm appropriate device position and the cable is then unscrewed for device release, keeping slight tension on the cable to maintain position.

TECHNICAL TIP

**Closing the PDA with occluder: A window-shaped ductus may be more effectively closed with an Amplatzer septal occluder (AGA Medical Corporation, Golden Valleys, MN) or CardioSEAL STARFlex device (Nitinol Medical Technologies, Boston, MA). The technique is similar to that described above for the Amplatzer PDA duct occluder device.

Post-placement assessment
Repeat hemodynamic measurements are then performed with particular attention to pressure measurements in the LPA, MPA, transverse arch, and DAO to assure no obstruction to the proximal LPA or DAO has occurred. A final angiogram through the pigtail catheter in the proximal thoracic DAO is performed in the lateral projection (35 cc at 35 cc/sec) to assess final positioning and closure. Some leak through the Amplatzer duct occluder device is expected as fibrin deposition on the fabric for complete closure occurs over hours (Figure 29-8).

COARCTATION

Coarctation is most often a discrete narrowing of the proximal descending thoracic aorta just distal to the origin of the left subclavian artery at the site of the ductus ligamentum. It makes up 7% of all patients with congenital heart disease

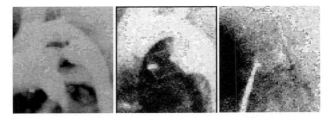

Figure 29-8: Lateral angiograms of PDA before, during and after Amplatzer duct occluder device closure.

and results in upper extremity hypertension, left ventricular hypertrophy, and eventually ventricular failure if left untreated. It should be considered during the initial evaluation of systemic hypertension and can easily be diagnosed on physical examination by decreased femoral pulses with a delay compared to radial pulses and blood pressure differential between the arms and leg. Often a 2/6 systolic ejection murmur can be heard at the left upper sternal border and over the left back. The narrowing is due to thick intimal and medial ridges that protrude posteriorly and laterally into the aortic lumen.[29] Intimal proliferation and elastic lamina disruption occur distal to the ridges due to the high velocity jet impact on the distal aortic wall. Cystic medial necrosis with disarray and loss of medial elastic tissue occurs commonly in the adjacent aorta and may extend to the ascending aorta as well. It is this abnormality that may lead to late aneurysm formation. The body's compensatory response to coarctation is the development of vessels that bypass the obstruction, collateral vessels from the innominate, carotid, and subclavian arteries that connect to the thoracic aorta below the level of the coarctation, often connecting through the intercostal arteries. Enlargement of the intercostal arteries due to this collateral flow is the mechanism for rib notching seen on chest radiograph in adult patients with severe native coarctation.

Balloon dilation for treatment of coarctation was first performed in the early 1980s in children with good success in both native and postoperative recoarctation.[30] Its efficacy in adults was found to be similar to that in children.[31–33] However, there remained a small but significant failure rate, with residual gradient greater than 20 mmHg in approximately 15% of patients treated. Stent implantation for repair of coarctation was performed sporadically in the early 1990s in children, being first reported in adults in 1995 with very promising results.[34] Since that time stent repair has become the treatment of choice for coarctation in many centers due to the improved success rate and low restenosis rate, although controlled trials are not available.[35] Procedural success has been reported in >95% of patients with residual obstruction of less than 20 mmHg.

Recurrent stenosis has been extremely rare, occurring in less than 5%, always in younger patients and generally mild. Complications have been reported in up to 20% and include aneurysm, perforation, stroke, and death.[35–39] In addition, femoral artery complications including arteriovenous fistula and pseudo-aneurysm have been reported associated with the larger arterial sheaths required for the procedure.

Indications: Any coarctation with a gradient of >10 mmHg and significant upper body hypertension or left ventricular hypertrophy without additional cause should be treated. For mild coarctation it is imperative to use stent implantation to assure complete resolution of the mild obstruction. Mild coarctations with <20 mmHg gradient without hypertension or LV hypertrophy should be considered for stent repair if collaterals are present or the patient has an abnormal blood pressure response to exercise. Patients with coarctation gradients of >20 mmHg at rest should be repaired.

Contraindications: Patients with coarctation gradients <20 mmHg with no evidence of collateral flow, hypertension, LV hypertrophy, or abnormal blood pressure response to exercise do not need treatment. Patients with significant hypoplasia and obstruction of the transverse aortic arch in the area of the origin of the carotids should be excluded. Stent repair with jailing of the carotids may be appropriate in the rare patient at extremely high surgical risk, but for the majority of patients with this lesion surgical repair should be performed. Any patient with an existing aneurysm should also be cautiously considered. The use of covered thoracic stents may have a role in this setting although there is limited data at present.

The procedure: The equipment available for angioplasty and stent repair of coarctation has improved significantly over the last 20 years. Balloons that are specifically designed for large stent implantation and stents that have adequate radial strength at sizes appropriate for an adult thoracic aorta are only recently available. Currently there are three large stent designs, two stainless steel and one of platinum, that can reach diameters of 18 to 25 mm with adequate coverage and radial strength appropriate for treatment of coarctation (Tables 29-2, 29-3).

Pre-procedure evaluation/management: A complete physical examination including upper and lower extremity blood pressure measurements is essential. Echocardiography may be helpful in confirming the diagnosis if the physical examination is unclear; however, echo often poorly defines the anatomic detail of the obstruction and frequently overestimates the degree of obstruction. Anatomical definition of the coarctation prior to catheterization is critical to determine the best approach for treatment. Patients with hypoplastic transverse arch or a "kinked" high third arch may respond poorly to stent repair and may best be treated surgically. MRI with magnetic resonance angiography is currently the best technique

Table 29-2
Comparison of PFO and ASD devices

Device		Frame	Material	Sizes	Delivery sheath
Amplatzer PFO		Nitinol wire	Polyester fabric	18, 25, 35	9
ASD				4–40	6–12
Button PFO		Teflon coated stainless steel wire	Poly-urethane foam	25–30	7–9
ASD				25–60	9
CardioSEAL		MPN35	Polyester fabric	17–40	10
Guardian Angel		Nitinol wire	Polyester fabric	18–30	10
Helix		Nitinol wire	PTFE	15–35	9
PFO Star		Nitinol wire	Ivalon plug	15–35	10

for defining the arch anatomy and can give functional data including estimation of degree of obstruction based on blood velocity at the site and percent of collateral flow, an excellent indication of the physiologic significance of the coarctation.[40] In addition the MRI gives accurate anatomic detail of the size, location, and length of coarctation so that appropriate equipment including dilation balloon and stent sizes are planned in advance. A CBC and type and cross is obtained for the procedure. Blood is kept available in the cath lab during balloon dilation and stent implantation. Usual protocols for antiplatelet, anticoagulant, anesthesia and antibiotic prophylaxis are suggested in Table 29-1. Additional IV narcotic, fentanyl, is given immediately prior to balloon dilation or stent implantation as aortic stretch caused a moderate amount of pain acutely. Patients who are taking antihypertension medications continue those the morning of the procedure. Short acting IV beta blocker is given immediately after balloon dilation or stent implantation if significant acute hypertension develops.

Table 29-3
Comparison of large stents used for coarctation and PA stenosis

Stent		Stainless steel wall thickness (in)/ Max. diameter	Delivery sheath 16 mm balloon (Fr)	Cell design	Flexibility	Radial strength
Genesis		0.0095 20 mm	8	Closed omega hinges	Excellent	6
IS-LD		0.0076 24 mm	10	Open	Good	4
Palmaz 8 series		0.0055 18 mm	10	Closed diamond	Poor	6
10 series		0.0095 25 mm	10	Closed diamond	Rigid	8

TECHNICAL TIP

**A note of caution: This procedure can have relatively high rates of significant complications that can be reduced by careful patient selection and operator experience; however, in hospital cardiothoracic surgical availability to address emergencies is mandatory.

Defining the anatomy

Right and left heart catheterization is performed in routine fashion. Because of the large sheath size required in the artery for this procedure, suture closure of the femoral artery is recommended, so be sure the sheath insertion site is appropriately superior. Cardiac index should be measured either with saturation or thermodilution techniques. This is essential both prior to and after balloon dilation or stenting to properly interpret the degree of stenosis measured across the coarctation. Pressure pullback across the area of coarctation is recorded.

TECHNICAL TIP

**Measuring the gradient across the coarctation: Remember the pressure gradient across the coarctation depends primarily on the cross-sectional area of the lesion, its length, and the amount of flow crossing the lesion. Severe coarctations may have very little pressure gradient from AAO to DAO if there are substantial collateral vessels limiting the flow through the lesion. Despite collateral vessels this obstruction remains a significant increased work load for the LV and stimulus for upper body hypertension.

An angiogram is performed in the distal transverse arch using a marker pigtail catheter to allow for accurate measurements. The AP camera should be angled 15° LAO and 10° caudal combined with a straight lateral projection with an injection of 35 cc at 35 cc/sec. Careful measurements are then made of the distal transverse arch diameter, coarctation diameter, coarctation length, distal normal vessel diameter, distance from the left subclavian artery origin to the coarctation, and diameter of the left subclavian artery (Figure 29-9).

Choosing balloon and stent size

Balloon diameter should never exceed the smallest diameter of normal aorta surrounding the coarctation that the balloon may contact. In other words, the goal is to enlarge the coarctation to the size of the smallest contiguous normal aorta, not to stretch it larger than the normal diameter. Preferably the balloon should be at least 2.5 times larger than the coarctation diameter but not more than 3.5 times larger. Remember that if the wire and balloon tip are in the innominate or left

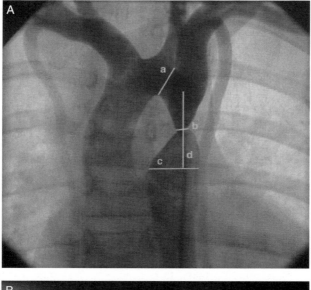

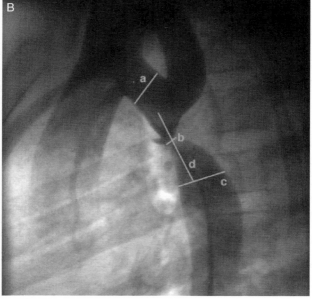

Figure 29-9: (A) AP angiogram of native coarctation with key measurements; a, transverse arch diameter; b, coarctation diameter; c, DAO diameter; d, coarctation length. (B) Lateral angiogram showing similar measurements.

subclavian artery for stabilization then the balloon diameter must not exceed the normal vessel diameter of the proximal innominate or subclavian. These guidelines will minimize the risk of aneurysm or rupture.

TECHNICAL TIP

**Sequential dilation of the coarctation: If the coarctation is severe with a diameter <¼ of the normal aortic diameter (for a normal sized adult with a 20 mm distal transverse arch that would be a coarctation diameter of 5 mm or less) then complete repair should be performed in two or three stages at 3-month intervals to allow adequate healing of the aorta in between procedures. The first procedure should be balloon dilation with stent implant and enlargement to 2.5 times the coarctation diameter (in the example given a stent would be implanted and dilated to 12 mm). Three months later the patient should have dilation of the implanted stent to the size of the surrounding normal aorta (in the example the stent would then be dilated to 20 mm).

Care must be taken to choose a balloon that is long enough to remain stable in the lesion but not extend around the arch or substantially into the head and neck vessels. Generally a 3 or 4 cm balloon length is optimal. The balloon should be of scratch-resistant material, preferably designed for use with stents. Remember that the stent will need to be mounted during the procedure so care must be taken not to damage the balloon during the mounting process. Some operators have advocated the use of a double balloon delivery catheter. This has an inner balloon 1/2 the diameter of the final outer balloon. The concept is the inner balloon allows a more uniform enlargement of the stent with minimal stent tip flaring and the ability to adjust stent position prior to final implant with the larger balloon in a more controlled manner. We have not found the balloons in a double balloon technique to offer any significant advantage over careful delivery with a single-lumen balloon; however, it adds complexity to coordinate inflation of both balloons sequentially.

The stent used should be able to reach a diameter appropriate for the normal aorta and the patient's size, which for most adults will range between 18 and 22 mm. The stent length should be kept as short as possible maintaining adequate length after foreshortening with dilation to completely cover the length of the lesion. Unnecessary stent length may be a disadvantage due to increased length of non-compliant aorta after implant that may influence blood pressure, particularly in response to exercise.

TECHNICAL TIP

**Advantage of MRI compatible stents: Although not readily available at present, platinum or Nitinol stents may be preferred over stainless steel stents due to their MRI compatibility allowing follow-up MRI assessment of these patients' coarctation site that is not possible after stainless steel stent placement.

Sheath and wire placement

Wire position is important to optimize balloon and stent positioning as well as minimize risk of complications. A relatively stiff exchange length wire should be used; we prefer an Amplatz wire with a short soft tip. The first choice for wire position is the left subclavian artery if there is adequate distance (1.5 cm) from its origin to the site of coarctation. This position is easy to obtain and allows for a straight balloon/stent course while minimizing wire/sheath/balloon exposure to the carotid arteries, thereby minimizing the risk of a neurologic complication. If the distance between the site of coarctation and the origin of the left subclavian is too short or the diameter of the proximal left subclavian is too small to accept the tip of the dilating/implanting balloon, then the wire should be placed in the right innominate and subclavian artery. This will usually allow for a reasonably straight balloon/stent course although it does mandate a wire and balloon immediately below the origin of the carotid arteries. If the right innominate cannot be used due to its small size or tortuous origin then an apex wire should be used and positioned in the LV apex.

TECHNICAL TIP

**Optimal wire position: Some operators have advocated positioning the wire in the ascending aorta. However, we have found this can lead to inadvertent cannulation of the coronaries or prolapse through the aortic valve resulting in significant ectopy. If wire placement in the LV is necessary, choose the shortest balloon possible to minimize the straightening of the aortic arch that will occur during dilation or stent implantation.

The sheath should be straight and long enough to reach the coarctation from the femoral artery. For stent implantation increase the French size of the sheath 1 or 2 above that recommended for the balloon alone (this will generally be 10–12F sheath size). To minimize the risk of a neurologic complication we prefer to keep the sheath at or below the area of coarctation, particularly if the wire is positioned in the right innominate or left ventricle. The sheath is continuously flushed with heparinized saline to minimize risk of clot formation.

Balloon and stent positioning

The stent is flared open on the table using an appropriate dilator to allow it to easily slip onto the delivery balloon (which is under negative pressure) without contacting the balloon material. The stent is hand-crimped onto the balloon and the negative balloon pressure released. The long sheath is positioned in the abdominal aorta and the stent balloon combination advanced to the tip of the sheath, allowing only the balloon tip to protrude. The sheath and balloon/stent system is advanced across the lesion and the sheath pulled back just below the coarctation. A hand angiogram through the sheath is then performed in the lateral projection to define the coarctation, and origin of the subclavian artery relative to the position of the stent. The stent should be centered on the coarctation with care taken so the proximal edge of the stent is distal to the origin of the subclavian artery.

TECHNICAL TIP

**No problem with subclavian jailing: The subclavian artery can be crossed and jailed if absolutely necessary to effectively stent the coarctation. Because the subclavian originates at approximately 90° to the aortic arch and the interspaces of these large stents are quite sizable, no obstruction will occur. There have been no late reports of either stenosis or distal thrombus following subclavian "jailing". However, daily aspirin is recommended for at least 12 months after implant if the subclavian is "jailed".

The sheath is retracted over the balloon catheter just to the proximal edge of the balloon. This way the sheath can help maintain balloon position during inflation to help prevent distal movement due to the force of the ejecting blood. This fact should be considered when positioning the balloon and stent prior to delivery by having the stent centered just proximal to the center of the coarctation. Inflation of the stent should initially proceed slowly until both ends of the stent are partially flared. The balloon's position can still be adjusted at this point if necessary. Full inflation is then performed taking care not to exceed the burst pressure of the balloon.

TECHNICAL TIP

**Post-dilation with high-pressure balloon: It is much better to postdilate a stent with a residual waist by placing a high-pressure balloon after initial implant than to attempt resolution of a residual waist by excessive pressure with the initial implanting balloon. Removal of a ruptured balloon from a freshly implanted stent can be problematic and the effectiveness of a post-implant high-pressure dilation is usually significantly greater than the initial implant dilation.

Post-placement assessment

Following balloon dilation or stent implantation, repeat hemodynamic assessment should be performed, including measurement of cardiac index by saturation or thermodilution techniques. Pressure pullback across the dilated and or stented coarctation should be performed with a Y adapter over a wire to maintain distal wire position and not disturb the site.

TECHNICAL TIP

**Accurate pressure gradient measurement: To get an accurate pressure measurement and optimal picture the wire used with the pigtail catheter should be downsized to a 0.025" Rosen or Amplatz wire once the pigtail catheter has been advanced well past the site of coarctation.

The pigtail catheter should then be advanced just proximal to the coarctation for an angiogram. Cameras should be kept with the AP angled 15° LAO and 10° caudal and a straight lateral projection with an injection of 25 cc at 25 cc/sec (rate and volume need to be reduced from initial picture to safely use the power injector with a wire and the Y adaptor). Additional views with different camera angles may be necessary if an aneurysm or extravasation of contrast is suspected on the initial post-implant angiogram.

PULMONARY VALVE STENOSIS

Pulmonary valve stenosis was first described by John Baptist Morgagni in 1761[41] and, although initially thought to be rare, makes up approximately 8–10% of all congenital heart disease. The pathology of congenital pulmonary valve stenosis is variable. In the most common form the valve is dome-shaped with two to four raphes present but no separation into valve leaflets.[42] Occasionally the valve may be diffusely thick with commissural fusion of one, two, or all three leaflets. In up to 15% of cases the valve is trileaflet but with dysplastic diffusely thickened cusps of myxomatous tissue without commissural fusion. This pathology is associated with valve annulus hypoplasia and commonly seen in patients with Noonan's syndrome.[43] Valve stenosis leads to secondary changes in the right ventricle consisting of right ventricular hypertrophy, and if severe, tricuspid regurgitation and right heart failure. The MPA becomes dilated due to the jet from the stenotic valve and on rare occasions this post-stenotic dilatation can extend into the proximal LPA. Patients are usually asymptomatic until the stenosis is severe, with presenting symptoms most typically exercise intolerance. The diagnosis is made on physical examination with an audible systolic ejection click and murmur heard loudest over the left upper sternal border. Confirmation and determination of severity is made by echocardiogram by estimating the gradient across the valve, the RV systolic pressure, and the RV wall thickness.

Indications: All patients with valvar pulmonary stenosis gradients >40 mmHg, or milder gradients with evidence of right ventricular hypertrophy, should have treatment with balloon dilation. There is no evidence that patients with mild pulmonary valve stenosis without evidence of right ventricular hypertrophy will benefit from balloon dilation. Dysplastic valve morphology and annular hypoplasia are independent predictors of poor response to balloon dilation. However, age and associated anomalies such as Noonan's syndrome are not.[46]

Contraindications: Patients with supravalvar narrowing of the main pulmonary artery can often appear on echo to have valvar pulmonary stenosis. This diagnosis can be difficult to differentiate angiographically due to the close proximity of the MPA narrowing to the pulmonary valve and a common association of thickened dysplastic valve leaflets (Fig 29-11). These lesions do not respond to balloon dilation and should be referred for surgical repair.

The procedure: Balloon dilation of valvar pulmonary stenosis was first described by Kan and associates in 1982, the first congenital lesion to be treated with balloon dilation.[44] The technique has remained unchanged since that time, although the balloon technology has progressed substantially to allow for faster, more effective, and lower risk procedures. Efficacy of balloon valvuloplasty in children and adults with congenital pulmonary valve stenosis is excellent, with procedural success in more than 95% and a residual gradient of <35 mmHg in over 75% of patients.[45–47] Complications occur in <5% and primarily relate to local femoral vein injury or transient ventricular ectopy although valve annulus rupture and death have been reported in children. Recurrence of stenosis with need for repeat intervention is necessary in <15 % of older patients with typical valvar stenosis. Mild insufficiency is commonly seen in up to 65% of patients after dilation but moderate or severe insufficiency is rare, seen in less than 7.[46]

Pre-procedure evaluation/management: A complete physical examination is important to rule out associated RV outflow obstruction. Surface echocardiogram should be complete to evaluate the pulmonary valve annulus, degree of stenosis, significance of RV hypertrophy by measuring wall thickness, RV pressure measurement, and any evidence of additional RVOT obstruction including infundibular, supravalvar, or branch stenosis. A 12-lead ECG is important at baseline to assess the degree of RV hypertrophy and monitor progress following balloon dilation. A CBC and type and screen is obtained for the procedure. Usual protocols for anticoagulant, antiplatelet, anesthesia, and antibiotic prophylaxis are suggested (Table 29-1). Additional IV narcotic, fentanyl, is given immediately prior to balloon dilation as pulmonary artery stretch causes a moderate amount of pain acutely.

Defining the anatomy

Right heart catheterization is performed in usual fashion using a 7F balloon tip wedge catheter through a femoral vein. Measurement of cardiac index using either saturation data or thermodilution technique is important to assess the significance of the valvar obstruction. A pressure pullback measurement should be obtained from MPA to RV to determine the systolic transvalvar gradient. An apex or Rosen 0.035" exchange wire is then positioned in the RV apex and the wedge catheter exchanged for a marker pigtail catheter for angiography of 35 cc at 35 cc/sec. The AP camera should be set with 15° of cranial angulation and the lateral plane in a straight lateral projection. Measurement of the pulmonary valve annulus can then be made in both planes (Figure 29-10) to guide balloon size determination.

Choosing balloon size

Balloon dilation can either be performed with a single or double balloon technique. There is no evidence that either technique offers a significant advantage regarding success, development of insufficiency, or recurrence of stenosis. A single balloon is technically less complicated but can be problematic for large pulmonary valve annuli. In experimental animal studies it has been shown that dilation with a balloon >150% the diameter of a normal pulmonary valve annulus can result in rupture.[48] In addition, there is reasonable clinical evidence in children and young adults with congenital valvar pulmonary stenosis that significant improvement in stenosis relief is achieved with balloon diameters greater than 100% of the annulus diameter.[49] Based on these observations the target balloon diameter should be 120% to 140% of the pulmonary valve annulus diameter. If a double balloon technique is used then two similarly sized balloons are used if possible to facilitate positioning.[50] The total circumference of the two balloons should equal 120% to 140% of the circumference of the valve annulus. The formula for calculating the double balloon diameter is:

Double balloon diameter = $1.2 \, \pi$ PV annulus diameter / $(2 + \pi)$

For example, a 22 mm pulmonary valve could either be dilated with a single 26 mm diameter balloon or two 16 mm diameter balloons. The balloon should be long enough to allow stable position across the RV outflow tract but not so long it protrudes into either the tricuspid valve proximally or a distal branch pulmonary artery. In animal experiment the majority damage due to balloon inflation occurs in the right ventricular outflow tract due to the proximal end of the balloon straighten-

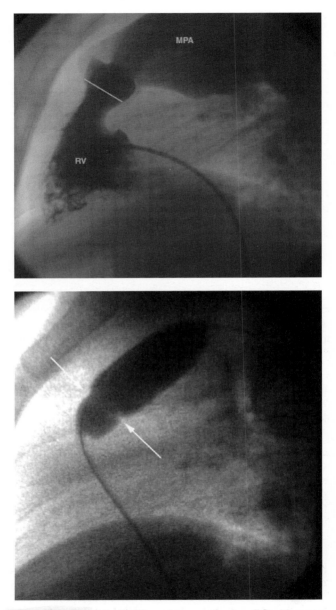

Figure 29-10: AP and LAT angiogram of valvar PS with measurements of valve annulus; lateral angiogram of balloon inflated with waist present (arrows). Notice this balloon is poorly positioned; the balloon should be centered on the valve for optimal dilation.

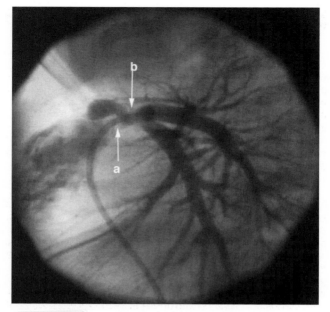

Figure 29-11: Lateral angiogram of supravalvar PS. Note the proximity of the tips of the valve leaflets (a) to the MPA narrowing (b).

ing anteriorly. Generally, balloons 4 cm long are adequate, although occasionally a 6-cm balloon is required to maintain position across the valve.

Sheath and wire placement
A long sheath is not required for pulmonary balloon valvuloplasty. An exchange length relatively stiff 0.035" wire such as a Rosen or Amplatz is positioned in the distal lower pulmonary artery using a 7 wedge catheter to obtain initial position. Either the left or right PA can be used, although the left provides a straighter course in most patients.

TECHNICAL TIP

**How to track the balloon across the valve: Take care to get very stable distal wire position in one of the lower segmental pulmonary arteries. This will facilitate tracking the balloon catheter across the valve and improve stability during inflation. If the balloon wedge catheter does not pass easily to a lower lobe vessel, use a directional wire to advance it into a desired distal branch. The tip of the wedge catheter can then be held in place in the distal vessel by gently inflating the balloon while advancing the exchange wire out the tip.

Balloon position and dilation

A road map from the lateral angiogram should be referenced to give landmarks for the pulmonary valve annulus position. The balloon is centered on the valve annulus and inflated to 6 ATM. Balloon movement during inflation is common, so the catheter must be maintained in position and the inflation recorded so that it may be reviewed. If the initial inflation did not result in complete resolution of the balloon waist centered on the valve then the balloon should be repositioned and the inflation repeated.

Post-dilation assessment

Following dilation the balloon catheter can be exchanged for the wedge catheter and right heart pullback hemodynamic pressure measurements repeated, including cardiac index measurement. The pigtail catheter is then placed in the RV for repeat RV angiogram in the AP and lateral projections to assess for dynamic RV outflow tract stenosis, aneurysm formation, or new onset tricuspid regurgitation. An increase in dynamic RV outflow tract obstruction after relief of significant valvar pulmonary stenosis is common and often causes significant residual gradient which can be confirmed on careful pressure pullback tracing and on the lateral angiogram. This residual dynamic obstruction will resolve gradually, with regression of the RV hypertrophy following valve obstruction relief.

PULMONARY ARTERY STENOSIS

Branch pulmonary artery stenosis is a rare congenital lesion in isolation but is often associated with complex congenital heart lesions following surgical repair, especially tetralogy of Fallot. Other associated lesions include truncus arteriosus or pulmonary atresia with ventricular septal defect after RV to PA conduit placement, transposition of the great arteries following arterial switch repair, and pulmonary artery sling after re-implantation. Branch pulmonary artery stenosis decreases perfusion to the affected lung and if severe, causes hypertension in the non-affected lung and right ventricle. Distal pulmonary artery stenosis promotes pulmonary insufficiency which compounds the decrease in cardiac output and increased workload on the right ventricle seen in these patients. Patients are often asymptomatic but may present with exercise intolerance.

Indications: The systolic gradient across branch pulmonary artery stenosis is, in isolation, a poor determinant of the need for treatment and can only be interpreted by also considering quantitative pulmonary flow data. Normal distribution of pulmonary flow is 55% to the right lung and 45% to the left lung. Patients with a reduction of ≥15% of flow or an absolute flow of <1 L/min/m² in the affected lung should be considered for stent repair. Patients with any degree of contralateral pulmonary artery hypertension, RV hypertension, or RV hypertrophy should be aggressively treated to prevent progression, as should patients with significant pulmonary insufficiency associated with the branch pulmonary artery stenosis.

Contraindications: Adult patients following repair of complex congenital heart disease such as tetralogy of Fallot or truncus arteriosus are complex, often with multiple anatomic, hemodynamic, and arrhythmia issues in addition to their branch pulmonary artery stenosis. It is critical these patients are evaluated completely and a comprehensive plan made, coordinated by a cardiologist familiar with congenital heart disease, and involving an electrophysiologist, cardiothoracic surgeon, and interventionalist. If surgical revision of the underlying repair is required, a surgical approach to the branch pulmonary artery stenosis may be preferable.

The procedure: Balloon dilation of branch pulmonary artery stenosis was initially described in 1983 by Lock *et al.*[51] However, only 50% of lesions responded with a significant restenosis rate.[52] With the availability of larger peripheral stents in the early 1990s and their application to pulmonary artery branch stenosis,[53] stent placement has rapidly become the treatment of choice in adults because of improved success and low restenosis rates. Shaffer *et al.* reported results in over 130 children and adults with postoperative branch pulmonary artery stenosis showing that in over 65% stent implantation increased lesion diameter by over 100%, with a median gradient reduction from 46 to 10 mmHg and RV to systemic pressure ratio reduction from 60% to 40%.[54] Long-term results have been excellent with restenosis rates <5%.[55] Complications are rare, occurring in less than 4% of cases overall, and include hemoptysis, aneurysm, perforation, refractory ventilation perfusion mismatch, and death.[54] Technical issues such as device malposition or embolization have been reported in <2% and are quite rare with recent improvements in balloon and stent technology.

Pre-procedure evaluation/management: A complete physical examination is important to rule out associated RV outflow obstruction. Surface echocardiogram should be complete to evaluate the significance of RV hypertrophy by measuring wall thickness, RV pressure measurement estimate and any evidence of additional RVOT obstruction including infundibular, supravalvar, or valvar stenosis. A 12-lead ECG is important at baseline to assess the degree of RV hypertrophy and monitor progress following stent repair. A nuclear pulmonary perfusion scan is critical to determine the functional significance of branch pulmonary artery stenosis and should be performed prior to catheterization to provide context for pressure measurement interpretation during the catheterization. A CBC and type and cross is obtained for the procedure. Usual protocols for anticoagulant, antiplatelet, anesthesia, and antibiotic prophylaxis are suggested (Table 29-1). Additional IV narcotic, fentanyl, is given immediately prior to balloon dilation with stent implantation as pulmonary artery stretch causes a moderate amount of pain acutely.

Defining the anatomy

Right heart catheterization is performed in usual fashion using a wedge end-hole or Multipurpose catheter, including measurement of cardiac index and pulmonary flow if residual left to right shunts are present. Both branch pulmonary arteries should be entered, including pressure measurements in the distal lower lobe segments. A stiff 0.035" exchange wire should be positioned in the distal pulmonary artery and the wedge catheter replaced with a marker pigtail catheter for a main pulmonary artery angiogram (30 cc of contrast at 35 cc/second). The AP camera should be angled approximately 30° RAO with the lateral camera orthogonal at 60° LAO and 10° caudal. This will profile the right pulmonary artery well in the AP projection and the left pulmonary artery in the lateral projection. Measure the affected artery including lesion diameter, vessel diameter proximal and distal to the lesion, and lower lobe segment origin diameter from the angiogram.

Choosing balloon and stent size

The goal of stent repair is to enlarge the stenosis to equal the diameter of the surrounding normal pulmonary vessel using the shortest stent possible that will completely cover the lesion. Distension of the lesion greater than the diameter of the surrounding normal vessel is not helpful. Intimal hyperplasia will result in the overdistended stent reducing intraluminal diameter to that of the surrounding vessel or even smaller. In addition, vessel overdistention may cause pain up to several weeks after implant. Excessively long stents are problematic due to difficulties advancing them through the tortuous RVOT during implantation and protrusion after implant into a segmental branch or main pulmonary artery. There are currently three stent types available and effective for treatment of branch pulmonary artery stenosis. The balloon used for stent delivery should be of scratch-resistant material and equal to or just slightly longer than the length of the stent (Table 29-3).

Sheath and wire placement

An appropriate sized long sheath, 2 French sizes above that recommended for the balloon alone, should be positioned in the right atrium over a stiff 0.035" exchange wire that has been positioned in the lower lobe pulmonary artery of the affected branch.

TECHNICAL TIP

**Stabilizing wire position in the pulmonary artery branch: Take care to get very stable distal wire position in one of a lower segmental pulmonary artery. This will facilitate tracking the stent through the tortuous RVOT into position. If a catheter does not pass easily to a lower lobe vessel for initial wire placement, use a directional wire to advance it into a desired distal branch for the stiff wire exchange.

Stent position and implantation

Because of the tortuous nature of the RVOT and MPA it is best to track the stent together with the long sheath through the RVOT and across the lesion. If the sheath is placed across the lesion when initially inserted, it will often kink upon removal of the dilator or when advancing the stent. To avoid this problem, leave the long sheath in the RA and advance the balloon/stent combination to the tip of the sheath until the distal edge of the stent is just covered by the end of the sheath while the tip of the balloon catheter protrudes. The sheath together with the balloon/stent is advanced over the wire as a unit through the RVOT and across the lesion in the proximal branch pulmonary artery.

TECHNICAL TIP

**Using a stiffer wire to track a stent: If tracking the sheath stent combination remains difficult, resulting in loss of wire position, exchange the 0.035" stiff wire for a super stiff 0.038" wire. This should be shaped by hand with a gentle curve in the distal 15 cm to conform to the RVOT and branch PA to allow positioning without excessive distortion of the heart.

The stent is centered on the lesion and the sheath retracted proximal to the proximal tip of the balloon. A hand angiogram should be performed through the side arm of the long sheath to define the stent's position in relation to the lesion, MPA, and upper lobe segmental artery (Figure 29-12). Once optimal position is confirmed, the stent is delivered using a pressure inflation device to achieve delivery pressures of up to 16 ATM, taking care not to rupture the balloon. Complete expansion of the stent with resolution of the waist is desired on the initial inflation.

Postdilation assessment

Following stent implantation it is critical to maintain distal wire position, both to facilitate assessment and address any complications if they develop. A catheter with both side and end holes such as a pigtail or Gensini catheter is advanced over the wire and positioned in the distal PA.

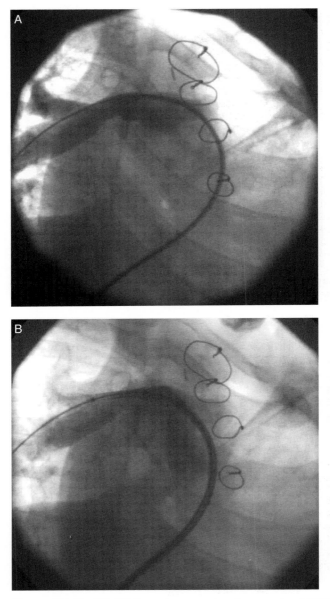

Figure 29-12: (A) RAO angiogram showing proximal RPA stenosis in a patient following tetralogy of Fallot repair. (B) RAO angiogram through delivery sheath confirming stent positioning prior to implantation. *(Continued)*

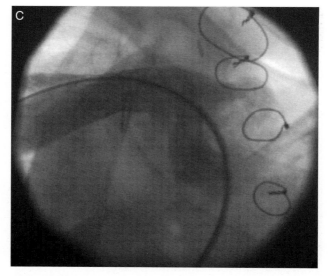

Figure 29-12: (C) Resolution of stenosis immediately after stent implantation.

TECHNICAL TIP

**Reshaping the pigtail catheter: If a pigtail catheter is used cut the tip so only a 90° curve remains. This will facilitate catheter manipulation over the wire and through the implanted stent.

Using a Y connector measure a pressure pullback across the stent into the main pulmonary artery and measure saturation in the main pulmonary artery to calculate pulmonary flow. An angiogram is performed through the Y adaptor with the side holes of the catheter positioned in the lumen of the stent. Camera angles should be the same as the initial angiogram with 20 cc of contrast injected at 20 cc/second with a maximal injection pressure of 600 psi. If the stent is incompletely expanded then repeat dilation with a high pressure balloon should be performed. If there is residual stenosis beyond the edge of the stent then placement of an additional stent will be necessary.

REFERENCES

1. Lock JE, Cockerham JT *et al.* Transcatheter umbrella closure of congenital heart defects. *Circulation* 1987; **75** (3): 593–9.

2. Bridges ND, Hellenbrand W *et al.* Transcatheter closure of patent foramen ovale after presumed paradoxical embolism. *Circulation* 1992; **86** (6): 1902–8.

3. Landzberg MJ, Sloss LJ *et al.* Orthodeoxia-platypnea due to intracardiac shunting: relief with transcatheter double umbrella closure. *Cathet Cardiovasc Diagn* 1995; **36** (3): 247–50.

4. Hagen PT, Scholz DG *et al.* Incidence and size of patent foramen ovale during the first 10 decades of life: an autopsy study of 965 normal hearts. *Mayo Clin Proc* 1984; **59** (1): 17–20.

5. Lechat, P, Mas JL, Lascault G *et al.* Prevalence of patent foramen ovale in patients with stroke. *N Engl J Med* 1988; **318**: 1148–52.

6. Du ZD, Hijazi ZM *et al.* Comparison between transcatheter and surgical closure of secundum atrial septal defect in children and adults: results of a multicenter nonrandomized trial. *J Am Coll Cardiol* 2002; **39** (11): 1836–44.

7. Martin F, Sanchez PL *et al.* Percutaneous transcatheter closure of patent foramen ovale in patients with paradoxical embolism. *Circulation* 2002; **106** (9): 1121–6.

8. Bruch L, Parsi A *et al.* Transcatheter closure of interatrial communications for secondary prevention of paradoxical embolism: single-center experience. *Circulation* 2002; **105** (24): 2845–8.

9. Wahl A, Windecker S *et al.* Percutaneous closure of patent foramen ovale in symptomatic patients. *J Interv Cardiol* 2001; **14** (2): 203–9.

10. Sievert H, Horvath K *et al.* Patent foramen ovale closure in patients with transient ischemia attack/stroke. *J Interv Cardiol* 2001; **14** (2): 261–6.

11. Beitzke A, Schuchlenz H *et al.* Catheter closure of the persistent foramen ovale: mid-term results in 162 patients. *J Interv Cardiol* 2001; **14** (2): 223–9.

12. Sam'anek M. Children with congenital heart disease: probability of natural survival. *Pediatr Cardiol* 1992; **13**: 152–8.

13. King TD, Mills NL. Nonoperative closure of atrial septal defects. *Surgery* 1974; **75** (3): 383–8.

14. Mills NL, King TD. Nonoperative closure of left-to-right shunts. *J Thorac Cardiovasc Surg* 1976; **72** (3): 371–8.

15. Hughes ML, Maskell G *et al.* Prospective comparison of costs and short term health outcomes of surgical versus device closure of atrial septal defect in children. *Heart* 2002; **88** (1): 67–70.

16. Chessa M, Carminati M *et al.* Early and late complications associated with transcatheter occlusion of secundum atrial septal defect. *J Am Coll Cardiol* 2002; **39** (6): 1061–5.

17. Suchon E, Podolec P *et al.* Cardiopulmonary exercise capacity in adults with atrial septal defect. *Acta Cardiol* 2002; **57** (1): 75–6.

18. de Lezo JS, Medina A *et al*. Effectiveness of percutaneous device occlusion for atrial septal defect in adult patients with pulmonary hypertension. *Am Heart J* 2002; **144** (5): 877–80.

19. Mitchell SC, Korones SB, Berendes HW. Congenital heart disease in 56,109 births: incidence, and natural history. *Circulation* 1971; **43**: 323–332.

20. Porstmann W, Wierny L *et al*. Closure of persistent ductus arteriosus without thoracotomy. *Ger Med Mon* 1967; **12** (6): 259–61.

21. Porstmann W, Wierny L *et al*. Catheter closure of patent ductus arteriosus. 62 cases treated without thoracotomy. *Radiol Clin North Am* 1971; **9** (2): 203–18.

22. Krichenko A, Benson LN *et al*. Angiographic classification of the isolated, persistently patent ductus arteriosus and implications for percutaneous catheter occlusion. *Am J Cardiol* 1989; **63** (12): 877–80.

23. Wang JK, Liau CS *et al*. Transcatheter closure of patent ductus arteriosus using Gianturco coils in adolescents and adults. *Cathet Cardiovasc Interv* 2002; **55** (4): 513–8.

24. Zhang Z, Qian M *et al*. Transcatheter closure in 354 pediatric cases of patent ductus arteriosus using five different devices. *Chin Med J (Engl)* 2001; **114** (5): 456–8.

25. Patel HT, Cao QL *et al*. Long-term outcome of transcatheter coil closure of small to large patent ductus arteriosus. *Cathet Cardiovasc Interv* 1999; **47** (4): 457–61.

26. Faella HJ, Hijazi ZM. Closure of the patent ductus arteriosus with the Amplatzer PDA device: immediate results of the international clinical trial. *Cathet Cardiovasc Interv* 2000; **51** (1): 50–4.

27. Bilkis AA, Alwi M *et al*. The Amplatzer duct occluder: experience in 209 patients. *J Am Coll Cardiol* 2001; **37** (1): 258–61.

28. Hong TE, Hellenbrand WE *et al*. Transcatheter closure of patent ductus arteriosus in adults using the Amplatzer duct occluder: initial results and follow-up. *Indian Heart J* 2002; **54** (4): 384–9.

29. Edwards JE, Christensen NA, Clagett OT *et al*. Pathologic considerations in coarctation of the aorta. *Mayo Clin Proc* 1948; **23**: 324–32.

30. Lock JE, Bass JC, Amplatz K *et al*. Balloon dilation angioplasty of aortic coarctations in infants and children. *Circulation* 1983; **68**: 109–16.

31. Morrow WR, Vick, GW 3rd *et al*. Balloon dilation of unoperated coarctation of the aorta: short- and intermediate-term results. *J Am Coll Cardiol* 1988; **11** (1): 133–8.

32. Tynan M, Finley JP *et al*. Balloon angioplasty for the treatment of native coarctation: results of Valvuloplasty and Angioplasty of Congenital Anomalies Registry. *Am J Cardiol* 1990; **65** (11): 790–2.

33. Paddon AJ, Nicholson AA *et al.* Long-term follow-up of percutaneous balloon angioplasty in adult aortic coarctation. *Cardiovasc Intervent Radiol* 2000; **23** (5): 364–7.

34. Diethrich EB, Heuser RR *et al.* Endovascular techniques in adult aortic coarctation: the use of stents for native and recurrent coarctation repair. *J Endovasc Surg* 1995; **2** (2): 183–8.

35. Zabal C, Attie F *et al.* The adult patient with native coarctation of the aorta: balloon angioplasty or primary stenting? *Heart* 2003; **89** (1): 77–83.

36. Harrison DA, McLaughlin PR *et al.* Endovascular stents in the management of coarctation of the aorta in the adolescent and adult: one year follow up. *Heart* 2001; **85** (5): 561–6.

37. Hamdan MA, Maheshwari S *et al.* Endovascular stents for coarctation of the aorta: initial results and intermediate-term follow-up. *J Am Coll Cardiol* 2001; **38** (5): 1518–23.

38. Marshall AC, Perry SB *et al.* Early results and medium-term follow-up of stent implantation for mild residual or recurrent aortic coarctation. *Am Heart J* 2000; **139** (6): 1054–60.

39. Suarez de Lezo J, Pan M *et al.* Immediate and follow-up findings after stent treatment for severe coarctation of aorta. *Am J Cardiol* 1999; **83** (3): 400–6.

40. Araoz PA, Reddy GP *et al.* MR findings of collateral circulation are more accurate measures of hemodynamic significance than arm-leg blood pressure gradient after repair of coarctation of the aorta. *J Magn Reson Imaging* 2003; **17** (2): 177–83.

41. Morgagni JB. *De Sedibus et Causis Morborum* (The seats and causes of diseases), vol 1. Remondini, 1761: 154.

42. Edwards JE. Congenital malformations of the heart and great vessels. In: Gould SE, ed. *Pathology of the Heart*. Charles C Thomas, 1953.

43. Koretzky ED, Moller JH, Korns ME *et al.* Congenital pulmonary stenosis resulting from dysplasia of the valve. *Circulation* 1969; **40**: 43–53.

44. Kan JS, White RI, Mitchell SE *et al.* Percutaneous balloon valvuloplasty: a new method for treating congenital pulmonary valve stenosis. *N Engl J Med* 1982; **307**: 540–2.

45. Teupe CH, Burger W *et al.* Late (five to nine years) follow-up after balloon dilation of valvular pulmonary stenosis in adults. *Am J Cardiol* 1997; **80** (2): 240–2.

46. McCrindle BW. Independent predictors of long-term results after balloon pulmonary valvuloplasty. Valvuloplasty and Angioplasty of Congenital Anomalies (VACA) Registry Investigators. *Circulation* 1994; **89** (4): 1751–9.

47. Mullins CE, Ludomirsky A *et al.* Balloon valvuloplasty for pulmonic valve stenosis – two-year follow-up: hemodynamic and Doppler evaluation. *Cathet Cardiovasc Diagn* 1988; **14** (2): 76–81.

48. Ring JC, Kulik TJ *et al*. Morphologic changes induced by dilation of the pulmonary valve anulus with overlarge balloons in normal newborn lambs. *Am J Cardiol* 1985; **55** (1): 210–4.

49. Radtke W, Keane JF *et al*. Percutaneous balloon valvotomy of congenital pulmonary stenosis using oversized balloons. *J Am Coll Cardiol* 1986; **8** (4): 909–15.

50. Mullins CE, Nihill MR *et al*. Double balloon technique for dilation of valvular or vessel stenosis in congenital and acquired heart disease. *J Am Coll Cardiol* 1987; **10** (1): 107–14.

51. Lock JE, Castaneda-Zuniga WR *et al*. Balloon dilation angioplasty of hypoplastic and stenotic pulmonary arteries. *Circulation* 1983; **67**(5): 962–7.

52. Ring JC, Bass JL *et al*. Management of congenital stenosis of a branch pulmonary artery with balloon dilation angioplasty. Report of 52 procedures. *J Thorac Cardiovasc Surg* 1985; **90** (1): 35–44.

53. O'Laughlin MP, Perry SB *et al*. Use of endovascular stents in congenital heart disease. *Circulation* 1991; **83** (6): 1923–39.

54. Shaffer KM, Mullins CE *et al*. Intravascular stents in congenital heart disease: short- and long-term results from a large single-center experience. *J Am Coll Cardiol* 1998; **31**(3): 661–7.

55. McMahon CJ, El-Said HG *et al*. Redilation of endovascular stents in congenital heart disease: factors implicated in the development of restenosis and neointimal proliferation. *J Am Coll Cardiol* 2001; **38** (2): 521–6.

INDEX

Note: References to figures are indicated by "f" and those to tables by "t".